Biology for Health

Applying the Activities of Daily Living

S. H. Cedar

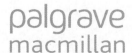

palgrave
macmillan

First published 2012 by
PALGRAVE MACMILLAN

Palgrave Macmillan in the UK is an imprint of Macmillan Publishers Limited, registered in England, company number 785998, of Houndmills, Basingstoke, Hampshire RG21 6XS.

Palgrave Macmillan in the US is a division of St Martin's Press LLC, 175 Fifth Avenue, New York, NY 10010.

Palgrave Macmillan is the global academic imprint of the above companies and has companies and representatives throughout the world.

Palgrave® and Macmillan® are registered trademarks in the United States, the United Kingdom, Europe and other countries.

ISBN: 978–1–4039–4547–1

This book is printed on paper suitable for recycling and made from fully managed and sustained forest sources. Logging, pulping and manufacturing processes are expected to conform to the environmental regulations of the country of origin.

A catalogue record for this book is available from the British Library.

A catalog record for this book is available from the Library of Congress.

10 9 8 7 6 5 4 3 2 1
21 20 19 18 17 16 15 14 13 12

Printed in China

This book is dedicated to my parents,
Sidney and the late Sylvia Cedar

Brief Contents

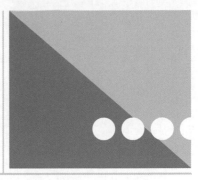

Full Contents

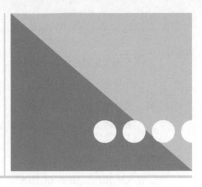

List of Figures

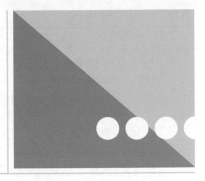

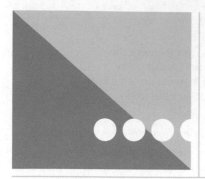

List of Tables

Acknowledgements

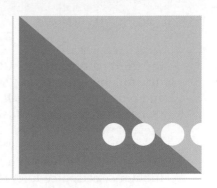

The achievement of anything in life is made much easier by excellent and inspiring teachers. I am indebted, therefore, to two magnificent teachers in an early stage of my life. Jane Lucas took me on although I did not even know the chemical names of the elements and got me through A Level chemistry in about five months. She made chemistry interesting and intellectual rather than boring or fact learning by rote. She was keen that there was understanding of what things meant and how they went together. She showed how the underlying principles beneath the reactions worked. Biology, unlike chemistry, has far fewer underlying principles, so there are many facts to learn. Ruth Popple made her A Level biology classes fun and engaging.

Due to both of them I entered university to study biochemistry, where I encountered even more inspiring teachers, including my personal tutor the crystallographer Professor Tom (now Sir Tom) Blundell, the microbial genetics lecturer Professor David Sherratt, the metazoan genetics lecturer Professor J. Robert Whittle, the cell biology lecturer Professor Chris Ford, the evolutionary biology lecturer the late Professor John Maynard Smith and countless other brilliant minds. I am also very grateful that during this time I obtained a scholarship to study in Massachusetts in the USA for one year, at a Liberal Arts university, keeping my other interests engaged, which show up as the epigraphs at the start of each chapter linking the science to the living!

On completion of my first degree I was very fortunate to secure a Wellcome Trust funded position to study for my PhD with the late haematologist and nanobiologist Professor Mike A. Horton, and my interest in stem cells continues to this day, including a recent sabbatical with Dr Stephen Minger in his Stem Cell Biology Laboratory at King's College London. After completing my PhD I had post-doctoral fellowships, an EMBO (European Molecular Biology Organisation) fellowship with the neurobiologist Professor H. (Mona) Soreq and an MRC (Medical Research Council) fellowship in control of gene expression with Professor Jamshed Tata.

Apart from carrying out research, I have been teaching biology and health for many years to university biology students and over recent years to those in the health field. It has been a pleasure teaching both groups of students, but for this book I am especially indebted to those in the health care arena. I have learnt a lot from them and hope that this book, in part a summary of my lectures and a reflection of my lecture style, will go towards feeding back what I have learnt and thanking them for the pleasure I have gained teaching them biology applied to health. I hope I have inspired some of them even a tiny bit as much as I have been inspired by some of my teachers.

No book is written alone, not even a single authored book. I need to thank all the people at Palgrave Macmillan for their enduring support, especially Jon Reed (now of jon reed consultancy) and Lynda Thompson; and a very large thankyou to Kate Llewellyn, who saw this through to completion. I should also like to thank the copy editor, Jo North, for editing the final version, and the design team at Palgrave Macmillan for interpreting my ideas into figures and for all their work on making this book look clear and legible. Finally I really need to thank my wonderful partner, Jyll Bradley, for so much encouragement and support.

The author and publishers would also like to thank the following for their permission to use third party material: Alfred Publishing Co. Inc. for the lyrics from 'Woodstock' – words and music by Joni Mitchell, Copyright © 1969 (Renewed) Crazy Crow Music, all rights administered by Sony/ATV Music Publishing, 8 Music Square West, Nashville, TN 37203. All Rights Reserved; iStockphoto and the individual contributors (see source line) for Figures 6.6, 8.17 and 10.6; World Health Organization for Tables 13.2 and 13.3 originally from WHO (2011) Factsheet no 310 *The top 10 causes of death* (updated June 2011) available at http://www.who.int/mediacentre/factsheets/fs310/en/index.html; and Cengage Learning for Fig 4.19 from Penfield/Rasmussen *The Cerebral Cortex of Man* © 1950 Gale, a part of Cengage Learning, Inc. www.cengage.com/permissions

Every effort has been made to trace all copyright holders but if any have been inadvertently overlooked the publishers will be happy to make the necessary arrangements at the first opportunity.

Introduction

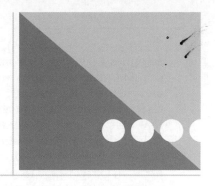

This book is intended to be an introductory text book for undergraduate students embarking on studies across the broad field of health, including courses such as nursing, health and social care, health studies, physiotherapy, nutrition, occupational therapy, podiatry, paramedic science, and sports and exercise science.

It covers many biological concepts and their application in health and how health can be guided by them. It shows the link not only between biology and health, but also between the breakdown in biological processes and the resulting ill health. In this book the theory within the biological processes is applied to health and to practices within health care such as assessments and treatments.

Biology is the study of living organisms, what they are made from and what they do. Investigating these areas involves the fields of chemistry, anatomy, physiology, biochemistry and biophysics, among other disciplines. Applying biology to health also incorporates clinical medicine and epidemiology as well as clinical technology, diagnosis and treatments. These ideas are interwoven in the book to show how all these areas interact in maintaining our biology and our health.

Biology also asks the question 'What is life?' or 'How are living things different from non-living things?' While many of us think we know what it is to be alive rather than dead, and the subtle difference between what it is to be alive rather than 'non-living' in the way an object such as a coffee cup is non-living (never having been alive), it is actually very hard to define what life is.

In biology we tend to talk about what living things are made of (anatomically) and what living things do (physiologically). What living organisms 'do' are called their **living processes**. These living processes include

- growing,
- reproducing,
- communicating,
- respiration,
- eating,
- eliminating waste,
- moving,
- metabolic processes,
- repairing and
- dying.

In the 1980s these living processes, the system properties of living organisms, were taken as a model for nursing by Roper, Logan and Tierney (1980, 2000) and called **activities of daily living (ADLs).**

The ADLs are

- maintaining a safe environment,
- communicating,
- breathing,
- eating and drinking,
- eliminating,
- personal cleansing and dressing,
- controlling body temperature,
- mobilising,
- working and playing,
- sleeping and
- dying.

While these activities formed the basis of a nursing framework in a patient-centred health care model they can be applied to other health disciplines.

These are the activities that we (adult) humans can do by ourselves when we are healthy and therefore independent of care. When our health is compromised some of these activities may also be compromised and we cannot undertake them; we become dependent on others for our care. Health care professionals therefore are often interested in ascertaining how able we are to undertake these activities, at levels appropriate to our age. For example, babies are highly dependent. There are developmental stages that they go through as they reach adulthood that can be marked by their being able to carry out these activities. The first time a baby walks or feeds itself or dresses itself are considered milestones in development into an independent adult. Not going through these stages is a symptom of something being amiss. Our physical health in adulthood, but also our mental health, may affect our ability to carry out these activities. For instance, when severely depressed we may lose interest in our physical being, not taking care of ourselves. We also assess others, such as those with learning difficulties or dementias, in terms of how many of these activities they can carry out. The activities of daily living have proved a very useful tool in assessing patient health, physically, mentally and socially.

Because of this and because these activities of daily living have their basis in the biology of living processes this book uniquely uses the Activities of Daily Living as the organising framework for all the biological explanations of how living organisms are in health and ill health. It shows how these activities, which we take for granted in our daily lives when we are fit and well, are governed in normal homeostasis and how they fail in ill health.

Guide to the book

Your health is linked to the ability to carry out activities of daily living and these in turn are affected by your biology. Everything that occurs in one part of the body impacts on all parts of the body. However, to understand biology it is easier to learn each part and process and then put them back together again to show how they connect and impact on the whole. This may sound like a reductionist approach, but by understanding the underlying biological processes we can build up to a truly holistic view of the body being composed of parts that must all interact correctly to enable the functioning human to enjoy their full potential, health. We can also then understand how something as complex as, say, a mental health condition, such as depression, may have an altered physiological process underneath it.

Biology tends to measure processes at the microscopic level. Health tends to measure outcomes at the performance level of ADLs. This book lays one discipline onto the other. It is organised so that each chapter covers an ADL and maps related biological living processes to the ADL. The chapters are mapped as follows:

- Chapter 1, 'Maintaining a Safe Environment', covers homeostasis.
- Chapter 2, 'Working and Playing', covers energy, chemicals and metabolism.
- Chapter 3, 'Growing and Developing', covers reproduction and growth.
- Chapter 4, 'Communicating', covers the nervous and endocrine systems.
- Chapter 5, 'Controlling and Repairing', covers the skin, body temperature and cell repair.
- Chapter 6, 'Moving', covers the skeletal and muscular systems.
- Chapter 7, 'Breathing', covers the respiratory system.
- Chapter 8, 'Transporting', covers the blood and cardiovascular systems.
- Chapter 9, 'Eating and Drinking', covers the gastrointestinal system and accessory organs.
- Chapter 10, 'Eliminating', covers the renal system.
- Chapter 11, 'Cleansing and Dressing', covers the immune system.
- Chapter 12, 'Sleeping and Healing', covers body rhythms, pain and pharmacology.
- Chapter 13, 'Dying', covers epidemiology, ageing and death.

Within each chapter the main body systems and homeostasis are introduced. In each chapter you will find **Health Connections** boxes linking the basic biological processes to a health condition, event or disease that illustrates the relevance of understanding the biology.

Information in biology and health needs to be universal and clearly understood so that it can be transmitted accurately. Due to this, much biology requires new, precise language. Key terms are highlighted in the text in **bold** and main discussion points are in *italic* to aid learning.

As everything in biology is interconnected many body systems can be dealt with in a number of ways; for example, the skin could be seen as a regenerating organ, an organ of temperature control or an organ of body defence. I have chosen a particular ADL for which to introduce each system, but to highlight the connections, you will find **Chapter Reference** boxes across the chapter which offer links to further discussion.

The figures are closely linked to the text as I am aware that different students have different ways of processing information. There are summary boxes of the main points throughout the chapters and at the end which should act as prompts for recall. In an information-driven age where it is hard to discern meaning or relevance the aim of the text is to move the reader to understanding and linking conceptual ideas in biology to health care.

Each chapter starts by placing the activity in the **environments**, both the external and internal ones, in which we find ourselves. In a world increasingly taking a global view on health, conservation, sustainability and resources, it seemed logical to do so. It also places us as a species in the environment in which we must survive and thrive. These environments, internal and external, are the ones we must sustain to sustain ourselves; we have a vested interest in each.

Our biology and our health vary with our age and lifestyle and each chapter links each ADL to these drivers: see the sections entitled 'Lifespan'.

The book ends with the chapter 'Dying'. Health professionals must face the fact that clinical interventions can temporarily prevent dying, but in the end dying is an ADL that all life meets.

Health care professionals are trained to be able to carry out assessments of ADLs and take many measurements. Nowadays there is a blurring of roles and the health care professionals of the future will need to be able to do more than carry out these functions; they must understand what the function shows and why they need to take a particular measurement. Knowing this will allow them to make decisions as to

- who needs a particular intervention,
- when they need it and
- why they need it.

Without understanding the underlying principles and concepts and the links between systems and events, health care professionals would be limited in their careers and remain reliant on other people's decision-making.

To be able to do this requires linking health to biology, the underlying physiology. This is the intention of the book, enabling the health care professional of the future to

- manage patient needs,
- lead team members and
- make clinical decisions.

Showing the underlying science I hope will make the causes and treatments of diseases clearer and reveal some of the ways in which clinical decisions are reached.

References

Roper, N., Logan W. W. and Tierney, A. J. (1980). *The Elements of Nursing*. Oxford: Churchill Livingstone.

Roper, N., Logan W. W. and Tierney, A. J. (2000). *The Roper–Logan–Tierney Model of Nursing: Based on Activities of Living*. Edinburgh: Elsevier Health Sciences.

Maintaining a Safe Environment

> *We are stardust,*
> *We are golden,*
> *We are billion year old carbon*
> *And we've got to get ourselves*
> * back to the garden.*
>
> **Joni Mitchell* (1943–),**
> **Canadian musician, songwriter**
> **and painter**

Introduction: A safe environment as an activity of daily living

Much is made nowadays of **Health** and **Safety**. There is legislation for it. There are experts in it. There are courses on it. But do we actually think about the link between these two words health and safety and why we need to join them?

In 1888 the makers of matches in London went on strike because of the disease they were prone to: 'phossy-jaw', a disease that turned their skins yellow and caused their hair to be lost in a form of bone cancer. The disease was caused by the phosphorous in the matches they made. The match-girl strike was a famous moment in Health and Safety policy linking a safe work environment to health. In the late nineteenth century boys were sent up chimneys to sweep them clean and suffered in later life from breathing problems and cancers. Workers were and are often bullied into doing dangerous jobs and carrying out unsafe practices. Health and Safety executives, while often annoying to some of us, have been instrumental in protecting all of us from bad work practices.

We live in two environments: our insides – what is beneath our skin – and the outside world. These constitute our internal and external environments. For all of us to survive and thrive and to be healthy we need a safe external environment. A safe external environment is one which, amongst other things, provides shelter from the elements, sustenance and protection from infection in the form of clean water and food, as well as some limits on traumatic events such as road or rail traffic accidents and injuries from work.

All of these safety issues reflect our need to maintain our biological selves against

- **injury,**
- **infection** and
- **environmental variables.**

However, the external environment is not always safe. What is it in our biology that makes us all so vulnerable to damage and to the vagaries of the external world?

The body is made up of millions of small units called cells. Cells can only exist in a very narrow range of environments; they are intolerant of large or prolonged changes to the optimum conditions, also called variables, which a cell can tolerate.

Health Connection

Work and environment

When a patient comes to a clinic they are often asked as part of their history what their job is. This is because certain jobs are associated with certain diseases. All of a person's history may help to explain and work out what is wrong with the patient.

While cells are very sensitive to changes, in contrast living things, organisms, which are made of cells, can exist in a fairly hostile environment.

To survive they carry out a remarkable process: they maintain their own internal environment within a fairly narrow range of variables. This maintenance is not done *for* the cells of the organism; it is done *by* the cells. This process of self-maintenance of internal variables and conditions is called **homeostasis** and is the basis of all the physiological processes of the body, the processes that the body carries out.

We have the ability to adjust internal conditions to remain within an environment tolerable for our cells. In ill health we often cannot adjust our internal environment to maintain it within the range that our cells can tolerate. If we cannot return to a normal range for a variable it may affect our cells to such an extent that they die. If too many cells die, we die. Medical or clinical intervention tries to adjust our internal environment back to within normal ranges.

In this chapter some key concepts in biology and health will be discussed. These include

- **homeostasis,**
- **internal and external environments** and
- **biological organisation.**

This chapter links to Chapter 2, 'Working and Playing', which

- looks at some of the variables that must be maintained;
- looks at the normal ranges for each variable;
- introduces how each variable alters during normal daily activities;

Box 1.1 Homeostasis

The word 'homeostasis' comes from the Greek:

- HOMOIOS – means something that is like or similar to;
- STASIS – means something that is standing or static.

So homeostasis (pronounced home-ee-oh-stay-sis) means trying to stay the same. The human body needs to maintain the integrity of its

- structure – or anatomy – what it is made of;
- function – or physiology – what it does.

Homeostasis is the maintenance of a safe, optimum internal environment within a narrow range for a number of conditions or variables in the face of fluctuating external environments. It is carried out by physiological processes discussed below.

- introduces some of the clinical observations and skills that are used to measure these variables;
- discusses links to homeostasis, health and ill health.

These chapters act as an introduction to the processes and mechanisms that will be discussed in detail in the later chapters.

▶ **Health Connection**

Vital signs

Vital signs are internal conditions that are measured by health care professionals to ascertain whether a patient is healthy, i.e. whether their internal conditions are within the normal range. See page 62 for a full list.

Living processes

It is very hard to come up with a definition of life, what it is and what distinguishes living from non-living things. The distinction between living and non-living things, by which we mean things that have never been alive (your car, the plate your food is on, for instance) as opposed to dead things which *used* to be living, is a concept, an idea, that underpins much of what is called natural philosophy, the branch of philosophy that all the sciences emerged from as subject areas about 2500 years ago. Biology is the science that studies living organisms. Because life itself is hard to define, biology defines living organisms by what they *do* rather than what they *are*.

Both living things and non-living things are made of material substances, matter, which is composed of atoms. In this respect what we are made of hardly distinguishes us from non-living things. In fact, the study of what we are made of could be left to the same scientists who study what everything is made of, chemists and physicists. What distinguishes the living from the non-living is not therefore material substance, but biological living processes – what organisms do.

These biological living processes include activities such as

- growing,
- feeding,
- moving,
- reproducing,
- excreting and
- dying.

As mentioned above these are what healthy independent living organisms *do*. So biology and health are intimately linked.

In the health field these living processes are called **activities of daily living (ADLs)**. They are what healthy people can carry out and are used to assess the state of a patient's independence and health. The ADLs are listed in the box below.

Box 1.2 Activities of daily living

The activities of daily living (ADLs) include

- maintaining a safe environment,
- working and playing,
- growing and developing,
- communicating,
- controlling,
- moving,
- breathing,
- transporting,
- eating and drinking,
- eliminating,
- cleansing and dressing,
- sleeping and
- dying.

These are the activities that this book will explore as they inform much of health care and provide the link between biology and health. The activities will also be looked at as ones that maintain and are maintained in homeostasis. The changes that occur during changes in **lifestyle** such as during physical activities or sleeping will be explored, as will changes during **lifespan** from birth to old age. They will all be put within the context of the variables that affect them and that they in turn affect.

The link between our biology and our health can be made even clearer if we think of homeostasis and ADLs (see box below).

Health Connection

Homeostasis and ADLs

Healthy, independent organisms maintain their *own* homeostasis, while those we think of as having failing health cannot maintain their homeostasis and thus they cannot maintain the cells of which they are made. When this maintenance is compromised we define an organism as unhealthy or ill. If the organism cannot repair itself it may die. The alternative is that the organism becomes *dependent* on others, particularly those in health care professions.

When we are in good health we don't notice that we are, in fact, maintaining ourselves, feeding ourselves, moving ourselves, communicating, breathing and all the other activities of daily living (ADLs). We only tend to notice when things go wrong.

Homeostasis is used as a measure of health in biomedicine. If homeostasis fails it is a measure of ill health and leads to clinical intervention.

In the biomedical model of health, diagnosing is the analysis of a problem and what is *causing* it and is carried out to ascertain which part of us is not fully functioning and maintaining itself. When that is done treatment is carried out to correct what is wrong. This is the basis of clinical intervention and treatment so that we can return to being fully homeostatic and functioning as healthy, *independent* people.

Health, homeostasis and independence are therefore linked in the biomedical model of health.

Losing the ability to carry out one of the ADLs may impact on one or many of the others. For instance, losing the ability to move prevents or reduces the ability to fetch food or water and therefore may lead to health problems such as malnutrition or dehydration.

The environment

There are two environments that affect living organisms:

- the *external environment* – the universe in which all life exists;
- the *internal environment* – the body that living things create and maintain.

The external environment

While we all wish for a safe environment, the environment in which all living organisms exist, the external environment of this planet Earth or what we call nature, is indifferent to our survival. It is passive, and merely *permissive* of our being here. For example, some compounds on this planet, such as lead and uranium, are quite dangerous to us. Volcanic eruptions and earthquakes are evidence that this is not a benign planet. However, as living organisms we adapt to what is available on this planet to sustain our lives and to thrive. We are made from the materials found on Earth, which appear originally to have come from the 'big bang'. The atoms we are made of made something else before us and will make something else when we are gone. We are a sort of recycling system and you will see in Chapter 9, 'Eating and Drinking', that we eat other organisms or their products and then eliminate what is waste for us but fodder for another organism!

The external environment is not set or constant; it varies between places and fluctuates at different times. Temperatures change, air composition changes, pressure changes, humidity changes and we must cope with all of these changes and the alterations to all these variables (things that can vary) if we are to survive and thrive.

For example:

- Changes in the external environment may affect our health.
- Changes in the types of pollen from flowers in the external environment may cause us to have allergies.
- Changes in air composition may cause breathing difficulties such as asthma. Changes in pressure may not only make our ears 'pop' but may cause circulatory problems, as seen in deep vein thrombosis (DVT).
- Changes in external temperature affect our body temperature; we become too hot or too cold and need to adjust our temperature to avoid damage to our cells which would result in ill health.

Chapter Reference

All these variables and how they are measured are discussed further in Chapter 2, 'Working and Playing' (see p. 35).

The internal environment

Wrapped around the outer edge of our bodies is a tissue so familiar that we forget that it is a living entity – skin. It forms a barrier between us and the external environment. Everything contained within it is part of our internal environment. This is composed of many different chemical materials, discussed in Chapter 2, 'Working and Playing'. Some of our inside environment is solid, some liquid and some gas. All of it is adapted to be able to carry out the functions of our bodies, which in turn allow us to carry out the activities of daily living. Disrupting the

- chemical,
- physical or
- biological

internal environment affects our health. We therefore invest a lot of effort in maintaining our internal environment in the face of an external environment which we cannot control and which varies constantly. Homeostasis is thus central to biology and health.

While we cannot really control the external environment to make it safe for our survival, through physiological mechanisms described in this book we try to make our own internal environment safe for our survival, our health, to maintain it within acceptable ranges.

Homeostasis and health: Linking the external and internal environments

To understand how we maintain a stable internal environment we can look at the problem in parts:

- What internal environment are we trying to maintain?
- Why are we trying to maintain it?
- How do we maintain a constant or stable internal environment?
- What happens when we don't maintain this stable internal environment?

The internal environment that is maintained

The internal environment operates around a narrow range for each variable.

The variables (in **bold** below) that need to be controlled around strict ranges include

- the correct **water** balance – called osmosis – for the movement of substances around the body;
- the correct **salt** concentrations – also called electrolytes or ions – for the correct movement of substances around the body and for chemical processes to occur;
- the correct **acid** and **base** levels – called pH – for chemical processes to occur;
- the correct **sugar** levels – for energy synthesis;

- the correct **nutrient** levels – for growth and maintenance;
- the correct **temperature** levels – for chemical processes to work;
- the correct **chemical** levels – for chemical processes to work;
- the correct **oxygen** levels – for energy to be synthesised;
- the correct **carbon dioxide** levels – for blood gases to be maintained;
- the correct **protein** levels – for growth and development;
- the correct **cell numbers** – for body maintenance and development;
- the correct **size** – for growth.

Health Connection

Changes in our internal environment

Changes in our internal environment can have drastic effects on our health. For instance, changes in the amount of blood in our body due to blood loss can cause shock and even death, while increases in blood volume can cause high blood pressure. This in turn affects all the components of our body, the cells and chemicals that make up our body and their ability to function, which in turn affects our health.

Why we try to maintain homeostasis

We need to maintain our internal environment; otherwise adverse effects can occur if we become, for example, too

- hot – proteins congeal;
- cold – metabolism stops;
- dry – blood transport stops;
- wet – blood pressure is high and nutrients are diluted;
- acidic or alkaline (basic) – metabolic processes can't occur;

- high or low in electrolytes – transport, metabolic processes and nerve conduction are affected.

All of these variables will be explained in subsequent chapters.

Homeostasis is a mechanism that maintains optimum internal conditions for cells and therefore maintains our health.

How homeostasis is maintained

To maintain any system one needs to know what is happening, if there are changes, and how to alter the system in an ordered, measured way to its optimal conditions. Homeostasis does all of that to maintain a suitable internal environment by carrying out three general processes:

- **recording** what is happening to each *variable*. There is no possibility of maintaining homeostasis unless it is known what is to be maintained and if it has fluctuated (changed) at all from where it should be;
- **collecting** and monitoring this information to *coordinate* a response. Any change that is recorded needs to be collected into a central area so that a coordinated response can be made rather than an erratic, disorganised response which could further endanger the internal environment;
- **responding** with an appropriate behaviour. An appropriate response must be made to the variable that has fluctuated rather than randomly responding to change.

Step 1: Each variable is measured. This is done by specific receptors, cellular devices that are tuned to a particular condition, *modality*, and receive, measure or detect any fluctuations from their set point. For example, just as a room thermostat is set to a particular temperature, so in the body there are cellular receptors tuned to a particular temperature, 37°C. These temperature receptors, with their specialist functions, are called thermoreceptors. Any fluctuation from 37°C is noted and a signal sent to the monitoring area.

Step 2: The monitoring and coordinating area for all the signals from the various receptors is in the brain, in an area called the hypothalamus. It is the control centre for homeostasis. Many of the responses are brought about by the autonomic nervous system, although some involve the voluntary nervous system or the endocrine system. Any changes detected by receptors are sent to this area, which coordinates and controls an appropriate response.

Chapter Reference

The endocrine and the nervous systems are discussed in Chapter 4, 'Communicating' (see p. 102).

Step 3: This control centre then sends signals to the body to bring about the correct response or **effect**. The response is brought about by an **effector**, bringing a particular effect into being, for example an increase or a decrease in temperature. This response must be brought about by changes in the internal environment, heating ourselves up or cooling ourselves down, for instance. There are various effectors depending on the response required.

The receptor therefore measures the input of a signal, the coordinating area takes all the inputs and decides what output is needed and then sends a signal to an effector which generates the appropriate response or output.

Box 1.3 General features of homeostatic control

1. Receptors detect a change.
2. Control centre receives signals of a change.
3. Effectors change behaviour.

Receptors are constantly measuring the variable they are tuned to, such as temperature, water levels or pH levels. These can change any moment and receptors are good at detecting

change, rather than detecting a variable that doesn't vary (is constantly the same).

The control centre is constantly receiving information from all the receptors about the state of all the variables and constantly coordinating responses.

Health Connection

Homeostatic control centre

The control centre for homeostasis is in the brain. Damage to the brain can affect this area, and if so coordinated and appropriate responses can be affected. This damage can come about through many causes, such as trauma to the brain, infections and **pathologica**l (disease causing) disorders. An uncoordinated or inappropriate response would affect homeostasis, and the internal environment would be compromised. This is turn would affect all the processes of the body.

The effectors are often trying to counterbalance a change. For example, if you are too hot, the appropriate effector will try to make you cooler. If you are too cold, the appropriate effector will try to make you warmer. The effector is therefore working in the opposite direction to the signal. This is an example of *negative feedback*.

Negative feedback

Imagine you are standing upright. You sway to the left, but your sense of balance brings you back to the centre. You sway to the right, but again your body brings you back to the centre. This is the way that negative feedback works. It doesn't matter which direction the change is in, too much or too little, it is opposed by the body, which tries to bring it back to where it was, in this case bringing you back to your centre. Negative feedback is where *changes are opposed*.

Temperature levels are also controlled in this way. If you think of a room thermostat set at 20°C, when the temperature of the room decreases below 20°C the thermostat receives or detects the information and sends it to a control centre which sends information to the boiler to carry out an effect, in this case to increase the heat (turn on the heating). When the temperature increases to the set point the thermostat, which, continues measuring the temperature sends the information to the control centre, which sends information to turn off the heating. In a human being if the temperature varies too much from 37°C mechanisms are switched on to restore the temperature (Figure 1.1).

> ### Chapter Reference
> Temperature regulation is discussed in Chapter 5, 'Controlling and Repairing' (see p. 142).

Positive feedback

Positive feedback leads to a greater departure from the original level. It operates by measuring the current state in your body of a variable, for example water levels, and comparing it to the desired level your body should be at. The difference between the two is the error. In positive feedback the error is increased. It *reinforces change*.

If you think about the swaying body again, in positive feedback if you sway from the centre to the right, positive feedback increases the sway until you fall over – it reinforces the change. If you sway to the left it reinforces that too until you fall over to the left.

If you were dehydrated you would become more dehydrated, rather than drinking and becoming less dehydrated. Positive feedback amplifies the situation, reinforcing the change rather than opposing it.

For example: Would you use positive feedback for controlling temperature? What would happen if you did? If you were hot you would get hotter and if cold you would get colder. Not very useful for these variables and homeostasis!

Positive feedback is used in a few control mechanisms of the body when if a process starts you don't want to suddenly stop it; you want it to continue until complete.

Both negative and positive feedback require the same homeostatic mechanism: a detector, a control centre and effectors.

> ### Health Connection
>
> #### Positive feedback
> Blood clotting and uterine contraction during labour are both under positive feedback rather than under negative feedback.
> Once blood clotting starts it proceeds (reinforces the change direction) until the area is completed.
> With uterine contraction again it proceeds until the foetus is born. If it was under negative feedback, as the contraction started it would be opposed and the foetus would not be pushed out. Positive feedback allows processes, once started, to proceed to completion. It is goal-oriented.

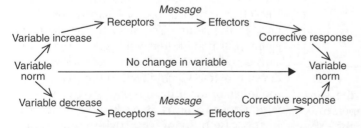

FIGURE 1.1 **Negative feedback**

Feedforward

We are also capable of **feedforward**, which means anticipating our needs or a potential disturbance to homeostasis. For example, when we eat dry food we anticipate becoming dehydrated so we drink at the same time, before we actually become dehydrated.

Motivation

Negative and positive feedback and feedforward all help to maintain homeostasis. They are also all parts of actions we carry out to maintain our internal environment – for example, drink water, move to a warmer place, eat food. We often do these actions without realising that we are being prompted, *motivated*, to do so to maintain our homeostasis. Homeostatic mechanisms have occurred internally, for example monitoring water levels, releasing hormones to alter thirst or to alter water absorption by the kidneys, but what you notice is your **motivation** to behave in a certain way.

Chapter Reference

Motivation and hormones are discussed in Chapter 4, 'Communicating' (see p. 102).

Water balance is discussed in Chapter 10, 'Eliminating' (see p. 282).

What happens when homeostasis is not maintained?

If homeostasis is not maintained the body strays too far away from the limits in which it can survive and flourish. This threatens health and can lead to death.

Ill health is when your body is not behaving homeostatically. It has been challenged and cannot effect the appropriate change. We can intervene clinically or medically at this stage to restore the internal environment if the patient cannot restore their own environment independently. In fact that is the main purpose of medical intervention, *restoring homeostasis*.

Health Connection

Dehydration – water input and output

Patients who have lost fluids need the fluid to be replaced to avoid dehydration. Much water is lost from our bodies in urine. We can measure the amount of fluid that is lost in urine and we can measure how much fluid a person has drunk or replaced in their bodies. These observations are made to avoid the patient becoming dehydrated, resulting in, among other conditions, altered blood pressure.

Health Connection

Signs, symptoms and diagnosis

When we are ill and seek medical help we tend to present ourselves to the health professional with signs and symptoms of an illness. Signs are measurable and observable, such as blood cell counts, temperature and skin rash. Symptoms are subjective reports by the patient and are more general, such as pain, fever and nausea.

The health professional must then **diagnose** (work out) what these signs and symptoms indicate (show) by

- finding out which variable is outside the correct range (temperature, pH, etc.);
- discovering, through appropriate investigations (such as blood pressure measurements, urine sample chemical analysis), what is causing the system to malfunction;
- deciding on the appropriate treatment to remove the cause of the problem or adjust the body by clinical intervention so as to restore the homeostasis of the body.

Box 1.4 Summary – Homeostasis

The environment in which we live is constantly fluctuating. We must maintain our own internal environment, which is different from the external environment and can also fluctuate due to changes in our daily activities.

To maintain our internal environment, to keep it suitable for us to survive, we have receptors. Each receptor can measure a particular variable, such as temperature or water levels or blood pressure. The measurement obtained must be sent to a control centre and the control centre must decide what to do and send signals to effectors to effect a change in our behaviour to maintain homeostasis.

Change can be brought about by

- negative feedback, where the change in a variable is opposed;
- positive feedback, where the change in a variable is reinforced (or increased);
- feedforward, where there is anticipation of need.

Detailed mechanisms of homeostasis will be discussed in each ADL chapter.

Levels of organisation

To study how living organisms survive and flourish, biology divides itself into separate levels of explanation based on size. We can start from the lowest level and work up to the whole organism (Figure 1.2):

- **atoms and elements,**
- **molecules,**
- **organelles,**
- **cells,**
- **tissues,**
- **organs.**

At the lowest level, atoms, elements and molecules, some basic chemistry is needed to understand why they are important in biology and health and how they work in compounds such as nutrients and drugs. We need to look at what they are made of, the material, and how they react, the energy. This will be discussed in Chapter 2, 'Working and Playing'. In this chapter we will look at the organisation at the biological level: cells, tissues and organs.

The biology of life

Cells and organelles

Cells are probably one of the hardest entities to describe and to imagine. It is the cell that defines life and is life. We are our cells. We started out as one fertilised egg cell with material donated by our mother and our father in a unique combination that makes us. This fertilised egg then went on to grow and divide, taking in nutrients to grow and then divide to make more and more cells. We humans are composed of about 10^{13} cells – that is a 1 with 13 noughts after it, or 10 trillion. When cells develop in the embryo they differentiate; that is, they become different from each other. They alter shapes and functions to carry out what is needed in the animal to which they belong, in this case humans. Cells can join together to form tissues and organs, all the anatomical structures that carry out the physiological functions to keep the individual alive by keeping the cells that the individual is made of alive.

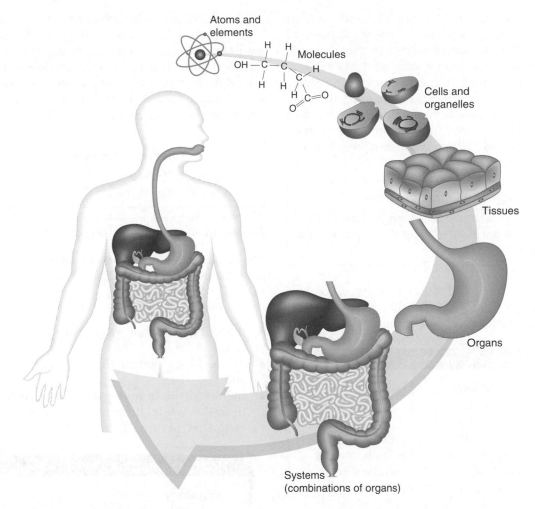

Atoms and elements

Molecules

Cells and organelles

Tissues

Organs

Systems (combinations of organs)

FIGURE 1.2 **Levels of organisation**

Chapter Reference

Development is discussed in Chapter 3, 'Growing and Developing' (see p. 64).

Cells are the basic functional units of life. They are the smallest discrete functional units that are able to be described as alive. Cells carry out a number of chemical reactions, taking what they need from their surroundings, food and water for example, converting these into what they need to carry out their living processes and producing waste products which they must excrete. These reactions are part of what are called metabolic reactions and mean that the cell is like a little chemical factory manufacturing all that it needs to maintain itself and its surrounding cells and to maintain their internal conditions.

The chemicals making up a cell are large organic molecules such as carbohydrates, fats, proteins and nucleic acids. Cells obtain these chemicals from food, so without food, which contains those chemicals called nutrients, the cell cannot survive. Some of the chemicals from food are used to replace worn-out parts of the cell and some are converted to energy in the form of another chemical called ATP. Energy is used for transporting substances, chemicals, into and out of the cell and for cell movement and metabolism, the processes needed to keep the cell alive. All of the processes carried out by a cell to keep itself alive are called cell **metabolism**.

Chapter Reference

Chemicals, nutrients, energy and metabolism are discussed in Chapter 2, 'Working and Playing' (see p. 35).

The structure of cells, their form, is part of their anatomy. The processes that cells carry out, their functions, are part of their physiology.

Health Connection

Pathology

When the anatomy or physiology of a cell alters from normal it can cause an imbalance in homeostasis and lead to disease. This is the area of pathology – the study of disease. If it is a physiological malfunction the area of study is pathophysiology.

The structure of cells

Cells have an outer membrane which forms a boundary and keeps the contents of the cell in and most other things out. This membrane is permeable to water and fats, but not to sugars and proteins, which must be actively transported into the cell. Active transport is discussed below.

Inside a cell are various small organs, called organelles, and other structures that help to carry out the function of the cell. The main purpose and function of a cell is to be alive

and to maintain itself through various metabolic processes. This takes energy, which cells get from converting food such as sugars into a chemical form of energy called ATP. The energy is used for transport of substances into and out of the cell (discussed below) and for the many chemical reactions needed by the cell.

Chapter Reference

Energy and ATP are discussed in Chapter 2, 'Working and Playing' (see p. 35).

Organelles and structures inside the cell

The main organelles and other structures inside the cell, their location and function are listed below.

The three main areas of a cell are

- the cell membrane, which surrounds the cell,
- the nucleus, usually in the centre of the cell, and
- the cytoplasm, a watery–salty liquid inside the cell where all the other main structures, organelles, of the cell are found floating.

Health Connection

Histology

Cells can be taken from a patient (by a procedure called a biopsy) to be examined. As cells are very small and not visible to the naked eye they can be magnified under a microscope. The cells are first stained with various chemicals to highlight the anatomical structures for viewing. The study of cells in a clinical setting is performed by histologists and is a branch of pathology.

The cell membrane is also called the plasma membrane. It is made of two layers of lipids (fats) which have a chemical phosphate group attached, so the layers are also called a bi-layer of phospholipid. There are proteins attached to either the internal or external surface of the membrane as well as proteins embedded through the membrane. These proteins are often involved with transport of substances into and out of the cell. Proteins are discussed below. Lipids are hydrophobic, disliking or repelling water, while the phosphate molecules are hydrophilic, being attracted to water (Figure 1.3).

Chapter Reference

Chemicals such as lipids and phosphates, and proteins and their properties, such as hydrophobicity, are discussed in Chapter 2, 'Working and Playing' (see p. 35).

The **nucleus** is a large structure within the cell. It has its own membrane surrounding it, the nuclear membrane, similar to the plasma membrane of the cell. It is thus separated from the rest of the cell. It contains long structures called **chromosomes** containing a material called **DNA**. This DNA is our genetic material, with coding sequences called genes. Genes

contain the instructions for how to assemble proteins. Chromosomes are a mixture of the genetic material and scaffolding materials made of proteins and sugars that protect the DNA and help it in its function. Also within the nucleus is a large body called the nucleolus, which also contains a form of genetic material used in making ribosomes – the structures that make proteins from genetic material. The nucleus thus contains this DNA, which is the instruction material for assembling proteins.

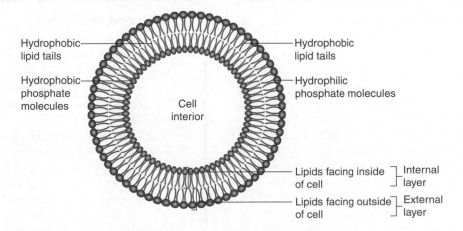

FIGURE 1.3 Cell membrane showing lipid phosphate bi-layer

Most of the functions of the cells are carried out by proteins. The instruction manual for assembling proteins, the genes, is very precious: if they are damaged by being in the cytoplasm, the instructions on how to make proteins are lost. So genes are kept separate from the cytoplasm area, where all the metabolism of the cell, its survival, is happening. Keeping it separate from the rest of the cell inside a nucleus is a way of protecting the genetic material.

Not only does the genetic material tell the cell how to make proteins, but it tells future cells how to make proteins. It is part of the generation of new cells; hence the words genes, genetics and generation all have the same root.

Chapter Reference

Genes, genetics, DNA and protein assembly are discussed in Chapter 3, 'Growing and Developing' (see p. 64).

Organelles

Within the cell are a number of specialised structures – organelles. Each of these carries out a particular specialised function or activity. The nucleus is one such organelle. Below are examples of others.

Health Connection

Genes and proteins
The genes are the instructions for how to assemble proteins. Any damage to the genes compromises our ability to make proteins (it is called a mutation). To avoid damage the genes are kept separately from the rest of the cell behind an extra layer of protective membrane, the nucleus. Damage can still occur from the external environment, such as ultraviolet (UV) rays of sunlight, or by the ingestion of toxic chemicals, the lack of essential nutrients or extreme temperatures.

Ribosomes are structures in the cytoplasm but are not strictly organelles, as they are not bound by a membrane, which other organelles are. They are the site where proteins are manufactured. This illustrates how the various functions inside cells are compartmentalised to different areas and organelles, each with its own specialist function. The nucleus holds the instructions for how to assemble proteins, but the ribosomes are the actual place of manufacture and assembly, the factory floor. If the ribosomes make a mistake in assembling a protein, there will be one bad protein, but the next one will follow the genetic instructions. Ribosomes may be free inside the cytoplasm, but are usually attached to **endoplasmic reticulum**, discussed below.

The **cytoplasm** is a watery fluid in which organelles and other structures exist within the cell. The fluid is composed of water and salts (electrolytes). The organelles carry out various functions and the cytoplasm is a favourable environment for these functions (Figure 1.4).

The **cytoskeleton** is a fine network of proteins that supports and gives shape to the cell.

Mitochondria are organelles involved in producing energy for the cell; they are often referred to as the 'powerhouse of the cell'. They oxidise glucose into ATP molecules. They contain their own genetic material.

Health Connection

Mitochondrial diseases
Since mitochondria have their own genetic material they can have mutations that are unique to mitochondrial genes. Many metabolic disorders are linked to mutations in mitochondrial DNA.

We inherit our mitochondrial genetic material solely from our mothers. Forensic and anthropological scientists can use this to trace us back to our foremothers. This can also help in establishing mitochondrial disorders that might be inherited and cause disease.

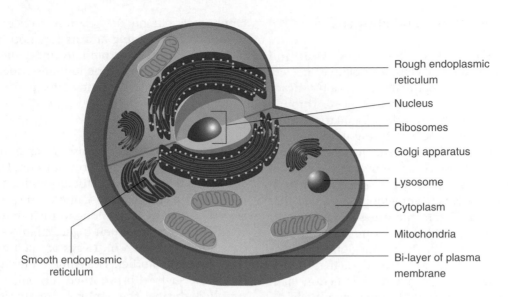

FIGURE 1.4 A generalised diagram of a cell showing the cell membrane, cytoplasm and organelles, including the nucleus and mitochondria

The **Golgi apparatus** is a stack of flat sacs of substances like the plasma membrane. These sacs are involved in packaging substances inside the cell and transporting them around the cell in vesicles, small sac-like bubbles of membrane in the cytoplasm, either for use by the cell or to be released from the cell.

The **endoplasmic reticulum** comes in two kinds, smooth and rough.

The **smooth endoplasmic reticulum** is a series of tubes which makes cholesterol, a steroid-based substance found in membranes and other steroid-based substances, such as some hormones, and which is involved in detoxifying drugs.

The **rough endoplasmic reticulum** has ribosomes attached to the tubes and allows transport of proteins around the cell.

Lysosomes are vesicles which contain enzymes that digest worn-out parts of cells and foreign substance that have invaded the cell, such as bacteria.

Some cells have **microvilli** projecting from the external side of the cell membrane. These increase the *surface area* of the cell, the amount of the cell on the edge or surface rather than deep within the cell. Increased surface areas allow for easy cell transport, discussed below.

They are particularly found on cells in the small intestine of the gastrointestinal tract.

Some cells have extensions from their cell surface that are involved in moving the cell along or moving substances along the outside of the cell. These **cilia** are found on cells such as follicles and ovary cells and in the respiratory system, discussed in Chapter 7, 'Breathing'.

Health Connection

Cells and death

All the organelles of the cell have particular functions. If they fail in their function the viability and health of the cell is compromised and it may die. Cells that are failing are encouraged to die by a process called **apoptosis** so that poorly performing cells do not continue to use up the resources of the body and potentially harm the other cells of the body. If too many cells are poorly performing our health is at risk. If too many cells die our life is at risk.

Cell sizes, shapes and lifespans

Cells come in different shapes, sizes and lifespans. Red blood cells, for example, are very small and have a particular shape, a biconcave disc, which allows them to squeeze through narrow blood tubes called capillaries. They have lost their nucleus during development. The nucleus is where genetic material is stored. The genetic material is the instruction manual of how to make proteins. The main protein in red blood cells is haemoglobin, a protein that carries oxygen from the lungs to all the cells of the body. Red blood cells are full of haemoglobin. However, if the haemoglobin proteins become worn out and need replacing, the red blood cell does not have the instruction manual of genetic material to tell it how to do so. So the red blood cell gradually decays and dies. New red blood cells are constantly being made to replace dead ones.

This illustrates a few things about cells:

Cell shape

Although we tend to show a cell as a generic round cell, cells come in different shapes to suit the function they carry out. In biology a lot of emphasis is put on the relation between the structure of something and its function, a bit like good design. Structure falls under the category of anatomy and function falls under the category of physiology (Figure 1.5).

Cell size

Cells have different sizes, also an anatomical feature, to suit their function. For example, the size of the female gamete, the unfertilised egg, and the size of the male gamete, the sperm, are very different. This is due to their different roles. Bird eggs are much bigger than human eggs. This is because bird eggs are laid externally from the mother. The embryo must grow inside the shell with no other nutrients being supplied during the embryo's maturation, merely warmth from the parent during incubation. Humans are mammals and grow via a placenta linking the mother's nutrient supply to that of the embryo, providing continuous nourishment. Not all the necessary nutrients therefore have to be included at fertilisation. With normal cells of the body there is also a range of size reflecting the function of the cell. Red blood cells are very small and liver cells are very large, reflecting their different functions. Red blood cells have one function, carrying oxygen. Liver cells carry out many metabolic functions.

It is useful to think about sizes in order to understand what cells look like and how complex they are, containing all the subcellular organelles within them (see Table 1.1).

Cell lifespan

Cells have different lifespans. Red blood cells live some 120 days. Brain cell neurons live throughout your life. Liver cells are replaced as needed. You can have a large part of your liver removed and it will grow back. Blood cells are also constantly replaced. Scientists would like to know the mechanism for getting cells to re-grow, part of the remit of stem cell and regenerative medical research, so that we could re-grow damaged brains and hearts.

> ### Health Connection
>
> **Haemolytic anaemia**
> Changes in shape can affect the ability of a cell to carry out its role (function). Red blood cells are usually biconcave discs, but in one particular disease, **spherocytosis**, the red blood cell takes on the shape of a sphere (hence the name of the disease). Because of this change of shape the cell's ability to carry out its function (the transport of oxygen) is severely compromised, which results in a condition called **haemolytic anaemia**. This will be discussed further in Chapter 7, 'Breathing'.

Box 1.5 Sizes of human beings

- Humans tend to be measured in the standard unit of metres. The average human is about 1.8 metres (1.8 m), or just under 2 metres.
- 1 metre is made up of 100 centimetres ('centi' is the Latin prefix for 100).
- 1 metre can also be described as being 1000 millimetres. In other words a centimetre has 10 millimetres in it.
- To visualise this look at a 1 m ruler marked with 100 centimetres, each composed of 10 millimetres.
- If a human is 1.8 m tall they are 180 centimetres (180 cm) or 1800 millimetres (1800 mm).
- Even though humans are about 1.8 m tall, inside of them are many metres of intestines and hundreds of metres of DNA.
- Cells are microscopic because they cannot be seen with the naked eye and must be magnified by a microscope. They tend to be a millionth of a metre long, or a thousandth of a millimetre.

Table 1.1 Some measurement sizes for comparison

1 m (= 1 metre, which is 1000 millimetres or 100 centimetres)
3 metres, length of a nerve cell of a giraffe's neck
1.8 metres, average height of a human
1 mm (= 1 millimetre, which is a 1/1000th of a metre or 1/10th of a cm)
120 mm, diameter of an ostrich egg (a dinosaur egg was much larger)
1 µm (= 1 micrometre, which is a millionth of a metre or 1/1000th of a millimetre)
100 µm, human egg
90 µm, amoeba
10–100 µm, most plant cells
10–30 µm, most animal cells
9 µm, human red blood cell
3–10 µm, the nucleus
3 µm, mitochondrion
2 µm, *E.coli* – a bacterium
1 µm, diameter of human nerve cell process
1 nm (nanometre, 1 nm = 1/1000th of a micrometre)
200–500 nm, organelles such as lysosomes
150–250 nm, small bacteria such as Mycoplasma
100 nm, large virus
11 nm, ribosome
10 nm, thickness of cell membranes
2 nm, diameter of a DNA alpha helix
0.8 nm, amino acid
0.1 nm, diameter of a hydrogen atom

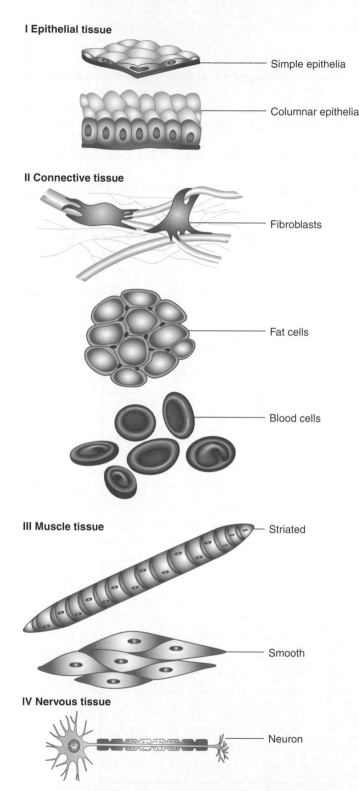

I Epithelial tissue

Simple epithelia

Columnar epithelia

II Connective tissue

Fibroblasts

Fat cells

Blood cells

III Muscle tissue

Striated

Smooth

IV Nervous tissue

Neuron

FIGURE 1.5 A variety of cell shapes suited to the functions which they carry out

Transport into and out of the cell

There are millions of different organisms on this planet. Humans represent just one type. Organisms such as amoebas and bacteria are made of a single cell. They are called unicellular organisms. All of their functions of life, growth and death are carried out in that one cell.

We humans are made of millions and millions of cells; we are multicellular. All of these cells have gone through a process called differentiation where during development different types of cells have developed into shapes suitable for carrying out the various functions needed to keep the whole multicellular animal, us, alive. Some cells become liver, some heart, some bone, for example. All of them look different from one type to another and do different things – processes. But all of these cells, whether from unicellular organisms or multicellular organisms, need to keep themselves alive and that requires replacing worn-out parts and obtaining energy. All of these functions of each cell are called cellular metabolism. Every cell needs to do this to maintain itself. It is part of what is called the housekeeping of the cell, apart from its specialist functions to do with the particular type of cell it has become during differentiation. Housekeeping and cellular metabolism require getting chemical substances such as carbohydrates and proteins and oxygen to each and every cell. Once at the cell these substances then have to cross the plasma membrane into the cell. Waste products and other substances have to be removed from the cell. At the membrane there is, therefore, traffic of

Chemotherapy

Chemotherapy is used in cancer treatments to kill growing cancer cells, but it also can kill any growing cells. Normal cells that are growing and dividing would be affected by chemotherapy, such as blood and skin in other words those cells with shorter lifespans which are constantly being replaced are most vulnerable.

Box 1.6 Summary – Cells

- Cells are microscopic entities.
- They have an outer boundary – a membrane.
- They contain a watery fluid – cytoplasm.
- In the cytoplasm float organelles.
- Organelles carry out specialised functions (activities).
- Cells can only survive in a limited range of conditions.
- If the condition varies too much the cell will die.
- If too many cells die, we die.
- Homeostasis attempts to keep the internal environment suitable for cellular activity and survival.
- Cellular activity alters the internal environment and is discussed in later chapters.

substances into and out of the cell. This is called cell transport.

Different substances have different ways of crossing the membrane, the lipid bi-layer. As the bi-layer is made of a fat-like substance, other fats are more able to cross the bi-layer than are non-fats. For example, oils and vinegars (a non-fat) are hard to mix in a sauce called 'vinaigrette', which is a salad dressing. Likewise fats and non-fats are hard to mix in cells and

across cell membranes; the maxim is 'Like dissolves in like.' However, non-fats need to be transported into and out of the cell across the plasma membrane. There therefore need to be transport mechanisms for doing this.

There are various ways of moving substances across the cell membrane. Below are three main ones:

- **Diffusion** (or **passive diffusion**) moves substances down a concentration gradient from high to low.
- **Active transport** (and all active systems) requires energy to move substances against a concentration gradient.
- **Osmosis** is the movement (diffusion) of water.

Diffusion

It is one of the rules of the universe that physicists have observed that substances tend to go from areas of high concentration to areas of low concentration. They do this without any help. This has to do with increasing disorder and is called entropy. It forms the basis of one of the laws of thermodynamics and links living things with the energies of matter found throughout the cosmos.

Imagine a vacuum flask, a flask with nothing in it, not even air, into which you allow some blue gas. The gas will diffuse into the whole flask, not collect all together at the entrance. It will go from an area of high concentration, where you let it into the flask, to an area of low concentration until it has diffused throughout the flask and the blue molecules of the gas are evenly spread out.

The problem is getting substances to go from low concentration to high concentration, which is sometimes needed in living organisms. This requires energy to move the substances against their natural tendency. This energy is obtained from cellular metabolism, and this mode of transport that takes energy is called active transport.

In Figure 1.6 there is little of the substance oxygen (O_2) inside the cell and more of it outside. The O_2 therefore moves down its concentration gradient from high outside to low inside until it is the same on each side (called equilibrium).

The other substance, carbon dioxide (CO_2), would move in the opposite direction down its concentration gradient from high concentration inside the cell towards the low concentration outside the cell.

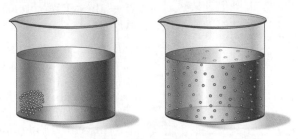

Diffusion of substance

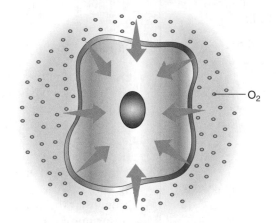

Diffusion into a cell

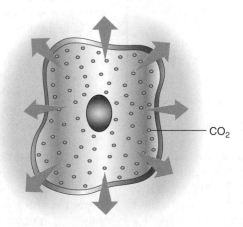

Diffusion out of a cell

FIGURE 1.6 **Diffusion**

Facilitated diffusion

Facilitated diffusion is a form of passive diffusion, but it differs in that this diffusion is *mediated* (helped) by proteins embedded in the plasma membrane. These proteins either

- allow the substance to move through specific pores in the membrane (channels) or
- bind the substance that is to diffuse across a membrane to transport or carrier molecules, which bind to the substance on one side of the membrane and release it on the other side.

Both of these methods facilitate the diffusion.

Active transport

Active transport is transport that requires energy to move a substance. It describes moving substances against their concentration gradient, moving them from low concentration to high concentration, rather than the other way by diffusion.

Most substances, whether moving by diffusion or by active transport, cross the membrane at specific places where proteins, or channels exist for them. The movement is often very specific, a protein in the membrane only binding or transporting one type of chemical (Figure 1.7).

Engulfment

Engulfment is where the membrane of the cell surrounds particles to form a vesicle. This vesicle is a small sac formed by budding off from an existing membrane. The substance inside the vesicle is then transported either within the cell or across the cell membrane.

Vesicles can

- transport substances from one structure to another within cells;
- take substances from the fluid outside the cell (extracellular fluid) – **endocytosis**;
- release substances into extracellular fluid – **exocytosis** (see Figure 1.8).

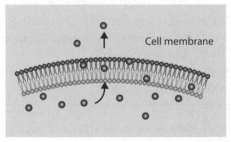

Passive diffusion

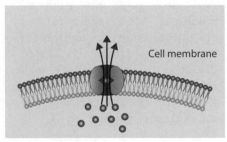

Facilitated passive diffusion

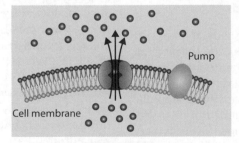

Active transport:
Substance pumped
against concentration gradient

FIGURE 1.7 Passive, facilitated and active transport compared

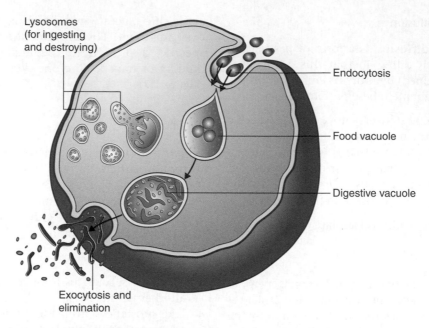

Lysosomes
(for ingesting
and destroying)

Endocytosis

Food vacuole

Digestive vacuole

Exocytosis and
elimination

FIGURE 1.8 Endocytosis (taking in) and exocytosis (eliminating)

Health Connection

Pharmacology

Pharmacology is the study of medicines. Most medicines that act on cells must be transported into cells by diffusion, facilitated diffusion, active transport or engulfment to have an effect on the cell. How drugs get into cells is part of the study of pharmacology.

Water, osmosis and body fluids

Water is the major fluid in the body. It forms part of the transport medium, blood, and the medium in which substances such as nutrients can dissolve in and around cells. It is a very good solvent, allowing many solutes, particularly hydrophilic (water loving) solutes, to be carried or dissolved. Keeping the correct hydration levels is very important for bodily functions. Too little water and blood pressure drops due to lack of blood volume. Too much liquid and blood pressure rises due to too much blood volume. The kidneys help to control the levels of water in the body and this is another example of homeostasis.

Chapter Reference

Water levels are discussed in Chapter 9, 'Eating and Drinking' (see p. 241) and in Chapter 10, 'Elimination' (see p. 282).

Blood pressure is discussed in Chapter 7, 'Breathing' (see p. 184).

The movement of water into and out of cells is called osmosis. Water moves, by osmosis, from areas of high solvent (water) concentration to areas of low solvent concentration. In other words, water moves from areas with lots of water and few solutes to areas with little water and lots of solutes. Water thus moves down its concentration gradient. Osmosis is a kind of diffusion.

The effect of water movement on other substances, though, is to change them from being diffuse to concentrated and those that were concentrated become diffuse.

The fluids in the body can be found in various compartments:

- *intracellular*, i.e. inside the cell;

- *extracellular*, i.e. outside cells, such as blood, plasma, lymph, cerebrospinal fluid;
- *intercellular* or *interstitial*, i.e. between cells.

All cells of the body are in contact with extracellular fluid, from which they obtain the chemicals they need. We operate all our reactions in a watery fluid both inside and outside of our cells. Any chemicals (gases, nutrients from food) that we bring into our bodies from the external environment must therefore be moistened to be suitable for our cells.

Health Connection

Water and health

Water and hydration are vital for human life. Dehydration is a major problem in many environments, particularly hospital settings and when patients cannot re-hydrate themselves. Hydration is discussed further in Chapter 9, 'Eating and Drinking' and in Chapter 10, 'Elimination'.

Health Connection

Replacing water

When replacing fluids that are lost by a patient either we can give water to drink or by infusion (into a vein) we can deliver saline (a water and salt solution at a strict osmotic balance to match that of the plasma of the blood). Water that is drunk is usually a mix of water and salts at a low concentration and is rapidly mixed with the contents of the stomach into a solution containing other substances. We cannot infuse pure water into a vein as this would alter the osmotic pressure of the surrounding cells, causing them to swell and burst.

In Figure 1.9 salt is at a high concentration and water is at a low concentration on the right, while water is at a high concentration and salt at a low concentration on the left. Water will diffuse from high concentration on the left to low concentration on the right by osmosis until both sides have similar concentrations of salt and water; they are then said to be in equilibrium. This is a dynamic state where the number of salt atoms or water molecules moving from

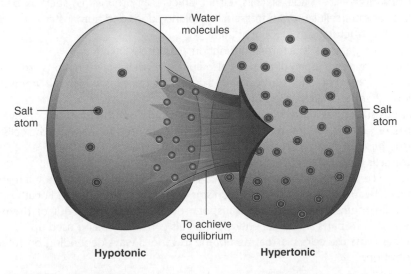

Hypotonic

Hypertonic

FIGURE 1.9 Osmosis

left to right is equivalent to the number moving right to left. This is a very important concept in biology, chemistry, physics and therefore in health. In health we are in dynamic equilibrium with our environment. In ill health we are not.

Tissues

In the above sections a cell has been described. Organisms composed of one cell are unicellular. Organisms composed of more than one cell are multicellular. Humans are multicellular organisms. The cells of our bodies come together to form large structures that carry out the functions (physiology) of our bodies. These functions are to keep the individual cells of the large organism, us, alive.

The cells we have talked about so far have been generalised cells. Our bodies are made of many cells and many different types of cells. During development, cells differentiate into different types of cells. Differentiated cells join together to make large structures called tissues.

These in turn can be part of even larger structures called organs.

Chapter Reference

Development and differentiation are discussed in Chapter 3, 'Growing and Developing' (see p. 64).

Each of the cell types in Table 1.2 has the features described for the general cell – a membrane, cytoplasm and organelles. Each of the cell types differs from other cell types by the shape of the cell or the inclusion of extra organelles or the exclusion of organelles or specialised proteins. These specialised cells can then form groups of specialised cells called tissues, which can in turn carry out specialised functions such as covering the body (epithelia) or transporting substances (blood). The cells in the group can be held together tightly, as in epithelia, or loosely, as in fat, cartilage, bone and blood. They can have other characteristics that group them together such as being contractile (muscle) or conducting electricity (neurons).

Box 1.7 Summary – Cells and transport

- Living organisms are made of cells, either unicellular organisms, such as bacteria and amoebas, or multicellular organisms, such as plants, dogs and humans.
- Cells are the structural and functional unit.
- In biological organisms structure and function are closely linked.
- The shape, size and lifespan of cells are also linked to what their functions are.
- Cells are composed of various subcellular structures, organelles, which are themselves made of various chemicals, such as fats and proteins.
- The various structures inside a cell, the organelles, carry out the functions of the cell.
- All of the organelles and transport methods of cells are used to maintain the cells' metabolism – the functions cells carry out to keep themselves alive.
- Different cells have different lifespans.
- If a cell from certain areas of the body dies it can be replaced, but others cannot. If many cells die all at once, the functions of the entire organisms may be compromised and death may occur.
- To maintain themselves cells must transport substances into and out of themselves, to replace worn-out parts and make energy, which is constantly being used up.
- Substances cross the cell's plasma membrane in various ways depending on solubility and concentration.

Table 1.2 Cell types, locations and functions

Cell group	Function	Features	Examples
Epithelial cells	Barriers, absorption, secretion	Tightly bound between cells	Linings of organs such as digestive tract, skin
Epithelial – hormone producing cells	Cell communication (indirect via blood)	Secrete chemical messages	Thyroid, adrenal, pituitary glands
Connective – support cells	Maintain body structure	Produce specialised extracellular material such as elastin	Bone, cartilage
Connective – adipose cells	Physical protection, heat insulation	Most of cell volume is fat	Under skin, around organs
Connective – blood cells	Transport oxygen, defence	Haemoglobin protein in red blood cells carries oxygen; immunoglobulins label foreign particles	Red and white blood cells
Muscle cells	Movement	Contractile	Skeletal muscle, heart muscle, smooth muscle
Neuron cells	Cell communication (direct, cell to cell)	Electrical potential	Nerves
Germ cells	Reproduction	Haploid chromosome numbers	Egg, sperm

To simplify categorisations, the cells that form the adult can be grouped together into four types of tissues based on their anatomy (what they look like) and their physiology (what they do). These four types of tissues are

- **epithelial** – tissues that make linings and tight junctions between cells, such as lining the digestive tract or forming the outer layer of skin;
- **connective** – tissue that makes support and transport structures with loose junctions and matrix material in between the cells. They can be solid or fluid such as bone, tendons and blood;
- **muscle** – tissue that can be made to contract, such as cardiac, smooth, voluntary;
- **nervous** – tissue that can conduct an electric impulse or support tissues that are electrical such as neurons and glia.

Each of these four types of tissues has further subdivisions.

Epithelial tissues are subdivided according to whether there is a single layer of cells (simple) or multiple layers of cells (squamous) and whether the shape of the cells is cuboidal, columnar or a mix (transitional). Different subdivisions occur in different areas of the body so that the appropriate anatomical type is matched to the physiological need. For instance, areas that need to protect the body, such as the skin, are stratified to contain many layers so that damage to the outer layers that are in contact with the outside environment does not affect the inner layers that are in contact with the internal environment of the body; areas that need to absorb oxygen, such as in blood capillary vessels, are formed from just one layer (simple). Areas that secrete enzymes, such as in the digestive tract, are also composed of one layer of epithelium (simple) while areas that need to absorb nutrients from the digestive tract and transport them to the blood are also simple, but need to have additional surface areas called villi to allow for fast absorption. The shape (anatomy) of a tissue reflects its function (physiology).

Connective tissue cells are subdivided into bone, cartilage, blood, dense and loosely packed cells. These too reflect their function. Bone is hard, giving rigidity and protection to the soft underlying organs of the body. Blood is composed of loosely packed cells in a liquid that allows the tissue to move around the body as a transport medium.

Muscle tissue cells are subdivided into skeletal or voluntary (attached to and moving the skeleton), cardiac (in the heart pumping blood) and smooth or involuntary (in organs moving substances such as food through the digestive tract). All muscle cells can contract and relax in response to electrical stimulation from nervous tissues.

Nervous tissue cells are subdivided into those that carry information, neurons, and those that support neurons, glial cells. Neurons carry electrical signals while glia provide a skeleton-type structure for neurons and move nutrients and waste to and from the neurons.

Health Connection

Tissues and cancers

Different cancers are categorised by the tissue from which they originate. The commonest cancers also describe their tissue of origin; carcinomas are from epithelial tissues and sarcomas are from connective tissues.

Organs

Collections of cells form tissues and tissues can then be formed into organs. An organ is a collection of specialised tissues that performs a specific function, such as skin providing a boundary around the body, kidneys filtering and excreting waste products from blood, lungs bringing air in from the external environment to the internal environment and the heart pumping blood around the body.

Chapter Reference

Each organ and its role in an activity of daily living are discussed in the chapters of this book.

Organs are usually composed of more than one tissue type. For example, the heart has an outer covering of connective tissue that holds it in the chest (thorax), a middle layer of muscle tissue that contracts to pump (or squeeze) blood through tubes and an inner layer of epithelial tissue that holds the liquid blood.

Some organs are composed mainly of two tissue types, such as skin, which has an outer epithelial layer and an inner connective layer. There are other types of organs called membranes (not the plasma membrane of a cell) which are also formed of two tissue types, discussed below.

Very few organs are composed of one tissue type. One such organ is called a gland. It is composed of epithelial tissue cells. Epithelial tissues can form linings or barriers and absorb or secrete. Glands are organs that secrete substances and epithelial cells are used in areas of the body where secretion takes place, such as in the gastrointestinal tract (passageway) or the urinary tract.

Glands

As mentioned above, most organs of the body are formed from various types of tissue. **Glands** are formed from just one type groups of epithelial cells which produce specialised secretions.

There are two types of glands, exocrine and endocrine (Figure 1.10), both secreting substances, but into different areas:

- **Exocrine** glands have ducts secreting fluids and chemicals into body cavities.
- **Endocrine** glands release chemical secretions called **hormones** into the blood.

Box 1.8 Summary – Tissues

While there are many different types of cells in the body they are categorised into four tissue types:

- Epithelial tissue cells make watertight linings.
- Connective tissue cells support and carry.
- Muscle tissue cells move and pump.
- Nervous tissue cells transmit information.

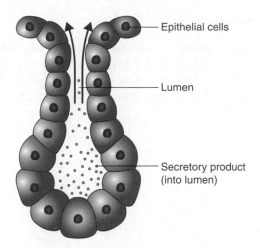

Epithelial cells

Lumen

Secretory product (into lumen)

FIGURE 1.10 **Exocrine gland. This is formed of simple epithelial tissue which allows easy diffusion of a substance out from (secretion) the cells**

Membranes

The membranes discussed below are not the plasma membrane of a cell, but a membrane that surrounds tissues and organs. These membranes are thin, sheet-like structures covering and protecting body surfaces, lining body cavities and covering the inner surface of hollow organs such as the gastrointestinal (GI) tract (the digestive tract along which food passes as it is broken down) and the respiratory passage, where air travels from the outside in.

These membranes are formed by sheets of epithelial tissue and their supporting connective tissue. They are very similar to, and include, skin. Their function is to cover or line internal structure or cavities or to protect surfaces.

There are three main types of membrane (Figure 1.11).

Mucous membranes

These are also called mucosae. They are moist membranes. Mucosae consist of epithelial cells and their secretions. The secretions are called mucus. Mucus accumulates in the epithelial cells, which swell full. The cell empties its contents to the free surface. The filled epithelial cell looks like a goblet and is known as a goblet cell. The mucus functions to protect surfaces from mechanical and chemical damage and traps foreign particles. Mucous membranes are found at all cavities that open to the exterior.

Mucosae are found in the

- respiratory tract – see Chapter 7, 'Breathing';
- gastrointestinal tract – see Chapter 9, 'Eating and Drinking';
- genitourinary tract – see Chapter 10, 'Eliminating'.

Mucous membranes can also be adapted for absorption – the taking in of substances – or secretion of substances such as mucus.

Chapter Reference

Mucous membranes are mentioned again in chapters referring to the activity in which they play a part. For instance, the mucous membrane involved in digestion is discussed in Chapter 9, 'Eating and Drinking' (see p. 241).

Serous membranes

These membranes are also called serosa. The serosa secretes a watery fluid called serous fluid. The serosa forms a double layer of cells of loose areolar connective tissue lined by simple squamous epithelial tissue. These two layers form

- a parietal layer – lines cavities;
- a visceral layer – surrounds organs.

The layers are separated by serous fluid. Serous fluid is secreted by epithelial cells and allows the two layers to glide across each other. The serous membrane thus prevents friction.

Serous membranes line cavities that do not open to the exterior and are found in

- plueral thoracic cavity and lungs;
- pericardium – pericardial cavity and heart;
- peritoneum – abdominal cavity and organs.

Chapter Reference

Serous membranes again appear in other chapters. For example, serous membranes surrounding the thoracic cavity are discussed in Chapter 7, 'Breathing' (see p. 184).

Synovial membranes are a type of serous membrane found lining joint cavities and surrounding tendons.

They secrete synovial fluid as a lubricant, as is often found around joints and cartilage of the skeleton.

Cutaneous membrane

This membrane forms the integumentary system, which contains the skin and accessory tissue such as hair and nails. This is formed of an outer epithelial layer and an inner connective

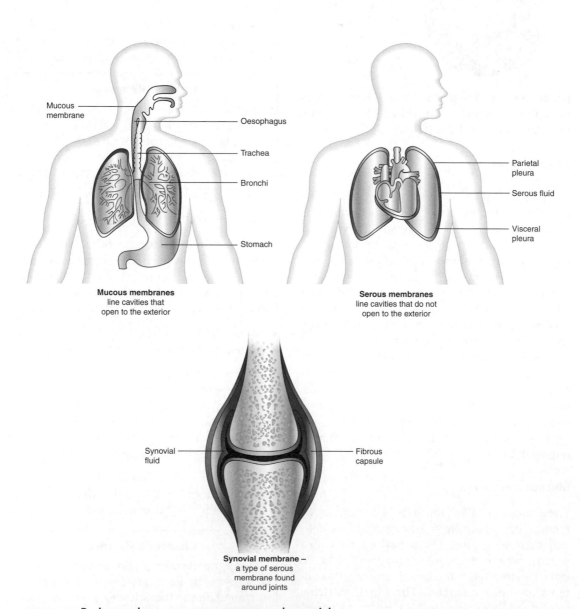

FIGURE 1.11 **Body membranes: mucous, serous and synovial**

tissue layer. The outer layer is mainly dry, with a large amount of keratin protein in the cells. The skin and nails help to form a protective barrier between the internal and external environments and play a part in controlling body temperature and maintaining a safe environment by excluding invading foreign organisms such as bacteria and viruses.

Chapter Reference

The skin is discussed further in Chapter 5, 'Controlling and Repairing' (see p. 142) and Chapter 3, 'Growing and Developing' (see p. 64). Avoiding infection is discussed further in Chapter 11, 'Cleansing and Dressing' (see p. 299).

Repair of tissues

As with other homeostatic mechanisms of the body, the number of cells we have in a tissue is regulated by the number we need. If cells are damaged they are replaced during a process called **tissue repair** or **wound healing**. During tissue repair cells are regenerated, i.e. generated again, by cell division from a pool of cells called stem cells. These are cells that are long living in the body, but provide daughter cells that are short living. The daughter cells have more specialised functions appropriate to the tissue in which they occur. For instance, damage to epithelial cells will cause epithelial stem cells to make daughter cells that will replace the damaged cells. These daughter cells will in turn be liable to damage and will be replaced again by regeneration.

Some tissues are more able to regenerate after damage than other tissues. Some tissues cannot regenerate similar cells and replace lost cells with **scar tissue**, which is formed from fibrous connective tissue. This scar tissue cannot carry out the normal function of the appropriate tissue and the function of the tissue is therefore compromised.

Tissues that regenerate easily:

- epithelial tissue and
- fibrous connective tissue.

Tissues that regenerate poorly:

- skeletal muscles.

Tissues that regenerate mainly with scar tissue:

- cardiac muscle and
- nervous tissue.

Chapter Reference

Tissue repair is discussed further in Chapter 3, 'Growing and Developing' (see p. 64) and Chapter 5, 'Controlling and Repairing' (see p. 142).

Organs and systems

Cells do not operate independently; they operate in groups, tissues, which in turn form organs. Organs operate to maintain the physiology of our bodies; our living processes need

---

Health Connection

Cancer

The tissues that can repair easily, epithelial and connective, are also the tissues that are most prone to cancerous growths. Epithelial tissue forms carcinomas, while connective tissues form sarcoma-type cancers. Each time a cell divides to form new cells there are chances that the copying of the genetic material, DNA, could be inaccurate and cause a mutation. This in turn could cause abnormal growth, a characteristic of cancers. Common cancers are in tissue that has a higher turnover of cells due to cells wearing out and being replaced by new cells. This will be discussed further in Chapter 3, 'Growing and Developing'.

to maintain our internal environment and keep our cells functioning.

Organs are fairly discrete structures both anatomically and physiologically. Some organs are composed of only one type of tissue; for example, glands are composed of epithelial tissue. Some organs are composed of two types of tissue; for example, skin is composed of epithelial and connective tissue. Most organs are composed of a number of tissues; for example, the heart has an inner epithelial layer lining the tubes and cavities, a middle layer of muscle tissue that carries out the pumping mechanism and an outer layer of connective tissue anchoring the heart to the chest wall.

Organs can in turn be part of organ systems (body systems) where two or more organs work together to carry out a function; for example, the stomach, intestines and pancreas work together to digest food. These systems work together to carry out the living processes of the body, for example to digest food into nutrients, to transport those nutrients to cells for metabolic processes and to remove waste.

These systems then work together to form the whole person.

Each of these organs and systems is discussed in chapters throughout this book (see Table 1.3).

Table 1.3 Organs and systems

System	Organs and cells	Chapter
Reproductive	Gonads (ovaries, testes), genitals (vagina, penis), uterus, placenta	3
Endocrine	Endocrine glands (pituitary, pancreas, adrenal, gonad)	4
Nervous	Brain, spinal cord, nerves, neurons, glia	4
Integumentary	Skin, hair, nails, sense receptors, sweat glands, oil glands	5
Skeletal	Bone, joints	6
Muscular	Muscles, tendons	6
Respiratory	Lungs, nose, trachea, bronchioles, diaphragm	7
Transport (circulatory)	Blood, lymph, heart, vessels	8
Digestive	Mouth, teeth, stomach, intestine, liver, pancreas	9
Excretory (elimination)	Renal, kidneys, bladder	10
Immune (lymphatic)	White blood cells, thymus, spleen, nodes, tonsils	11

Health Connection

A community of cells

We have started with cells, progressed to tissues and now are looking at the organs and body systems. It is hard to think down to the cellular and fluid levels to see that most of what affects a large organ or system starts at a small cellular level, a cell not having what it needs and therefore not acting in the normal physiological manner, which then affects the cells around it, which then affects the whole person. We may be multicellular, but we are really a community of cells each affecting and being affected by the other cells.

Health and illness

When a patient presents with a problem it is often associated with an organ and therefore has an effect on a whole system, which affects the whole body and person, making them 'feel ill' in general.

During health our bodies work as a cohesive whole. If cells start to malfunction they can affect the organ in which they are, which in turn affects entire body systems and can result in illness. Cells act independently, but exist in cooperation to maintain homeostasis in health. Any malfunctions can therefore affect our health. The functioning cells, tissues, organs and systems are therefore studied by biologists, who then inform our understanding of health.

Anatomical orientation: Cavities and the organisation of the body

Finally, the tissues and organs are found in various locations in the body. These locations can be categorised or described in a number of ways.

There are detailed anatomical descriptions to make locations precise and orienteering accurate. Below are some common anatomical terms and their meanings:

- superior – above,
- inferior – below,
- anterior – in front of,
- posterior – behind,
- medial – on the inner side of,
- lateral – on the outer side of,
- proximal – close to,
- distal – farther from,
- superficial – at the body surface,
- deep – away from the body surface,
- dorsal – to the front,
- ventral – to the rear,
- rostral – to the head and
- caudal – to the tail.

The body can be divided, simply, into three areas:

- head,
- trunk and
- appendages (arms and legs).

It can also be divided into cavities (from the word cavernous or cave) or gaps, which identify where organs can be found. The six cavities are (also see Figure 1.12)

- cranial,
- thoracic,
- pleural,
- pericardial,
- abdominal and
- pelvic.

Anatomical terms

Anatomical terms help us to navigate around the body and are used clinically to be precise about where an injury, intervention or treatment occurs.

The position on a body can also be described by regions (body areas) (Table 1.4).

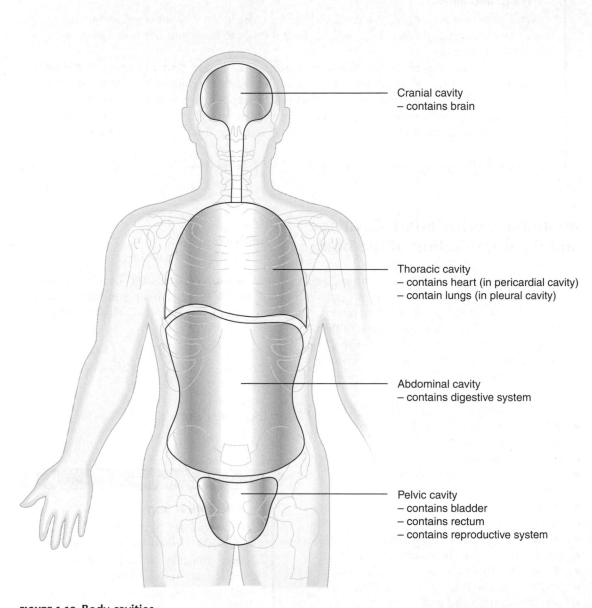

Cranial cavity
– contains brain

Thoracic cavity
– contains heart (in pericardial cavity)
– contain lungs (in pleural cavity)

Abdominal cavity
– contains digestive system

Pelvic cavity
– contains bladder
– contains rectum
– contains reproductive system

FIGURE 1.12 Body cavities

Table 1.4 Anatomical terms and their body regions

Anatomical term	Body regions
Abdominal	Anterior body trunk inferior to ribs
Axillary	Armpit
Brachial	Arm
Digital	Fingers, toes
Femoral	Thigh
Inguinal	Area where thigh meets body trunk; groin
Oral	Mouth
Nasal	Nose area
Pelvic	Area overlying the pelvis anteriorly
Sternal	Breastbone area
Thoracic	Chest
Umbilical	Navel
Cervical	Neck region
Deltoid	Curve of shoulder formed by deltoid muscle
Gluteal	Buttocks
Lumbar	Area of back between ribs and hips
Occipital	Posterior surface of head
Sacral	Posterior area between hips

Conclusion: Maintaining a safe environment

We live in an indifferent external environment in which we coexist with many other species of organisms all trying to survive and thrive. In a multicellular organism such as humans, our cells coexist in a community, each one trying to survive and thrive as well as contribute to our total survival; each competing and cooperating to increase its individual and our collective chances of living. Variables, by their nature, vary. Those in the external environment we cannot really control, but we must control the internal ones to maximise our chances of survival and keep ourselves as safe as possible. Homeostasis is the mechanism that measures our variables, reports any changes and motivates us to maintain optimal conditions. When all of this is in place our internal environment is relatively safe and we are healthy and able to carry out all the ADLs that allow us to interact with our environment and be alive.

Chapter Summary

- This chapter introduces the concept of homeostasis (self-maintenance).
- Homeostasis allows biological living processes to be carried out to maintain the organism.
- In health homeostasis allows us to maintain our own internal environment so that we may carry out the needed activities of daily living (ADLs) that allow us to function.
- The external environment fluctuates and is not ideal for our bodies.
- Our internal environment fluctuates due to metabolic processes.
- All living processes are carried out to maintain our internal environment.
- Homeostasis links our internal needs to the external environment.
- Homeostasis links our health to our safety.
- We are formed from cells and have formed all the cells of our bodies using the raw material of the universe, chemicals.
- Cells have a plasma or cell membrane, cytoplasm and organelles.
- Differentiation is a process that allows cells to have variety from a generic type.
- Different cells vary in their shape, size and lifespan.
- Different types of cells form different types of tissues.
- We have many types of cell, but they are categorised into four types called tissues.
- These four types are epithelial, connective, muscle and nervous.
- The four types have different anatomical shapes from the generic cell.
- The anatomical differences allow different physiological functions (processes) to be performed.
- The large organs of our bodies are formed from tissues which are formed from cells.
- Organs carry out the functions of our bodies in groups called systems.
- Some organs are formed of *one* tissue type only; e.g. glands are made from epithelial tissue.
- Other organs are made of *two* types of tissue, e.g. membranes, skin.
- Most organs are made of many tissue types; e.g. the heart is made mainly of cardiac muscle, but also has connective tissue, and the inner tubes with blood flowing through are lined with epithelial tissue.
- Surrounding many organs are membranes that protect and hold organs in place.
- The body can be oriented through descriptive terms to help locate tissues precisely.

Working and Playing

Chapter Outline

- Introduction: Working and playing as activities of daily living
- Levels of organisation
- Chemicals: Energy and reactions
- Energy and ATP
- Conclusion: Working and playing
- Chapter summary

All work and no play makes Jack a dull boy

James Howell (1659) Historian and writer

Introduction: Working and playing as activities of daily living

There is a very famous saying that is applied to business transactions, but in fact is based on some fundamental laws of physics: *There is no free lunch in the universe*. In physics it points to the fact, for example, that there are no perpetual-energy machines. Making energy, such as electrical energy, requires using another energy source, such as the burning of fossil fuels (oil or coal). You cannot synthesise energy you can only *transfer* it from one substance to another. In biology we also cannot create energy from nothing; we *release* it from one source and *transfer* it to another. The source from which we obtained the energy then no longer has that energy. Just like a bank account: once you take money out to put it somewhere else (a shop or another account) the original money is no longer there. There is no free lunch in the universe; everything has a *cost* associated with it and *work*, using energy, must be done to achieve what is needed.

In biology if you want to transport chemicals around the body you either have to make substances that will act as transporters (which takes energy to do) or use up a lot of energy to move substances (active transport as we saw in Chapter 1, 'Maintaining a Safe Environment'). If you want to move yourself around it takes energy. If you want to escape from a predator you need to run, which takes energy. And what's more you have to make the energy that you need to carry out all the activities that consume energy; it doesn't arrive without effort. To maintain your homeostasis takes energy.

We measure the energy we make and consume in *calories* (in science we use the *joule* instead). These measurements are assessing how much energy there is in a substance. Energy can then be released from a substance and used to do *work*, and work allows us to rest and *play*.

We all strive to achieve a balance in our lives between work and play. If we cannot make energy we cannot function at all; we cease to work. Our muscles will not move, our lungs will not fill with air and our blood will not circulate – we will die. Energy is vital for our survival and we have to work to make it so that we can use it do work! This chapter looks at how we enable ourselves to make the energy we need for all our activities, whether they are work or play.

To understand how we can work and play we must first understand what we are made of, the atoms, elements and molecules of our bodies and some of the most important chemistry of the body.

Levels of organisation

The internal environment

We mentioned the internal environment in Chapter 1, 'Maintaining a Safe Environment'. The internal environment is the safe environment we are trying to maintain. We are adapted, through a process called **evolution**, to be able to survive in a variety of conditions; we are self-maintaining, but we must adjust our living processes to cope with the variety of environments we encounter and our day-to-day needs. The external environment in which we live varies all the time and we must do work to survive in it, to maintain our internal environment safely, in homeostasis, in the appropriate ranges, to keep our internal environment at optimal conditions. Failure to do that results in ill health and even death. This chapter will look further at what our internal environment is made of and reactions needed to keep it healthy.

> **Chapter Reference**
>
> Evolution is discussed in Chapter 3, 'Growing and Developing' (see p. 64) and in Chapter 13, 'Dying' (see p. 340).

We are composed of the same material substance or *matter* as the external environment in which we live. This matter is composed of *chemicals*. Chemicals obey the laws of nature in their behaviours and thus we must obey these same laws of nature, of physics and chemistry, like any other composites of chemicals. We living things seem to be quite rare in the universe. This may be due to how complex we are or to what we are made of. The most abundant chemical in the Earth's crust is *oxygen*, while the most abundant in the universe is a chemical called *hydrogen*. Oxygen is the most abundant chemical in us as it appears not only as a gas, oxygen, but also as part of water.

The famous TV science-fiction programme *Star Trek* got it right when it said that we are '*a carbon-based life form*'. The chemical carbon forms the basis of many of the substances that give us structure: the cell membranes, the foods we eat and need, the proteins that carry out our functions. Carbon, however, is not the most the most abundant chemical on this planet; in fact carbon's nearest relative, silicon, a chemical that forms the basis of sand and glass, is one of the most abundant chemicals, but we are not made of it. There must be something about carbon, therefore, that makes it more suitable as a material for living processes than silicon or some other more abundant chemicals found on this planet. We shall discuss carbon chemistry below as it forms the basis of most organic chemicals and living organisms.

> **Chapter Reference**
>
> What we are made of and how it behaves ultimately affects our health and will be discussed more fully below.

Apart from obeying the laws governing the material from which we are made we also obey laws relating to the energy we consume. It takes a lot of energy to maintain our physical body structures and our ability to carry out activities. For our cells to function we have to obtain the energy which they use. Plants can take basic raw chemical matter and combine it with sunlight through a process called **photosynthesis** to synthesise the more complex material they need. Animals cannot photosynthesise. We spend a lot of our time finding and making energy. As with other animals, we get our energy from food. Food is composed of chemicals which contain energy and these foods and energy are ultimately from plants that have captured sunlight and converted it into sugars. So we all rely on plants and sunlight, ultimately, for our food and energy needs and thus for our survival. The chemicals that we consume help to provide nutrients and energy and thus maintain homeostasis.

Our internal environment is therefore influenced by the external environment, such as amount of sunshine, water and its quality, air gases and their quality, chemicals and nutrients available, other organisms and the plant life of the planet. We are not alone and we interact with the planet and all its contents to maintain ourselves in health.

Chapter Reference

Food is discussed in Chapter 9, 'Eating and Drinking' (see p. 241).

Homeostasis is discussed in Chapter 1 'Maintaining a Safe Environment' (see p. 1).

Chemicals: Energy and reactions

In Chapter 1, 'Maintaining a Safe Environment', we looked at different levels of organisation from the cell to the whole organism. The chemical world looks at the smallest levels of organisation – what matter is made of, **atoms** and what they *do*, and *reactions* due to energy changes. This echoes the anatomy (structure) and physiology (processes) of living organisms, which is not wholly surprising given that the cells and tissues are ultimately made of atoms and that they therefore have behaviours that are governed by the behaviour of atoms. This is called a *reductionist view*, that we are based on our anatomy and physiology and our anatomy and physiology are based on atoms and reactions. Atoms are the focus of this section.

All material substances found in the universe are, by definition, made of matter, and matter is made of chemicals. Chemistry is the study of these material substances and how these substances combine to make other materials, for instance how carbon combines with other chemicals to make sugar.

At the lowest level of chemical size are **atoms**. All matter is composed of atoms and these atoms can combine to make larger substances called **molecules** and very large molecules found in biological systems called **macromolecules.**

Atoms and elements

Atoms exist in about 110 different types called **elements**. However, in living organisms only

---

Box 2.1 Lifespan – atoms and cells

Atoms are billions of years old, mainly created at the start of the universe. You literally are stardust. Cells, as discussed in Chapter 1, 'Maintaining a Safe Environment' vary from hours to days old, with a very few lasting a lifetime. We are therefore composed of young cells, but old atoms. We recycle the atoms to make new cells. Lifespans are, therefore relative; humans are young in terms of the universe, old in terms of our atoms, and various ages in terms of other humans and our time on Earth.

---

a few types of elements occur. The elements which predominate in biological systems are

- carbon (C),
- hydrogen (H),
- oxygen (O),
- phosphorus (P),
- nitrogen (N) and
- sulphur (S).

There are also trace amounts of other elements, such as

- calcium (Ca),
- sodium (Na),
- potassium (K),
- magnesium (Mg),
- iron (Fe) and
- chlorine (Cl).

In fact 96% of the human body is made of just four elements: carbon, oxygen, hydrogen and nitrogen (see Table 2.1).

All elements are made of atoms. The difference between each element is in slight variations in the atoms of which it is made.

All atoms, from whichever element, have some similarities in structure. They have a central area called (like the one found in a cell) a **nucleus**, around which are **shells** or **orbits** rather like a planetary arrangement with the sun at the centre and planets circling around (see Figure 2.1).

Table 2.1 Elements occurring in the human body by percentage

Symbol	Name	Percentage of human body weight
O	Oxygen	65.0
C	Carbon	18.5
H	Hydrogen	9.5
N	Nitrogen	3.3
Ca	Calcium	1.5
P	Phosphorus	1.0
K	Potassium	0.4
S	Sulphur	0.3
Na	Sodium	0.2
Cl	Chlorine	0.2
Mg	Magnesium	0.1
Trace elements	Boron (B), Chromium (Cr), Cobalt (Co), Copper (Cu), Fluorine (F), Iodine (I), Iron (Fe), Manganese (Mn), Molybdenum (Mo), Selenium (Se), Silicon (Sn), Tin (Sn), Vanadium (V), Zinc (Zn)	0.01

All atoms are composed of *subatomic* particles. There are a number of types of particles, but only three are of interest here:

1. **Protons (p^+)** are particles with a positive charge. They are contained in the nucleus of the atom.
2. **Neutrons (n^0)** are neutral particles with no charge, but add mass to the atom. They are contained in the nucleus of the atom.
3. **Electrons (e^-)** are particles with a negative charge. They are contained in **orbits** or **shells** which circle around the nucleus.

In a **neutral atom**, an atom with no net electric charge, the number of protons is the same as the number of electrons. For instance, if an element has an atom with six protons the element will also have six electrons. The number of positive protons will be equal, therefore, to the number of negative electrons and there will be no net charge – the element's charge will be neutral.

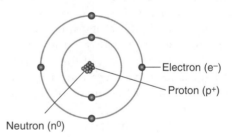

FIGURE 2.1 **A typical element, carbon. Element number 6 with six protons and six electrons. Carbon also has six or seven neutrons in the nucleus**

Neutral atom: proton number = electron number

While all elements are made of atoms the difference between the 110 elements is characterised by the number of protons each has, its **proton number**, also called its **atomic number**. (We shall discuss the neutrons and electrons in Figure 2.1 in a moment.) Because we are usually talking about neutral atoms, the number of protons is equalled by the number of electrons, so we don't tend to mention the electrons when saying which element we are talking about. Each element also has a name, but it is the proton number which tells us more about the element. The name is given a **symbol** (shorthand) for convenience. Sometimes the symbol is not obvious. It may be due to another element starting with the same letter so they both cannot have the same symbol or because the element is known also by another name, often a Latin name. The atomic number, on the other hand, is simple and unique to the element.

Atomic number = number of protons in atom = element (and its name)

For example:

- Element 1 has one proton (element 1 is named hydrogen, symbol H).
- Element 2 has two protons (element 2 is named helium, symbol He).
- Element 3 has three protons (element 3 is named lithium, symbol Li).
- Element 11 has 11 protons (element 11 is named sodium, symbol Na).
- Element 17 has 17 protons (element 17 is named chlorine, symbol Cl) etc.

The atomic number is one of the ways atoms are organised and grouped together in a table. You may not be used to graphs and tables, but tables are just ways of representing things such as variables. For example, we can use an attendance table (register) where the names of the people are written in one column and how often they attend is written in another column. The elements can be written in a table. The table that you may have seen in school organises the elements in their ascending atomic number so that element 1 (with one proton) is before element 2 (with two protons). It is thus a convenient way

of listing the elements by counting up how many protons they have and arranging them in ascending order from 1 to 110. The table is called the **Periodic Table of the Elements** and lists all the elements in the universe from 1 to 110.

The Periodic Table of the Elements

The Periodic Table of the Elements lists all 110 elements, as seen in Figure 2.2.

If you read it from left to right it starts with element 1, hydrogen (H); then all the way over on the other side is element 2, helium (He); then the next row down is element 3, lithium (Li), then element 4, beryllium (Be), then element 5, boron (B), then element 6, carbon (C) and so on. The elements are written by their symbol for shorthand, rather than their full names. However, they are arranged in increasing proton (atomic) number. There are a couple of exceptions to the layout, which make the numbers jump from 57 to 72 and from 89 to 104. These are the rare earth metals, also called the lanthanide and actinide series, which are depicted in the figure in grey (elements 58–71 and 90–103 respectively).

The reasons that there are groups and columns with number 1 on one side and number 2 on another will be explained below.

As discussed, atoms are a form of matter or material; they have substance. However, the material that makes up atoms, the protons and especially the electrons, has very little substance. There is a third particle, the **neutron**, that adds mass to atoms and is important in the atomic weights of the elements. Neutrons have little impact on the chemistry that we shall discuss here, but are important in the chemistry of **isotopes**, which are varieties in which an element occurs.

Very few of the elements occur in biological systems so there are very few that need to trouble us in this book! We are concerned with the main elements found in biological systems, as mentioned above, in Table 2.1.

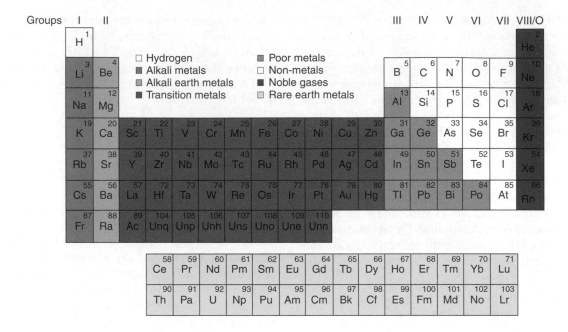

FIGURE 2.2 **Periodic Table of the Elements**

Box 2.2 Summary – Elements

- There are 110 elements in the universe.
- All elements are all composed of atoms.
- The elements can be listed in a table.
- The elements can be numbered from 1 to 110.
- The number of an element is its atomic number.
- The atomic number is a function of how many protons the element has.

remained as separate elements there would only be 110 types of material in the universe. However, elements tend to join together to form molecules and macromolecules. This allows there to be many types of substances, also called *compounds*, in the universe.

If this is hard to imagine think of the English language. There are many words (compounds) in the language, but if you broke them down into their constituent parts there are

Chemical bonds, electrons and ions

While there are 110 known elements in the universe there are millions of different types of material substances. If all of these elements

only 26 – the letters (elements) of the alphabet. Any English word can be composed of only these letters; the same with compounds. If you break down the compounds into their constituent parts they are composed of the elements above.

The Periodic Table shows the elements in ascending order of atomic (proton) number. It also has *columns* of elements *grouped* together. These elements have been lined up in this way because they behave in similar fashions. While, so far, we have only discussed the protons, the changing behaviour of elements in the groups seen in the table is due to how their *electrons* are arranged. This in turn affects how they join with other elements to form molecules and macromolecules.

If we look at the right-hand side of the Periodic Table there are a group of elements in **red** called the **noble gases**. These elements are also called the **inert gases**. Inert means that they have a tendency to remain the same. These elements are very unreactive, meaning that they do not like to combine with each other or with any other element to form more complex compounds. If all elements behaved like inert elements there would be, as mentioned above, only 110 types of things in the universe. Most elements are not like these and are reactive.

If we look at the arrangements of the *electrons* that surround the protons of an atom we shall start to see why some are unreactive and some are very reactive.

Electrons are contained in shells that orbit around the nucleus of the atom. Shells are numbered from the innermost shell, the one closest to the nucleus, outwards (see Figure 2.3).

Each shell has a set number of electrons it can contain:

- The first shell, innermost shell, can contain a maximum of *two electrons*.
- The second shell can contain a maximum of *eight electrons*.
- The third shell can contain more than *eight electrons*.

If you look at the first inert gas, helium (He), it is element number 2. It therefore has two protons and two electrons. Electrons tend to fill the shell nearest the nucleus first before filling the next shell. Both electrons fill shell number one, which can contain a maximum of two electrons. There is no space for more and the shell is complete.

The second inert gas is neon (Ne), element 10. It has 10 protons and 10 electrons. Two of the electrons will fill the first shell and then the other eight electrons will fill the next shell, which can contain a maximum of eight electrons. Both the first and second shells are thus filled.

The third inert gas is Argon (Ar), element 18. It has 18 protons and 18 electrons. Two of the electrons fill the first shell. Eight of the electrons fill the second shell and the last eight electrons fill the third shell. All three shells are thus complete (Figure 2.4).

The outer shell of an element is called a **valence shell**. In inert elements their valence shells are complete. This arrangement gives us a clue as to why these elements have such inert behaviour. Complete shells appear to confer stability to an element – they don't want to change. This is the reason they are so unreactive. Inert gases can be used in areas where we don't want a reaction, such as in light bulbs (neon lights for example) that we don't want to explode.

If we look at element 11, which is called sodium (chemical symbol Na), we can see how its electrons are arranged. Element 11 has 11 protons and 11 electrons. Two of the electrons are in the first shell, eight are in the second shell and the eleventh is all by itself in the third shell as there is no room for it in the first two shells.

It would appear that to be stable and *inert*, not changing or combining, an element has to have complete shells. For sodium to have complete shells would require it to lose that one electron that is alone in its outer shell. Then it would have a complete first and second shell. If it loses one electron it remains atomic number 11 with 11 protons, but now it only has 10 electrons. There is thus one more proton (11) than there are electrons (10). This atom of sodium is no longer neutral; it has a charge on it, a positive charge of one. It is no longer called an atom of sodium; it is called and **ion**

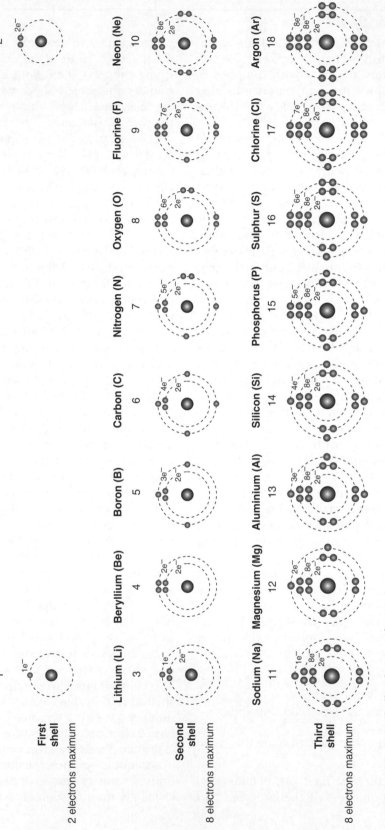

FIGURE 2.3 Electron shells of some elements

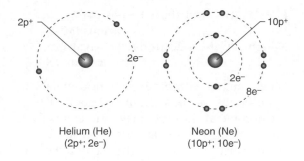

Helium (He)
(2p⁺; 2e⁻)

Neon (Ne)
(10p⁺; 10e⁻)

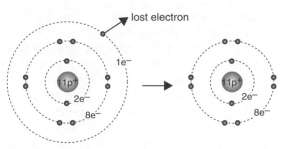

FIGURE 2.5 **Sodium atom loses an electron to become a sodium ion**

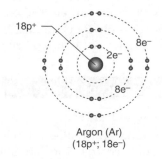

Argon (Ar)
(18p⁺; 18e⁻)

FIGURE 2.4 **Inert elements**

of sodium – in this case a positive ion, a **cation**. Ions are therefore atoms with electrical charges, either positive or negative (Figure 2.5).

If we look at element 17, which is called chlorine (chemical symbol Cl), we can see that is has 17 protons and 17 electrons. The electrons are arranged as follows:

- two electrons in the first shell,
- eight electrons in the second shell and
- seven electrons in the third shell.

For chlorine to behave like an inert gas the easiest solution to complete its third shell would be by the addition of one electron (rather than lose seven electrons). It would still have 17 protons if it did that, but it would now have 18 electrons. There would therefore be 17 positive charges in the atom, but 18 negative charges, a net charge of one negative charge. It is no longer a neutral atom of chlorine, but an ion of chlorine, in this case a negative ion, an **anion**.

In **ions**, therefore, there are a different number of electrons to protons.

Box 2.3 Summary – Atoms and ions

- All elements are composed of atoms.
- Atoms contain protons (positive) and electrons (negative).
- Neutral atoms have equal numbers of protons and electrons.
- Each element has a unique number of protons (atomic number) and therefore of electrons (when neutral).
- Ions are not neutral atoms.
- In ions atoms do not have equal numbers of protons and electrons.
- In ions the numbers of electrons change.
- Cation = atom – electron.
- Cations have more protons than electrons (the element has lost electrons). Cations have a positive charge.
- Anion = atom + electron.
- Anions have fewer protons than electrons (the element has gained electrons).

Anions have a negative charge: Ionic bonds

Where does chlorine get its extra electron from to make it a negative anion? Well it may well take the one that sodium wishes to lose. When it does that sodium becomes positively charged and chlorine becomes negatively charged. Opposites attract, so the positive sodium cation is attracted to the negative chlorine anion. These two elements come together to form a compound. They are held together by these ionic attractions where their outer valence shells form what is called an **ionic bond** between them. If one element forms a bond with another element it has formed a **compound**. This means that there can be more than 110 types of matter in the universe; there can be compounds of many different types of elements. The compound formed in this case is **sodium chloride**, which we know as common table **salt** (Figure 2.6).

Metals, salts and electrolytes

Looking at the Periodic Table most elements on it are called **metals**. Metals are elements that lose electrons to form **positive cations**. The non-metals on the right of the table tend to gain electrons to form negative anions.

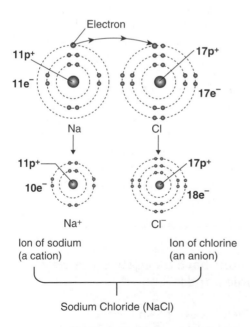

FIGURE 2.6 **Electron transfer and ionic bonding in sodium and chlorine**

Metals (M) – electron (e⁻) = positive
cations (M⁺).
Non-metals (N) + electron (e⁻) = negative
cations (N⁻).

When metals combine with non-metals in ionic bonds such as the metal sodium with the non-metal chlorine, they form compounds called **salts**, and salts can form large ionic molecules called salt crystals. They tend to be very hydrophilic and dissolve in water into their ionic parts. The dissolved ions are then called electrolytes as they give an electric charge (+ and –) to the solution. Salts are also formed from acid–base reactions, discussed below.

Health Connection

Ions, salt and water

Ions are atoms with either a positive or negative charge. They are able to dissolve in water and when they do so they are called electrolytes, giving the water an electrical charge. Electrolytes play a vital role in the fluids of our bodies in health, in our diets (as minerals or salts) and in many medicines and will be discussed in further chapters.

This is partly why we are able to have electrical charge flow through us.

Groups

The Periodic Table is not just organised in ascending order of proton numbers; as mentioned above, the elements are also grouped in *columns* with similar *properties*.

On the left-hand side are group 1 elements – hydrogen (H), lithium (Li), sodium (Na), potassium (K) etc. All group 1 elements have one electron in their outer ring and tend to lose that *one* electron when making compounds to form 1+ cations. They are then written in their ionic forms as, for example:

H^+
Li^+
Na^+
K^+

All group 2 elements, such as beryllium (Be), magnesium (Mg), calcium (Ca), have two electrons in their outer ring, which they tend to lose to form positive cations with *two* positive charges on them.

They are then written in their ionic forms as, for example:

Be^{2+}
Mg^{2+}
Ca^{2+}

If we ignore the middle of the table between group 2 and group 3, the **transition elements** such as copper (Cu) and iron (Fe), we can see a group that starts with boron (B) and aluminium (Al). These elements have three electrons in their outer shells and would like to lose all *three* electrons to become:

B^{3+}
Al^{3+}

It takes energy to remove electrons so the elements that only need to lose one electron can do so more easily than those that need to remove three electrons. Sodium is thus a very reactive element and forms compounds readily, which is why you do not find pure elemental sodium around the place – it has reacted with other elements. Aluminium is less reactive and thus can be isolated and used in pure elemental form such as coating foils and cans, forming a barrier and not easily reacting with elements such as oxygen at room temperature.

On the other side of the table the elements in the group with fluorine (F) chlorine (Cl) and bromine (Br) have seven electrons in their outer shell and would like to gain *one* electron

to become negative anions. They would then be written as:

F^-
Cl^-
Br^-

If we look at the group with oxygen (O), sulphur (S) and selenium (Se) they all have six electrons in their outer shell and would like to gain *two* electrons to complete that shell. They would then be anions with two negative charges:

O^{2-}
S^{2-}
Se^{2-}

Finally, the group with nitrogen (N) and Phosphorus (P) in it have five electrons in their outer ring and would like to gain *three* electrons to complete the ring. They become negative anions:

N^{3-}
P^{3-}

The **ion charge** + or – of the element is written *above* the element.

Health Connection

Electrical ions

If our heart stops we can be electrically stimulated to cause it to start again in the same way a car can be 'jump-started' when its battery has gone flat. We can also be electrocuted if we touch a live wire. Both of these are due to having electrical elements in us, called ions.

Chemical formulas

In chemical formulas we write the ratio of one element to the other. For example:

$CaCl_2$ has one calcium for every two chlorines. $MgCl_2$ has one magnesium and two chlorines. NaCl has one sodium and one chlorine.

Box 2.4 Groups of ionic forming elements

Metals:

Group 1 lose one electron   Form a 1^+ cation
Group 2 lose two electrons   Form a 2^+ cation
Group 3 lose three electrons   Form a 3^+ cation

Non-metals:

Group 7 gain one electron   Form a 1^- anion
Group 6 gain two electrons   Form a 2^- anion
Group 5 gain three electrons   Form a 3^- anion

The *ratio* of how many of one element combine with another element is written *below* the element.

When we write $CaCl_2$ (calcium chloride) we are saying that there is one calcium for every two chlorines. That is because calcium has two electrons it wants to lose from its outer shell, but chlorine only has room for one electron in its outer shell of seven so another chlorine is needed to 'mop up' the second electron from calcium. We can write it with the ion charge on it:

$$Ca^{2+} Cl^-_2$$

This formula means that calcium loses two electrons to make a cation with two extra positive charges, while chlorine is able to gain one electron to make an anion with one extra negative charge. However, the other electron is still available from calcium so another chlorine atom is needed. Now both electrons from the calcium are attached, one to each chlorine, and the calcium and the chlorine each has a 'complete' outer shell. The chemical formula is a quick way of saying all of this!

Elements can thus appear as neutral, uncharged atoms such as Na and Cl or as charged ions such as Na^+ and Cl^-.

The compounds these elements form through ionic bonds are called **salts** and tend to be *soluble* in water (**hydrophilic**, meaning loving water) and thus **dissolve** in water. **Ions**, also called **electrolytes** when dissolved in water, are thus charged versions of atoms, and are important in biology.

While elements can join together through ionic interactions, not all elements will do this.

Health Connection

Chemical formulas and drugs

Often we need to replace chemicals lost in the body either during healthy living or during a trauma or illness. When we replace chemicals clinically we may use drugs. Drugs have an active part that we want, but may also be attached, chemically, to inactive (inert) chemicals or to carrier chemicals. The full chemical formula shows all the parts that are in a drug and the ratios of each part.

Covalent bonds

The Periodic Table has a number of columns in it. If we ignore the transition elements between groups 2 and 3, we can count across eight groups. We have already said that group 1, with sodium in it, has elements with one electron in their outer shell which they tend to lose, while elements in group 7, such as chlorine, have seven electrons in their outer shell and tend to gain one electron. In the middle are group 4 elements, and the most important one for us is element 6, **carbon** (C). As carbon is element number 6 or atomic number 6, carbon has six protons and six electrons. The electrons are arranged:

- two electrons in the first shell,
- four electrons in the second shell.

This presents a conundrum. To have complete shells either carbon needs to gain four electrons in its outer second shell or lose the four electrons in its outer second shell to have a complete first shell. Both possibilities are unlikely. It takes a lot of energy to move an electron and the likelihood of moving four is very remote. So instead carbon *shares* electrons in its valence shell and forms bonds called **covalent bonds**. Carbon is not the only element that can form covalent bonds, but this gives it many properties that allow it to form what we call 'organic molecules', which form the basis of life. It can also form covalent bonds with other elements (Figure 2.7).

This has very important implications for how carbon behaves. Chains and rings of carbon form the basis of what is called organic chemistry, which eventually is part of biochemistry, the chemistry of life. We, as they say, are a 'carbon-based life form' because of the chemistry of carbon.

Carbon can *share* electrons with other carbon atoms and with other elements, such as oxygen or hydrogen. Sometimes when forming these molecules there are still spare electrons that are not fully involved in a bond. These electrons can make double bonds for example:

- Single carbon to carbon bond   C–C
- Double carbon to carbon bond C=C

Double bonds can have various effects on a molecule; the commonest one we see is in *saturated* and *unsaturated* fats. Saturated fats have no double bonds: all the electrons form single bonds; the molecule is saturated. Unsaturated fats have one or more double bonds. This affects how the molecule lines up. Saturated fats can form long lines of carbon and hydrogen atoms and lie next to each other. Due to this they can often be *solid* at room temperature. Unsaturated fats have kinks in them due to the double bond and the molecules cannot line up next to each other. They tend to be *liquid* at room temperature. Chefs like saturated fats as they don't burn so easily; they are solid and then heat up to liquid. Health professionals prefer unsaturated fats as they do not appear to block blood vessels as easily as saturated fats. So knowing about bonds can help us understand cooking and health!

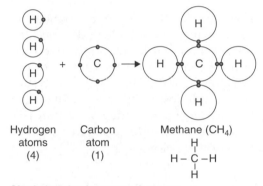

Hydrogen   Carbon   Methane (CH_4)
atoms   atom
(4)   (1)

$$H-\overset{\displaystyle H}{\underset{\displaystyle H}{C}}-H$$

Single bonds share two electrons

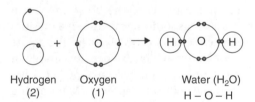

Hydrogen   Oxygen   Water (H_2O)
(2)   (1)

H – O – H

Single bonds share two electrons

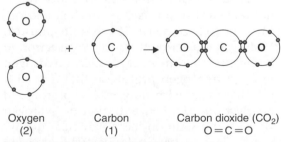

Oxygen   Carbon   Carbon dioxide (CO_2)
(2)   (1)   O=C=O

Double bonds share four electrons

FIGURE 2.7 **Examples of covalent bonds**

Chapter Reference

Fats will be discussed in Chapter 9, 'Eating and Drinking'.

Artherosclerosis and blood vessels will be discussed in Chapter 8, 'Transporting'.

Chemicals and foods

You are what you eat. As you use up chemicals in your body each day you need to replace them. The chemicals you replace them with must be similar to the ones you are made of. Most of our foods are carbon based; carbohydrates – which actually means carbon, hydrogen and oxygen – proteins and fats and are all carbon based and therefore part of organic chemistry.

Box 2.5 Summary – Chemical bonds

- Elements form bonds with each other to complete their outer (valence) shell.
- Some elements lose or gain outer electrons to form ions.
- These ions can then form ionic bonds with other elements.
- Negative ions form ionic bonds with positive ions.
- Some elements share their outer electrons to form covalent bonds.

Polar and hydrogen bonds

Some covalent bonds are *non-polar* – the electrons that form the bond are evenly distributed between the two atoms.

Some covalent bonds are *polar,* where the electrons forming the bond are not evenly distributed between the two atoms, each pulling or pushing away the electrons with different forces so that one atom becomes slightly positive and one slightly negative. These types of bonds have a slight polarity to them but not as much as an ionic bond. They are much weaker (easier to break apart) than ionic bonds. Other types of weak bonds are *hydrogen bonds,* where the one electron of hydrogen is not lost, but moves towards an element with a strong positive charge, leaving the hydrogen slightly negative. While all of these are weak bonds in themselves, they are *cumulative* (they add up); the more there are of them in a molecule the more stable the molecule is against disruption from the environment.

Many biological compounds are composed of huge molecules held together in covalent bonds. The molecules fold over one another into three-dimensional (3D) shapes.

In covalent bonds some elements pull or push electrons towards or away from themselves making the covalent molecule polar. They are held together by polar, non-polar or

hydrogen bonds. These give great stability to the 3D structure. Many biological molecules, such as enzymes and hormones, derive their properties from their 3D shape and will be discussed below. Altering the 3D shape results in the molecule losing its activity. Hydrogen bonds play a large part in the 3D structure of a molecule. Three-dimensional structures will be discussed further below.

Hydrogen ions and pH

Dissolved in the fluids of the body are a variety of ions such as sodium, calcium, magnesium and chlorine. Some are involved in electrolyte and water balance which is very important for the movement of substances around our bodies and is discussed in Chapter 1, 'Maintaining a Safe Environment', and in Chapter 10, 'Eliminating'.

Hydrogen can form ions in two ways. It has one electron in its valence shell and can gain one to become H^-. This is quite unusual. Hydrogen tends to lose its solitary electron to become **H^+** to form what is called a **hydrogen ion** or a **hydrogen proton**, as that is what it is: a hydrogen with only its one proton and no electron. The concentration of hydrogen H^+ ions in a solution has a particular quality called the **acid–base balance**. Acids are solutions with lots of H^+ (hydrogen ion protons) in them, while bases are elements with fewer

H$^+$ in them. Bases are often defined as solutions with lots of **OH**$^-$ ions in them. This is due to the nature of water, which can become slightly **polarised** (see above) and therefore ionic.

$$H_2O \leftrightharpoons H^+ + OH^-$$

The amount of H$^+$ ions in a solution can be measured on a scale called the **pH scale**. The pH scale runs from 1 to 14. Acidic solutions have low pH from 1 to 6. Alkalis have a pH from 8 to 14. The very high and the very low pH solutions tend to be dangerous, very caustic soda or very strong acids. In the middle at pH 7 the solution is said to be neutral.

Acids in general are molecules that can release hydrogen ions. They are sometimes called **proton donors**. Bases are molecules that are sometimes called **proton acceptors**. When acids and bases react together they form water and a salt in a neutralisation reaction (Table 2.2).

Many fluids of the human body, such as *blood*, *urine*, *lymph*, have a pH near neutral, ranging from 6.8 to 7.2 and most of the cells of the body can only operate around this neutral pH. There are exceptions to this; for example, inside the *stomach* the pH is very acidic at about pH 2. Because of this the cells lining the stomach are covered in sticky *mucus* to protect them from the extreme pH.

Health Connection

Activity and pH

The pH of body fluids has a large impact on the behaviour of cells and reactions. The pH in the stomach is very low and acidic. This affects the cells lining the stomach and the contents of the stomach. Only certain enzymes (discussed below) can function in this pH. The skin secretes fluids with acids in to kill bacteria. Blood proteins function best at a near-neutral pH.

Table 2.2 The pH scale. This scale goes from 0, which is very acidic, to 14, which is very alkaline or basic

Acid or Alkaline (basic)	pH	Examples
Very acidic	0	Battery acid
	1	Hydrochloric acid, gastric acid
	2	Lemon juice
Acidic	3	Vinegar, grapefruit juice
	4	Tomato juice
	5	Black coffee
Weakly acidic	6	Milk, urine
Neutral	7	Distilled water
Weakly alkaline	8	
	9	Toothpaste
	10	Milk of magnesia
Alkaline	11	Ammonia
	12	Soapy water
	13	Bleach, oven cleaner
Very alkaline	14	Drain cleaner, caustic soda

The pH levels of our bodies are maintained at their correct level as part of homeostasis. Detectors in the body are sensitive to changes in pH and correct it if it strays outside normal parameters. The main organs involved in maintaining body pH are the kidneys. They help to maintain pH levels by secreting or absorbing H+ ions.

Many functions of the body are carried out by **proteins** (discussed below) and particularly by a type of protein called an **enzyme**. Proteins are especially sensitive to pH. Any deleterious or prolonged changes to pH can have serious consequences for proteins and enzyme actions.

Health Connection

Blood gases and pH

Most systems in the body work within very strict pH ranges. If fluids are not in their appropriate pH range it is an indication that there is something wrong which needs correcting. If the pH varies too much the body cannot carry out its chemical functions. Observations on pH, usually looking at blood gases, are very important in clinical practice.

Health Connection

Stomach problems and pH

When your digestion is 'upset' after eating certain foods it is often a sign that the food has caused a pH imbalance. Many of the medications offered rebalance the pH of the stomach or small intestine.

Water

While we discussed separating water into its constituent parts above to affect pH, water itself is not ionic, but covalent. Because oxygen tries to pull electrons towards itself to fill its outer valence shell, oxygen becomes slightly negative

Health Connection

Salts and nutrition

The elements that form positive ions (cations) are also called metals. They can combine with non-metals such as chlorine to form ionic compounds called salts. Some salts, such as sodium chloride, potassium chloride, magnesium chloride, are essential for our health. They maintain the osmotic balance of our internal fluids, such as cytoplasm, and allow the transport of needed chemicals (nutrients) around the body. Other salts, such as mercury based salts, are dangerous. Mercury is used in thermometers and blood pressure gauges, but should never be ingested or inhaled.

(electronegative), while hydrogen becomes slightly positive (electropositive). In water it means that although the association between oxygen and hydrogen is covalent, there is a slight charge on the molecule, a **dipole**, which means that the water has a **polarity** to it. This allows ionic compounds to be able to dissolve in water and to carry charge through it – beware of electrical appliances near water.

Characteristics of water:

- Water is composed of two atoms of hydrogen to one atom of oxygen and is written in chemistry by the formula H_2O.
- The pH of distilled (pure) water is 7, right in the middle of the pH scale, and water is said to have a neutral pH, neither acidic nor basic.
- Water is the basis for many fluids of our body, as many substances will dissolve in it and can be transported in it.
- Water thus acts as a **solvent** in which many substances, chiefly ionic compounds, can dissolve.
- Ionic substances are water loving, **hydrophilic**, using water as their solvent.
- Non-ionic substances such as fats, oils and lipids are **hydrophobic**, water hating.

Safety, cleanliness and detergents

Fats are a good source of energy and therefore of food. Waste fats must be removed from surfaces to avoid bacterial **growth** and *slippery* surfaces. Because fats don't dissolve in water they are hard to remove from articles such as floors and plates. **Detergents** are designed to have two ends, a **hydrophobic** end that attaches to fats and a **hydrophilic** end that attaches to water. Detergents can thus remove fats in a watery solution such as washing up liquid.

Water

As so many substances can dissolve in water, water is described as the universal solvent of the body. Our bodies are composed of about 60% water. Nearly all our chemical reactions occur in a watery solvent. All the chemicals and gases we take into our bodies are, therefore, moistened or dissolved in water to allow for metabolism to occur.

Without enough water the transport of substances fails and the ability to carry out chemical reactions is severely reduced. This is part of the phenomenon called dehydration, which has such serious health consequences if not quickly corrected. Most of us can survive days without food, but only a few days without water.

Reactions

When atoms or molecules form bonds they combine together. This is called a **synthesis** reaction. When molecules break apart it is called a **decomposition** reaction.

$$A + B \rightarrow C \rightarrow A + B$$
Synthesis   Decomposition

Forming bonds is an **endothermic** reaction; it requires an *input* of energy to make the reaction occur. Breaking bonds between atoms is an **exothermic** reaction; energy is released as an *output*.

To carry out any reactions in the body energy is either needed or released. Some reactions release energy. Some reactions require energy. The energy released from one reaction can be used to fuel another reaction.

Metabolism is a balance of all the chemical reactions of the body, those that need energy and those that release energy. The making and releasing of energy is usually related to the making and breaking of ionic or covalent bonds and this is to do with the movement of electrons. Thus the movement of electrons in ionic and covalent bonds is the basis of chemical reactions. The synthetic reactions where bonds are formed are also called **anabolic** reactions and the reactions where bonds are broken are also known as **catabolic** reactions (Figure 2.8).

Metabolism, energy and diet

Our metabolic rates are a measure of how in balance we are with our inputs of food and our outputs of energy and work. If we put in more food than we use to carry out metabolic reactions the food is stored as fat. If our metabolic reactions use more energy that we acquire in our foods we use up surplus fat and can start to degrade our own body tissue such as muscle, including cardiac muscle. This can lead to severe problems, as seen in starvation and **anorexia nervosa**, an eating disorder which results in severe malnutrition and the catabolism of body tissue to release energy from the molecules in the tissues to be used for vital reactions in the body.

Anabolic reactions
Synthetic reactions where bonds are formed

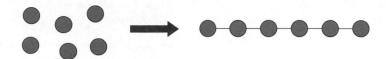

Catabolic reactions
Decomposition reactions where bonds are broken

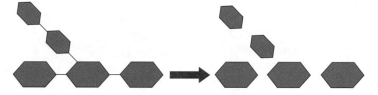

FIGURE 2.8 **Anabolic and catabolic reactions**

Energy and ATP

Energy is required by all living cells to perform the living processes. We are used to energy in the form of coal or gas. These are *fossil fuels*, using previously alive organisms and the energy contained in the carbon atoms that made them. There are other forms of energy, such as sunlight, which is used by plants to make food. While plants can harness the energy of the sun we cannot get our energy directly from sunlight and must consume the food made by plants to release the energy (*calories*) stored in the food. Food is thus a form of *stored energy*. Living systems such as humans can store and utilise a particular chemical form of energy. The chemical that we can use and store is called **adenosine triphosphate (ATP)** and comes from the chemical oxidation of glucose, in other words the combining of oxygen with glucose to make ATP. The glucose comes from food. The oxygen comes from air. We need a digestive system to extract the glucose from food. We need a respiratory system to extract the oxygen from air. We also need a transport system to move the glucose and oxygen to every cell in the body. There they are transported into the cells and utilised in the mitochondria of the cell to make ATP. This ATP is then used for all the functions of the cell and therefore of the body.

Chapter Reference
ATP is discussed in Chapter 9, 'Eating and Drinking' (see p. 241), and in Chapter 7, 'Breathing' (see p. 184). Food is discussed in Chapter 9, 'Eating and Drinking' (see p. 241).

Once glucose and oxygen have combined to make ATP the ATP is used for a variety of processes. When glucose and oxygen combine to form ATP there are also waste products, by-products, made. These waste products are carbon dioxide and water, which must be removed from the cell. Carbon dioxide is expelled by the respiratory tract. Water levels are controlled by the kidney. To outline what happens in the body a **chemical equation** can be used. This shows on one side the starting substances (the **reactants**) and on the other side the **products** that have been synthesised from those reactants.

Glucose + oxygen = ATP + carbon dioxide + water
Reactants ⟶ Products

ATP (Figure 2.9) is synthesised and used all the time, so a constant supply of glucose and oxygen is needed by the cells. Waste products are also synthesised continuously in this process and must be removed via the blood to the sites of exit from the body. This is why we started the

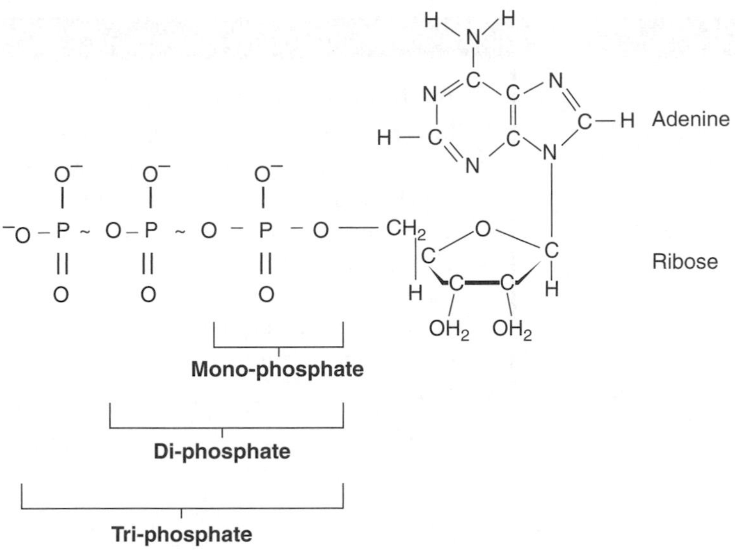

FIGURE 2.9 **ATP. Adenine triphosphate is a nucleotide made up of adenine (a nucleoside), ribose (a sugar) and phosphate (PO$_3$)**

chapter with the saying 'there is no free lunch in the universe'. We must make energy to fuel our activities and it takes energy to make energy!

When using up ATP one of the phosphates is released. As that happens, energy (E) stored in the bond is released:

Catabolic reaction:
ATP ⟶ ADP + P + energy
Adenine~P~P~P ⟶ Adenine~P~P + P + energy
Adenine triphosphate becomes adenine diphosphate + phosphate + energy

The energy released is used for anabolic reactions.

When ATP is synthesised from ADP (adenine diphosphate) and phosphate, energy (E) is consumed, used, to make the high energy bond in ATP.

Anabolic reaction:
Adenine~P~P + P + energy ⟶ Adenine~P~P~P
Adenine diphosphate + phosphate + energy become adenine triphosphate

The energy used is from a catabolic reaction.

The amount of energy released above in the catabolic reaction is exactly the same amount of energy consumed above in the anabolic reaction.

As shown above energy is used in converting ADP to ATP, while energy is released for driving reactions by liberating the energy held in the third phosphate bond. When that happens ATP becomes ADP and must be re-synthesised. ATP is synthesised in the mitochondria of the cell, the powerhouse of the cell for all metabolic reactions of the cell.

Chapter Reference

The removal of waste will be discussed in Chapter 10, 'Eliminating' (see p. 282).

Health Connection

ATP and airways
We have very little ATP stored. We must, therefore, constantly make it. It is then constantly used in reactions. To make ATP requires a constant supply of oxygen and glucose. We can store surplus glucose. We cannot store surplus oxygen. We obtain oxygen from air via our lungs. Therefore we must have a continuous supply of oxygen. If we stop breathing the supply of oxygen ceases. If this occurs we are no longer able to make ATP. In emergency situations the **airways** that connect the external environment containing oxygen to our lungs are always checked to ensure that air and oxygen can reach our lungs so that ATP can be synthesised. Without ATP there is no energy for reactions and we die.

Temperature and heat

At a constant temperature, for example room temperature, chemical matter can be in different **physical states** (gas, liquid, solid).

- Air is a *gas*.
- Water is a *liquid*.
- Salts are a *solid*.

These states, gas, liquid and solid, are called the **phases** of a substance.

Temperature reflects the amount of **kinetic energy**, the energy of movement, a substance has. The molecules in gases move more than those in liquids, and the molecules in liquids move more than those in solids.

Gases have more kinetic energy than liquids, and liquids have more kinetic energy than solids.

Different substances have different states due to the amount of energy they possess. This energy can be due to their different **heats**. Different substances have different heats, even at room temperature.

Heat reflects the total energy of the system, which is to do with its kinetic energy and other energies such as how complex or simple a substance it is and how random or organised it is. We measure heat in **joules** or **calories**. These measures are the ability to do *work*; energy allows us to work and play.

In health we tend to measure temperature in **degrees Celsius** (°C):

- Zero degrees Celsius (0°C) is the freezing point of water, when liquid water becomes solid ice; that is, it changes phase.
- The boiling point of water is 100°C, when water changes from liquid to gas.

Temperature is a number that is related to the average kinetic energy of the molecules of a substance. When a molecule has no kinetic energy it is at a temperature called **absolute zero**. For all elements this measure is −273°C, or 273 degrees below the freezing point of water. This number is also called zero degrees on the **Kelvin** scale of measurement. If temperature is measured in Kelvin degrees, then this number is directly proportional to the average kinetic energy of the molecules.

Chemical processes require energy for them to occur. The energy often comes from heat. We heat things up to make processes happen or cool them down to slow them. Chemical reactions may also create energy, often in the form of heat.

We carry out chemical (or biochemical) reactions all the time. This is called our **metabolism** – the chemical reactions our cells carry out, such as converting glucose and oxygen into energy. During metabolic reactions heat can be *produced* or *consumed*. If heat is produced it can be transported away from the site of the reaction, the cell, and passed into the blood. The blood is then warmed up. The blood transports this heat around the body and keeps our bodies at a constant internal temperature of around 37°C. We need to be maintained at this temperature because we can only carry out metabolic reactions at that temperature. It is one of the problems we have: maintaining our temperature requires surplus heat from reactions to keep us warm. Another problem is that all our reactions occur at 37°C. Cars burn fuel (petrol) at *hundreds* of degrees in air (oxygen) to make energy. We have to do the same reaction – fuel (glucose) burnt in oxygen – to make energy (ATP) at **37°C**. In other words there is a limit to how hot we can be. Because of this we need special molecules called **enzymes**, discussed below, for our metabolism to occur.

Chapter Reference

Heat is discussed further in Chapter 5, 'Controlling and Repairing' (see p. 142).

Enzymes are discussed below and again in Chapter 9, 'Eating and Drinking' (see p. 241). Energy is discussed further in Chapter 5, 'Controlling and Repairing', and in Chapter 9, 'Eating and Drinking'.

Health Connection

Fever

Extreme temperatures in patients can be a sign of infection. Fever helps the body to rid itself of the infection and is therefore a part of the homeostatic response to infection. However, prolonged changes in temperature affect the proteins and thus the cells of the body and can cause more damage than good. Patients are often thus cooled down to reduce their temperature by applying cool materials, particularly to the back of the neck to cool the blood going to the brain.

Macromolecules and nutrients

Molecules can assemble together to form large molecules, **macromolecules**, which can then fold up to have a three-dimensional shape to them. Many macromolecules are based on the element carbon.

Carbon

As mentioned above, what is especially interesting about the element carbon is that its atom can join together with other carbon atoms to form

- long chains of carbons, found in foods such as **fats** and **lipids**, or
- rings, found in foods such as the **sugars** glucose and fructose.

Polymers are large molecules usually formed by joining together basic units. If we imagine a long word it is a polymer of simple letters.

Sugars can exist as simple ring compounds of carbon, oxygen and hydrogen called **monosaccharides**. Monosaccharides, single sugar units, can in turn join together to form large chains of rings, **polysaccharides**, which are macromolecule **polymers** of sugars. These polymers of sugars are also called **carbohydrates**, for example starch and cellulose.

Carbon can also form large structures with another element, nitrogen, to form molecules called **amino acids**. In biological systems only about 20 amino acids occur, with names such as glycine, tryptophan, phenylalanine and leucine. These amino acids can join together to form **polymers** called **peptides** and **proteins.**

Carbon and nitrogen in another ring formation can also form macromolecules that carry all our genetic information, information that instructs us how to make proteins. This macromolecule is called **DNA**.

Chapter Reference

Genes, DNA and genetics will be discussed in Chapter 3, 'Growing and Developing' (see p. 64).

From very few chemicals many different macromolecules can be formed. These macromolecules help to form us, our food and other organisms. A lack of them, or too many of them, can cause illness. Many illnesses are caused by lack of or too much of certain foods. Foods are composed of chemicals, so we can measure the chemicals we have consumed to see what is missing or is present in too high a quantity.

The large starch carbohydrate in Figure 2.10 is a polysaccharide (many saccharide sugars). The individual units are monosaccharide sugars.

Triglycerides have three long lipid chains held together. If they are depicted with single lines between the carbon atoms these denote *single* bonds and fat is **saturated**. If there are *double* lines between the carbon atoms these denote a double bond and the fat is **unsaturated** (as there are spare bonds to which hydrogen, for example, could bind). Single and double bonds are discussed in the context of covalent bonds above (Figure 2.11).

The phosphate end in Figure 2.12 (red) is polar and hydrophilic and will dissolve in watery solvents. The other end is non-polar and hydrophobic. The lipid bi-layers of cells are composed of two rows of this fat. This structure suggests how molecules can or cannot cross the plasma membrane and why some substances will passively diffuse in and out of the cell while others need facilitated transport.

Cholesterol is a fat found in the plasma membrane of cells. Cholesterol is also a fat that is the basis of steroid hormones (Figure 2.13).

Balancing equations

When we write a reaction such as

Glucose + oxygen = carbon dioxide + water + ATP

Reactants $\longrightarrow$ Products

we need to account for the precise chemical forms of the molecules if we are to *balance* the equation so that there are equal numbers of starting (reactants) and finishing (product) material. Glucose has 6 carbon atoms, 12

Health Connection

Diet and macromolecules

In a normal balanced diet we need a mix of various macromolecules to maintain our health. These macromolecules are broken down into their constituent parts (nutrients) during digestion, absorbed into our blood and transported to our cells, where they are assembled into the macromolecules needed by our bodies.

hydrogen atoms and 6 oxygen atoms in it while oxygen exists as a molecule, O_2. This means that the reaction above is in fact as shown in Figure 2.14.

Nutrients

Nutrients enable cells to functions. The main types of nutrients are:

- proteins,
- carbohydrates,
- fats,
- water,
- vitamins,
- minerals (salts) and
- nucleic acids.

Some of these nutrients are macromolecules formed from basic subunits. Some are more complex macromolecules, such as proteins. Some are small, simple chemicals such as ionic salts.

The body, using the gastrointestinal tract, breaks the large macromolecular food particles into smaller particles which are then absorbed into the transport medium, blood, and taken to all the cells of the body, where the particles are used in cell metabolism.

Thus nutrients are digested into their constituent parts, chemicals, which are used by the body to make its structures (anatomy) and carry out its functions (physiology). We are therefore

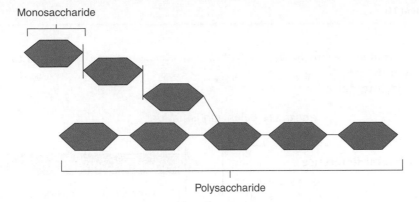

FIGURE 2.10 **Sugar and carbohydrate macromolecule**

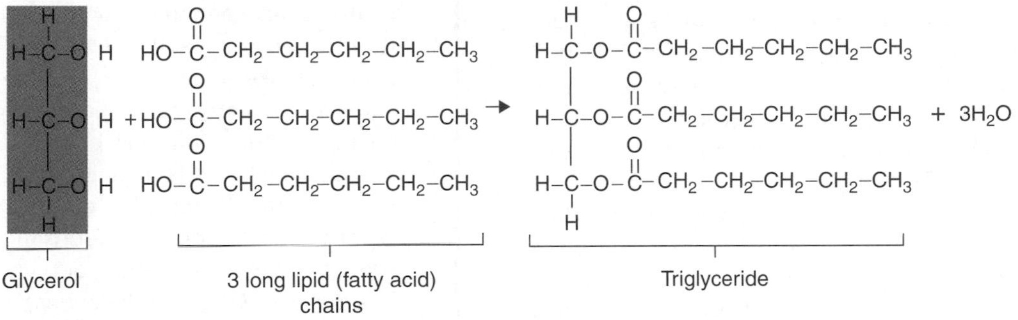

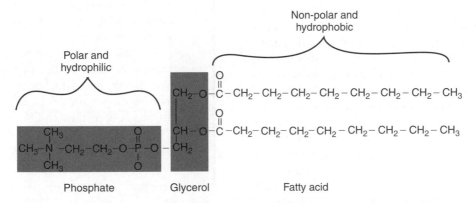

FIGURE 2.11 **A triglyceride fat**

FIGURE 2.12 **A phospholipid molecule as found in the plasma membrane (see also Fig 1.3)**

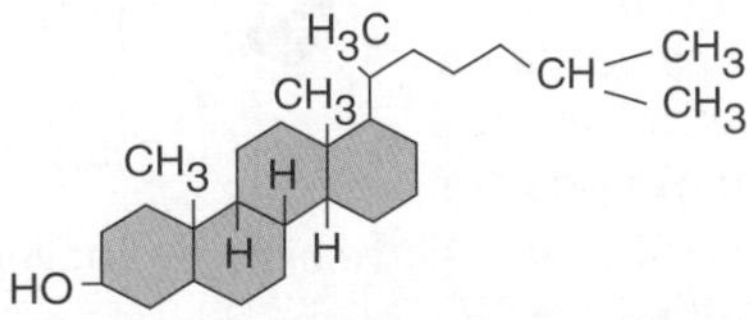

FIGURE 2.13 **Cholesterol**

linked to the external environment, which we use to maintain our internal environment.

$$C_6H_{12}O_6 \quad + \quad 6O_2 \quad \longrightarrow \quad 6CO_2 \quad + \quad 6H_2O \quad + \quad ATP$$

| Glucose | Oxygen gas | | Carbon dioxide | Water | Energy |

FIGURE 2.14 Balancing equations

Chapter Reference

Nutrients and food will be discussed in Chapter 9, 'Eating and Drinking' (see p. 241).

Enzymes

To carry out many functions in biology molecules and macromolecules need to be converted from one form to another. In chemistry there are certain substances called **catalysts** that help in this conversion. In biology these substances, biological catalysts, are called **enzymes**. One very important feature of enzymes is that they alter substances but the enzymes themselves remain unchanged.

Enzymes are a variety of proteins. Proteins are three-dimensional: they have a shape. The 3D shape of enzyme proteins helps them bind substances, similar to a key fitting a lock. If the shape of the enzyme changes it cannot bind substances. There are many enzymes, each like a particular key which will only fit its particular lock. Once the molecule fits the enzyme the enzyme alters it, like turning the key, and then the altered molecule pops out again as it no longer fits the enzyme. Enzymes may convert substances, for example one type of fat to another, or break large sugar macromolecules into small sugar molecules. By binding to a substance enzymes allow us to carry out many reactions that otherwise would require very high temperatures, which in turn would require vast energy input. Enzymes thus *lower* the amount of energy needed to carry out a chemical reaction, the **activation energy**. Besides converting one macromolecule to another type, nearly all metabolic reactions are carried out by enzymes. How these special enzyme proteins are synthesised has fascinated molecular biologists for many years (Figure 2.15).

Health Connection

Metabolic diseases, enzymes and genes

Enzymes are a type of protein and the instructions for how to make proteins are encoded by genes. If you have a faulty gene and cannot make a particular enzyme you cannot carry out a particular chemical conversion. This can have serious effects on your health and cause many metabolic diseases where fundamental metabolic processes cannot be carried out.

The disease **PKU** (phenylketonuria) is one where a person does not have a particular enzyme (called phenylalanine hydroxylase) and cannot convert one small part of a protein, an **amino acid**, into another amino acid (in this case the amino acid phenylalanine to the amino acid tyrosine). Because of this, phenylalanine builds up in the body and becomes *toxic waste* and interferes with the homeostasis of the body. PKU is a serious disease and all newborns are tested for the presence of the functioning enzyme.

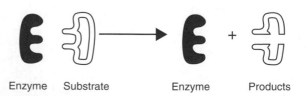

| Enzyme | Substrate | | Enzyme | | Products |

FIGURE 2.15 Enzyme aided reactions

Protein shape and structure

When molecules fold up into three-dimensional shapes the folding is very specific. This is particularly true for proteins. The folding relies on the units of which the macromolecule is made. In proteins units of amino acid molecules are held together in a long chain. The order of the units affects the folding of the chains such that a protein with a chain consisting of, for example, tryptophan, glycine, glycine, leucine, glycine, alanine, valine will have a different shape from a protein consisting of a string of amino acids in the order glycine, glycine, leucine, tryptophan, tryptophan, leucine, leucine. The order of the amino acids is important in the same way that the order of letters is important in words. With words, sounds and meanings are made; with proteins shapes and functions are made.

There are about 20 main amino acids that make up proteins in humans. There are various ways of categorising them. For example, some are called 'essential amino acids' that we cannot synthesise and must, therefore, consume in our diet (within the proteins we eat).

Essential amino acids (from diet):

- isoleucine,
- leucine,
- lysine,
- methionine,
- phenylalanine,
- threonine,
- tryptophan,
- valine and
- histidine (semi-essential).

Also essential in children:

- cysteine,
- tyrosine and
- arginine.

Non-essential amino acids (we can synthesise):

- alanine,
- arginine,
- aspartate,
- asparagine,
- cysteine,
- glutamate,
- glutamine,
- glycine,
- proline,
- serine and
- tyrosine.

We may also categorise them into physical types:

- aromatic (carbon rings),
- positively charged,
- negatively charged,
- non-polar or
- polar.

Health Connection

Amino acids and diet

Some amino acids are called **'non-essential'**, not because we do not need them, but because we can manufacture them in our own cells. The non-essential amino acids are alanine, arganine, aspartate, cysteine, glutamate, glycine, proline, serine, asparagine.

Eight amino acids are **'essential'** amino acids; we cannot manufacture them so we must consume them in our diets. Without them we suffer malnutrition and cannot make the proteins we need for our cells to function. The essential amino acids are phenylalanine, isoleucine, leucine, lysine, methionine, threonine, tryptophan and valine.

Additionally some amino acids are required in the diet of infants and growing children: cysteine, tyrosine, histidine and arginine.

Diet is discussed in Chapter 9, 'Eating and Drinking' (see p. 241).

Box 2.6 Amino acids

- There are many ways of categorising amino acids.
- **Amino acids** get their name because they contain a molecular group called an **amine** (NH_3) and a molecular group that is an acid group, called a carboxy **acid** (**COOH**). So we get amine-acid or amino acid.
- The amino acids vary depending on the molecules, called side chains, on the side of the main amino group.
- Eight amino acids have non-polar hydrophobic side chains.
- Two amino acids are acidic with carboxy acid side chains.
- Three amino acids are basic with amine side chains.
- The rest are polar and hydrophilic (water loving).

Box 2.7 Summary – Homeostasis, shape and function

- The shape and function of proteins is dictated by the order of the amino acids. The same amino acids in a different order would make a different protein shape, which would have a different function – just like the order of letter in a word, GOD versus DOG for example.
- Shape is very sensitive to changes in pH and in temperature. For example, when you boil an egg, what changes inside the egg to make it go solid is a protein in egg white called albumin. As the egg is heated the albumin changes shape and it goes hard. You cannot 'unboil' an egg. In other words you cannot restore the shape of the albumin molecules by putting the boiled egg into a cool environment. Our proteins also change shape if we get too hot, which is one reason we monitor temperature. As many of our reactions of metabolism are carried out by enzymes, changing heat not only results in loss of water, which affects our osmosis and water balance, but also results in our enzymes altering shape irreversibly. As their actions rely on their recognising shapes by their own shapes, they can no longer function. This is an elegant example of the link between the shape (anatomy) of our bodies and the functions (physiology) of our bodies. If we change the anatomy the physiology no longer works.
- Enzymes, and proteins in general, are particularly sensitive to changes in pH. Most of our body fluids are around a neutral pH of about 6.8–7.4. Outside of this range proteins change shape and no longer function.
- We are made of the same material, chemicals, as the external environment in which we find ourselves. We re-fashion it to suit our internal environment to maintain our anatomy and physiology so as to carry out our activities of daily living, which in turn allow us to survive and thrive.

Health Connection

Hydrogen bonds, hydrogen ions, pH and health

As mentioned, many molecules are given shape by hydrogen bonds which have a slight polarity (charge) on them, even in covalent molecules. This is due to hydrogen being able to move its one electron towards another element or bring another electron towards itself to complete its electron shell. A change in pH will have an effect on hydrogen bonds in a molecule, which will have an effect on the stability and shape of the molecule and therefore on its activity. A change in pH, therefore, can have a serious effect on physiology, which is why pH is closely monitored in health settings. The smallest element can have a large effect on our health.

The physical type influences how the amino acid behaves and therefore the form of the protein. Because of how proteins fold up in 3D, in some proteins hydrophilic groups will be on the outside of the protein, while in other proteins hydrophobic groups will be on the outside. This will affect their behaviour and how they react in the main fluid, plasma, of our bodies. The shape therefore has an effect on behaviour; the form affects the function.

Health Connection

Patient observations

Two very important measurements are often carried out on patients, *temperature* and respiratory or *blood pH*. Both of these have severe effects on our health and independent functioning and need to be restored to normal ranges by clinical interventions.

Chapter Reference

Metabolism will be discussed further in Chapter 9, 'Eating and Drinking' (see p. 241).

Health Connection

Molecules, reactions and homeostasis

We saw that large molecules can have a 3D shape to them. Changes in pH or temperature can affect the shape of molecules. If their shape is altered, enzymes, for example, may not recognise them and will not be able to bring about appropriate reactions. Enzymes may also be affected by changes in temperature and pH. Metabolism is thus affected, which then affects the internal environment, having severe effects on homeostasis. Thus changes in pH or temperature can have effects down the line on living processes and activities of daily life.

Health Connection

Normal ranges

Our bodies have requirements for various chemical substances and physical parameters, such as pH and temperature. In health our normal range for these is measured so that in ill health these requirements, called variables, can again be measured to ascertain any fluctuations outside the normal range and help in the diagnosis of the cause of the malfunction.

Most health professionals spend time measuring variables such as temperature, gas pH, blood pressure, pulse rate, heart rate and urine volumes. The values are noted to see if they fall outside the normal range. This normal range has been ascertained by measuring many healthy people and averaging their readings. So each variable is being compared to what is expected in a healthy person. Any variable that is outside that range indicates a problem with the homeostasis of that variable. This indicates where a problem may be occurring. It gives an objective measure and a close link to where the problem may be occurring. Signs and symptoms can be too general, while vital signs may help to pinpoint the problem and aid diagnosis (Table 2.3).

Table 2.3 Vital signs

	Normal value	Normal range	Approximate non-lethal limits
Oxygen (pp mmHg)	40	35–40	10–1100
Carbon dioxide (pp mmHg)	40	35–40	5–80
Sodium ion mMole/L	142	138–146	115–175
Potassium ion (mMole/L)	4.2	3.8–5.0	1.5–9.0
Calcium ion (mMole/L)	1.2	1.0–1.4	0.5–2.0
Chloride ion (mMole/L)	108	103–112	70–130
Bicarbonate ion (mMole/L)	28	24–32	8–45
Glucose (mMole/L)	85	75–95	20–1500
Body temperature (°C)	37.0	36.0–38.0	18.3–43.3
pH	7.4	7.3–7.5	6.9–8.0
Blood pressure	120/80	110–120/70–80	110/65

Notes:

Normal ranges of common variables in adults.

This table shows normal ranges for many variables in health. Note should be taken that measurements are done on resting individuals and changes occur during exercise that would move these variables outside their normal range. In the healthy individual these values should then return to the normal range after rest.

Newborns and infants have different ranges.

Variables are measured in a variety of ways depending on their state – solid, liquid or gas – for example, their concentration (amount per litre), degrees on a temperature scale, or on a pH scale.

Conclusion: Working and playing

In the words of a rather famous chocolate bar advertisement, to be able to 'work, rest and play' requires energy. We convert matter, especially chemical bonds, into energy to fuel the metabolism of our bodies. If we don't have the appropriate chemicals we cannot fuel the body. We obtain these chemicals in our diet. If we cannot make any part of the machinery that converts energy, such as enzymes, again we fail to make the energy. Life is very precarious and we work hard to preserve it. To do so requires our ability to carry out all the ADLs and to carry them out requires energy! There really is no free lunch in the universe.

Chapter Summary

▲ Material substances, matter, are made of chemicals. Chemicals are made of atoms. Atoms can be neutral (uncharged) or charged, in cases where there are more or fewer electrons than protons. If charged they are called ions. There are about 110 different types of atoms in the universe, called elements.

▲ We are composed of the matter of the universe, stardust!

▲ This matter is composed of chemicals.

▲ We make ourselves from this and maintain ourselves using this.

▲ Humans and other living things on this planet are made from a few of these elements. Carbon is the main element we are made from. Carbon can make long chains and rings with itself. Carbon can make rings with nitrogen and other elements.

▲ Food is made of large macromolecules of carbon rings or chains. Carbohydrates are polymers of sugars. Lipids are polymers of fats. Proteins are polymers of amino acids. We are mainly polymers of carbon units; the units are fats, sugars, amino acids and nucleic acids, with a few small molecules such as salt.

▲ The fluids found in our body contain a large amount of water. Water is a solvent for many substances in our bodies and provides the basis of transport of substances around our body. pH is a measure of how acidic or basic (alkaline) a fluid is and is a measure hydrogen ion concentration. Water has a pH of 7. Many of our body fluids have a pH of 7.2–7.4.

▲ Our bodies carry out metabolic reactions synthesising (anabolism) and degrading (catabolism) substances. Metabolic reactions involve chemical reactions and require or release energy.

▲ Most of the metabolic reactions in our bodies are carried out by enzymes. Enzymes are made of protein. Enzymes are biological catalysts. Enzymes alter substances but the enzymes themselves remain unchanged.

▲ Temperature and pH can affect the shape of molecules by altering weak bonds.

▲ Many molecules, including enzymes, need to maintain their shape for their function.

3 Growing and Developing

By nature all men are alike; it is their habits that separate them.

Confucius (551–479 BCE), Chinese thinker and social philosopher of the Spring and Autumn Period

Chapter Outline

- Introduction: Growing and developing as activities of daily living
- The external environment
- The internal environment
- Why we grow and develop
- Our foundations: Structure and function
- Inheritance: Translation, transcription, replication and the genetic code
- The reproductive system
- Development and differentiation
- Stem cells
- Lifespan changes
- Conclusion: Growing and developing
- Chapter summary

Introduction: Growing and developing as activities of daily living

Personal growth and development are normal activities of humans; they have even become industries with companies and consultants telling us how to grow or develop as humans or as organisations. Growth or increase is seen as a good thing. Development is seen as a sign of experience and expertise. Most of us will grow from our childhood sizes to adulthood and develop into mature humans. These are normal activities. There are some individuals whose physical growth or whose mental development is limited. This restriction is often due to **congenital** development in the womb or due to **genetic** changes. There are many diseases that have a genetic component to them and many diseases that have a developmental component to them. Genetic alterations or congenital alterations can affect our health and our ability to carry out other activities of daily living. Both genes and development will be discussed in this chapter.

In biology, growing and developing have a physiological significance to do with

- cell numbers,
- size and
- development of functions.

All of these also impact on our *self-maintenance*, the ability to have the correct numbers of cells and the correct types of cells, and on our ability to *repair* ourselves after cellular trauma.

We grow from a single fertilised egg cell. We continue through life to grow and hopefully develop from childhood to maturity. Not only we do grow, but we pass on bits of ourselves to found the next generation. To do this we engage in sexual reproduction.

We have sex for a number of reasons: to express love, to procreate, to release emotions, to bond and to please are among some of these reasons. Sex is an activity of daily living and the ability to enjoy sex throughout adult life affects not only our ability to procreate, but also many emotional attachments. In older age and in care environments this ADL may be compromised and this may have deleterious effects on our feeling of well-being and closeness to loved ones.

To be able to choose whom we have sex with is, in many ways, a *necessity* and also a *luxury* – a necessity particularly if sex is being done for procreation because, being *mortal*, having a limited lifespan, procreation may be one way to have some stake in immortality, passing on part of yourself, your genes, to the next generation. Choice is a luxury because in many cultures, even today, one cannot choose whom one can have sex with. Choosing one's partner assumes that there is mutual consent. How do we choose our partners and what purpose do our choices serve? When do we choose our partners and how do we reach this stage of development? These are some of the questions addressed in this chapter. However, this is a biology book, not a psychology book, so the central theme will be the biology of sex and generation and the processes related to this that allow the activities of growth and development.

Chapter Reference

Mortality and death are discussed in Chapter 13, 'Dying' (see p. 340).

The external environment

Biology is part of the natural sciences, which have sprung up from natural philosophy, the curiosity about the universe and our place in it. There are a number of take-home messages that we need to be aware of in the way that science views this planet and the environment we live in.

The external environment is totally indifferent to our being here; it is merely permissive. We can survive in it because we are *adapted* to it, but it does *not* adapt to us. There may be other planets on which we can survive. However, they too would be indifferent to us. Only we think we are important! So we find ourselves here on this small rock in the middle of a very large universe and we should be aware of how insignificant we are. The interesting thing

about us is that we are *alive* and that seems to be different from merely being a collection of chemical, or passive materials to which things happen. It is this difference that sets the *living* apart from the *non-living* (things that have never been alive). Living, organic beings are made of the same stuff, matter, as non-living beings such as the rocks on which we find ourselves. The non-living matter and energy on this planet are conducive to our being here, but it takes an enormous amount of effort for us to sustain ourselves in this environment. We must make and use energy to build and maintain ourselves. Luckily for us the generous environment unwittingly provides for our every need. However, our lives affect the external environment: we alter the environment we live in and that could be for good or bad. If we pollute and destroy with our waste, the environment will not sustain us or our offspring. We should take care of our environment because without it we cannot survive and thrive. In this environment we must *compete* with each other and other organisms for our needs. Sometimes we *cooperate* with others for our needs. With whom we cooperate has been the basis of some of the science of genes and **natural selection**.

Chapter Reference

Matter and energy are discussed in Chapter 2, 'Working and Playing' (see p. 35).

The internal environment

There has, for many years, been a debate between two main camps as to which has the most influence on who or what we are: **nature** or **nurture**; in other words whether we are the consequences of our biology, *nature*, or whether we are the consequences of the environment, *nurture*. The biological nature debate has centred on our genes and especially one theory, the **selfish gene**; the nurture debate has centred on our upbringing. There are good and bad parts to each side, but the bad sides are very bad! In the genetic debate the bad side has led to theories such as **eugenics**, which started in the nineteenth century as a good idea to stop ill health – the public health of its day. It ended with Nazism, the ideology of the superiority of the Aryan race and sterilising people with learning difficulties. The genetic debate continues because we can see the consequences of having genes that do not work; they can cause debilitating diseases. However, the opposite is less clear; having a particular version of a gene may prevent you having a disease and the gene may help carry out a certain physiological function, but it doesn't confer health. Health appears to be more complex and to involve life choices. The nurture debate is often the domain of sociology and centres on our lifestyles and especially on poverty. However, it often ignores our biology and the impact of our choices on our bodies. In biology the debate is not as polarised; the nurture side becomes part of the internal, biological environment in which genes exist and the products of genes, proteins, affect the environment of the gene itself in a feedback loop, as seen in homeostasis. The other processes in and of the body all affect the internal environment and are affected by it, and in turn we affect the external environment, the domain of the conservation biologists.

Why we grow and develop

We are **mammals**. All mammals, such as dogs, cats, horses and whales, share some common features. These include the type of skin we have, being **warm-blooded** (**homeotherms**), being suckled when first born on **mammary glands**, reproducing sexually (possessing what are called **gametes**, eggs and sperm) and most importantly having our **embryos** develop internally rather than being egg laying.

Having our embryos develop internally has advantages and disadvantages. The embryo is protected and is born in a fairly developed state rather than developing in an externally laid egg, which is vulnerable to predators. However, there is a limit to how big the embryo can be, due to the birth canal, and there is a limit to how developed it can be too. Carrying a growing and developing embryo, **pregnancy**, entails very large metabolic and physiological costs to the mother.

Once we are born we therefore need to grow to our mature size and develop to a state in which we can repeat the process that our parents have carried out, reproduction. To grow requires cell numbers to increase, and to develop requires the maturation of cells to adult structures, particularly the maturation of our gametes in structures called **gonads**.

Our foundations: Structure and function

In the beginning we started our existence in two parts: an **egg** and a **sperm**. By chance, out of the thousands of eggs our mother possessed and out of the millions of sperm our father made, one particular egg and one particular sperm joined to make a new individual. That moment, **conception**, is when the unique set of genes that are part of what makes each individual slightly different from another individual are united. While society, particularly western society with its emphasis on the individual, implies that we are unique (and therefore, we think, interesting!), in biological terms the differences between us are very small, in fact minute. We are alarmingly similar to one another and very closely related. We need to be, and we need to have many similarities so that we belong to the same species, *Homo sapiens*, human beings, and are able to carry out the many processes of life. If the genes vary too much they may compromise the viability of the developing organism.

We are a mix of *conservation* (maintaining a similarity) and *diversity* (differences). The mix of genes from egg and sperm, female and male, makes each one of us similar to our parents and yet slightly different. This process of conservation and diversity is significant to biological evolution, the process by which new species arise. Our similarities bind us together as a species. Our differences may divide us into new species, some of which will survive and thrive and some of which will disappear from the planet before being well established. The randomness of our existence is quite amazing! The more biology you learn, the more surprised you should be that you as an individual are here and that we as a species are here.

> **Chapter Reference**
>
> Reproduction and embryo development are discussed later in the chapter (see pp. 86–94).

Our foundations – Functions, proteins and amino acids

We are made of cells. Each cell has to maintain itself and carry out various functions, such as importing food molecules, exporting waste and synthesising new parts to replace old parts. To do this requires work, in the form of energy, and machinery, in the form of **proteins**. There are many types of proteins carrying out various functions, such as

- enzymatic, e.g. catalase, peroxidase,
- hormonal, e.g. insulin, glucagon,
- neurotransmission, e.g. GABA,
- growth factors, e.g. insulin and
- transportation, e.g. haemoglobin, albumin.

In fact, most of the functions of the body are carried out by proteins. There are tens of thousands of different proteins that are found and synthesised in the human body.

Proteins and amino acids

We eat proteins in our foods and digest them by breaking them down into their constituent parts, called **amino acids**. The amino acids are then transported to all the cells of the body, where each cell can reassemble the amino acids from digested food into the proteins required by the cell. As discussed in Chapter 2, 'Working and Playing', there are about 20 types of amino acids found in human proteins. Some of them are essential in our diet and some are non-essential as we can synthesise them.

Essential amino acids (from diet):

- isoleucine,
- leucine,

> **Chapter Reference**
>
> Cells are discussed in Chapter 1, 'Maintaining a Safe Environment' (see p. 1). Proteins are discussed in Chapter 2, 'Working and Playing' (see p. 35) and in Chapter 9, 'Eating and Drinking' (see p. 241).

Health Connection

Proteins
Proteins carry out most of the functions of our cells. If they are altered by outside effects such as pH, heat or pressure their three-dimensional shape, as discussed in Chapter 2, is altered and they no longer carry out their function. If their three-dimensional shape is altered by changing the arrangement of amino acids they again may not be able to carry out their function.

- lysine,
- methionine,
- phenylalanine,
- threonine,
- tryptophan,
- valine and
- histidine (semi-essential).

Also essential in children:

- arginine,
- cysteine and
- tyrosine.

Non-essential amino acids (we can synthesise):
- alanine,
- arginine,
- asparagine,
- aspartate,
- cysteine,
- glutamate,
- glutamine,
- glycine,
- proline,
- serine and
- tyrosine.

All amino acids, as their name implies, have an *amine group*, NH_3, and an *acid group*, COOH. They can then have side chains that are hydrophobic or hydrophilic, acidic, basic or neutral. Their names are often rendered in shorthand, such as proline being Pro and tryptophan being Typ.

Health Connection

Amino acids and food labels

Often foods and food supplements will label their contents. Protein-rich foods may label which amino acids they contain as some are essential amino acids which the body cannot synthesise and which must be consumed from an external source (see below).

Proteins can be very big and complex, made of many amino acids, or very short, **peptides**, made of a few amino acids. Some are made of a large variety of the 20 possible amino acids and some are made of very few types of amino acids. Thus the differences between proteins are

- the numbers of amino acids they have;
- the order in which the amino acids appear in a protein;
- the variety of amino acids they have.

In Figure 3.1 the same four amino acids (met, pro, typ, val) joined in different orders form different peptides (small proteins).

This is comparable to the English language. In English there are 26 constituent parts to all the words that appear: the alphabet. From those 26 parts we can construct thousands of words, some with many different letters, some with just a few, some big, some small and all dependent on the order of the letters. For example, we can use the same three letters to make two different words due to the order of the letters. The letters D G O can be arranged to spell DOG or GOD. Proteins also rely on the order of the amino acids. Change the order and you have a different protein.

Each cell needs to make its own proteins to do the work of keeping the cell alive, so each cell receives amino acids from the breakdown of proteins by the gastrointestinal tract. How does each cell know how to assemble the amino acids into the proteins it needs?

Each cell makes the proteins it needs from the amino acids supplied by the cell or from the diet through a process called **translation.**

Inheritance: Translation, transcription, replication and the genetic code

Translation

There are about 10 trillion cells in the human body. Each cell needs to be able to make the tens of thousands of proteins it needs. Cells need a way of assembling amino acids in the correct order into all the different proteins. The problem therefore is in knowing how to do this. With any manufacturing system, there is a *blueprint* of how to put things together. Cells need a blueprint, a simple code, for assembling amino acids into proteins.

Cells have found a simple way of assembling complex proteins from the 20 amino acids. They have found a coding system for the 20 amino acids that requires only four parts. These four parts that code for how to translate 20 amino acids into thousand of proteins are called **nucleic acids (NAs)**; specifically they are called **deoxyribose nucleic acid, DNA.**

Nucleic acids are composed of carbon, hydrogen, oxygen and nitrogen; they are similar to amino acids in composition, but their structure is different.

DNA is composed of these nucleic acids in the form of **nucleotide bases**. Nucleotide bases have carbon and nitrogen rings with phosphate

---

Pro-Val-Met-Trp $\Longrightarrow$ Peptide A
Val-Pro-Trp-Met $\Longrightarrow$ Peptide B

FIGURE 3.1 **Protein amino acid order**

groups attached. There are four nucleotide bases found in DNA (Figure 3.2):

- A = adenine,
- G = guanine,
- C = cytosine and
- T = thymine.

The four nucleotide bases of DNA must assemble 20 types of amino acids into thousands of proteins. We need a way of going from a simple nucleic acid code to a complex string of amino acids and a diverse number of arrangements of those amino acids into many protein types.

The code stands for, replaces, the amino acids. How can four DNAs code for 20 amino acids? If each nucleotide base stood for one amino acid, the code would only replace four amino acids. For example:

> If adenine stood for lysine,
> if thymine stood for glycine,
> if cytosine stood for glutamine and
> if guanine stood for threonine,
> What stands for proline?
> What stands for serine?
> What nucleic acid stands for each of the other 16 amino acids?

We have run out of nucleic acids for the other 16 amino acids. So obviously each nucleic acid cannot replace an amino acid.

If the amino acids were grouped together in words of two letters we could make many more words. In fact with four letters (A, T, C and G) we can make 16 two-letter words: AA, TT, CC, GG, AT, TA, AC, CA, AG, GA, CG, GC, TC, CT, TG, GT. This is because there are four DNAs and they can be combined as two-letter words by this piece of maths:

> If there are four DNA letters: ACTG,
> and two letters in each word,
> the number of combinations that are possible or the number of words that can be made are:
> four × four (4 × 4) = four squared (4^2) = 16.

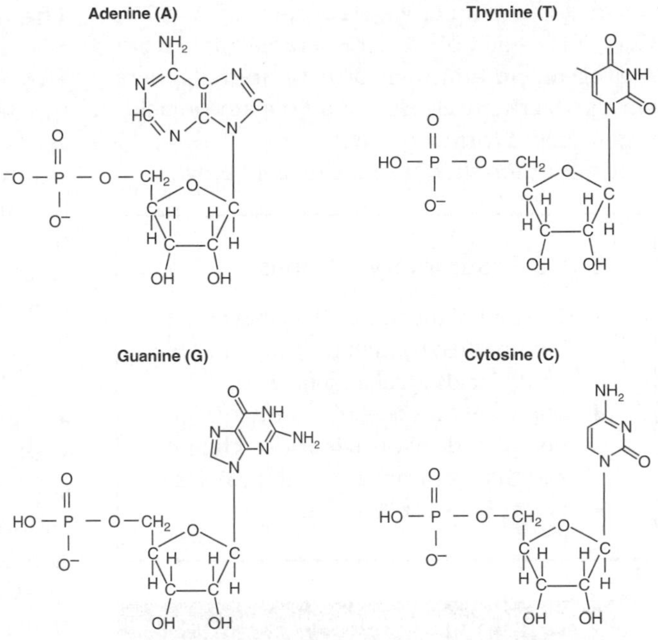

FIGURE 3.2 **The four nucleotide bases found in DNA**

In English:

> With 26 letters, the number of possible two-letter words (e.g. at, me, us, we)
> = 26^2 = 26 × 26 = 676 two-lettered words.

With four types of DNA letters making two-letter words we can make 16 two-letter words. We need to make at least 20 words for all the 20 amino acids we need to replace with a simple code.

If we try it with three-letter words, each composed of any three of the four nucleic acids, we have

> Four (DNA types) cubed (number of letters in word) = 4^3 = 4 × 4 × 4 = 64 three-letter words.

The code for translation is therefore three-letter words. We have some *redundancy*, spare 'back-up', in the code where an amino acid can be coded for by more than one three-letter DNA word. Each DNA word is called a **codon**. The codon is not alone. Just as there are lots of words here joining together to make this sentence so the codons make words, amino acids, that join together to make a sentence, a protein.

So, for example, we have AAT, TTA, GTA, CGT, TTG, each of which is a three-letter word coding for an amino acid. If we join all these words together we can join all the amino acids together and form a protein.

Codons are shown in Figure 3.4 below.

Box 3.1 Summary – Genes

- The part of the nucleic acid that codes for a protein by dictating the order of amino acids is called a gene.
- The genetic code is a sequence of genes made of nucleic acids – chemicals that get translated into proteins.
- Genes code for proteins.

Health Connection

Redundancy and homeostasis

The concept of redundancy is important in biology, particularly developmental biology.

In most environments, work or play, it is very hard to have the exact number of something for any situation or eventuality. In biology we can make too little of something or too much; it is very hard to make exactly the right number of cells or enzymes or hormones. Too little means we won't function. Too much means we have waste. So in biology waste is more tolerable than lack. In the case above we have redundancy, where one vital chemical can be coded for by more than one codon.

In health and homeostasis we tend to have a range rather than an exact amount. So we can have an amount within a range. Generally in health too much is as bad as too little; too much of a drug (overdose) is as bad as too little. Our health range has fairly strict limits.

The genetic code and genes

The order of the nucleic acids determines the three-letter words that are the codons, 'little codes'. These codons can be *translated* into another language, amino acids. So the four codons capable of making 64 three-letter words can code for another language, the language of amino acids and therefore of proteins. In the language of nucleic acids there are also 'grammar' signals.

Codons can be used for

- amino acids or
- instructions.

Some of the codons are translated, not into amino acids, but into *instructions* such as 'start translation', which is equivalent to a capital letter at the beginning of a sentence. Other codons are equivalent to a full stop, halting translation. There is, therefore, a signal to start translating from nucleic acids, and then the sequence of nucleic acids that follows dictates which amino acids are to be joined in which order to form a protein, and then at the end there is a stop signal. From the start to the stop is, therefore, the genetic code for a protein, and that is called a **gene**.

That genes code for proteins is one of the cornerstone concepts in biology and is also one of the most misunderstood (along with evolution by natural selection), which is why it is important to emphasise it here. You will hear many incorrect versions of this, but again, *genes code for proteins*. Not for behaviours or strategies or health or ill health, but for proteins! They are chemical entities. They are made of nucleic acids. They are a simple instruction manual of four parts that allows the assembly of 20 different chemicals into thousands and thousands of functional other chemicals called proteins. So when you hear a parent say their child's talent for playing the piano is inherited, via their genes, you may wonder about the link between a protein and a behaviour, between nature and nurture. Not having a particular gene can cause ill health and will be discussed below.

Transcription and ribose nucleic acid, RNA

In the discussion above DNA has been shown to code for and be translated into amino acids. In fact DNA does not directly translate and assemble proteins. There is an *intermediate* molecule called **RNA** (**ribose nucleic acid**).

DNA is first copied, by a process called **transcription**, into a mirror image, but in the chemical RNA. This occurs in the nucleus, where the DNA is held. The entire gene that codes for a protein is transcribed into an RNA as a long string called a **messenger RNA** (**mRNA**) carrying the message of how to assemble amino acids into a protein. The strings are part of a longer string, the genetic code, which contains genes, the sections of code that will be made into, transcribed into, mRNA. These mRNAs will then be translated into proteins.

The translation occurs on ribosomes in the cell cytoplasm, while the genetic code is contained in the nucleus. mRNA molecules thus come out of the nucleus into the cytoplasm. The cytoplasm contains many chemicals, some of which degrade mRNA. However, if the master code, the DNA, is protected in the nucleus, the degradation of mRNA, part of the assembly machinery, is not so worrying as it can be replaced by transcribing the highly protected DNA.

There are two differences between RNA and DNA:

1. In RNA the sugar part of the molecule is **ribose** sugar not deoxyribose sugar.
2. In RNA the nucleic acid **uracil (U)** is substituted for the nucleic acid called thymine (T).

The four nucleotide bases of RNA are

- A = adenine,
- G = guanine,
- C = cytosine and
- U = uracil.

To see how we go from DNA to amino acids we shall simplify by calling all the amino acids by numbers instead of names and work with a protein that consists of only four amino acids to avoid complexity. If

- AGG means amino acid 1,
- GAA means amino acid 2,
- TAA means amino acid 3 and
- TCT means amino acid 4,

then if we assemble those amino acids in that order we shall make protein *A*. If

- GAA means amino acid 2,
- TAA means amino acid 3,
- TCT means amino acid 4 and
- AGG means amino acid 1,

then if we assemble those amino acids in that order we shall make protein *B*.

In these two examples these are the same codons in a different order, and therefore the *same* amino acids are assembled in a different order to make a *different* protein. As with words in English, the order of the letters matters; for example, the word BAN is made from the same letters as NAB, but the different order of the letters denotes a different word and a different meaning.

In biology this is a very important concept: the *order of things*, particularly the *order of subunits*. The same subunits such as amino acids or sugars in a different order make different proteins and carbohydrates. Not only do the orders matter, but the order of the subunits dictates the three-dimensional shape and therefore folding up of large molecules. The three-dimensional shape dictates the function of the molecule. If you alter an amino acid you alter the shape and therefore the function. This is another important concept in biology: the *shape* affects the *function*.

Health Connection

Transcription, translation and proteins

Transcription, the copying of DNA into RNA, and translation, where RNA codons are translated into amino acids and hence proteins, are both carried out by proteins. There are enzymes that transcribe and others that translate and polymerise amino acids into proteins. So to make proteins we need proteins. All the functions of our cells are carried out by proteins and are part of homeostasis.

Box 3.2 Summary

In translation we go from very few nucleic acids and progress to very complex organisms:

- 4 Deoxyribose nucleic acids (ATCG);
- 4 Ribose nucleic acids (AUCG) – by transcription;
- 20 amino acids – by translation;
- 10^3 (thousands) proteins – by assembly on ribosomes;
- 10^{13} (trillions) cells;
- Functions of cells and organs;
- Activities of daily living.

With very few nucleic acids we can assemble all the amino acids found in humans into all the

Chapter Reference
The three-dimensional (3D) shape of molecules is discussed in Chapter 2, 'Working and Playing' (see p. 35). The cell and its organelles are discussed in Chapter 1, 'Maintaining a Safe Environment' (see p. 1).

Box 3.3 Summary

- Amino acids are coded for by three-letter nucleotide 'words' called a codon.
- A string of codons with a start reading and stop reading at either end is a gene.
- A gene dictates the order for the assembly of amino acids into proteins.
- Genes code for proteins.
- Different codons can be used for the same amino acid – redundancy.
- Going from a gene into a protein requires first DNA in the nucleus to be transcribed into RNA and then the RNA to be translated into amino acids on the ribosomes in the cytoplasm.
- DNA is the instruction manual of how to put amino acids into the correct sequence.
- The process of assembling the amino acids is carried out in the cytoplasm by RNA on ribosomes.

proteins we need. This is the beauty and simplicity of the genetic code and its translation from nucleic acids into proteins.

Once we understand how translation is done we have one further problem. Every cell in our body needs to be able to translate a simple code into complex and diverse numbers of proteins. If one of my skin cells can make a protein I would probably need many of my skin cells to be able to make that protein. So not only can we translate codes, but we can pass on how to assemble proteins into every cell. This is done by a process called **replication.**

Replication: copying the instruction code

Every cell in our body needs to be able to make proteins; therefore nearly every cell in our body needs to have the instruction manual, DNA. The DNA we have in our body (**soma**) cells is identical to the DNA in the very first cell that made us, the fertilised egg cell. In theory, therefore, any DNA in us from the nucleus of any cell of our body is the same as any DNA from any other cell in our body and is the same as our first cell.

For all the DNA in all our cells to be identical requires an accurate copying mechanism. In the 1950s the structure of DNA was established by two scientists, James Watson and Francis Crick, in Cambridge, England. Once the physical structure of the molecule was understood, how it got copied into every cell of the body became clear; the basic science made the function clear.

Unlike the single long strand of a messenger RNA molecule, deoxyribonucleic acid is two long strands wound around each other to form a **double helix**. This double helix is organised by **complementary bases**, where one base in one chain is always opposite a particular base in the other chain, preserving the order of the gene in each chain. These then form **complementary strands**. The bases are organised as follows:

- Adenine on one strand is always opposite thymine on the other strand.
- Guanine on one strand is always opposite cytosine on the other strand.

This is written in the shorthand

- A = T
- T = A
- G ≡ C
- C ≡ G

What hold the complementary strands together are hydrogen bonds, with A–T having two hydrogen bonds while G–C has three hydrogen bonds.

Chapter Reference

Hydrogen bonds are discussed in Chapter 2, 'Working and Playing' (see p. 35).

In the example below we are looking at a small section of DNA in a very long strand, and the dashes ------ represent other, *flanking* nucleotides (also known as **bases**) on either side of the example sequence which would be too numerous for us to follow what is happening. So we are taking a 'snapshot' of a part of DNA.

If one strand of DNA is in the order, for example,

------ A T T G C C G T A T A A G C C T G G A ------

then the complementary strand will be

------ T A A C G G C A T A T T C G G A C C T ------

to form a complementary double helix:

------ A T T G C C G T A T A A G C C T G G A ------
------ T A A C G G C A T A T T C G G A C C T ------

Now if we want to make replicas of this, we can use each strand as a **template** to make new strands (Figure 3.3):

------ A T T G C C G T A T A A G C C T G G A ------
Original strand (OS)

------ T A A C G G C A T A T T C G G A C C T ------
Complementary OS

Each original strand (OS) is then copied to make new strands:

------ A T T G C C G T A T A A G C C T G G A ------

OS as template

------ T A A C G G C A T A T T C G G A C C T ------

New strand (NS)

------ A T T G C C G T A T A A G C C T G G A ------

NS

------ T A A C G G C A T A T T C G G A C C T ------

OS as template

When the replication is complete this results in four strands of DNA; the upper strands are identical complementary pair strands to the original (parent) double helix, and the lower two strands are identical complementary pairs to the original complementary pair.

In this case we can see how we *conserve* the order of the DNA and hence the genes and proteins that we are made from in every cell in our body.

The strands have a *direction* to them due to the phosphate groups and hydroxyl groups on the DNA: they are said to be anti-parallel. Because of this, one end of the strand has a 5' phosphate group (the ' sign is called **prime**) and the other end has a 3' hydroxyl group. One strand is then said to be in the 5' phosphate to 3' hydroxyl direction, written as **5' to 3'** direction, while the other strand is in the **3' to 5'** direction. This has an effect on the mechanism of replication, which is done in one continuous direction 5' to 3' on one strand and in small sections on the other 3' to 5' strand due to the nature of the enzyme carrying out the replication. Also, transcription and therefore translation into a protein occur from just one of the strands.

5'------ A T T G C C G T A T A A G C C T G G A ------3'
3'------ T A A C G G C A T A T T C G G A C C T ------5'

Sometimes the wrong nucleotide, also called a base, is inserted. When this happens there is an enzyme that *proofreads* and corrects the mistake, cutting out the wrong base from the strand and inserting the correct one.

Sometimes the proofreading doesn't work and the wrong base is thought to be the correct one, so the correct complementary base is cut out and a wrong base inserted. When this occurs a single point, just one base pair, is now different and the gene in which this occurs is **mutated**.

Sometimes the copying is incorrect:

------ A T T G C C G T A T A A G C C T G G A ------

OS as template

------ T A A **T** G G C A T A T T C G G A C C T ------

NS with MUTATION

Usually the mistake is rectified and a **C** put in where the **T** is. But sometimes the mistake is not rectified and an **A** is put into the complementary strand where the **mutant T** is:

------ A T T **A** C C G T A T A A G C C T G G A ------

OS + MUTATION

------ T A A **T** G G C A T A T T C G G A C C T ------

NS with MUTATION

Human DNA contains 3×10^9 nucleotide bases (three billion bases) in each strand, so copying all of this into every cell of the body is quite a challenge, especially as you are composed of about ten trillion (10^{13}) cells. Given that many cells die and are replaced during one day of your life and each of these cells needs all the bases in the DNA to be copied into new strands, in **DNA synthesis** the chances of having a mishap are immense!

DNA is synthesised at a very rapid rate. About 250 million pairs of bases can be replicated in several hours, with 50 nucleotides per second per replication fork on each strand of DNA. Due to this the chance of putting in the incorrect base is high! The *rate of DNA mutation* is calculated as 10^{-4} to 10^{-6} mutations per base pair per generation, that is a 1/10,000 to 1/1,000,000 chance that a base will be mutated in each replication or cell cycle. It must be remembered that there are 3×10^9 bases, so some bases are mutated.

Mutations and alleles

Mutations can be

- *good*, in that a better protein is made;
- *bad* and cause problems if a functioning protein cannot be made;

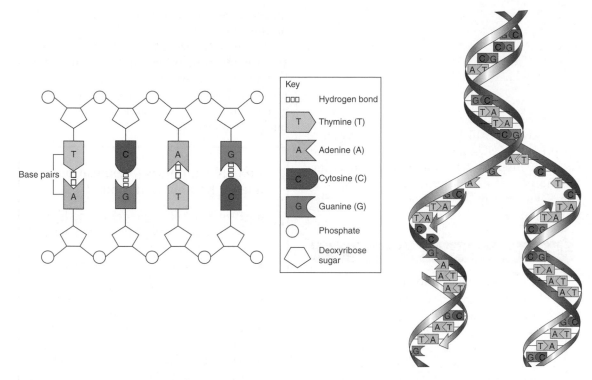

FIGURE 3.3 **DNA. The DNA molecule is made of two complementary strands. The strands replicate by separating and using each strand as a template for a new strand**

- *neutral* and have no effect on the function of a protein.

Health Connection

Mutations and disease

Many serious diseases are thought to be single point mutations where one base is substituted for another, which then causes a different amino acid to be inserted into a protein. Most of the metabolic diseases, where an enzyme is missing or the body lacks an anchoring protein that holds skin to its underlying tissue, for example, are thought to be single point mutations. As there is so much DNA in a cell, locating the problem, the gene responsible, its *position* in the DNA and the *base* that is mutated is not a simple task.

Because mutations can occur every time the DNA is replicated there are many *versions* of each gene. Each version is called an **allele**, and each allele either makes a functioning version of the gene, a non-functioning version or one that is similar to the 'original' functioning type (i.e. it works as well as the original type). The original functioning type is called the **wild type.**

Because the gene is making a particular protein, a single point difference will be an *allelic difference,* making the same protein, but in a slightly different form. The change affects a codon. Sometimes it affects the amino acid inserted and sometimes it doesn't, because there is redundancy in the genetic code where one amino acid may be coded for by more than one codon, as discussed above. So the change may still code for that amino acid, a neutral mutation.

As an example, in the genetic code the amino acid leucine (Leu) is coded for by the following codons:

UUA
UUG
CUU
CUC
CUA
CUG

If UUA were mutated to UUG the amino acid leucine would still be inserted correctly into the protein. If UUA became UCC instead serine would be inserted. Now this may not affect the function of the protein or it may have a serious effect. Either way it would be an allelic variation (Figure 3.4).

Health Connection

DNA sequences and diseases

Not only can a base change, but it may or may not have an effect on a protein or function. Having the entire sequence of all our DNA, therefore, does not always tell us if we have the functioning proteins and metabolic pathways. Having a different allele does not mean we will get a disease. We sometime have to look from a disease backwards to see if there is a gene involved.

Haploid and diploid

Many organisms are **haploid**, meaning that they have *one* copy of each gene in their body. Most higher organisms, including humans, are **diploid**; we have *two* copies of every gene.

The versions, alleles, of each gene may be **homozygous**, identical, so that there are two identical alleles, or they can be **heterozygous**, non-identical.

```
------ AAATTTGGGCC ------
------ TTTAAACCCGG ------      Gene A allele 1   Protein A

------ AATTTTGGGCC ------      Gene A allele 2   Protein A''
------ TTAAAAGGGCC ------
```

Here there are two versions, alleles, of the same gene. They result in Protein A and another version of Protein A, Protein A'', which may or

may not be a functioning version depending on the codon.

As we have two copies of every gene, we are diploid; if the other copy codes for a functioning protein we may not suffer from the non-functioning copy. Being diploid, like the genetic code, gives us *redundancy*, a back-up if one gene doesn't function.

Box 3.4 Summary – Replication, alleles, haploid and diploid

- Every cell needs the genetic code to tell it how to assemble amino acids into proteins.
- The genetic code is held in the DNA of the cell.
- The DNA must be able to be replicated into every cell of the body.
- When it is replicated mistakes can be made – mutations.
- Mutations can be good, bad or indifferent (neutral).
- Genes come in varieties called alleles.
- We have two copies, diploid, of every gene.
- The two copies we have of each gene may be homozygous (identical) or heterozygous (different).

Health Connection

Disease genes and other factors

Most diseases are caused by a number of genes interacting with an environment. They are **multifactorial**, having a number of factors that affect them.

Packaging, chromosomes, X and Y

We have thousands of genes and they are composed of thousands of bases (nucleic acids). To hold them in the nucleus in some order our genes are contained on long strands of DNA

Second base in codon
(second letter)

		U	C	A	G	
First base in codon (first letter)	U	UUU ⌐Phe UUC ⌐ UUA ⌐Leu UUG ⌐	UCU ⌐ UCC ⌐Ser UCA ⌐ UCG ⌐	UAU ⌐Tyr UAC ⌐ UAA Stop UAG Stop	UGU ⌐Cys UGC ⌐ UGA —Stop UGG —Trp	U C A G
	C	CUU ⌐ CUG ⌐Leu CUA ⌐ CUG ⌐	CCU ⌐ CCC ⌐Pro CCA ⌐ CCG ⌐	CAU ⌐His CAC ⌐ CAA ⌐Gln CAG ⌐	CGU ⌐ CGC ⌐Arg CGA ⌐ CGG ⌐	U C A G
	A	AUU ⌐ AUC ⌐Ile AUA ⌐ AUG	ACU ⌐ ACC ⌐Thr ACA ⌐ ACG ⌐	AAU ⌐Asn AAC ⌐ AAA ⌐Lys AAG ⌐	AGU ⌐Ser AGC ⌐ AGA ⌐Arg AGG ⌐	U C A G
	G	GUU ⌐ GUC ⌐Val GUA ⌐ GUG ⌐	GCU ⌐ GCC ⌐Ala GCA ⌐ GCG ⌐	GAU ⌐Asp GAC ⌐ GAA ⌐Glu GAG ⌐	GGU ⌐ GGC ⌐Gly GGA ⌐ GGG ⌐	U C A G

Third base in codon
(third letter)

Amino acids

Ala = alanine	Gln = glutamine	Leu = leucine	Ser = serine
Arg = arginine	Glu = glutamate	Lys = lysine	Thr = threonine
Asn = asparagine	Gly = glycine	Met = methionine	Trp = tryptophan
Asp = aspartate	His = histidine	Phe = phenylalanine	Tyr = tyrosine
Cys = cysteine	Ile = isoleucine	Pro = proline	Val = valine

FIGURE 3.4 **The genetic code**

called chromosomes. Each gene of a diploid pair is contained on different chromosomes.

We are composed of about 35,000 gene pairs. Because there are so many genes they cannot all be contained on one chromosome pair. The answer is to have more than one chromosome.

Humans have **23 chromosome pairs**, making 46 chromosomes in total. Of these, chromosomes 1 to 22 are called **autosomal**:

- chromosome 1 is the largest;
- chromosome 2 is the next largest;
- chromosome 3 is the next largest, and so on to
- chromosome 22.

Chromosome 23 is known as the **sex chromosome**. Chromosome 23 comes as a pair with a slight difference, where chromosome 23 can be X or Y.

- In females there are two copies of chromosome 23 in the X version; females are **XX**.

- In males there is only one copy of chromosome 23 X; the other one is chromosome 23 Y; males are **XY**.

Health Connection

Chromosome numbers and karyotype

The number of chromosomes and their appearance can be investigated in what are called metaphase spreads to see that they are the normal human numbers and sizes. The 23 pairs are written as 46 chromosomes with the sex chromosomes described to denote the gender. This is a karyotype (Figure 3.5).

The normal female karyotype is 46 XX.

The normal male karyotype is 46 XY.

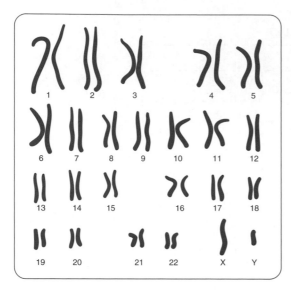

FIGURE 3.5 **Metaphase spread of human chromosomes**

In Figure 3.5 the 22 pairs of autosomal chromosomes 1–22 (44 autosomal chromosomes) can be seen, and the 23rd pair, the sex chromosomes, are separated. The figure here is of a male, XY. His **karyotype**, the number of chromosomes he has, is normal (23 pairs) and is written as **46 XY**.

Replication and cell division

We have seen above how DNA

1. contains the instructions for protein synthesis;
2. is replicated or synthesised into each cell of the body.

Health Connection

Chromosome disorders and karyotypes

We have seen that a change in one base pair or nucleotide in a gene can alter the amino acid inserted into a protein and therefore alter the function of that protein. There are human diseases where the number of chromosomes is altered.

Entire chromosomes carrying thousands of genes can also cause ill health. In some diseases we find

- an extra chromosome: the chromosome is no longer a pair (diploid) but now has three chromosomes;
- a missing chromosome of a pair (haploid);
- part of a chromosome missing or duplicated or moved (translocation).

In fact anything that can go wrong may go wrong.

- **Down's syndrome** is a chromosomal disorder where chromosome 22 has three copies instead of two. Those with Down's syndrome have a karyotype 47 XX or 47 XY depending on whether they are female or male.
- **Turner's syndrome** is a disease where one of the sex chromosomes is missing and children have the karyotype 46 X0. They are female, as they have no Y chromosome, but they do not have the full complement of XX.
- Some leukaemias (blood cancers) have translocations of a chromosome, the **Philadelphia chromosome**.

The mechanism for how the karyotype is changed will be discussed below.

Human Genome Project

The Human Genome Project (HUGO) has read and noted all the bases in the entire collection of human chromosomes, the human genome. The aim of this is to be able

- to compare humans with other species, to trace evolution;
- to compare humans with other humans to see relationships;
- to compare humans with other humans to see mutations;
- to trace mutations and diseases with the intention of gene therapy – the replacement of 'faulty' genes with wild type (normal) genes.

Cells have two major periods of growth and activity:

- **interphase** – during which cells
  - grow in size and
  - carry on metabolic processes;
- **cell division** – during which cells
  - replicate themselves and
  - produce more cells for growth and repair processes.

Before a cell divides into two new cells there are two stages DNA goes through:

- replication – DNA synthesis and
- mitosis – separation of chromosomes.

The DNA is replicated and then goes through a process called **mitosis** to *separate* the new chromosomes into the new cells. DNA is synthesised by semi-conservative replication (see above), where each old strand of the double helix serves as a template for a new strand. Each cell therefore inherits one old strand and one new strand. If the cell synthesised without separating the chromosomes we would go from

being diploid to tetraploid (4 copies) to having 8 copies then 16 (doubling). So DNA synthesis is linked to chromosome separation and cell division to form new cells.

The mechanics of **mitosis** are illustrated in Figure 3.6.

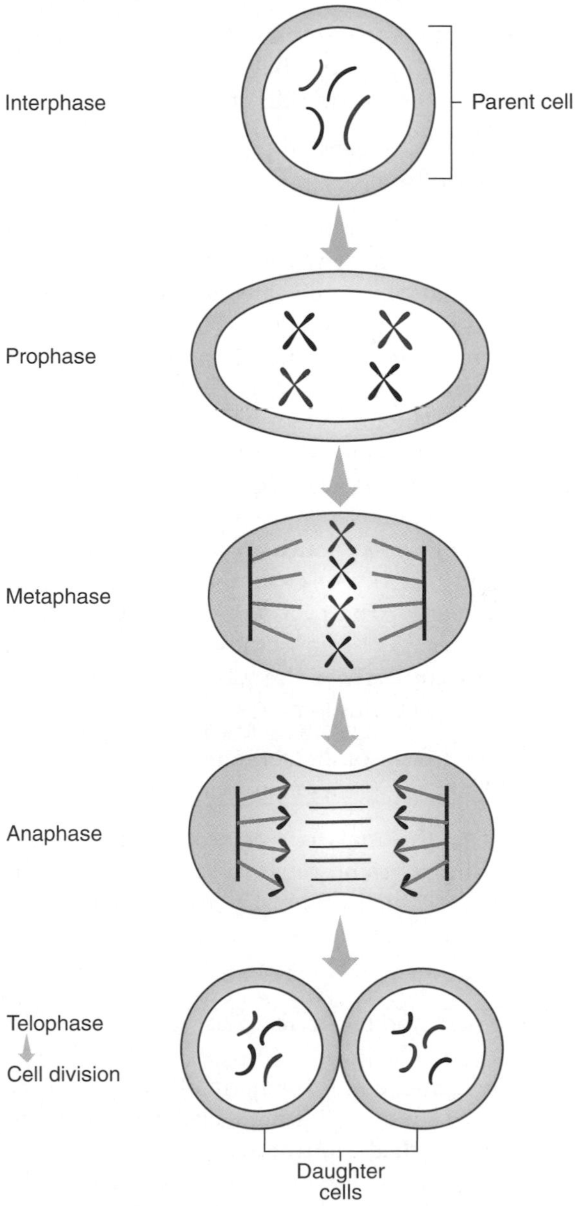

FIGURE 3.6 **Mitosis**

Sex

Biologically, sex is part of sexual reproduction and is a function of our genetic inheritance. Our cells, the cells of our bodies, somatic cells, are diploid. We have a set of cells, however, that only have one copy of each gene; they are haploid. These cells are our germ cells, reproductive cells; they germinate the next generation (our words in biology have roots that link them together). Our germ cells are

- **oocytes**, or eggs, in females and
- **sperm** in males.

These cells go through an extra round of DNA separation into new cells, **meiosis**, where the diploid chromosomes are separated and each oocyte or sperm ends up as haploid, with just one chromosome, rather than two.

There are various stages of replication and division. The important point in meiosis is the *reduction–division,* where the diploid chromosome number is reduced to the haploid chromosome number.

When we reproduce sexually we pass on our haploid number of chromosomes, *23 chromosomes,* rather than *23 pairs* of chromosomes. The other 23 chromosomes to make a diploid human come from the person we reproduce with. We are thus a mix of

- 23 chromosomes from our mother and
- 23 chromosomes from our father.

Together this makes 23 pairs of chromosomes.

Which chromosomes of each pair we get is random. Which one of the pair we pass on is random.

Dominant and recessive

Many genes come in many alleles, versions. Some of these alleles are called **recessive** and some are called **dominant**.

If a gene is recessive both copies need to be the same for the effect to be felt. For instance, if a gene makes a protein and we have a faulty version in one of our diploid copies, it may be

Health Connection

Chromosomal abnormalities and congenital disorders

During mitosis the chromosomes should part equally and be distributed into the new cells. Sometimes this does not occur and one cell can end up with more than 23 pairs of chromosomes. For example, instead of chromosome 21 being diploid it can end up having three copies, with the sister cell only having one copy – unequal distribution. Extra copies of chromosomes are as dangerous as too few.

During meiosis there should be an equal reduction in the number of chromosomes to the haploid number so that each egg or sperm has 22 pairs of autosomal chromosomes and if an egg an X chromosome (22 X) or if a sperm cell either an X or a Y chromosome (22 X or 22 Y). If there is not an equal reduction in numbers of chromosomes to the haploid number some cells may have none of one chromosome and three of another. If these cells are passed on during sexual reproduction the developing embryo will have an unequal number of chromosomes in every cell of its body. In some cells this may have an enormous effect. This unequal reduction–division in meiosis is increasingly seen in ageing egg cells. Diseases such as Down's syndrome and Turner's syndrome can result. Older mothers (after the age of 35) are offered screening of their embryo; however, many object to abortion.

sufficient that we are able to make the protein from the other, non-mutant copy. Being diploid gives us a back-up. This gene would be recessive.

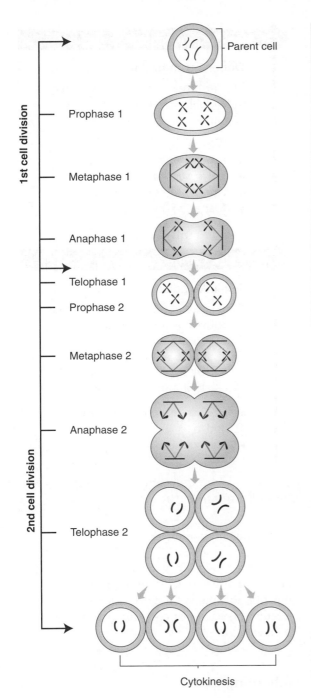

FIGURE 3.7 **Meiosis**

We would need both copies to be faulty so that no functioning protein would be made to have an effect.

Box 3.5 Summary – Chromosomes and cell division

- We have many genes.
- Genes are contained on chromosomes.
- Chromosomes are passed on to new cells during replication of DNA.
- The chromosomes are separated (segregated) during mitosis.
- Somatic cells have the diploid number of chromosomes.
- Germ cells have the haploid number of chromosomes.
- Germ cells go through an extra process, meiosis, to reduce the number of chromosomes to the haploid number.

Health Connection

Genetic diseases

If we have a genetic disease, a gene caused by a mutation, we can pass it on to our offspring during meiosis when we form our germ cells. A germ cell gets passed on to our offspring and if it contains the faulty gene our offspring may suffer the disease. We are diploid and if our partner passes on a functioning copy of the gene our offspring may not get the disease. This will depend on whether the gene is recessive or dominant.

If a gene is dominant and is making a version of a protein that is harmful, just one copy of that gene would have the effect and cause us health problems.

In a diploid cell with two chromosomes there are two versions of each gene. Here we are looking at just one gene A on one chromosome and A' on the other chromosome.

If A is the normal (wild type) gene and A' is the faulty gene, in a recessive mutation one of the pair, A, is working and enough protein can be made for the cell to function.

In a dominant mutation A′ harms the cells.

> ### Health Connection
>
> #### Recessive disorders
>
> In recessive disorders both parents carry one copy of the faulty gene. This gene is then passed into an egg and a sperm. The chance of an egg with a particular faulty gene coming together with a sperm with the same faulty gene is 1 in 4. If this occurs, both copies of the gene are recessive and the child has the disease. Examples of recessive disorders are
>
> - cystic fibrosis,
> - sickle cell anaemia,
> - Tay Sachs disease and
> - phenylketonuria (PKU).

Sex-linked genes

Apart from different recessive and dominant versions of genes, genes can also be sex-linked. Any gene that is on the X chromosome can appear as a recessive or a dominant gene, as with genes on autosomal chromosomes. If you are an XX female you can inherit two versions of the genes on the X chromosomes and they can be two different alleles or the same. However, males only receive one X chromosome. The Y chromosome is not complementary, or half of a diploid pair. So if there is a mutant gene on a male's X chromosome he does not have another version on his Y chromosome. These genes are therefore called sex-linked. Females pass on their X chromosomes to their male children and a male may inherit either of the two X chromosomes. If one of them has a lethal recessive gene on it, his mother is carrying the gene but has the normal, wild type allele on the other chromosome so she does not suffer from the disease. If one

> ### Health Connection
>
> #### Dominant mutations
>
> In dominant mutations every individual has an affected parent. Examples of dominant disorders are
>
> - achondroplasia,
> - polycystic kidney disorder,
> - Huntington's chorea and
> - Marfan's syndrome.

> ### Health Connection
>
> #### Sex-linked diseases
>
> There are a number of disorders that are caused by recessive genes on the X chromosome where the mother is a carrier and some of her male children will inherit the allele from one of the two X chromosomes, such as
>
> - Duchenne's muscular dystrophy and
> - haemophilia.

of her male children inherits the mutant allele he will suffer from the disease.

Genotype and phenotype

What type of gene we have, our **genotype**, affects what we look like and how we function, our **phenotype**. We are not exactly sure of the alignment, as genes code for proteins not for behaviours.

Inheriting genes

We are diploid animals. We can only pass on one copy (haploid number) of each gene. We cannot choose which of our two copies of each gene we pass on. Our chromosomes randomly segregate during meiosis to form our egg and

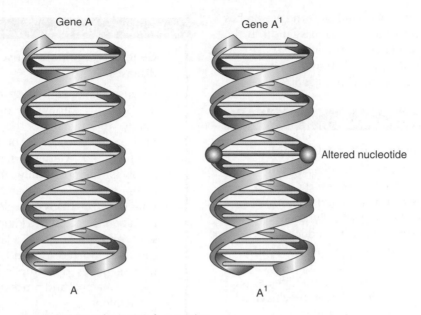

Gene A   Gene A^1

Altered nucleotide

A   A^1

FIGURE 3.8 **Dominant and recessive**

sperm (germ) cells. All of us are carrying about six recessive lethal mutations which would kill our offspring if our partners passed on similar genes. One of the sayings in molecular genetics is '*The greatest invention for the human race is the bicycle.*' What we mean is that we can get on our bicycle and go to the next village, town or county and out-breed, rather than in-breed! In-breeding with sister–brother mating, as practised by royal lines in ancient times such as the Pharaohs of ancient Egypt, resulted gradually in 'pure-bred' offspring, meaning that both versions of a gene were *identical* (homozygous), as seen in selective breeding in animals. It also resulted in many deaths and diseases of childhood due to recessive mutations.

To look at an example we shall discuss an invented or imaginary gene for eye colour which we shall call E.

E is a gene, the normal, wild type gene that makes brown pigment in eyes.

e is a recessive mutant version that does not make the brown pigment.

If we inherit E on one chromosome and e on the other our *genotype* is written E/e.

Our *phenotype* is brown eyes. One copy of E is sufficient. It is dominant over e.

If we inherit e from one parent and e from our other parent our *genotype* is e/e.

Our *phenotype* is blue eyes because we lack the gene to make the brown pigment.

If we substitute fibrosis, say, for eye colour we see that recessive mutations can cause debilitating diseases if both copies that are inherited are recessive and lethal.

Health Connection

Cystic fibrosis

Cystic fibrosis is a recessive autosomal disease, meaning that we need both copies in our somatic cells to be the cystic version to have an influence and that the gene is on an autosomal chromosome, not a sex X or Y chromosome. The gene is carried as one copy by 1 in 22 people of European origin.

With dominant genes the person carrying the gene will also have the condition. If the dominant gene is expressed (felt) early on and is lethal it may result in the death of the person with the gene. This death may occur before the person has reproduced, so the gene is not passed on. If the gene is expressed later the person may have had children. In dominant conditions the chances of passing on the gene to offspring is 50%.

Health Connection

Huntington's disease (chorea)

This is a dominant disease, but it has a late onset where the effects are seen later in life, usually from about 40 onwards. By then the person may have reproduced and passed on the disease to their offspring. This adds to the burden on the person suffering the disease, who will wonder whether they have passed on the gene causing it.

Health Connection

Diseases

Because genes code for proteins not behaviour there are problems in trying to link a gene to an illness or to health. A few diseases are caused by a single gene mutation such that the functioning protein, often an enzyme, is no longer made and a particular metabolic pathway can no longer be carried out. PKU is an example of this.

Generally diseases are multifactorial, having many causes. A gene alteration, mutation, can be one of the factors, but it would require other factors such as lifestyle factors to see the disease develop. Some diseases are due to chromosomal abnormalities during the formation of the egg or sperm. Some are congenital due to problems during embryonic development.

Health Connection

Genetic screening against diseases

Because genes can cause disease, if a gene is known to run in a family members of the family may be screened or embryos may be screened. Genetic screening involves taking family histories to see who is a carrier and who a sufferer, which helps to decide if the condition is recessive, dominant or sex-linked. If the gene is known it can be compared to wild type and disease genes by sampling some genetic material and processing it in a laboratory.

Evolution, nature and nurture

The theory of **evolution** sought to explain how different species came into being. The theory of genetics and genetic replication provides a mechanism for it. The DNA containing the genes has mutations. The ones which make a more successful protein are passed to all cells and, through reproductive advantages, to all members of a species, while the ones that are bad for a cell are not passed on to other cells or to other members of the species. Those that are passed on may lead to a gradual change in the individuals in a group, who may eventually become a different species. This is evolution by natural selection, where the trait that is being selected for has a genetic component. For single gene mutations this appears possible, and new species arise through these changes.

There is also evolution by selective breeding. This is where we breed together flowers, for example, that have a particular characteristic we want, such as one having scent and one having colour. Breeding a male and female flower together would provide offspring some

> ### Health Connection
>
> #### Gene therapy
>
> One idea for treatment of genetic disorders is **gene therapy**, where a functioning copy of the faulty gene is inserted into the DNA. Technically we can put genes into DNA. Our problem is which cell to put it into.
>
> Many or all of our somatic, body, cells may have the problem, and as there are ten trillion of them it is not feasible to replace the faulty gene in each of them.
>
> There are alternatives to this:
>
> - Screen fertilised eggs, once the sperm has fused with the egg, to see if the faulty gene is being passed on. The screening process is carried out in some forms of **in-vitro fertilisation (IVF)**, where the egg is removed from the female and fertilised in a test tube (in vitro). When this is done, before the fertilised **zygote** is implanted, the genes can be screened and any faulty embryos not implanted. There are tremendous ethical implications to this form of clinical intervention.
> - Replacing faulty genes in embryos is not allowed due to the fact that it would influence every cell in the embryo's body. Huge ethical issues surround this concerning altering the human genotype, diversity and differences.

of which carry both characteristics, scent and colour. We have also selectively bred animals such as dogs, horses and domestic farmed animals.

There are problems with natural selection and genes:

- Natural selection selects organisms, not genes; it cannot see inside the cell, so the trait or characteristic must be inherited.
- Genes code for proteins, not behaviours. So it is hard to explain behaviours, such as hunting, by genes.
- We do not know how we go from genes to whole organisms and whether genes cause this or are the vehicle for it.
- Saying that one gene gives behavioural advantages and another disadvantages leads to eugenics.

However, the link between genes and natural selection currently explains much of our understanding of biology and biological processes and makes the argument for our nature having a large part to play in who we are.

> ### Health Connection
>
> #### Eugenics
>
> In the nineteenth century a scientist called Galton wanted to breed humans selectively to remove disease from the population. He thought that diseases were caused by the genes we possess. His idea brought forth eugenics, a theory that was seen in its worse form in Nazi Germany in the 1930s. Taking a theory in science into a political arena is not recommended. His theory also has not stood the test of time, as many diseases are caused by microbial infections and environmental damage.

Reproduction

We have organs for carrying out each of the ADLs of our bodies and maintaining homeostasis. There is, however, one event in our lives we cannot avoid regardless of our homeostasis and health or health care and clinical interventions, namely death. While death removes us from the planet we can leave a trace of ourselves behind, a sort of immortality, by reproducing and bearing children.

Because we are a species that reproduces sexually (rather than asexually like bacteria) our children inherit half of their genetic material from each parent, but combine these to be diploid offspring with the human characteristics of our genes (nature) and due to our environments, our nurture. Being able to reproduce ourselves is an activity of daily living and is carried out using our reproductive systems. All the systems of our bodies are identical in males and females apart from the **reproductive system**, which in fact defines whether we are male or female.

Health Connection

Sex and death

In former times there was a large cultural link in poetry between sex and death, with sex being described by some poets as a minor death. Now we think of sexual reproduction as a way of passing on our genes to future generations.

The reproductive system

Male and female body systems and organs are identical, as are their ADLs. The only differences between males and females are in the reproductive system. We have different **gonads**, primary sex organs.

- In males the gonads are testes.
- In females the gonads are ovaries.

The gonads produce **gametes**, also called germ or sex cells, and secrete hormones. As mentioned above the gametes are

- sperm in males and
- ova (eggs) in females.

Male reproductive system

The production of sperm gametes in males occurs in the testes. There are two testes in males. They are a series of ducts, accessory organs and external genitalia.

The duct system includes

- epididymis,
- ductus deferens and
- urethra – the tube through which either sperm or urine travels to the exterior.

The accessory organs are

- seminal vesicle,
- prostate gland and
- bulbourethral gland.

The external genitalia include

- penis and
- scrotum.

The scrotum is a divided sac of skin outside the abdomen. Its function is to maintain the testes at 3°C lower than normal body temperature to protect sperm viability.

The penis delivers sperm into the female reproductive tract. It is divided into a number of structural regions:

- shaft,
- glans penis (enlarged tip) and
- prepuce (foreskin), a folded cuff of skin around the proximal end, often removed by circumcision.

Sperm production

The production of sperm cells begins at **puberty**, around 12 years of age, and continues throughout life. It occurs in the **seminiferous** tubules. **Spermatogenesis**, the production of sperm, takes 64–72 days.

The **spermatogonia** (cells that form sperm) undergo rapid mitosis to produce more spermatogonia cells before puberty. On each division one of the spermatogonia remains as a spermatogonia and the other cell becomes a primary **spermatocyte**. This unequal division is part of **stem cell differentiation** and

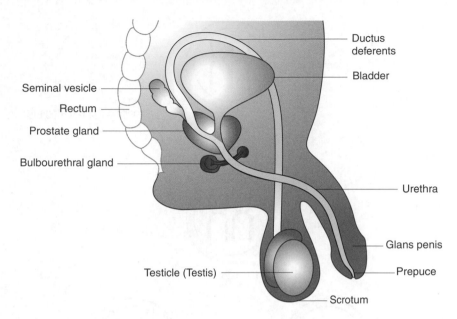

FIGURE 3.9 **The male reproductive tract**

is discussed below. A hormone – follicle stimulating hormone (FSH) – modifies spermatogonia division. The primary spermatocytes undergo meiosis to produce haploid **spermatids**. These then go through **spermiogenesis**, the genesis of sperm.

Sperm cells are haploid, as are eggs. They therefore have to be able to deliver DNA to the egg. Sperm are the only human cell with **flagella**, extensions of the membrane that act to move the cell along. Sperm have three main regions:

- head – which contains DNA (haploid chromosome number) covered by the acrosome,
- midpiece and
- tail – the flagellum that propels the sperm along.

Female reproductive system

The production of oocytes, eggs, in the female occurs in the **ovaries.**

The ovaries are composed of ovarian follicles, which are sac-like structures containing

- oocytes and
- follicular cells.

As in the testes there are a series of duct-like structures. The ducts include

- the **fallopian** (uterine) tubes and
- the **uterus**.

These ducts are where the sperm meets the oocyte.

The uterine/fallopian tube

This is the area which the oocyte travels through once released from the follicle in which it develops. The oocyte is then either fertilised or lost through the menstrual cycle. The tube provides a site for fertilisation. There are fimbriae along the distal end of the fallopian tube, which are finger-like projections that receive the oocyte. Cilia inside the uterine tube slowly move the oocyte towards the uterus, which takes 3–4 days.

Uterus

The uterus consists of the following:

- body – main portion,
- fundus – area where uterine tube enters and
- cervix – narrow outlet that protrudes into the vagina.

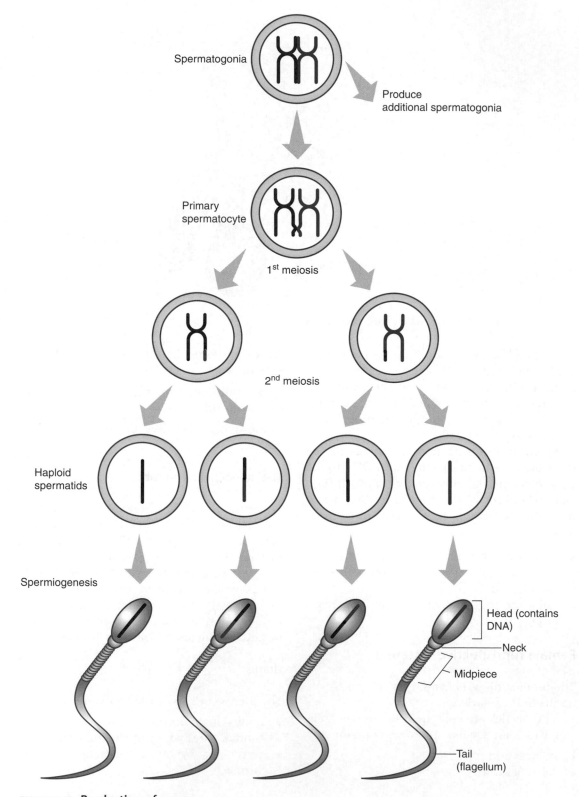

Spermatogonia

Produce additional spermatogonia

Primary spermatocyte

1st meiosis

2nd meiosis

Haploid spermatids

Spermiogenesis

Head (contains DNA)

Neck

Midpiece

Tail (flagellum)

FIGURE 3.10 **Production of sperm**

The uterus is located between the urinary bladder and rectum. It is a hollow organ. Its main function is to receive and retain a fertilised egg.

The endometrium layer, the inner layer, allows for implantation of a fertilised egg and sloughs off if no pregnancy occurs (menses).

The myometrium layer, the middle layer of smooth muscle, extends from the cervix to the exterior of the body, running behind the bladder and in front of the rectum. This functions as the birth canal and receives the penis during sexual intercourse.

Health Connection

Pregnancy and bladder control

Because the embryo develops in the uterus, which runs behind the bladder, as the embryo grows it pushes into the bladder, causing the stretch detectors of the bladder to send signals that the bladder is full. The bladder is discussed further in Chapter 10, 'Eliminating' (see p. 282).

Production of oocytes (eggs)

Unlike males, females are born with all the eggs they will ever possess. The ability to release eggs begins at puberty, around age 12. This means not only that there is a limited supply of eggs – female reproductive ability ends at **menopause**, at around 50 – but that the oocytes age. This can lead to some of the problems of congenital chromosomal disorders with incomplete meiosis discussed above.

Menstrual cycle and oocyte maturation

The production of the oocyte is through a process called **oogenesis.** During this the oocytes are matured in the developing ovarian follicles. The oocytes themselves start as **oogonia**, which are found in the developing foetus. These oogonia undergo mitosis to produce primary oocytes. The primary oocytes are surrounded by cells that form primary follicles in the ovary. Oogonia no longer exist by the time of birth as all have become oocytes. These are inactive until puberty.

The immature oocyte is contained in the primary follicle. The follicle and oocyte mature in the Graafian (vesicular) follicle. Follicle stimulating hormone (FSH) causes some primary follicles to mature. Meiosis, a reduction–division, starts inside maturing follicles, producing a secondary haploid oocyte or **ovum**, and the other cell of the division is referred to as the first **polar body.**

At ovulation the egg is mature and the follicle ruptures, releasing the oocyte. The ruptured follicle is transformed into a **corpus luteum.** This occurs about every 28 days. Meiosis is completed after ovulation only if fertilisation occurs and sperm penetrates the oocyte. If this occurs two additional polar bodies are produced.

Health Connection

Conception and the menstrual cycle

The release of the oocyte and the formation of a receptive uterus are under hormonal control. The timing of conception is thus quite fine; there are only a few days in which the released oocyte (egg) can be fertilised and implant.

During the production of oocytes (see Figure 3.11) the critical part is the production, by meiosis, of haploid oocytes or ova.

In both males and females the important part of the process is the production of haploid gametes by meiosis, a reduction–division. An oocyte and sperm can then fuse, fertilisation, to form a diploid offspring carrying a haploid set of chromosomes from each parent. These join together to form the diploid zygote, which then copies the diploid chromosomes into every cell

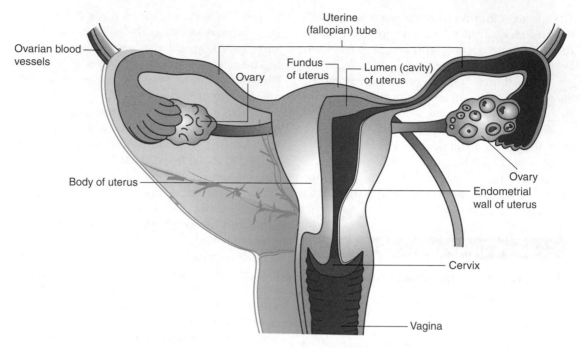

Ovarian blood vessels

Uterine (fallopian) tube

Ovary

Fundus of uterus

Lumen (cavity) of uterus

Body of uterus

Ovary

Endometrial wall of uterus

Cervix

Vagina

FIGURE 3.11 **Female reproductive tract**

of its body. The genes from your parents that you receive at fertilisation are therefore the same ones that you have in every cell of your body. You then pass on half of your genes (a quarter of each of your parents' genes) when you create the next generation. Some of the gene pairs you receive will be in an identical version, allele, from your mother and father, homozygous. Some will be different, heterozygous. You are a mix of conserved genes and diverse alleles.

Health Connection

Dizygotic twins

While one oocyte (egg) is usually released for potential fertilisation at each ovulation, sometimes two are released. If both are fertilised they may each develop into an embryo. They would then form two zygotes and be dizygotic twins, siblings that are born at the same time.

Development and differentiation

Embryonic development

Once the haploid sperm and ovum are formed in the male and female respectively the possibility of forming the next generation occurs. To do this four main stages occur:

- fertilisation,
- embryonic development,
- foetal development and
- childbirth.

Fertilisation

Fertilisation or conception is when the haploid genetic material of the sperm and the haploid genetic material of the oocyte combine. The resulting (diploid) cell is called a zygote. Generally only one sperm can fertilise an oocyte. There is a timing window during which fertilisation is possible:

- The oocyte is viable for 12 to 24 hours after ovulation.
- Sperm are viable for 12 to 48 hours after ejaculation.

Sperm cells must make their way to the uterine tube for fertilisation to be possible. Membrane receptors on an oocyte pull in the head of the first sperm cell to make contact. The membrane of the oocyte does not permit a second sperm head to enter. Once fertilisation has occurred the oocyte undergoes its second meiotic division.

Embryonic development

Once the DNA from the sperm and oocyte have fused, the first cell, the zygote, of the new individual is formed. A series of rapid mitotic cell divisions then takes place, **proliferation**, while the zygote is in the uterine tube. The zygote (or the ball of cells it is becoming) moves towards the uterus during this period.

Health Connection

Monozygotic (identical) twins

If during the first division of the embryo into two cells the cells come apart, they can each go on to form an entire embryo. Each embryo will be genetically identical to the other as they have been formed from one zygote – monozygotic (identical) twins. Even so, there are often subtle developmental differences due to the position of one embryo or the other, so there may be individual differences.

During this early stage the embryo is not implanted into the uterus; it is floating and being wafted along towards the uterus. The divisions it is going through to produce many cells are without growth. The mother has laid down a store of nutrients for the first week, pre-implantation, and the cells that are formed gradually deplete this supply. This time is called **cleavage**, as the large zygote cleaves, or divides, into many smaller cells.

The zygote becomes an embryo, the stage of development from the start of cell division until the ninth week of development. At the 16 cell stage the embryo enters the uterus and continues dividing. By the end of the first week after fertilisation the embryo has formed a ball of cells with a central watery area, a **blastocyst**, and used up all the nutrients of the oocyte. It must now implant into the uterus and form a **placenta**. The placenta will allow the developing embryo to obtain nutrients from its mother's blood supply. All mammals form placentas: this is one definition of being a mammal, such as a cat, dog, horse, camel, whale or human. The other defining characteristic is mammary glands for the newborn to suckle.

Health Connection

Implantation, miscarriage and menstruation

Many embryos fail to implant in the first week and thus cannot obtain nutrients for continued growth. The uterus will not make the hormones needed to maintain a pregnant uterus without the implantation of an embryo. The embryo will cease to thrive and will be flushed out of the uterus during menstruation. This would be such an early miscarriage that the woman may not realise she was pregnant.

The late blastocyst, the ball of cells with a central watery fluid, implants in the wall of the uterus by day 14.

The blastocyst is a ball-like circle of about 100 cells. There are two main areas to the blastocyst:

- **trophoblast** – the outer ring of cells, which forms the placenta;
- **inner cell mass (ICM)** – the inner ball of cells which form the embryo.

Ectopic pregnancy

Sometimes the zygote fails to implant correctly into the uterus, but implants into the fallopian tube instead, causing an ectopic pregnancy. This can be extremely dangerous for the mother.

The placenta

- forms a barrier between mother and embryo (blood is not exchanged);
- delivers nutrients and oxygen;
- removes waste from embryonic blood;

- becomes an endocrine organ (produces hormones) and takes over for the corpus luteum and produces
  - oestrogen,
  - progesterone and
  - other hormones that maintain pregnancy.

The blastocyst also secretes human chorionic gonadotropin (HCG) to produce the corpus luteum to continue producing hormones.

Development after implantation involves the following stages:

- Chorionic villi (projections of the blastocyst) develop.
- The blastocyst cooperates with cells of the uterus to form the placenta.

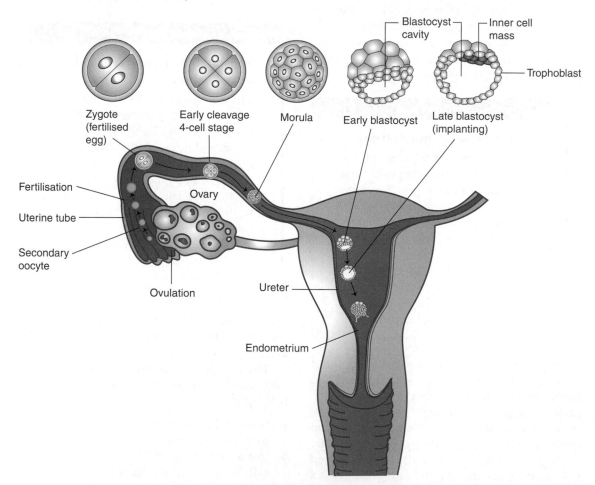

FIGURE 3.12 **The early stages of zygote proliferation before implantation into the uterus**

- The embryo is surrounded by the amnion (a fluid-filled sac).
- An umbilical cord forms to attach the embryo to the placenta.

The inner cell mass, ICM, produces all the cells of the body, the **primary germ layer**. We humans and many vertebrates (animals with a vertebral column) are composed of three germ layers:

- **ectoderm** – outside layer, which goes on to form
  - nervous system and
  - epidermis of skin;
- **endoderm** – inside layer, which goes on to form
  - gastrointestines,
  - mucosae,
  - glands and
  - many internal organs;
- **mesoderm** – middle layer, which goes on to form
  - muscles and
  - somites.

The cells of the ICM, therefore, must *differentiate*, become different from one another, to form all the different cell and tissue types that make up the functioning organs of the body.

The embryo must, therefore, produce more cells, by proliferation, and produce many types of cells by differentiation. The adult human has about 206 cell types, all derived from the original zygote and all containing the same genetic material that was present in the zygote by DNA replication.

The process of differentiation and cell development is discussed below under stem cells.

Foetal development

The embryo becomes a foetus at the beginning of the ninth week of gestation (post-fertilisation). At this stage all the organ systems are formed, if rudimentary and not fully functioning. From this stage onwards the foetus goes through growth and organ development.

Childbirth (parturition)

The main events of childbirth are described as **labour**. Labour is a series of events that expel the foetus from the uterus or birth canal. It begins with a rise in hormone levels causing uterine (muscular) contractions which help to expel the foetus.

- The placenta releases prostaglandins.
- The pituitary gland releases oxytocin.
- The placenta releases oestrogen.

As mammals we also produce the hormone prolactin to aid milk production.

> ### Health Connection
>
> #### Congenital abnormalities
> Foetal development and the formation of a fully functioning foetus require millions of cells being produced, differentiating to form structures and being in the correct place at the correct time. Any alterations to this and to the schedule can result in congenital abnormalities, development problems in the womb, resulting in a foetus with some altered structures. Cleft lips or missing limbs can occur, for example.

> ### Chapter Reference
> Hormones are discussed in Chapter 4, 'Communicating' (see p. 102).

There are three stages to labour:

1. **dilation**, during which
   a. The cervix becomes dilated.
   b. Uterine contractions begin and increase.
   c. The amnion containing the foetus ruptures.
2. **expulsion** of the foetus from the birth canal, during which
   a. The foetus passes through the cervix and vagina (birth canal).

b. Normally 'crowning' is seen, where the head is delivered first.
3. **placental stage**, during which
   a. The placenta is delivered or expelled from the uterus.

Health Connection

Caesarean section

Sometimes there are problems with the delivery of the foetus through the birth canal and a Caesarean section must be performed, where the pelvic wall is cut and the foetus delivered through the opening.

Stem cells

During normal mitotic cell division DNA is synthesised and then the four copies of each chromosome (tetraploid) are divided equally between two new cells. The daughter cells contain the same DNA as the parent cell. Each time a cell divides it forms two new cells and they go on to each form two new cells.

Clones of cells are formed (see Figure 3.13) during cell division by the replication and division of chromosomes so that the daughter cells are identical, genetically, to the parent cell.

With stem cells there is an unequal division, but it is not of the DNA. This is divided as in any other cell division. However, instead of both new cells becoming daughter cells, with stem cells one replaces the parent cell while the other becomes a daughter cell. The daughter cell goes on to make more daughter cells while the stem cell repeats the process, with one new cell always becoming a stem cell, replacing the parent. This is a process seen in every tissue compartment of the body. The stem cell has three properties:

- It is immortal.
- It remains a stem cell (undifferentiated).
- It provides a proliferative pool.

The stem cell supplies a pool of daughter cells. The daughter cells go on in development to differentiate into functional end cells. Differentiation is the process where cells become different from one another. They contain the same genes, but they do not express (transcribe and translate into proteins) all the same ones. So kidney cells express kidney specific genes, while skin expresses skin specific genes. This is what makes all the tissues and organs different from one another. Added to that the daughter cells become mortal functional end cells; they have a limited life expectancy varying from hours to days to a lifetime.

Chapter Reference

Lifespan of cells is discussed in Chapter 1, 'Maintaining a Safe Environment' (see p. 1).

This process allows a separation of immortal, proliferative stem cells and mortal, functional cells. The functional cells are disposable and get damaged doing their jobs. The stem cells are more protected in an inner environment, a stem cell niche.

Health Connection

Stem cells and cancer

It is now thought that most cancers are caused by an aberration in the control of the growth of stem cells. Instead of stem cells replenishing lost cells, they continue to grow unabated.

Stem cells and development

There are various types of stem cells:

- totipotent stem cells,
- embryonic stem cells, which are pluripotent,
- somatic stem cells, which are multipotent, and
- induced pluripotent stem cells, which are pluripotent.

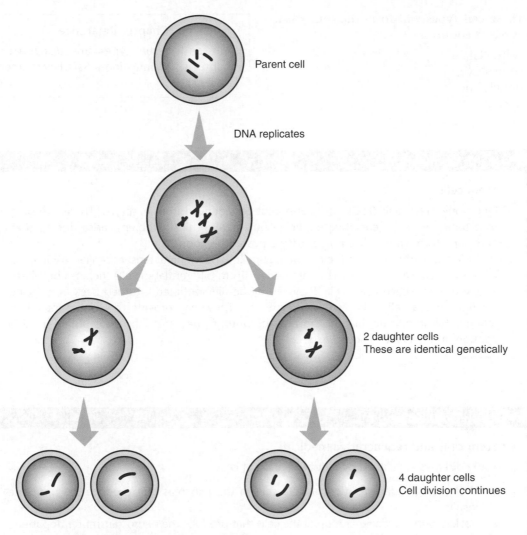

FIGURE 3.13 **The formation of clones of cells**

In each tissue of the body are **somatic stem cells (SSCs)**, cells of the body soma, which supply cells for replacing worn-out cells. These are also called **multipotent stem cells** as each of the cells supplies daughter cells that can be of various types within a tissue. For example, in the bone marrow there are SSCs which provide daughter cells that will be red blood cells, white blood cells and platelets. In other words the SSCs form daughter cells with multiple potentials.

At the moment of fertilisation the zygote is a **totipotent** stem cell: it will form all the types of cells of the developing embryo. However,

this is a short-lived cell type and very soon the cells of the zygote at the blastocyst stage form an inner cell mass (ICM). The cells of the ICM are **pluripotent**, not as potent as the totipotent zygote, but more potent than the multipotent SSCs. These pluripotent stem cells (PSCs) are also called **embryonic stem cells (ESCs)**. These PSCs or ESCs will form all the cell types of the body:

- ectoderm,
- endoderm and
- mesoderm

in the embryo.

These cell types will form the four tissue types of the adult:

- epithelial,
- connective,
- muscle and
- nerve.

Chapter Reference

Cells and tissue types are discussed in Chapter 1, 'Maintaining a Safe Environment' (see p. 1).

Health Connection

Stem cells

Embryonic stem cells (ESCs) are pluripotent cells derived from embryos. There are many uses for them in regenerative medicine but many ethical problems arise due to their derivation from very early embryos (day 6 post-fertilisation).

Induced pluripotent stem cells (iPSCs) appear to have characteristics similar to ESCs, but with fewer ethical problems. They are derived from differentiated cells such as fibroblasts, a type of connective tissue cell. They can be de-differentiated – turned back from being a differentiated cell to be an 'early' type cell. They may provide the source for future regenerative medicine, but, at the time of writing, they are difficult to obtain in high enough numbers for clinical use.

Health Connection

Stem cells and regenerative medicine

Many diseases are caused by a degeneration of cells.

- **Diabetes** is a degeneration of beta cells in the pancreas that produce the hormone insulin.
- **Parkinson's** is a degeneration of the cells that produce the neurotransmitter dopamine in the basal ganglia of the brain.

Some diseases are caused by trauma.

- In **myocardial infarction** the muscle cells of the heart (myocytes) are starved of oxygen due to problems in the cardiac circulation and therefore die. Once dead they are not replaced.

All of these diseases need new, working cells. Some of these diseases are treated by **transplants**, but there is a shortage of suitable donors of organs. Stem cells may provide a source of new cells instead. SSCs are restricted in what they can become and are hard to grow. ESCs have been seen as a better candidate cell type as they are easier to grow, have the potential, with the correct growth medium, to become any cell type and have fewer immunological rejection reactions. However, there are ethical objections to using ESCs. Recently a pluripotent stem cell type has been made called induced pluripotent stem cells which may provide the answer for **regenerative medicine** in an ageing population.

In other words as we go through development to form functional cells our cells become gradually more *restricted* in their potential and what they can become.

Health Connection

In-vitro fertilisation (IVF)

Some couples have problems conceiving embryos and go through IVF, where oocytes are removed from the female and fertilised with sperm from the male in a dish (in vitro meaning in glass, although most sterile dishes tend to be plastic nowadays). A successfully fertilised oocyte (not all will be fertilised) is then reintroduced into the uterus (womb) for **implantation** into the uterus and development into a foetus. The success rate is quite low for this procedure.

The couples undergoing this procedure do so for a number of reasons. Low sperm count in the male may be overcome by increasing the chance that the sperm and oocyte will meet. Conception problems in the female may be due to blocked fallopian tubes. There may also be an inherited genetic disease in the family. IVF allows for **genetic screening** before the fertilised oocyte is reintroduced into the uterus. Any embryo with the faulty gene can be excluded from reintroduction. There are, of course, many ethical problems beyond the discussion here.

Health Connection

Screening for chromosomal abnormalities: Amniocentesis and chorionic villi sampling

Both of these are prenatal (pre-birth) diagnosis methods for analysing chromosomal abnormalities such as Down's syndrome or Turner's syndrome.

In amniocentesis a small amount, about 20 ml, of amniotic fluid is extracted from the amniotic sac that surrounds the developing foetus. This fluid contains some foetal tissue, and the foetal DNA is examined for genetic abnormalities. This procedure can be carried out at 15–20 weeks usually, but there is a low risk of miscarriage.

Chorionic villi sampling can be done about four weeks earlier than amniocentesis, but has a higher risk of miscarriage. This technique involves the sampling of chorionic villi from the placenta. It also allows chromosomal diagnosis as well as gene sampling.

With both methods any abnormalities can be reported to the parent(s) and the choice of whether to abort the foetus is then discussed. This presents many ethical dilemmas to all of those involved.

Lifespan changes

Pregnancy

At the same time as the foetus is developing and being born the mother is pregnant! Pregnancy is the period from conception until birth and puts a large burden on the health and homeostasis of the mother.

There are many anatomical changes of the mother during pregnancy, such as

- enlargement of the uterus,
- accentuated lumbar curvature and
- relaxation of the pelvic ligaments and pubic symphysis due to production of relaxin.

There are also *physiological* changes occurring, such as to the

- gastrointestinal system,
- urinary system,
- respiratory system and
- cardiovascular system.

There is thus a large physiological cost to the mother as well as a metabolic cost. An additional 400–450 calories are needed in the diet as some nutrients are taken by the growing embryo.

> **Chapter Reference**
>
> Calories and nutrition are discussed in Chapter 9, 'Eating and Drinking' (see p. 241).

Health Connection

Changes affecting body systems during pregnancy

Gastrointestinal system

- Morning sickness is common due to elevated progesterone.
- Heartburn is common because of organ crowding by the foetus.
- Constipation is caused by declining motility of the digestive tract.

Urinary system

- Kidneys have an additional burden and produce more urine.
- The uterus compresses the bladder.

Respiratory system

- Nasal mucosa becomes congested and swollen.
- Vital capacity and respiratory rate increase.

Cardiovascular system

- Body water rises.
- Blood volume increases by 25–40%.
- Blood pressure and pulse increase.
- Varicose veins are common.

All these body systems will be discussed in subsequent chapters.

Gender

Gender has taken on many meanings. It is often used to denote roles rather than genetics. In biology the gender we have, male or female, is determined at fertilisation by the presence of the sex chromosomes:

- Males have XY sex chromosomes.
- Females have XX sex chromosomes.

Females can only pass on X chromosomes while males can pass on X or Y chromosomes. The gender you have is therefore dependent on which sperm from your father fertilised the egg. If he passes on a sperm with 22 X chromosomes you will be female. If he passes on a sperm with 22 Y chromosomes you will be male.

Puberty and the development of gonads

We humans are not born able to reproduce. Our gonads are formed early in the embryo, from about the eighth week.

In the embryo the testes form in the abdominal cavity and descend to the scrotum one month before birth. The determining factor for gonad differentiation is testosterone. Without it we are female.

The reproductive system organs do not function until puberty, which usually begins between ages 10 and 15.

- Sperm production starts during puberty and continues throughout life.
- The first menses usually occurs about two years after the start of puberty.
- Most women reach peak reproductive ability in their mid-20s.

While males do not make sperm until puberty females are born with all their oocytes. These are in a suspended state and begin maturation and release for fertilisation from puberty onwards, one at a time.

Health Connection

Gametes, mutations and damage

Sperm are not made until puberty and the testicles are sensitive to chemical or radioactive chemicals, which may affect the sperm produced.

Any damage or removal of the follicles or fallopian tubes can have long-term effects on fertility in females as the eggs are already present at birth.

Puberty and gender

We mentioned gender above in biological terms. It is also seen in the roles of hormones. Both males and females have hormones and very few hormones are involved in sexual maturity. Most are involved in metabolism and cell growth. Gender is also seen in the roles allocated to males and females. These are usually taught or conditioned by learning from birth,

Health Connection

Gender, chromosomes and realignment

While chromosomally males are XY and females are XX there are some people who have one chromosomal gender but have different gender or genital alignment. Some XX females have male characteristics and some XY males have female characteristics. The chromosomes may not match the gender as gender is a more fluid characteristic relying on embryonic development, hormonal levels and behavioural stereotyping.

Some people will have **gender realignment surgery**, where their *external* physical sexual characteristics will be altered to the gender they feel they are. Males having gender realignment with the removal of the testes will become sterile and unable to reproduce. They will not go through the regular female cycles and will need supplementary hormones. Females having gender realignment can remain fertile if they wish. They too will need hormone treatment.

and by puberty there are various expectations based on societal roles. These may reflect some biological basis, but may also be more political or ideological than biological. At puberty bodies mature and develop and gender becomes more apparent. Some people have problems fitting into the roles ascribed to them and feel uncomfortable with their bodies. This can be because of nurture, expecting people to behave in certain ways, or because of nature: some people have altered chromosomal genotypes (untypical male or female), and some people have altered hormone receptivity because of which the hormone does not switch on the entire 'gender' array of biological events so that puberty is incomplete. Some people feel that they were born in the wrong gender's body. Whether this is nature (genetic and developmental) or nurture (expectations and behaviours by parents, society and self) is not known.

Menopause

This occurs when ovulation and menses (menstruation) cease entirely and ovaries stop functioning as endocrine organs.

There is no equivalent of menopause in males, but there is a steady decline in testosterone.

> **Health Connection**
>
> #### Menopause, hormones, fertility and sexuality
>
> For many people hormone levels can affect their feelings of desire and sexuality. This can also be seen in those with mental health problems or on medications that can lower **libido**, the desire for sex. Both male and female hormone levels change during development and ageing. However, each person is different and it should not be assumed that desire and sexual needs disappear in the elderly. Fertility and sexuality are different from one another, and lack of ability to be fertile does not mean that a person has lost their libido.

Regeneration, repair and replacement

This chapter has looked at **generation**, the ability to make from new. Regeneration, the ability to grow anew, is seen in tissue repair and replacement. This will be illustrated in Chapter 5, 'Controlling and Repairing'.

> **Health Connection**
>
> #### Menopause and hormone replacement therapy
>
> Because hormone levels alter during the menopause they can affect the menstrual cycle as well as other physiological and psychological states. Hormones can be supplemented or replaced if they are lacking to help stabilise the normal levels in hormone replacement therapy, HRT.

Conclusion: Growing and developing

We grow and develop from a fertilised egg to a full-grown adult and are then capable of passing on our genes to future generations. We are not able to reproduce throughout our lives: for the first 12 or so years we are immature, and our fertility decreases as we grow older.

Our ability to grow and develop may be compromised by our genes and chromosomes. Our ability to reproduce is not guaranteed as many people have fertility problems.

While growing and developing are ADLs, they are not rights. Should growing and developing be compromised by our biology there are many treatments. However, there are also many ethical issues in this area of our health.

Our biology makes us all different from one another. As the epigraph at the start of the chapter says 'by nature [genetics] all men are alike'; it is our behaviour, habits and practices (nurture) that separate us. How genes link to behaviour is a field of interest for many scientists, psychologists, anthropologists, sociologists and health professionals and, more dangerously, a problem for politicians and governments.

Chapter Summary

- Genes are a simple language to code for proteins.
- Proteins carry out the functions of the cell and the body.
- We pass on the entire repertoire of proteins that we need, the human genome, into every cell of our body through replication and into future generations through reproduction.
- Each time we replicate our genetic material, DNA, we can make mistakes (mutations).
- Mutations can be good, bad or neutral.
- We are diploid.
- Our gametes are haploid.
- We make haploid gametes and pass on half of our genetic material through sexual reproduction.
- The other half of the genetic material comes from the other parent of our offspring.
- Pregnancy allows the embryo formed from the sperm and egg during conception to develop internally.
- Puberty is the age at which we become able to reproduce future generations.
- We continue throughout life to repair our bodies.
- We regenerate and generate!

Communicating

CHAPTER 4

We are what we think. All that we are arises with our thoughts. With our thoughts we make the world.

Buddha (*c.*563–483 BCE), Nepal

Chapter Outline

- Introduction: Communicating as an activity of daily living
- The environment
- The nervous system
- Organisation of the nervous system
- Cellular communication
- The endocrine system
- Changes during lifespan and lifestyle
- Conclusion: Communicating
- Chapter summary

Introduction: Communicating as an activity of daily living

Nowadays we often hear the term 'communication skills', by which we mean having the ability to communicate well with other people. Some of us cannot communicate with others due to poor communication skills, presumably part of poor social skills, not being able to interact appropriately with others. Some of us cannot communicate with the external world due to our mental state; being depressed often leads to being withdrawn. Some of us cannot communicate with the outside world due to damage either to parts of our brain or to parts of our muscles. Not being able to communicate with the external world, being 'locked in', is one of our biggest dreads. We are social animals and speech and non-visual communication are part of how we form communities. These aid our survival and social needs.

Biologically, there are many forms of communication. Not only can we carry out external communication, one to another using a variety of forms such as speech, writing, hearing, seeing, touching and making gestures, but we also have a wealth of internal communications between parts of our body so that they can act together as a whole. These rely on chemical signals and **receptors** that are able to detect the signals. In fact all communication is reliant on a message or signal going out in some form (chemical or physical) and a receiver that is able to pick up or detect the signal and then make some meaning out of it.

Communicating is a vital activity of daily living. Without being able to communicate externally with the world we feel cut off. Without being able to communicate internally between tissues and cells, our community of cells, us, ceases to function properly and our health is severely impaired.

The environment

Communicating and the external environment

How do we know the world or even know our own small personal world? We think we are in control, but the only thing we control is our *perception*, the way we see and interpret the messages we receive. Really, we know what we have trained ourselves to know and we are limited by the messages we are capable of receiving (tuned into). Just like a radio antenna we can only pick

> ### Health Connection
>
> #### Communication and mental health
>
> There are many issues that can affect communication. Our mental health is one of them. If we are depressed or suffering from another mental health disorder we may find it impossible to face talking with others, or we may be in an internal world that has altered perceptions and therefore altered ways of communicating. I, the sufferer of the altered mental state, may think that I am communicating normally and that it is you, the carer, that is unable to understand because of your poor communication skills.

> ### Health Connection
>
> #### Sensory impairment and the external environment
>
> Some people do not have the full range of senses. They may, for example, lack the ability to detect light (visual impairment) or sounds (hearing impairment). There are clinical devices and interventions that can aid their internal environment, such as hearing aids. While we cannot change all of the external environment, there are changes we can make to some of the external environment, such as bumps on the surfaces of pavements near road crossings or loop hearing aids in theatres, that make parts of the external environment more enabling and accommodating and allow those with a sensory impairment to remain independent and healthy – able to carry out the full range of ADLs.

up signals within a certain *range* and within a certain *frequency*. There are many signals that we do not have the receptors for and cannot detect. Having intelligence has allowed us to make devices that can detect these signals and 'translate' them into a signal we can 'read'.

A famous behavioural scientist once described the animal he investigated, the spider, and its behaviour: If the spider sees something bigger it should run away to avoid being preyed on, if it sees something smaller it should run towards it and eat it, and if it sees something about the same size it should try to mate with it! We need to know what is happening in the external world to aid our survival, to find food, shelter and mates, and to avoid being food. We are capable of perceiving fragments of the external world as signals that are interpreted by our internal world to give meaning and affect outcomes that aid our survival. If we get it wrong we can die.

Communicating and the internal environment

For all the cells of our body to work together as one whole organism they must coordinate and control their functions to bring about homeostasis, maintaining the inner environment. To do this, communication is needed. In any large organisation a lack of communication leads to parts of the organisation working separately to their own ends without regard for the aims of the whole. The same applies with a complex organisation such as a human. Communication in living organisms is carried out at a number of levels and by a number of means. Cells communicate with their neighbours, tissues communicate with organs and there are structures dedicated to communication, such as the **endocrine system** with overall responsibility for outputs to organs and the **brain** with responsibility for monitoring inputs and initiating outputs.

How do we know what is going on? When we are dehydrated we feel like having a drink, but how do we know we are thirsty? If we are to maintain our temperature at 37°C how do we know what temperature our bodies are? How do we know when to eat? Where does the sensation of hunger come from? How do we know when to urinate? Where does the sensation of having a full bladder come from? In fact, all the actions we take, that we think we are in control of, are *motivated*, meaning we carry out the actions that will keep us alive and maintain our homeostasis and our health. So much for free will!

Just as in homeostasis, we must first *receive a signal*; we then *interpret* the signal and *integrate* any other relevant signals and then mount a *response*. All of this communication is under the control of the **nervous** and **endocrine systems**, which help to *monitor* our internal environments and bring about an *appropriate response* to it and to our external environment.

Chapter Reference

Homeostasis is discussed in Chapter 1, 'Maintaining a Safe Environment' (see p. 1).

In this chapter we shall first discuss the nervous system and then the endocrine system.

The nervous system

The nervous system *controls and coordinates* all the activities of the body, *monitoring* the internal environment, *controlling* homeostasis, as well as *monitoring* the external environment so that you can make the appropriate *response*. It gathers information inwards as input, called **sensory (afferent) information**, as in having a sensation, and sends information outwards as output, called **motor (efferent) information**.

The nervous system and its cells communicate with other cells of the nervous system and cells of the **voluntary** or **skeletal** and **involuntary** or **smooth muscles** as well as with **secretary glands**, both **exocrine** – glands that secrete into ducts such as the bile duct – and **endocrine** – glands such as the pituitary gland that secrete substances called **hormones**, chemical messengers, into the blood.

The nervous system initiates **electrical impulses** or *messages* called **action potentials**

which are carried along neurons. The neurons transmit electrical information very rapidly. The output from a neuron can affect voluntary skeletal, cardiac or involuntary smooth muscles, causing them to contract (shorten), or it can affect the output of endocrine glands to make them secrete hormones. The output can also affect other neurons.

Health Connection

Homeostasis and communicating

The nervous and endocrine systems monitor signals in the external environment (outside world) and in our internal environment. They then coordinate appropriate responses. Any damage to these systems, such as trauma to our nervous system (particularly brain and spinal cord) or cancers of our endocrine system, therefore disrupts our ability to survive and our ability to maintain homeostasis. This may lead to our not being able to keep our internal organs functioning correctly and can result in our death.

Chapter Reference

The motor output to voluntary muscles is discussed in Chapter 6, 'Moving' (see p. 163).

Cells of the nervous system

The nervous system is composed of billions of functional cells. There are two main types of cells of the nervous system:

- **Neurons** conduct electrical information.
- **Glia** support neurons and the nervous system.

The cells of the nervous system, particularly the neurons and the extended parts of neurons, *projections*, are contained in the brain, spinal cord and periphery of the body.

The neurons conduct electrical impulses, also called action potentials. The information travels in two parts of the neuron:

- **Dendrites** input information to the cell body.
- **Axons** output information from the cell body.

Both dendrites and axons are *membrane projections* from the cell, similar to cilia or flagella.

Chapter Reference

Cell structure is discussed in Chapter 1, 'Maintaining a Safe Environment' (see p. 1).

There are *many* dendrites on a neuron, but only *one* axon.

Neurons are the functional cells of the nervous system, moving information around the nervous system. Neurons are often arranged in groups, called nerves.

A neuron is a cell, with all the general features of a cell as outlined in Chapter 1, 'Maintaining a Safe Environment'. Neurons are specialised cells that are *differentiated* from the generic cell. They have an area called a cell body that contains the nucleus and other organelles. In addition, they have extensions from the cell membrane, axon and dendrites.

The anatomy of neurons reflects their physiological function. Neurons receive and transmit electrical information. They receive information, input, on dendrites and transmit information, output, on a single axon. Large nerves containing axons are called nerve tracts. The electrical information travels in *one direction* only from the cell body towards the terminus (see Figure 4.1).

Action potentials

The cells of the nervous system, neurons, are like any other cell in that they must take substances in to maintain them and excrete waste products. They produce proteins such as enzymes to help in their own metabolism.

Health Connection

Electricity

Because our nervous system runs on electrical information and sends electrical signals to muscles we can be electrocuted. Accidental contact with high voltage or currents can alter our own electrical conduction and make it stop. Likewise, if our muscles have stopped they can be innervated, stimulated, by an electrical impulse. This is seen in **cardiac arrest**, where the cardiac muscle has stopped contracting and thus the heart is no longer pumping blood. We can also take electrical readings from the heart, such as e**lectrocardiograms**, and from the brain.

They are surrounded by a lipid membrane and it is this membrane that is specialised in a neuron.

Neurons have many dendrites bringing information into the cell and one long axon taking information out. The axon may branch to form many **axon terminals**. Electrical action potentials run along the dendrite and axons in one direction. At the axon terminal the action potential stops and causes the release of **neurotransmitter** molecules into the **synapse**, gap. Axons are often covered by a fatty insulating material called **myelin**. This is made by glial cells, such as **Schwann cells**, which wrap themselves around the axon. Between the myelin are gaps called **nodes of Ranvier**.

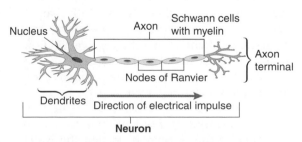

FIGURE 4.1 Neurons, axons and dendrites

The membrane is composed of fatty lipids and is, therefore, hydrophobic ('water hating'). It does not allow the passage of ionic substances, which are hydrophilic ('water loving'), such as ions or electrolytes, but does allow other hydrophobic substances such as fats across. Due to this the membrane can be used to conduct electricity.

Health Connection

Electrical disturbances and death
Because our neurons conduct electricity, any external source of electricity can interfere with the neuron. We can, therefore, be electrocuted to death. Conversely we can sometimes be electrically stimulated to life if our electrical conduction has ceased.

Chapter Reference
Ions or electrolytes are discussed in Chapter 2, 'Working and Playing' (see p. 35).

Ions have an electric charge on them. Sodium, potassium, calcium and magnesium ions, for example, are positively charged, while a chlorine ion is negatively charged. If one has a large amount of positive charge on one side of a membrane and a large amount of negative charge on the other side of a membrane there is a difference in charge across the membrane, called a **potential difference**, which can be measured in volts. This is similar to having a large amount of a substance on one side of a membrane and very little of it on the other. The substances tend to diffuse down their concentration gradient. With charged substances, the ions tend to diffuse down their **electrical gradient** so that the positive will flow towards the negative and the negative towards the positive. This flow, or current, of electrical charge can be measured in amps.

Imagine a tank of water (see Figure 4.2) separated from an empty tank by a tube with a stopper. If the stopper is opened the water will flow (a current of water) until both tanks

Chapter Reference
Diffusion and concentration are discussed in Chapter 1, 'Maintaining a Safe Environment' (see p. 1).

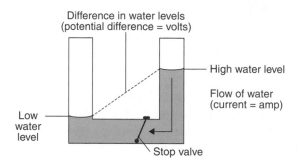

FIGURE 4.2 **Water flows as a current from high concentration to low concentration, similar to diffusion**

have the same amount of water. Water will not suddenly flow just into one tank up to the top. Before the water was released from the full tank there was a difference between the two tanks, a potential difference. Once the water is equal in both tanks there is no potential difference. When the full tank had the tap opened the water flowed out and the potential difference was converted into a **kinetic (movement) difference**, a current. This is the principle of the hydroelectricity station. Water at a great height flows over and as it falls it generates kinetic energy which can be used to turn a turbine and generate electricity.

Once the water is the same in both tanks, the kinetic energy, the flow that forms a current, stops. To maintain this flow one tank must be higher, have a difference, than the other, and the first tank would need refilling. This difference between the two tanks is a potential difference that allows the flow. To reinstate this potential difference would require pumping the water back out of one tank and into the first tank. The amount of energy that is consumed pumping the water out is exactly the same as the amount of energy generated when the water flowed. This is a *law of the universe*:

energy cannot be made or destroyed; it can only be converted from one form to another. This is why, when we use up energy pumping muscles or in active transport, we must make more energy, or release the energy contained in food. We are converting various forms of *energy* to do *work*.

The neuron uses ions instead of water. It loads positive ions on one side of the membrane (outside the cell) and negative ions on the inside of the cell. Remember, this is like pumping water uphill: it takes a lot of energy to pump positive ions out and negative ions in by active transport. Both sets of ions want to run down (passive diffusion) their electrical gradient and down their concentration gradient.

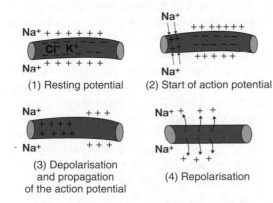

(1) Resting potential

(2) Start of action potential

(3) Depolarisation and propagation of the action potential

(4) Repolarisation

FIGURE 4.3 **Resting potential and action potential of an axon**

The membrane of the neuron has pumps in it (Na^+/K^+ ATPase pumps) that move, by active transport, ions across the membrane against their **concentration gradient**. This sets up a concentration gradient and because the ions are charged +/– this causes an electric gradient across the membrane called the **resting potential.** The resting potential is where there is a **polarisation** of ions, positives on one side and negatives on the other side of the membrane. When a signal (current) is sent, pores open and ions cross, **depolarising** (losing the different polarities) the membrane so that the axon is no longer polarised. To send another signal the axon must be **repolarised** by pumping ions out across the membrane.

This difference across the membrane is called the **membrane potential** or the resting potential. In fact it is not resting as it takes a lot of ATP energy to pump ions against their gradients. This pumping is done by ATPase pumps situated all along the membrane or axon. In biology words with 'ase' on the end denote enzymes. The ATPase enzyme uses ATP energy to pump ions by active transport. The membrane potential gives the neuron the *potential to act*, in this case to send an electrical impulse, the action potential, along the membrane. When a signal is received by a neuron that excites the neuron to send an action potential, pores in the membrane of the axon open, allowing the movement of ions across. As the ions move the voltage drops and a current flows along the axon. This depolarisation travels along the axon towards the axon terminus as the action potential.

Once a pore has opened and allowed ions to flow it closes for a **refractory period**. During this time the ATPase pump continues to pump ions against their concentration and electrical gradient, maintaining or repolarising the membrane.

Health Connection

Ion channels and anaesthetics
Anaesthetics are a class of drug that reduces the sensation of pain in a patient, allowing surgery and dentistry to be performed. One form of anaesthetics used especially in dentistry works to block the ion channels in the membrane of neurons. This prevents the electrical signal travelling. Pain and touch sensations are therefore reduced.

The conduction of electricity relies on ions, the charged version of atoms, and voltage. The hard work of the nervous system is setting up the ability to use electricity, not the actual conduction of electricity. The nervous system uses 20% of the available oxygen and glucose to make ATP energy as it is a high consumer of energy. The brain is very vulnerable to lack of oxygen or starvation.

Myelin

Some neurons are **myelinated** (covered in glial cells that produce fats, myelin, as insulators). Myelinated neurons conduct electricity, action potentials, faster than non-myelinated neurons.

Myelinated axons transmit action potentials faster than non-myelinated axons due to the position of the pores that allow the movement of ions across the membrane during the electrical impulse, depolarisation. In myelinated axons these pores are concentrated in the gaps between the myelin sheath; the gaps are called the nodes of Ranvier. The impulse thus leaps from node to node in myelinated axons rather than travelling along the entire length as in non-myelinated axons.

Synapses and neurotransmitters

Neurons take messages from one neuron to another or to a muscle or gland, depending on

the type of neuron. Between neurons and their target are gaps called synapses. Neurons do not conduct electricity across these synapses. Instead, when the action potential reaches the end of an axon, called the axon terminal, the action potential causes chemicals at the terminal to be released into the synapse. These chemicals are called neurotransmitters. They are stored in **vesicles** in the axon terminal. The chemical neurotransmitters cross the synapse and bind to receptors on the target cell. The chemicals cause a reaction in the cell that binds them (Figure 4.4).

At the terminus of an axon are vesicles containing neurotransmitters. When an action potential reaches the terminus it causes the vesicles to secrete the neurotransmitter into the synapse. This signal transmitter molecule

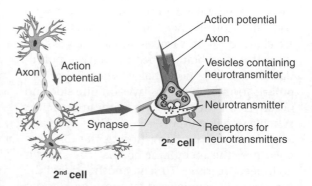

FIGURE 4.4 The synapse

then binds to specific receptors on the next cell, causing a change in ion concentrations in that next cell. If that next cell is a muscle it will contract. If it is a neuron it may excite it or inhibit it.

Each neuron synthesises its own neurotransmitter which characterises the type of neuron that it is. Chemicals that are released by a neuron in response to an action potential are thus neurotransmitters. Some of the same chemicals can be released from an endocrine gland as a hormone, discussed below.

Once the neurotransmitter has bound to the receptor in the next cell, the downstream receptor, it is destroyed by enzymes so that the effect is short-lived. The bound transmitter has an effect on the downstream cell. If it is a muscle cell forming a neuro-muscular junction, the neurotransmitter acetylcholine is released and the muscle contracts.

If the receptor is on another neuron, that neuron can be

- *excited* and produce its own action potential, relaying the message onwards;
- *inhibited*, stopping the message going further.

This is because each neuron has many inputs, up to a thousand, on its various dendrites, but only one output on its axon. The output is either an action potential or no action potential, *all or nothing*. The inputs are summed for excitatory and inhibitory.

- If there are more excitatory inputs than inhibitory inputs this causes the membrane to depolarise and an action potential to travel along the axon.
- If there are more inhibitory inputs than excitatory inputs this prevents the depolarisation of the axon.

This may seem strange, but all day long we are receiving millions of signals and cannot react to all of them. Thus we can receive many inputs and decide (sum up) whether to react.

Many neurotransmitters are amino acids or quite basic chemicals. It is where they are released from and the effect they have on the ion channels that cause the next neuron (downstream) to open or close its ion channels and hence to have an action potential or not (Table 4.1).

Table 4.1 Examples of neurotransmitters

Transmitter Molecule	Site of synthesis
Acetylcholine	Central nervous system (CNS), parasympathetic nerves
Serotonin 5-hydroxytryptamine (5-HT)	CNS, chromaffin cells of the gut, enteric cells
GABA	CNS
Glutamate	CNS
Aspartate	CNS
Glycine	Spinal cord
Histamine	Hypothalamus
Adrenaline (epinephrine)	Adrenal medulla, some CNS cells
Noradrenaline (Norepinephrine)	CNS, sympathetic nerves
Dopamine	CNS
Adenosine	CNS, peripheral nerves
ATP	Sympathetic, sensory and enteric nerves
Nitric oxide, NO	CNS, gastrointestinal tract

Health Connection

Pharmacology and the synapse

Pharmacology is the study and use of chemicals, drugs, that can produce a therapeutic effect. Many drugs work at the synapse to interfere with electrical transmission to either block it or to induce it to produce the desired effect. Pharmacology is discussed further in Chapter 12, 'Sleeping and Healing' (see p. 324).

Health Connection

Nicotine

Nicotine acts as a nerve stimulant, akin to a key opening a lock. It mimics the body's own neurotransmitter nicotinic acetylcholine and binds to receptors for this neurotransmitter. These receptors are located throughout the body in the brain and in the adrenal glands and release adrenaline and noradrenaline hormones. These hormones raise heart rate and blood pressure.

Box 4.1 Summary – Neurons and electrical transmission of information

- Neurons are cells that carry electrical impulses in the form of action potentials.
- To do this they must first establish a resting potential, a potential to carry an impulse.
- The resting potential uses concentration gradients where there are positive ions on the outside of the membrane of the axon and negative ions on the inside.
- To establish the resting potential, active transport that uses ATP must pump ions against their concentration gradients.
- The action potential carries ions in by diffusion and a current flows along the axon.
- Nodes of Ranvier allow the action potential to jump from node to node and speed up the action potential. The nodes are between myelin sheaths. Myelinated neurons thus have quicker action potentials than non-myelinated neurons.
- The action potentials release neurotransmitters at the axon terminus.
- The neurotransmitters enter a synapse, the gap between neurons or between neurons and effector cells.
- Neurotransmitters bind to their receptors and excite or inhibit the next neuron.
- Action potentials are all or nothing; once activated they run at the same strength along the axon.
- While action potentials are all or nothing (on or off) their frequency can increase to denote a stronger stimulus.

Organisation of the nervous system

We divide the nervous system into

- central nervous system (CNS);
- peripheral nervous system (PNS):
  - somatic nervous system and
  - autonomic nervous system (ANS).

The CNS will be discussed later. The PNS has two main functions:

- It inputs (incoming) information from the periphery of the body.
- It outputs (outgoing) information to the periphery of the body.

The inputs to the PNS come from the senses and are thus called **sensory information**.

The outputs from the PNS go to muscles and glands and cause an effect. These outputs are thus called **motor outputs** that go to *effectors* (muscles or glands).

The *motor pathways* to the voluntary muscles of the soma (body) and the face cause muscle contraction and movement.

The motor output can also go to the involuntary system via a part of the nervous system called the **autonomic nervous system (ANS)**, which controls the smooth involuntary muscles around the organs of the body and the glands (Figure 4.5).

The divisions of the nervous system in Figure 4.5 are not real, but constructed to enable us to study and understand how information is categorised and acted upon. Sensory information comes in to the central nervous system and motor information comes out from the CNS to either the somatic nervous system or the autonomic nervous system.

The PNS

The peripheral nervous system (PNS) brings information, in the form of electrical impulses (action potentials), from the inside and external worlds and takes information out to the periphery. Information brought from the periphery is sensory (afferent). Information taken out to the periphery is motor (efferent). Action potentials are discussed later.

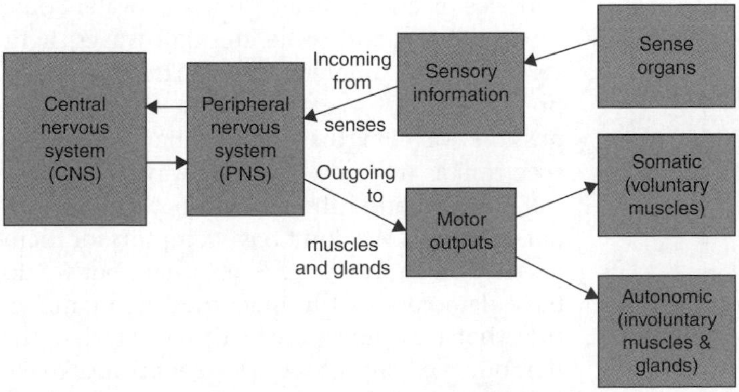

The action potential or electrical impulse travels in one direction from the cell body to the axon terminus. This is important for separating incoming and outgoing information in the entire system. Due to this neurons can be

- sensory or
- motor.

Neurons that bring information in from the periphery towards the centre of the body and nervous system are called **sensory neurons**.

Neurons that take information out towards the periphery of the body are called **motor neurons**.

The difference between a sensory and a motor neuron depends on the arrangement of the cell and its axons (Figure 4.6).

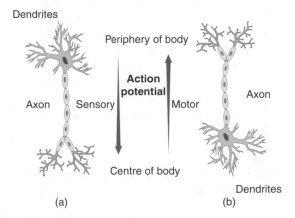

FIGURE 4.6 **Sensory and motor neurons**

Neuron (a) in Figure 4.6 is sensory, bringing information from the periphery to the centre. Neuron (b) in Figure 4.6 is a motor neuron, bringing information from the centre to the periphery. Arrows show the direction of the electrical impulse.

Sensory or motor neurons are identical in the sense that they are taking their output along axons. The difference between them is whether the axon is running from the periphery to the centre, a sensory axon, or from the centre to the periphery, a motor axon.

FIGURE 4.5 **The divisions of the nervous system**

Funny bone

Many of us have had the sensation of banging our elbow and feeling tingling in our fingers and registering pain! We call it the funny bone even though the sensations are not very funny. One nerve tract, the ulnar, lies near the ulna bone at the elbow. If you bend your arm at a right angle and feel in between the two bones (ulna and radius) at the elbow you may stimulate the ulnar nerve. Messages registering touch and pain can run up to the brain and motor outputs to the fingers also run along the nerve. Stimulating the nerve and all its axons halfway between the brain and the fingers at the elbow by banging or pressing it confuses the impulses, which then start at the pressure point and radiate out each way.

The sense organs: Sensing the external environment

Energy comes in various forms, such as

- light,
- sound,
- chemical,
- mechanical and
- heat.

We are capable of deciphering these various forms of energy due to sense organs. Sense organs are specialised receptors tuned to a particular energy type; they have their own **sensory modality**, the energy they can detect and respond to.

- Light energy is detected by the sense of seeing.
- Sound energy is detected by the sense receptors for hearing.
- Chemical energy is detected by the senses of smell and taste.

- Mechanical energy is detected by the sense of touch and pressure.
- Thermal energy is detected by the sense of temperature.

All of these senses have sense organs that are able to detect a particular type of energy. For instance, the eyes are sense organs that are tuned to detect and to respond to light energy. Light (which is a form of electromagnetic radiation) may be shining all over your body, but only the receptors in your eyes are capable of detecting and responding to light energy. Likewise with sound: only detectors in your ear can hear sound waves. Sound, unlike light, is formed when air particles, the molecules in air, bounce off each other, oscillate. This is why, as the film *Alien* says, 'In space no one can hear you scream', because space is a vacuum with no air in it, so there can be no oscillations of air particles and therefore there is no sound. To smell, chemicals must be volatile gases at 37°C which can be detected by the chemical receptors, smell receptors, in our noses. Thus there are various forms of energy and there are various receptors, sense organs, for each type.

We humans tend to think that anything we detect is all there is to detect! We call the light that we can detect with our eyes the 'visible light spectrum', the spectrum being the range of wavelengths of light that our eyes can detect and respond to. In fact it is the 'human visible spectrum' as other animals can detect different wavelengths of light.

Wavelengths are the frequency which light particles or energy is at. Just as in water some waves are low and some are high waves, light also comes in different waves. These we interpret as colour. We know that the range of possible wavelengths is larger than the visible spectrum as we know there are wavelengths we call UV light and infrared light beyond our colour spectrum. We don't have receptors for them in our eyes so we cannot 'see' them, but we do have detectors in the machines we manufacture that can detect these other wavelengths that our eyes cannot see. These machines make them visible for our eyes. We are technologically capable of more than our biology!

Other animals can detect energies in different ranges than us. For example, a dog whistle is at a pitch higher than human hearing, which means dogs can hear in a range in which we cannot hear. So when we say 'visible light' what we really mean is 'human visible light'. This applies to all energies; we can detect them within a limited frequency. So the world we detect is the world we are capable of detecting, the world we have receptors for, but there is a larger world out there!

When the energy, be it light, chemical, sound or mechanical energy, reaches the particular sense organ that is tuned to it, the receptors in the organ detect the energy and *transduce* it. This means that they change it to a common form that the nervous system can interpret (they translate it). So while we have sense organs that are tuned to particular energies our nervous system needs all those variations transduced into one form, an electrical impulse called the action potential. The sense organs are thus receivers and transducers. When they receive the energy to which they are sensitive, receptors transduce that energy into an action potential. The action potential then travels along to the brain. All the energies from the external world that stimulate our senses are thus transduced or translated in an electrical signal. What we see, hear and smell are action potentials.

How we know how much energy is coming in, the *intensity*, and for how long is the same as how we detect pain, which is discussed in Chapter 12, 'Sleeping and Healing'.

Briefly, receptors can respond to the amount of energy (intensity of signal) coming in. They have a threshold under which they don't respond. When they reach their threshold they send an action potential along their nerve cell. If the intensity increases, they send more action potentials. An action potential is always of one size, it is said to be all or nothing. In other words it is on or not on. So a larger stimulus does not result in larger action potentials, but more frequent action potentials. This holds for all action potentials; the frequency can increase to reflect a larger stimulus.

Health Connection

Sensory damage
Damage to a sense organ will result in **sensory impairment**, the reduction in a sensory modality, the particular sense that is affected. This can affect communication. The fact that a person has a sensory impairment does not necessarily mean that any other brain or mental capacity is affected. For example, the famous and brilliant composer Beethoven was deaf.

Seeing

Light waves are a form of electromagnetic radiation. The eye contains receptors in an area called the **retina** that is sensitive to various wavelengths of light. Light is focused by the lens at the front of the eye. The light then falls on the retina at the back of the eye. In the retina the **rod receptors** detect black and white while the **cone receptors** detect colour. When the appropriate receptor detects the stimulus to which it responds it sends a nerve impulse to the visual centre in the brain.

Wavelengths of light are measured in nanometres (one thousand thousand thousandth of a metre, 10^{-9} m). Different receptors detect different wavelengths of light. For colour our cones can see between ultraviolet via blue, green, yellow and red to infrared. Our blue-detecting cones are stimulated by light at 420 nm wavelengths. Our red-detecting cones are stimulated by light at 600 nm wavelengths (Figure 4.7).

Light comes into the front of the eye, the cornea, which bends the light. It then passes through the pupil, which is within the coloured iris. This allows for changes in brightness and darkness by dilating and constricting. The light is then focused by the lens and through the vitreous humour, a jelly-like substance. The light is now reversed and inverted so the image is backwards and upside-down,

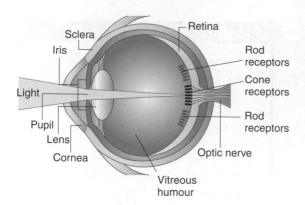

FIGURE 4.7 **The eye**

respectively. The image is then focused onto the back of the eye, the retina. This contains cells that are sensitive to light, rods and cones, which respond when particular light energies hit them. They then send electrical signals to their neurons, which are all collected into the **optic nerve.**

Health Connection

Retinopathies

The retina is susceptible to damage mainly from embolisms, clots and poor drainage of fluids.

Diabetic retinopathy occurs in Type 1 diabetes (insulin dependent) and Type 2 diabetes (not requiring insulin for treatment) due to damage to blood vessels blocking perfusion, blood flow, to the retina and retinal nerves.

Health Connection

Retinal detachment

A tear or hole in the retina allows fluid between the retinal cell layers to accumulate. This can push the retina away from its anchoring cells, detaching the retina. This results in a loss of vision.

Health Connection

Glaucoma

Glaucoma represents a group of disorders all due to an increase in the pressure inside the eye. If this pressure becomes very high it can damage the optic nerve, resulting in no signals being sent to the brain. Initially the main sign of this damage is detected by the patient as blind spots within their visual field, especially at the outer edges of the field of vision, called peripheral or side vision. As the damage to the optic nerve gets worse, the visual field can shrink, leading to tunnel vision or even loss of central vision, affecting a patient's ability to read. There appears to be a genetic link to this disease, but as yet no complete cure. Genes are discussed in Chapter 3, 'Growing and Developing'.

Hearing

Sound travels in the air as air waves. The ear has receptors that can detect these waves or oscillations and respond by transducing the waves into nervous impulses which are then sent to the brain. Waves enter the ear and cause the **eardrum** in the outer ear to vibrate. It passes on the vibrations to the bones of the middle ear. This causes movement of the **oval window**. The vibrations are passed to the inner ear, which contains the **cochlea**, a closed tubular structure containing fluid. This causes ripples in the cochlear fluid which disturb sensory hairs inside the cochlea. Each hair vibrates at a different frequency caused by different pitches. Each hair connects to a sensory neuron that sends an impulse to the auditory centre in the brain (Figure 4.8).

The outer ear collects sounds consisting of air waves. These vibrate the bones in the middle ear at various frequencies, depending on their pitch and volume. These vibrations then

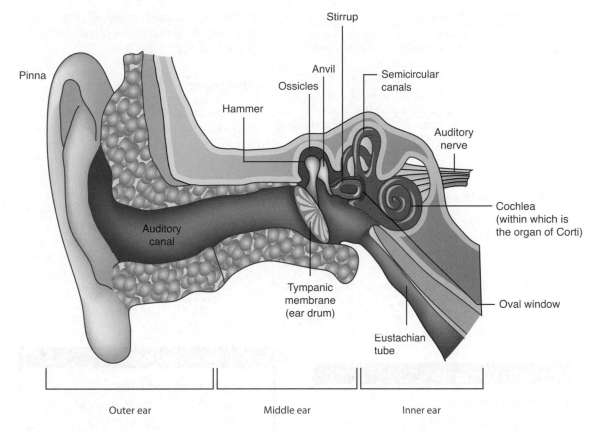

FIGURE 4.8 **The ear**

move the liquid in the cochlea of the inner ear, which in turn causes particular hairs to vibrate, each hair vibrating in response to a particular frequency received. The hairs are attached to nervous tissue and the vibrations are transduced into electrical impulses (Figure 4.9).

Health Connection

Hearing

The hairs of the cochlea are formed in the foetus. If they are damaged during life they can break. They do not re-grow and the sound that the hairs respond to is lost, with subsequent diminution of hearing. This is a problem especially for people working in loud environments such as amplified music.

Health Connection

Ear popping

Usually the air pressure on both sides of the eardrum is the same. If atmospheric pressure drops, such as in an aeroplane, there will be more air on the inside of the ear, which will then push against the eardrum, pushing it outwards. Swallowing, yawning and chewing can introduce external air into the Eustachian tube, which connects the mouth to the ear. This can make the ears pop.

Balance

Apart from the cochlea, the inner ear also contains semicircular canals, the **utriculus** and

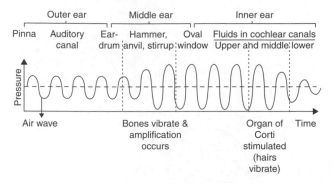

FIGURE 4.9 **Transduction of sound into vibrations in the inner ear**

sacculus, involved in balance. The semicircular canals contain fluid. At the end of the canals are swellings called **ampula** with sensory hairs embedded in jelly. When your head moves, the fluid moves and the **cupula** in the ampula moves. This is detected by the hairs and an electrical action potential is initiated.

> ### Health Connection
>
> #### Motion sickness
> The liquids in the semicircular canals of the ear and the vestibular apparatus can be overstimulated by constant motion. This can result in nausea and vomiting.

Tasting and smelling

Most of our sense of taste is in fact linked to our sense of smell. If you hold your nose and then eat, your sense of taste will be diminished. Our tongues have sense receptors on the sides of the **papillae**, small raised portions, of the tongue that can distinguish sweet, salt, bitter and sour, which is quite crude (Figure 4.10).

Our noses, however, have many sense receptors, **olfactory senses**, that can distinguish between many different chemicals. The chemicals must be in a *volatile* state, gaseous, so that they can filter into the air that enters our nose. When a chemical binds to its receptor it initiates an action potential that travels up a sensory nerve to our olfaction centre in the brain (Figure 4.11).

Other senses

We have more than the five senses without having to invoke 'extra-sensory' mysticism. These include internal receptors, **enteroceptors**, and receptors that tell us where our bodies, especially our limbs, are, measuring the stretch in them, **proprioception**. We also seem to have sense organs tuned to extreme noxious stimuli, **nociceptors**, detecting extreme heat or mechanical pressure. So we are composed of many detectors, each tuned to different stimuli.

> ### Health Connection
>
> #### Colds, smell and taste
> The tongue is quite basic in what it can taste. It has receptors for
>
> - sour,
> - sweet,
> - bitter and
> - salt.
>
> Most of the fine-tuning of taste is actually done by smell. We smell the chemicals in food and drink. If we have a cold the receptors in our noses are blocked by mucus and our sense of smell decreases, as does the taste of food.

> #### Chapter Reference
> Proprioception is discussed in Chapter 6, 'Moving' (see p. 163). Nociceptors are discussed in Chapter 12, 'Sleeping and Healing' (see p. 324).

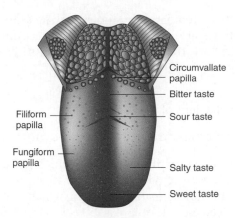

Circumvallate papilla

Bitter taste

Filiform papilla

Sour taste

Fungiform papilla

Salty taste

Sweet taste

FIGURE 4.10 **The tongue**

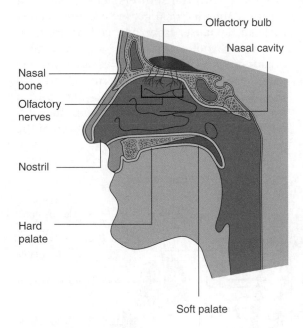

Olfactory bulb

Nasal cavity

Nasal bone

Olfactory nerves

Nostril

Hard palate

Soft palate

FIGURE 4.11 **The nose**

The ANS: Sensing and affecting the internal environment

Information can be taken as input from the internal environment through internal sense organs or receptors called **enteroceptors**. There are various types of enteroreceptors, each detecting its own particular energy, such as

- **thermo-receptors**, monitoring temperature;

- **baro-receptors**, monitoring blood pressure; and
- **chemical receptors**, monitoring particular chemicals, such as glucose levels or carbon dioxide levels.

Information from the internal environment helps to control homeostasis. The hypothalamus, a region of the brain, together with the pituitary endocrine gland, a gland that lies under the hypothalamus, takes this information as output via a separate part of the nervous system called the autonomic nervous system (ANS). This is generally involuntary. The electrical messages taken out by the ANS affect internal organs and glands, such as making the smooth (involuntary) muscles around blood vessels constrict or dilate. The ANS is divided into two: the **sympathetic**, which generally increases the effect on internal organs, and the **parasympathetic**, which generally decreases the effect on internal organs.

While the ANS has outputs to smooth muscle and cardiac muscle it also has outputs to the endocrine system of glands. These glands produce chemicals called hormones and secrete them into the blood. The main hormones released are those produced by the adrenal glands, which lie above the kidneys. These hormones are called adrenaline and noradrenaline. The release of these hormones in response to stimuli from the ANS happens in times of stress or emergency. They help in 'fight or flight' – whether we stand our ground in the face of a threat or run for cover. They help to mobilise glycogen, the storage form of glucose, from the liver, ready to be converted into the energy, ATP, needed in an emergency to allow the muscles to contract faster. These hormones help increase heart rate and thus the delivery of blood containing glucose and oxygen to muscles.

Chapter Reference

The endocrine system is discussed in more detail below (see p. 134).

There are other outputs from the ANS, for example to trigger salivation in response to the presence of food in the mouth, aiding digestion (Figure 4.12).

The ANS sends messages to increase or decrease activity in effectors. These effectors can be glands that secrete hormones or enzymes or send outputs onto involuntary, smooth muscle. The output is an **autonomic reflex**, discussed below.

The hypothalamus

The hypothalamus is a brain region that is in the central nervous system situated under the **thalamus** of the brain (see Figure 4.17 below). The pituitary gland of the endocrine system is attached to the hypothalamus.

The role of the hypothalamus is in the control of homeostasis. It is an important part of the limbic system, which is involved with emotions.

It receives inputs from internal receptors about the state of all the variables of the body, such as temperature and blood pressure. Its outputs are to the ANS and to the pituitary gland of the endocrine system, discussed below.

The divisions of the ANS

As stated above the ANS is divided into

- the sympathetic system, which tends to increase activity, and
- the parasympathetic system, which tends to decrease activity.

Each of the two branches of the ANS relies on different neurotransmitters, chemicals that transmit the electrical action potential across the gap, synapse, from one cell to another. The sympathetic branch of the ANS uses noradrenaline, mentioned above as a hormone when released from an endocrine gland into the blood. Noradrenaline is also able to be a neurotransmitter when released from the nervous system. The parasympathetic branch of the

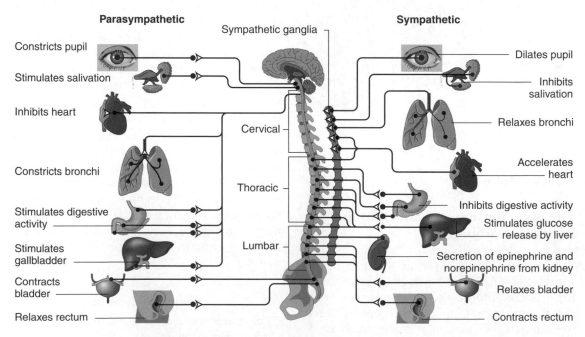

FIGURE 4.12 **The ANS and effectors**

ANS uses the neurotransmitter acetylcholine. There are variations in how these branches act on some target organs, but in general they use these two different neurotransmitters to bring about their effect.

Chapter Reference

Neurotransmitters, synapses and the action potential are discussed above (see pp. 104–110).

The somatic nervous system

Outputs to the somatic nervous system are onto voluntary, skeletal muscles and result in movement, discussed in Chapter 6, 'Moving'. These motor outputs are along motor neurons, which initiate muscle contraction and thus movement.

Motor outputs

There are a variety of possible motor outputs. The electrical output is onto motor neurons, which synapse onto voluntary muscle. Some of the outputs result in voluntary, conscious movement and some in **reflex** movement.

Chapter Reference

Motor output to voluntary muscle resulting in conscious movement is discussed in Chapter 6, 'Moving' (see p. 163).

Reflex movements

Our somatic nervous system can make voluntary muscles move by reflex. Reflex movement is:

* rapid,
* predictable and
* an involuntary response to stimuli.

The movement is brought about by a **reflex arc**. This is a route from a sensory neuron to an effector muscle via an intermediary neuron called an interneuron. It does not involve the decision-making centres of the brain.

There are two types of reflex movements:

* **autonomic reflexes** – where smooth muscles are regulated, such as
    * heart and blood pressure regulation,
    * regulation of glands and
    * digestive system regulation;
* **somatic reflexes**:
    * activation of skeletal muscles (Figure 4.13).

Reflexes link parts of the PNS together. A stimulus is detected by sense organs, which send information to peripheral sensory neurons, which carry the information to the spinal cord, a part of the CNS. The spinal cord can send information straight out to motor neurons, which then innervate voluntary skeletal muscles, generating movement.

Chapter Reference

Muscle movement is discussed in Chapter 6, 'Moving' (see p. 163).

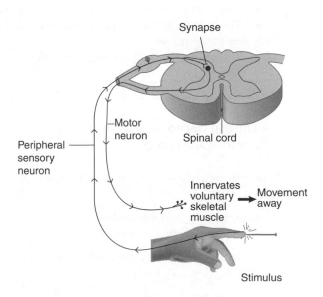

FIGURE 4.13 **Somatic reflex movement**

> **Health Connection**
>
> **Motor neuron disease**
>
> The inability to move muscles can be due to damage in the muscle or to damage in the motor neuron that initiates muscle movement. **Motor neuron disease (MND)** causes the gradual loss of function of motor neurons and thus the loss of movement. The person is still fully conscious, but may have communication problems due to poor muscle control, including of the muscles used in speech. The inability to move muscles does not necessarily affect other brain or mental functions. The famous and brilliant physicist Professor Stephen Hawking has MND, but still manages to publish insightful work on black holes and the formation of the universe. This decrease in verbal communication, together with the decrease in sensory communication for those with sensory problems, is being emphasised because many patients with these problems are treated as if they have a mental incapacity to think and understand rather than a sensory or motor malfunction. Much scientific work is focused on trying to repair the input and output pathways.

Box 4.2 Summary – peripheral nervous system

- The peripheral nervous system receives information from the external and internal environment.
- The information from the external environment enters from sense organs.
- The information from the internal environment enters from internal receptors.
- Both forms of information are sensory.
- Sensory information is brought to the CNS, where it is integrated and an effect is stimulated.
- The output is either to voluntary, somatic muscles or to involuntary muscles or to glands.
- The output to the voluntary muscles, the somatic nervous system, results in movement, a motor response.
- The output to the involuntary muscles or glands is part of the ANS. This helps to control homeostasis.

The central nervous system (CNS): Brain and spinal cord

As mentioned above the nervous system is divided into

- the peripheral nervous system and
- the central nervous system.

The **central nervous system (CNS)** is composed of

- the brain and
- the spinal cord.

Nerve tracts, bundles of axons, from the PNS enter (sensory) or leave (motor) the CNS either through the spinal cord or through the cranial nerves of the face.

The spinal cord

The spinal cord is a series of nerves joined to a central cord. The central cord relays information up to and down from the brain. The nerves contain sensory and motor neurons.

The spinal cord sorts electrical signals into incoming (sensory) and outgoing (motor). It

Box 4.3 Summary – nervous system

The functions of the nervous system include

- **sensory input from the external or internal environment,**
- **integration:**
  - to process and interpret sensory input and decide if action is needed, usually carried out in the CNS, and
- **motor output:**
  - a response to integrated stimuli
  - which activates muscles or glands.

Information is gathered by sense organs and taken along sensory paths to the CNS. There it is integrated with other information, such as memory, or signals from other senses and a response is mounted. This is seen as output to motor paths. The motor paths impact either on somatic, voluntary (skeletal) muscle or on autonomic involuntary muscle of internal organs or on glands.

Linking the sensory inputs from the PNS to the motor outputs to the muscles and glands is the central nervous system, which centralises all the information, integrating it into a coherent whole and initiating an appropriate response.

---

is divided into a number of bony **vertebrae**. The vertebrae protect the nerves of the spinal cord.

Health Connection

Spinal cord pain

Damage to the vertebrae can result in severe pain due to the bones pressing on the nerve tracts and causing electrical signals to be sent up to the brain (Figure 4.14).

Sensory signals from the PNS enter the spinal cord and motor outputs to the voluntary muscles exit. The messages enter and leave at the appropriate vertebra that contains all the information for that particular **dermatome** – area of the body (see below).

The spinal cord has white and grey matter. The white matter contains neurons that are insulated by a fatty substance called myelin while the grey matter is un-myelinated.

The nerves tracts entering the spinal cord contain both sensory and motor neurons, but

these become *separated* at the spinal cord. The sensory neurons enter the spinal cord at the back of it, the **dorsal** side, while the motor neurons exit the spinal cord at its more **ventral** side. Both the dorsal and ventral sides are in the central grey matter.

Between the sensory and motor neurons are neurons called interneurons. These interneurons relay signals up to the brain in the white matter (myelinated). Messages coming down from the brain to the spinal cord also travel in the white matter before being conducted to the ventral part of the spinal cord.

The spinal cord is segmented. A segment of spinal cord corresponds to a spinal nerve. This also corresponds to the segmentation of the vertebrae.

Each spinal nerve not only corresponds to a particular vertebra, but also corresponds to a particular area of the body called a dermatome.

Dermatomes

An area of skin from which all the sensory information enters one spinal nerve and thus one vertebra is called a dermatome (Figure 4.15).

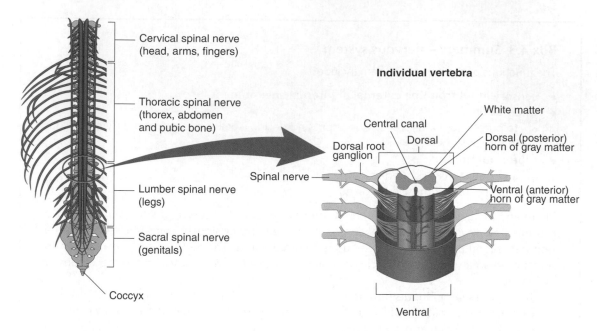

FIGURE 4.14 **The spinal cord**

Areas of skin have sensory neurons taking touch information into one particular region of the spinal cord. On our spinal cord we have a *topographic map* or representation of our body. Motor output from one segment of the spinal cord also exits to one dermatome.

The body is thus divided into a number of dermatomes. The sensory information from a particular area of skin or dermatome is thus preserved in one particular spinal nerve, which enters at one vertebral point. The topography of the body, its spatial arrangement, is therefore preserved in the spinal cord.

Health Connection

Spinal cord damage

Damage to the spinal cord results in impairment of sensation or movement. How much damage and where the damage is felt depend on which part of the spinal cord is affected. All information travels up and down the spinal cord in the white matter. If the damage is in the lower back, sensation from the lower limbs, or movement of the lower limbs, is affected. If the damage is higher up the spinal cord, not only will the areas of the spinal nerve for that segment be affected, but also any information from below or to below that spinal segment may be affected if the damage is severe. The higher up the spinal cord damage is done, the more of the periphery is affected. Breaks to the vertebrae of the neck, for example, may result in severe damage to the spinal cord at that segment and the blockage of transmission of electrical impulses from or to areas below that segment.

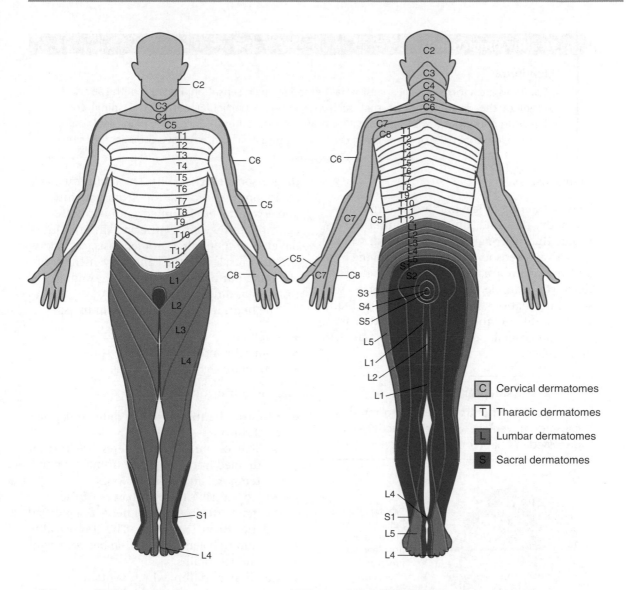

C 5	Clavicles
C 5, 6, 7	Lateral parts of upper limbs
C 8, T 1	Middle sides of upper limbs
C 6	Thumb
C 6, 7, 8	Hand
C 8	Ring and little fingers
T 4	Level of nipples

T 10	Level of umbilicus
T 12	Inguinal or groin region
L 1, 2, 3, 4	Anterior and inner surfaces of lower limbs
L 4, 5, S 1	Foot
L4	Medial side of great toe
S 1, 2, L 5	Posterior and outer surfaces of lower limb
S 1	Lateral margin of foot and little toe
S 2, 3, 4	Perineum

FIGURE 4.15 **Dermatomes**

Cranial nerves

Nerves entering or leaving the CNS from above the body, the head, do so via **cranial nerves**, rather than through the spinal cord. Cranial nerves carry sensory information from the head and motor information to the muscles of the head. For example, the optic nerve carries sensory information from the eyes to the brain, while motor neurons carry information from the brain to make the eyes move (Figure 4.16 and Table 4.2).

Chapter Reference

The motor outputs of the CNS to muscles, causing movement and reflex actions, are discussed in Chapter 6, 'Moving' (see p. 163).

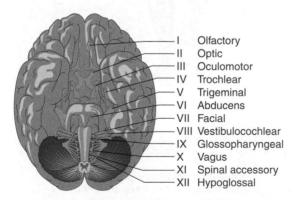

I	Olfactory
II	Optic
III	Oculomotor
IV	Trochlear
V	Trigeminal
VI	Abducens
VII	Facial
VIII	Vestibulocochlear
IX	Glossopharyngeal
X	Vagus
XI	Spinal accessory
XII	Hypoglossal

FIGURE 4.16 **Cranial nerves**

The brain

The brain is situated in the head under the skull bones. It is a soft tissue, protected by the skull bones, made up of billions of neurons and their associated glial cells. The brain integrates all incoming information from the internal and external environments and initiates an appropriate response, either making the internal environment alter, homeostasis, or making skeletal muscles contract and movement occur, changing our behaviour from, for example, sitting to standing or running.

The brain is made of three main parts:

- forebrain,
- midbrain and
- hindbrain.

The **forebrain** consists of

- **cerebral hemispheres** (a right and a left cerebrum):
  - The cerebral hemispheres are further divided into four lobes: frontal, parietal, temporal and occipital lobes.
  - Connecting the two halves of the cerebral cortex is a tract of nerve fibres called the **corpus callosum.** The corpus callosum transfers information between right and left brains.
- the **diencephalon**, which contains
  - the **thalamus**, which receives and relays information and initiates some responses, filters sensory information, senses pain;
  - the **hypothalamus** – part of the limbic system – which regulates hunger, thirst and body temperature. The hypothalamus is part of the ANS and outputs to the 'master switch' of the endocrine system, the pituitary gland, which lies just below the hypothalamus. Both the hypothalamus and pituitary are involved in homeostasis;

Table 4.2 Cranial nerves

Nerves in order	Modality	Major functions
Olfactory I	Special sensory	Smell
Optic II	Special sensory	Vision
Oculomotor III	Somatic motor Visceral motor	Moves eyelid and eyeball
Trochlear IV	Somatic motor	Turns eyes downward and laterally
Trigeminal V	Branchial motor General sensory	Muscles of mastication (chewing) Sensation of touch and pain for head/neck, sinuses, meninges and external surface of tympanic membrane
Abducens VI	Somatic motor	Turns eyes laterally
Facial VII	Branchial motor Visceral motor General sensory Special sensory	Controls most facial expression Secretion of tears and saliva Taste
Vestibulocochlear VIII	Special sensory	Hearing and balance
Glossopharyngeal IX	Branchial motor Visceral motor Visceral sensory General sensory Special sensory	Taste Senses carotid blood pressure
Vagus X	Branchial motor Visceral motor Visceral sensory Special sensory	Senses aortic blood pressure Slow heart rate Stimulates digestive organs Taste
Spinal Accessory XI	Branchial motor	Controls swallowing
Hypoglossal XII	Somatic motor	Controls tongue movement

- the **epithalamus**, which secretes melatonin, sets day/night cycle.

The **midbrain** is the smallest region of the brain. The midbrain

- contains areas such as
  - the basal ganglia, substantia nigra and red nucleus, which initiates movement,
  - the thalamus,
  - the hypothalamus,
  - the tectum and
  - the tegmentum;

- acts as a relay station for auditory and visual information;
- controls visual and auditory systems;
- controls eye movement.

The **hindbrain** consists of

- the **cerebellum** at the base of the brain, which is involved in balance and learnt movement, gait and posture,
- the **pons** and
- the **medulla.**

Often the midbrain and the pons and medulla of the hindbrain are referred to collectively as the **brain stem.** The brain stem, where the spinal cord enters and exits, is involved in wakefulness and has cardiac and respiratory centres as well as connecting to some cranial nerves. It contains the **reticular activating system (RAS),** which filters important and unimportant information from sensory input.

The cerebrum

The cerebrum is the outermost part of the brain, containing the motor, sensory, visual, audio cortex. The cerebral hemispheres are highly folded structures to increase the surface area within the confined space of the skull bones of the head. The folds are called **sulci** (singular sulcus) and appear on the surface, **cortex** (from the Latin meaning 'bark'). The sulci surround areas called gyri (see Figure 4.17).

There is a deep furrow which divides the cerebrum into two halves, known as the left and right hemispheres. The two hemispheres look mostly symmetrical yet it has been shown that each side functions slightly differently than the other. Sometimes the right hemisphere is associated with creativity and the left hemisphere is associated with logic abilities. The corpus callosum is a bundle of axons which connects these two hemispheres.

The cerebrum or cortex is the largest part of the human brain, associated with higher brain function such as thought and action.

The cerebrum can be divided into four anatomical **lobes,** which carry out different physiological functions (Figure 4.18):

- **frontal lobe** – regulates impulses, inhibitions, judgement, thinking, planning, and central executive functions; motor execution;
- **parietal lobe** – somatosensory perception;
- **temporal lobe** – language function and auditory perception, involved in long-term memory and emotion; integration of visual and somatospatial information;
- **occipital lobe** – visual perception and processing.

The cerebrum has areas connected with the senses, such as:

- gustatory area (taste),
- visual area,
- auditory area and
- olfactory area.

The forebrain demonstrates the link between anatomy and a physiological function. The cerebrum has specialised areas or regions where different functions are carried out, such as

- the **somatosensory** area or cortex, which receives impulses from the body's sensory receptors;
- the **motor** area or cortex, which sends impulses to skeletal muscles;
- **Broca's area,** which is involved in our ability to speak.

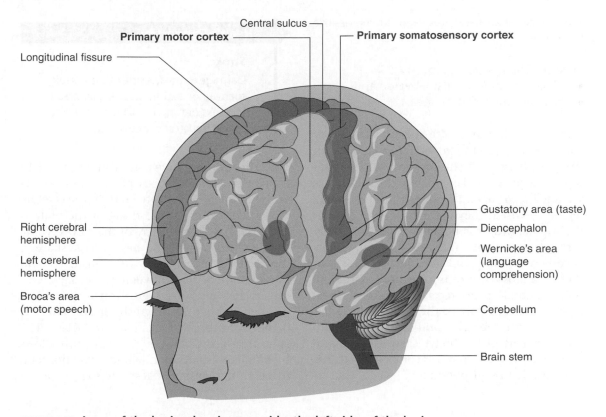

Central sulcus

Primary motor cortex

Primary somatosensory cortex

Longitudinal fissure

Right cerebral
hemisphere

Left cerebral
hemisphere

Broca's area
(motor speech)

Gustatory area (taste)

Diencephalon

Wernicke's area
(language
comprehension)

Cerebellum

Brain stem

FIGURE 4.17 **Areas of the brain, showing one side, the left side, of the brain**

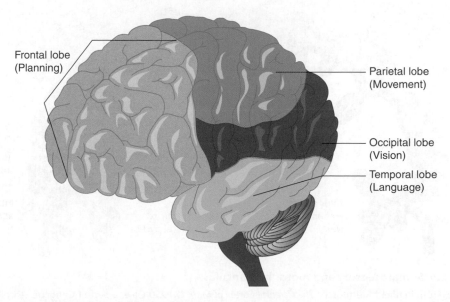

Frontal lobe
(Planning)

Parietal lobe
(Movement)

Occipital lobe
(Vision)

Temporal lobe
(Language)

FIGURE 4.18 **Lobes of the cerebrum**

There are also interpretation areas of the cerebrum:

- speech/language region,
- language comprehension region and
- general interpretation area.

Two interesting areas are the somatosensory cortex, which receives touch information from the periphery, and the motor cortex, which sends outputs to skeletal muscles. Both are arranged *topographically*, preserving the bodily region to which they correspond. Just as with the spinal cord, it is possible to plot the body across these regions (Figure 4.19). The difference between this and the spinal cord is that there is a cross-over of information so that the right cerebral cortex receives and sends messages to the left part of the body and the left cerebral cortex receives and send messages to the right part of the body. There is a somatosensory cortex and a motor cortex on both the right and left hemispheres.

Health Connection

Stroke
Damage to the *left* side of the cortex, such as occurs in stroke, will result in a loss of function to the *right* side of the body (and vice versa).

The other point of note concerning Figure 4.19 is that the size of the body part does not correspond to the area dedicated to it in the cerebral cortex. For example, the trunk of the body is large, but has a small share of the cortex, while the fingers are small and have a large share of the cortex. This is to do with sensitivity and the amount of fine movement we have. Our fingers are very sensitive to touch, for example, being able to distinguish, or discriminate, between cotton, wood, metal and glass. The large area of the brain dedicated to this allows such fine discrimination, while we do not tend to feel things with our backs and so less brain is

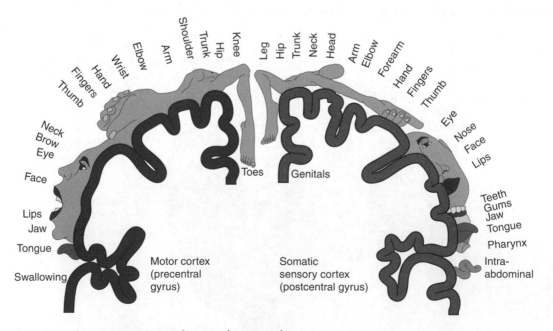

FIGURE 4.19 Somatosensory and motor homunculus
Source: From Penfield/Rasmussen. *The Cerebral Cortex of Man.* © 1950 Gale, a part of Cengage Learning, Inc. Reproduced by permission. www.cengage.com/permissions

dedicated to touch from the back. Likewise we can move many small muscles in our fingers to bring about fine movements, while we move large muscles in our back for big movements. The amount of muscle contracted by one motor neuron is called a **motor unit**. We have many small motor units in our fingers, faces and eyes making small movements, while the motor units in our backs are large; one motor neuron innervates (excites) many muscle fibres.

Health Connection

Two-point discrimination test

When we are touched by two points very close together we can usually tell when just one touches us or whether both points touch us. The two-point discrimination test involves putting either one or two points onto the skin to see if we can detect them or to determine whether there has been some sensory damage.

Speech

There are two aspects to speech. One is the physical mechanism in the larynx and the other is sentence construction and grammar, which happens in the brain. The larynx in the neck is involved in breathing and speech, or talking. The sounds that we emit are due to the alteration of the length of the vocal cords, a series of thin membranes which can be tightened or loosened to alter our pitch, just as in a musical instrument. Air flowing over these cords produces sound.

The brain has many areas associated with speech. Damage to any of these regions has various effects. The two main areas are named after those people that discovered them: Broca and Wernicke (see Figures 4.17 and 4.18). Damage to Broca's area results in problems of output of language, speech, while damage to Wernicke's area results in problems of processing auditory (sound) information such as speech.

Learning and memory

There appear to be many different memory systems in the brain, such as **short-term** or working memory, which enables us to remember something such as a telephone number while dialling, and **long-term memory**, which holds memories for a lifetime. There is also **episodic memory**, the ability to remember personal events or episodes that happened to us; **procedural memory**, the ability to remember procedures such as riding a bicycle; and **semantic memory**, general knowledge of the world, such as knowledge of words and how to use them. All of these memory systems may be held in different brain locations. The hippocampus, an area of the cerebral cortex, appears to be important in laying down memories.

Health Connection

Dementia

Dementia is a loss of cognitive (reasoning) function. It is seen mainly as loss of memory, especially short-term memory, where recent events are lost, but long-term memories remain. Much research is being carried out on this because it is seen more in ageing populations and our population is living longer. With a gradual loss of memory there is a concomitant loss of selfhood.

You cannot remember things that you have never encountered. So before you have a memory you must have a learning experience. Learning appears to alter the anatomy of the synapse (discussed below), making the connection stronger, perhaps reinforcing that we should 'use it or lose it'.

Consciousness

Damage to areas involved in memory, such as the hippocampus, and in speech, such as Wernicke's area, can leave a person unable to function normally. Their ability to communicate can be impaired as can their ability to comprehend information. This can be described as an altered consciousness. Damage to various regions of the brain can alter our cognitive functioning, our ability to think and reason. Gerald Edelman, a Nobel Prize winning immunologist, in 1989 proposed a way to describe **consciousness** and how we humans come to know ourselves and our universe. He proposed that conscious beings

- can categorise things;
- can distinguish between self and non-self;
- have memory systems that can re-categorise information as a result of experience.

The conscious self must rely on many brain areas to form a picture of itself and its world. The fact that it is a higher function of the large cerebral cortex of the human brain points to us being the most conscious species on the planet – currently!

Health Connection

Learning difficulties
If the brain is damaged congenitally, before or at birth, or it does not develop properly, the affected person can have a physical or mental disability. They may have difficulties learning and therefore in memory.

There are many congenital causes for this condition:

- lack of oxygen to the brain during birth,
- infection during foetal development,
- endocrine under-development due to the absence of thyroxin,
- maldevelopment of the skull and blood vessels of the brain preventing development,
- toxic effects such as lead poisoning, smoke or rhesus factor during foetal development, and
- congenital chromosomal damage such as in Down's syndrome.

Health Connection

Epilepsy
The temporal lobes are vulnerable to damage, often resulting in epileptic activity. When this occurs a number of neurons are active at the same time in the lobe, which can result in an epileptic seizure. Working memory is seldom affected, but long-term memory may be.

Health Connection

Coma
We can generally be aroused from sleep even though we are not fully conscious. Unconsciousness, such as in coma, is a state in which we are not arousable.

Health Connection

Parkinson's disease
Parkinson's disease is a disease that affects motor output to the voluntary skeletal muscle and hence affects movement. It is classified as a movement disorder. Muscles in people with Parkinson's often tremble. The **basal ganglia** in Parkinson's patients degenerate so that the electrical output is compromised. The basal ganglia use **dopamine** as a neurotransmitter, so treatment of Parkinson's is to replace dopamine. Due to the **blood–brain barrier** (discussed below) injected dopamine will not enter the brain, so dopamine is administered in the form of a precursor molecule, **L-dopa**, which is converted in the brain into dopamine.

Box 4.4 Summary – General functions of the three brain regions

- The cerebrum and forebrain is the highest part of the brain in location, development and function.
- It analyses symbolic information and gives rise to cognitive and intellectual abilities, reason, learning and thinking.
- The midbrain is a relay station sending sensory information to the higher brain and motor functions to the lower brain and spinal cord.
- The hypothalamus is involved in involuntary actions such as thirst, hunger and body temperature regulation.
- The lower or hindbrain and spinal cord deal with reflexes and learnt movement. The cerebellum coordinates learnt movement and balance.
- The medulla oblongata is involved in heartbeat and blood vessel constriction.

Health Connection

Alcohol

Alcohol can be absorbed partially from the stomach as well as from the small intestine. It can, therefore, enter our bloodstreams quickly. It is a depressant, slowing down the rate of nerve transmission. Excess alcohol consumption can be fatal, a fact not often known in the non-health-professional world. Twenty per cent of it is absorbed from the stomach directly into the bloodstream. The other 80% is absorbed from the small intestine. The liver breaks down alcohol (it takes one hour to break down one glass of wine). Excess alcohol that the liver is not breaking down travels in the blood to many organs, including

- brain stem, affecting the medulla oblongata, depressing heart rate and breathing;
- cerebellum, affecting balance and coordination;
- brain cortex, affecting sensation, perception, speech and judgement.

Protection of the nervous system

As the nervous system controls homeostasis, movement and behaviour it is the most important organ in our bodies. It defines us, and damage to it alters our ability to respond to our environment, our behaviours and emotions and our intellectual abilities of reasoning and thought. It therefore is very vulnerable and needs protecting from external and internal damage.

Bones

The brain is protected by the skull bones, while the spinal cord is protected by the vertebrae.

Meninges

Further protection is given by **meninges**, connective tissue that forms layers around the nervous tissue. There are three layers of meninges:

- dura mater – the outermost layer,
- arachnoid mater – a middle layer with a weblike structure, and
- pia mater – the innermost layer, which adheres to the surface of brain.

Cerebrospinal fluid (CSF)

In the centre of the spinal cord and in ventricles, gaps, in the brain is **cerebrospinal fluid**.

Cerebrospinal fluid is similar to lymph, a watery fluid. Some 750–1000 ml is produced each day, with about 150 ml circulating in the brain. It is produced in the choroid plexus in ventricles of the brain. CSF flows in the arachnoid and pia mater. This is called the subarachnoid space. CSF contains proteins, glucose, chloride ions and a few lymphocytes. It acts as

- a shock absorber;
- a source of nutrients and chemicals;
- a buoyancy medium, reducing brain weight by up to 97% – akin to floating in a pool (Figure 4.21).

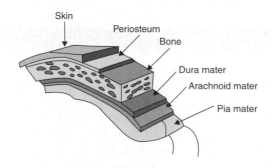

Skin
Periosteum
Bone
Dura mater
Arachnoid mater
Pia mater

FIGURE 4.20 **Meninges**

Health Connection

Brain damage
The skull bones and meninges help to protect the brain. Damage to an area of the brain through, for example, trauma can remove a function such as speech or vision or can alter a personality if the limbic frontal lobes are affected. While the bones can offer some protection any swelling of the brain during trauma will result in the brain pressing against the bones.

Blood–brain barrier

The brain is very vulnerable to damage. It has a high metabolic rate and thus substances are brought to it and waste removed from it at a high rate. While one would expect the capillaries of the brain to be highly permeable to substances passing in and out of the brain, in fact the capillaries of the brain are the least permeable capillaries of the body.

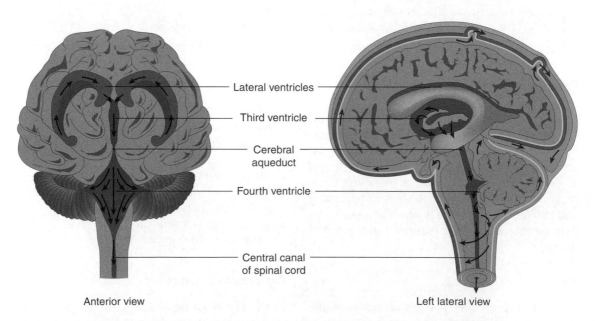

Lateral ventricles

Third ventricle

Cerebral aqueduct

Fourth ventricle

Central canal of spinal cord

Anterior view

Left lateral view

FIGURE 4.21 **Ventricles of the brain**

Meningitis

The disease meningitis can be caused by a micro-organism which grows in the meninges. To diagnose this disease fluid from the CSF around the meninges of the spinal cord is removed and the liquid, which should be clear rather than cloudy with infection, is analysed in a pathology laboratory.

These capillaries exclude many potentially harmful substances. However, they are less useful against substances such as

- fats and fat-soluble molecules,
- respiratory gases,
- alcohol,
- nicotine,
- anaesthesia and
- certain drugs.

The brain, spinal cord and peripheral nervous system allow very rapid communication, which helps to coordinate appropriate responses and aid homeostasis and survival. Any damage to the system can have profound physiological effects and profound effects on the individual as memory and learning are also situated in the nervous system. Damage to the brain can have effects on personality.

The disadvantage of the nervous system is that these very rapid transmissions can only occur along specific pathways, axons. There are other communication systems that are more diffuse, allowing messages to travel throughout the body. The disadvantage to these systems, the chemical transmissions discussed below, is that they are slower.

Cellular communication

All cells must communicate with one another in the community of cells that constitute the human body. They can do this because cells manufacture many products. Among these products are chemicals that can be used as neurotransmitters if they are released from a neuron or as messengers. Some are released between cells, while some travel around the body. They have an effect on cells as part of a signalling pathway, turning on or off processes in the recipient cell.

There are various types of chemical messenger:

- **autocrine** – work on the cell that produced them,
- **paracrine** – work on cells close by,
- **endocrine** – act as hormones, described above, and
- **neuroendocrine** – produced by neural tissue and released into the blood like a hormone to be transported to the target.

Cytokines are chemical messengers that act on target cells that have a receptor for them. They can be very potent at low doses; they behave in a manner similar to hormones and can work as mediators of hormone actions. There are many different types, such as tumour necrosis factor (TNF) and platelet derived growth factor (PDGF). Each of them, however, has a number of actions and may be synthesised by many different cell types.

Cellular communication and cancer

In a community of cells such as us humans, cell numbers are carefully balanced to replace those that are lost and those that are made. Usually this is controlled by cells sending signals between their neighbours. Many cancers are the result of cells not responding to the signals around them, particularly the signals that encourage or prevent growth. If this occurs the cells continue to grow beyond the numbers needed to maintain the organ or tissue.

There are many signal molecules between cells helping cells to act as part of a community rather than as lone operators. When cells cease to communicate or be sensitive to signals their growth and metabolism can be affected.

Cellular communication can involve complex processes of signal transduction and amplification through molecules acting as second messengers. They often rely on phosphorylation reactions similar to those seen with ADP to ATP. The pharmacological industry is interested in the detailed mechanisms to control cell growth and cell regeneration. Further discussion of pharmacology is in Chapter 12, 'Sleeping and Healing'.

The endocrine system of communication will now be discussed.

The endocrine system

The endocrine system is the body's second major controlling system, influencing the metabolic activities of cells. It consists of a number of endocrine glands, such as the

- pituitary,
- thyroid,
- parathyroid,
- adrenal,
- pineal, and
- thymus glands (Figure 4.22).

There are other tissues and organs that synthesise and secrete endocrine products, such as adipose cells, pockets of cells in the walls of the small intestine, stomach, kidneys, and heart. Some of the endocrine glands produce both endocrine and exocrine products.

Endocrine glands synthesise and secrete products, usually proteins or **steroids**, derived from a type of lipid, cholesterol. There are two types of glands: **exocrine glands** that secrete their contents into ducts, such as mucus secretions from glands of the gastrointestinal tract or digestive enzyme secretions from the exocrine part of the pancreas, and **endocrine glands** that secrete their contents, hormones, into the blood. Released hormones travel in the blood and can affect multiple sites. To have an effect the hormone must bind to its **target cell receptor**. Once the hormone is bound the receptor communicates this to the cell and an effect is initiated. This effect can be one of many functions.

The endocrine system of hormones affects

- growth and development,
- metabolism,
- reproduction,
- energy balance,
- fluid and electrolyte balance and
- response to stress.

Thus

- endocrine cells release a signal (hormone);
- the signal binds to a receptor;
- the receptor causes a change in the target cell if a hormone is bound to it (Figure 4.23).

An endocrine cell releases a chemical hormone. The hormone travels in the blood to the target cells. These cells have receptors for the

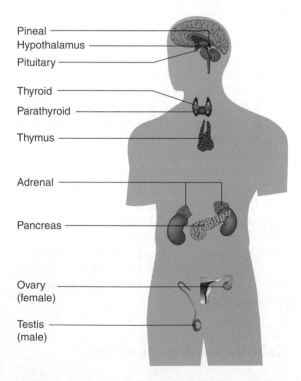

Pineal
Hypothalamus
Pituitary

Thyroid
Parathyroid

Thymus

Adrenal

Pancreas

Ovary (female)

Testis (male)

FIGURE 4.22 **Major endocrine glands secreting hormones into the blood**

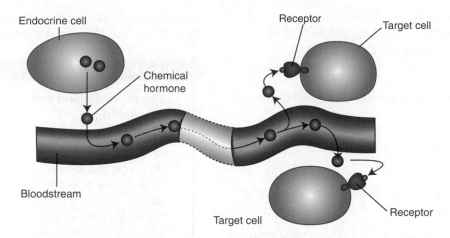

Endocrine cell

Receptor

Target cell

Chemical hormone

Bloodstream

Target cell

Receptor

FIGURE 4.23 **Endocrine hormone release, transport and action**

hormone. The hormone binds to the target cell and has an effect on that cell. The effect could be to make the cell grow, to stop it growing, to make the cell release other chemicals or to make the cell synthesise certain substances.

Control of hormone release

Most hormone release is regulated by negative feedback.

The stimulus for release of a hormone can come from one of three main sources:

- humoral stimuli – release of hormone in direct response to changing levels in the blood of chemicals such as nutrients or ions;
- neural stimuli – release of hormones due to action potential in a neuron;
- hormonal stimuli – release of hormones due to the action of another hormone.

The link between the brain and the endocrine system

While the brain and endocrine system are both able to communicate with cells of the body they also communicate with each other. The hypothalamus of the brain is the centre of homeostasis. It receives information about the internal state of the body. It sends outputs to the ANS and to the pituitary gland of the endocrine system, which lies immediately under the hypothalamus.

The hypothalamus secretes hormones that attach to either the anterior pituitary gland or the posterior pituitary gland.

Hormones and glands

There are many hormones secreted from various glands. Below is a sample of some of them.

Pituitary gland

This gland is controlled by inputs from the hypothalamus. The gland is divided into two parts:

1. The **anterior pituitary** releases hormones that affect the
    - thyroid gland,
    - adrenal cortex and
    - gonad (testis).

The hormones released by the anterior pituitary include:

- growth hormone,
- thyroid stimulating hormone (TSH),
- prolactin,
- adrenocorticotropic hormone (ACTH),

- gonadotropins:
  - follicle stimulating hormone (FSH),
  - luteinising hormone (LH) and
  - interstitial cell stimulation hormone (ICSH).
2. The **posterior pituitary** releases hormones that affect:
   - kidney tubules,
   - mammary glands and
   - uterine muscles.

The hormones the posterior pituitary gland secretes are:

- antidiuretic hormone (ADH) – reduces urine output,
- vasopressin and
- oxytocin – starts uterine contractions.

Health Connection

Anterior pituitary gland and growth hormone (GH) disorder

If there are changes in hormonal secretions growth can be affected.

- Hyposecretion of GH during childhood can cause pituitary dwarfism.
- Hypersecretion of GH during childhood causes gigantism.
- Hypersecretion of GH during adulthood causes acromegaly.

This shows that it is not only the amount of hormone secreted that can have an effect, but when it is secreted.

Thyroid gland

This gland is located in the neck region. It is the major metabolic gland, producing hormones that affect the rate of metabolism. They increase basal metabolic rate and heat production:

- thyroxine T4 – containing iodine, and
- triiodothyronine T3 – containing iodine.

The gland also produces another hormone, **calcitonin**, which functions in calcium metabolism.

Health Connection

The thyroid gland and metabolism

Some people suffer from an underactive thyroid, where too little thyroxine is produced. It can result in having a lower metabolic rate, being tired and gaining weight. Thyroxine supplement can be given to raise thyroxine levels.

Some people suffer from an overactive thyroid, where too much thyroxine is produced. Drugs to block this may be used.

Parathyroid glands

These are four small glands embedded on either side of the posterior surface of the thyroid gland. The release of the hormone **parathyroid hormone (PTH)** is controlled by humoral stimuli, not by the pituitary gland. PTH works with calcitonin hormone from the thyroid gland to maintain blood calcium levels within the normal limits of 9–10 µg/dL.

Calcium is needed for many body functions, such as bone growth and muscle contraction (Chapter 6) and heart contraction (Chapter 8). Calcium levels are controlled by two hormones working antagonistically (in opposite directions) to maintain homeostasis:

- calcitonin from the thyroid gland and
- parathyroid hormone from the parathyroid gland.

Calcitonin *lowers* blood calcium levels (the calcium is deposited in bone). It is released from the thyroid gland when blood calcium is high.

Parathyroid hormone *raises* blood calcium (the calcium is released from bone). Parathyroid hormone is released when blood calcium is low.

The pancreas

This is a mixed gland composed of both endocrine and exocrine gland cells (**acinar** cells). The endocrine gland cells are contained in a region of the pancreas called the **islets of Langerhans**. The islets are made up of three types of cell:

- α (**alpha**) **cells** – produce glucagon hormone;
- β (**beta**) **cells** – produce insulin hormone;
- δ (**delta**) **cells** – produce somatostatin hormone.

Insulin and glucagon are involved in glucose metabolism.

Insulin, glucagon and blood glucose

Immediately after a meal the blood sugar level rises as glucose is released from digested carbohydrates. The beta cells in the islets of Langerhans of the pancreas secrete **insulin** hormone in response to the high blood sugar, by a process of negative feedback. Insulin has the effect of lowering blood sugar level by enhancing the transport of glucose from the blood into the cells, muscles and adipose tissues for use with oxygen to make ATP energy. After energy needs are met, excess glucose is converted to glycogen and fat and stored in the liver. This process lowers the blood sugar level. (Insulin also stimulates the uptake of amino acids and protein synthesis.) During this *absorptive state* of digestion, with rising blood glucose the beta cells increase insulin release. This leads to greater uptake of glucose by cells and greater conversion of glucose to glycogen, with the result that blood glucose levels fall.

Glucagon is a hormone that is a potent *hyperglyaemic* agent, raising blood glucose. Its major target is the liver, where it promotes

- the breakdown of glycogen to glucose: **glycogenolysis**;
- the production of glucose from lactic acid and non-carbohydrates: **gluconeogenesis**;
- the release of glucose into the blood from liver cells, causing an increase in blood glucose level.

In the *post-absorptive state* falling blood glucose leads to the alpha cells in the pancreas releasing glucagon. This leads to the liver converting glycogen to glucose and the release of glucose into the blood. This results in a rise in blood glucose.

Blood glucose control is an essential requirement for brain and nervous tissue function as the brain and nervous tissue rely on glucose as their energy nutrient.

Health Connection

Diabetes mellitus

There are various forms of diabetes. Type I diabetes (early onset) requires the use of insulin. This is due to the loss or lack of beta cells in the pancreas and the subsequent lack of insulin. Late onset diabetes, Type II, may be due to increasing insensitivity to insulin and may be caused by environmental effects such as a diet high in sugar.

Adrenal medulla

This gland and its secretions were mentioned above when discussing the ANS.

The gland secretes adrenaline and noradrenaline.

Briefly, secretion of these hormones causes

- blood vessels to constrict;
- the heart to beat faster;
- blood to be diverted to the brain, heart and skeletal muscle.

Adrenaline is the more potent stimulator of the heart and metabolic activities.

Noradrenaline is more influential on peripheral vasoconstriction and blood pressure.

The adrenal glands, together with the hypothalamus, are involved in the stress response.

Adrenal cortex

The adrenal cortex synthesises and releases steroid hormones called corticosteroids.

Different corticosteroids are produced in each of the three layers:

- mineralocorticoids, which regulate water and electrolytes (mainly aldosterone);
- glucocorticoids (mainly cortisol);
- gonadocorticoids (mainly androgens, such as testosterone and oestrogen).

Health Connection

Adrenal cortex disorders

There are various disorders associated with the adrenal gland, such as

- **Addison's disease:**
  - results from hyposecretion of *all* adrenal cortex hormones;
  - signs and symptoms include bronze skin tone, muscles are weak, burn-out, susceptibility to infection;
- **Cushing's syndrome:**
  - results from a tumour in the middle cortical area of the adrenal cortex;
  - signs and symptoms include 'moon face', 'buffalo hump' on the upper back, high blood pressure, hyperglycaemia, weakening of bones, depression.

Chapter Reference

Homeostasis and negative feedback are discussed in Chapter 1, 'Maintaining a Safe Environment' (see p. 1).

Health Connection

ADH and blood pressure

Our kidneys, along with our cardiovascular system, are involved in maintaining blood pressure. People with high blood pressure are sometimes given a diuretic, whose effect is the reverse of ADH by encouraging copious urine production. This reduces the volume of the blood and therefore lowers blood pressure.

Health Connection

Cushing's syndrome

Cushing's syndrome can also be caused by overproduction of corticosteroids by the adrenal gland. This can be caused by a tumour in the adrenal or pituitary glands but commonly it is caused by using oral corticosteroids as a long-term treatment for inflammatory conditions. Corticosteroids are involved in the regulation of metabolism and play a part in salt and water balance and blood pressure. The excess corticosteroids disrupt these control mechanisms and can lead to hypertension, osteoporosis, diabetes mellitus and chronic heart failure.

Antidiuretic hormone (ADH)

This hormone is secreted from the pituitary gland in response to falling fluid levels of the body, or lowered blood pressure. This dehydration results in neurons sending messages to motivate drinking and in the release of ADH. The ADH binds to receptors in the kidney and reduces the amount of water excreted in the urine by altering the osmotic pressure in the kidneys. If less water is excreted more is maintained in the body, reducing dehydration and maintaining homeostasis. When the water levels increase ADH secretion is suppressed through negative feedback.

Sex glands

The sex glands vary depending on gender. In the female they are the ovaries and in the male they are the testes. The hormones they produce are needed in the development of the sexual characteristics of each gender and for the maintenance of the reproductive organs once full development is reached.

Many of the main sex hormones are steroid hormones, hence the name – sterone. They are all derived from the lipid cholesterol.

The testes in the male secrete **testosterone** hormone. This is the most important hormone of the testes and is the main male sex hormone or androgen. It is also found in females. It is produced in the interstitial cells of the testes.

The functions of testosterone include

- stimulating reproductive organ development;
- underlying sex drive;
- causing secondary sex characteristics:
  - deepening of voice,
  - increased hair growth,
  - enlargement of skeletal muscles and
  - thickening of bones.

The ovaries in the female secrete **oestrogen** hormone, which helps secondary sexual characteristics such as breast development and aids the onset of menstruation. They also secrete **progesterone** hormone, which assists in the normal development of pregnancy.

Oestrogens are produced by follicle cells in the ovaries.

The main functions of oestrogen are

- causing secondary sex characteristics such as:
  - enlargement of accessory organs,
  - development of breasts,
  - appearance of pubic hair,
  - increase in fat beneath the skin,
  - widening and lightening of the pelvis and
  - onset of menses (menstrual cycles).

The menstrual cycle

The menstrual cycle refers to the cyclic changes of the endometrium of the uterus. It is regulated by cyclic production of oestrogen and progesterone. It makes the uterus or womb ready for the implantation of a fertilised egg. If this does not occur the lining is lost through menstruation.

The stages of the menstrual cycle are

- menses (menstruation), where the functional layer of the endometrium is sloughed;
- proliferative stage, where there is regeneration of the functional layer;
- secretory stage, where the endometrium increases in size and becomes ready for implantation of a fertilised egg (Figure 4.24).

Progesterone

Progesterone is produce by the corpus luteum. It helps to maintain pregnancy. Production of progesterone continues until luteinising hormone diminishes in the blood.

Health Connection

Addison's syndrome

This is caused by insufficient levels of corticosteroid hormones in the blood, causing changes in body chemistry. The common cause of this is damage to the adrenal gland by an autoimmune disorder, in which the body attacks its own tissues. It is twice as common in females and can run in families.

The symptoms include tiredness, weakness, loss of appetite, weight loss, skin pigmentation similar to suntan, especially in creases of palms and on knuckles, elbows and knees.

In Addison's crisis excessive loss of salt and water leads to dehydration, extreme weakness, abdominal pain, vomiting, confusion, coma and death (if untreated).

Chapter Reference

The development of sexual characteristics is discussed in Chapter 3, 'Growing and Developing' (see p. 64).

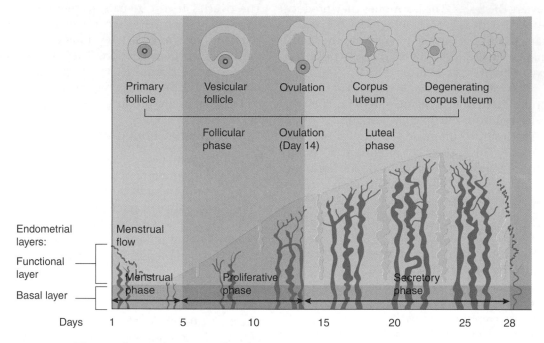

FIGURE 4.24 **The ovarian and menstrual cycle**

Other sex glands include the **mammary glands.** These are present in both sexes, but only function in females. They are modified sweat glands. Their function is to produce milk. They help give the name to the class of animal to which we humans belong, mammals, animals that feed their newborns via mammary glands.

Hormones are also released from cells within other organs (see Table 4.3).

Changes during lifespan and lifestyle

Whatever we consume in the way of food, drink or drugs has an impact on our internal environment and on our hormones. Feeling full or feeling happy relies on feedback from hormones to maintain our internal environment in homeostasis. Altering our state by drugs therefore affects our homeostasis.

Much pharmacology, the science of replacing or replenishing chemicals in our bodies, is interested in drugs that affect the nervous and endocrine systems.

We are not born fully formed and our nervous system and endocrine system do two things during development:

- They change, in that the nervous system and endocrine system develop.
- They change other organs and affect their development.

Table 4.3 Other hormone producing structures

Organ	Hormone
Heart	Atrial natriuretic peptide (ANP)
Gastrointestinal tract	
Stomach	Gastrin
	Serotonin
Duodenum	Intestinal gastrin
	Cholecystokinin (CCK)
Kidney	Erythropoietin
Skin	Cholecalciferol (pro-vitamin D3)
Adipose tissue	Leptin
Placenta	Oestrogen
	Progesterone
	Human chorionic gonadotropin
	Human placental lactogen

We alter our nervous system all the time by learning new things and committing them to memory. Our nervous system, while having axonal connections to the right outputs that are quite hardwired, also must display plasticity, the ability to store new memories.

Our endocrine systems go through rapid development around puberty when we become sexually developed and fertile, able to produce the next generation of humans. In middle age females go through **menopause**, when menses cease and they are no longer fertile, but are still able to continue all other functions. Males may also lose some of their fertility, with sperm from older males being less viable than those from younger males. Levels of sex hormones may also alter.

Conclusion: Communicating

Cells communicate with each other, as do all the systems of the body, to coordinate a response to incoming signals. The signals coming in affect sensory pathways, each signal having its own detection system. We are thus sensitive to many different signals. However, we cannot detect all signals across all frequencies. If we cannot detect something we cannot respond.

Communication requires the ability to detect and respond. Without it all our actions can become inappropriate or irrelevant, we cannot control our internal environment or we can become isolated from our external environment. Each cell of our multicellular body is part of something larger that needs to work as one. Or as the poet John Donne put it sublimely:

> No man is an island, Entire of itself. Each is a piece of the continent, A part of the main.
>
> *Meditation* XVII (1623)

Chapter Summary

▲ The nervous and endocrine systems communicate with the cells of the body to enable us to respond appropriately to changes in our internal environment (maintaining homeostasis) and our external environment (maintaining survival).

▲ The nervous system is a rapid, but localised, transmission system.

▲ The endocrine system is a slower, but diffuse, transmission system.

▲ The nervous system uses electrical impulses and neurotransmitters to send messages.

▲ The endocrine system uses hormones to send signals.

Controlling and Repairing

The part can never be well unless the whole is well.

Plato, classical Greek philosopher (c. 424–347 BC)

Chapter Outline

Introduction: Controlling and repairing as activities of daily living

We cannot control the external environment, which varies moment by moment, but we can control our internal environment by the processes of homeostasis, to make it as suitable as possible for the activities of our cells. Homeostasis, the control of our internal environment within set limits, is central to health. Controlling, therefore, is an ADL, allowing us to be independent organisms. If we go outside of the limits set for each variable, **damage** can occur. We have another system within homeostasis, repair, that allows us to rectify damage. Repair is linked to replacement of damaged cells. This chapter looks at both controlling our internal environment and our ability to repair ourselves.

To illustrate this, the chapter uses two features as examples:

- **controlling body temperature** and
- **controlling cell numbers**.

We shall first look at control of body temperature and then look at control of cell numbers

in damage and repair. The **skin** is used as the organ that best illustrates these principles.

Body temperature as an activity of daily living

How we feel about our temperature is quite a subjective measurement, for example, if you put us all in the same room some of us will feel warmer than others. In response to that feeling we will change our behaviours, some moving to warmer or cooler places, putting on or taking off clothing or drinking warm or cool drinks in an attempt to make ourselves feel comfortable. However, if we are healthy all of us have a similar temperature if measured objectively with a thermometer.

But what if we couldn't control our body temperature, and if we were subject to the vagaries of the external environment? How could we manage any other aspects of our biology and therefore our health? Our entire metabolism would be compromised; reactions would be slowed down if we were too cold and this would affect our ability to move muscles and make us more prone to predation by large predators. If we were too hot our proteins might unravel affecting all enzymatic reactions. We would sweat more and risk dehydration causing further metabolic and homeostatic imbalances.

Controlling our body temperature is therefore essential to our well-being and our health.

The environment

The external environment

We cannot control the weather. We are subject to what nature throws at us. Originally we only had our own bodies to protect us from the environment. We then discovered fire and could warm ourselves by burning fossil fuels. Thousands of years later we are still burning fossil fuels to keep ourselves warm and to provide energy.

The external environment of planet Earth has temperature ranges from −40°C (that is 40° below 0°) to 50°C on the surface of the planet. Underwater streams in the ocean, the interior of volcanoes and beneath the Earth's crust can have temperatures that are thousands of degrees centigrade.

> #### Chapter Reference
>
> **Temperature** is a measure of the **heat energy** in an object. This is mentioned in Chapter 1, 'Maintaining a Safe Environment' (see p. 1), but will be discussed further below (see p. 144).

The internal environment

Human populations are found living in temperatures varying from −40°C to +50°C and can cope with fluctuations of 35°C in a day. We are **homeotherms**, animals that maintain a *constant* internal temperature. Other animals, such as fish and reptiles, are **poikilotherms;** they have temperatures that *vary* with the outside **ambient** temperature. These animals must rely on the sun to warm themselves up. Animals that are homeotherms expend a lot of energy maintaining a constant temperature.

This activity of daily living (ADL) is under strict homeostatic control and allows us to live in various ambient temperatures. While the ambient temperature of the environment varies our bodies are maintained in a range of 35.6° to 37.8°C (96° to 100° F). Controlling body temperature is also called **thermoregulation**. It is an activity occurring normally all the time. In illness, especially during infections by microbial organisms or agents, our temperature may vary. We can survive fluctuations for a short period of time, but longer or extreme temperature variation can be deleterious and can result in death.

> ### Health Connection
>
> #### Temperature
> We measure the heat of a patient by their temperature. There are various ways to measure temperature and which method you use depends on the patient, the accuracy you need and the frequency you need to take the temperature. How often and why you are taking it depends on your interpretation of the health of the patient. You may be interested in heat loss or gain and you might be interested in the causes of these. This, together with other clinical data, will help you to diagnose the condition of the patient.

Why we control body temperature

Our body has many processes or ADLs such as

- digestion,
- nerve transmission,
- movement,
- growth,
- protection and
- communication.

These are carried out by proteins such as

- enzymes,
- neurotransmitters,
- transport proteins,
- antibodies and
- hormones.

Proteins are strings of amino acids. The order in which the amino acids are put together follows instructions from the genetic code. The protein once assembled does not remain in the form of a long string of amino acids, but folds itself into a *three-dimensional* (3D) structure. These 3D structures are sensitive to temperature and can be altered by high or low temperatures. The functioning protein, such as an enzyme, relies on its 3D shape to fit with its substrate. If this is altered it will no longer function. *Protein structure*, and thus *protein function*, is very *temperature sensitive*.

> **Chapter Reference**
>
> Genetics is discussed in Chapter 3, 'Growing and Developing' (see p. 64).

We must, therefore, maintain our internal environment at a temperature at which our proteins can maintain their 3D shape. For example, when we eat an egg for breakfast it is full of protein. The white of the egg consists mainly of the transport and osmotic balance protein **albumin**. When we boil the egg, the protein unravels and forms a solid structure with other albumin molecules. Once the egg is boiled, we cannot unravel the protein and put it back to its 3D shape. It cannot, therefore, function as albumin even though it consists of the amino acids in the correct order for albumin. We too cannot tolerate extremes of internal temperature for long as damage would be done to our proteins 3D structure that cannot be undone.

Health Connection

Differing normal body temperature

Our bodies have an internal temperature between 36°C and 38°C. Temperatures at the core of the body are different to temperatures at different locations. Rectal temperature is higher than oral temperature and skin temperature fluctuates. Temperature also changes during the day. It is lowest while asleep as metabolic needs are lower and muscle movements are also fewer.

Metabolism and thermoregulation

Heat

Heat energy or **thermal energy** is a form of energy related to the property of material objects, matter, and is related to the amount of energy they contain. The more energy they have the more heat they contain. This heat can be seen in a property called kinetic energy, the energy of movement. When a material object changes from solid to liquid the molecules or atoms which it is made up from move about more. So as objects become hotter they also have more kinetic energy and change in what are called phases from solid to liquid to gas. The amount of heat an object has can also be measured as temperature. We tend to think in terms of how we measure heat as the temperature of an object. Generally, solids have lower heat and temperature than liquids and liquids have lower heat and temperature than gases.

Heat can be *transferred* (moved) from one object to another in a variety of ways:

- **radiation** – transfer of heat in the form of electromagnetic rays such as infrared rays between a warmer object and a cooler one without physical contact;
- **conduction** – the heat exchange between two materials in direct contact, e.g. a chair, clothing, jewellery;

- **convection** – transfer of heat by the movement of a liquid or a gas between areas of different temperatures. Air or water in contact with body, e.g. cool air becomes warm against the body (conduction) and is moved away by convection currents;
- **evaporation** – conversion of a liquid to a vapour such as the daily loss of 300 ml from lungs and 600 ml from skin.

All of these can be used to warm or cool a body such as a human body.

> **Chapter Reference**
>
> Heat and energy are discussed in Chapter 2, 'Working and Playing' (see p. 35).

Making heat

As we must maintain ourselves at a constant temperature we must *generate* and *lose* heat as appropriate. Heat is a form of energy and we expend energy making it. Heat is generated by metabolic processes.

The food we consume contains **calories**. These are an indication of the amount of energy they contain. These calories are released from our foods during **catabolism**, the *breaking* of chemical bonds. It is the chemical bonds (ionic and covalent, for example) that contain the energy. Some of this energy can be used to do work. We can store the energy released from metabolic reactions as ATP (Figure 5.1).

ATP (as discussed in Chapter 2) has three phosphate groups: the terminal one contains a high energy bond, the penultimate one contains an energy bond and the first one contains some energy in its bond. ATP can, therefore, store and release energy. It releases the energy when ATP (triphosphate) becomes ADP (diphosphate) and can release more energy when ADP becomes AMP (mono-phosphate). It then needs to be

re-synthesised as ATP. The amount of energy released when ATP becomes ADP is exactly the same amount of energy needed to make ATP from ADP.

$$ATP \leftrightarrow Energy+ ADP + P$$

> **Chapter Reference**
>
> ATP is discussed in Chapter 2, 'Working and Playing' (see p. 35).

Work is a physical term meaning *energy requiring activity*. Examples of work are activities such as

- active transport,
- anabolic reactions (forming chemical bonds),
- muscle contraction,
- synthesis of new molecules and
- putting up shelves! (Figure 5.2).

Some of the energy we release from catabolism can be used to do work, but some of the energy is released as heat. The total energy used by the body at any unit of time is the **total energy expenditure**:

total energy expenditure = heat generated + external work done + heat stored

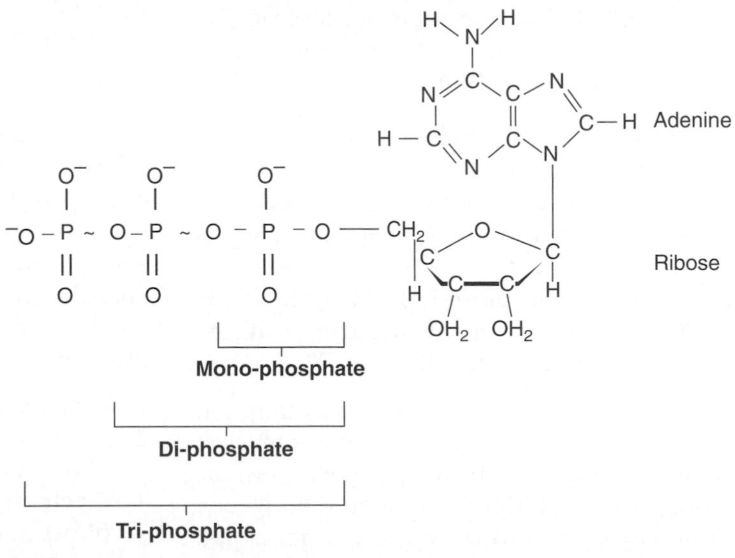

FIGURE 5.1 **ATP**

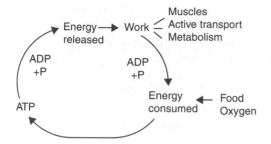

FIGURE 5.2 **ATP, energy, work and ADP**

We cannot store ATP, but we can store energy in the form of fat or glycogen for later use as the raw material for ATP synthesis.

Chapter Reference

The fate of surplus fats and glycogen are discussed in Chapter 9, 'Eating and Drinking' (see p. 241).

Much of the energy released during catabolism is **heat**:

Energy generated = energy used + heat released

The rate at which energy is used by our bodies is called our **metabolic rate.** Our **basal metabolic rate (BMR)** is the amount of heat produced by the body after fasting for 12 hours and at rest. It changes during our lifespan and between individuals. There are various factors that influence our BMR such as

- Surface area of the body – a small body usually has higher BMR;
- Gender – males tend to have higher BMR;
- Age – children and adolescents have a higher BMR;
- Thyroxin (hormone) production – the higher the amount of thyroxin produced the higher our metabolic rate.

We need to balance our energy consumption and our energy output to maintain homeostasis and to maintain our weight. If we consume more, excess, calories in our food than we use to do work, we will store the calories as fat. If we do more work than we generate energy

for, we will lose weight and can go into energy depletion, muscle wastage and death. Our **total metabolic rate (TMR)** is the amount of energy we need to consume to maintain our activities of daily living (ADL). Most of the energy we consume is released as foods are oxidised, but much of this energy escapes as heat.

Health Connection

Calories
Most of us need a calorie intake of about 1500–2000 calories per day, depending on how active we are. Pregnant women need an extra 400 calories per day.

Production of energy and heat

We consume energy during work. We must therefore produce energy ourselves. The energy we produce can then be used to fuel the energy we consume. We balance

- **catabolic reactions** – breaking chemical bonds and releasing energy with
- **anabolic reactions** – making chemical bonds which requires energy and storing it in the body.

As mentioned above, metabolic reactions produce energy and heat. There are a number of ways we can produce energy.

The main molecule we use to generate energy is glucose. It is catabolised and releases energy during its catabolism. The energy released can be stored as ATP. ATP acts as the energy currency of the cell and is coupled to anabolic (energy-using) cellular processes.

Glucose is broken down in a series of reactions:

1. **Glycolysis** – in the cytoplasm of the cell.
2. **Krebs** or **TCA cycle** – in the mitochondria of the cell.
3. **Electron transport** coupled to **oxidative phosphorylation** – in the inner mitochondria of the cell.

For each molecule of glucose completely catabolised, 36 molecules of ATP are formed.

One major route is by a process of **oxidation: reduction** reactions. Oxidation:reduction reactions involve the movement of oxygen, hydrogen electrons and protons and are discussed below.

> ### Health Connection
>
> #### Energy and ADL
> All day long we use up energy to perform ADL. We therefore need oxygen and glucose to make ATP. We can store surplus sugars, but we cannot store surplus oxygen. We must have a constant supply of oxygen. Any interruption in the supply is therefore detrimental to our health. This is why one of the first questions we ask in an emergency is 'Are they breathing?' and why we are so keen to keep the airways clear. For more on getting oxygen into our bodies, see Chapter 7, 'Breathing'.

Glycolysis

A process called glycolysis, involving the use of glucose from food, is one of the first parts of energy reduction. Initially we consume foods that contain carbohydrates. These are broken down in the gastrointestinal tract and the constituent parts of the carbohydrates, sugars, are released. Glucose is one such sugar. Glucose from the gastrointestinal tract is absorbed into the blood and transported to all cells of the body. There it is taken up, with the aid of a **hormone** called **insulin**, and used in a process called **cellular respiration**.

Glycolysis is a reaction that occurs in the **cytoplasm** of cells. Glycolysis is a stepwise conversion of glucose into **pyruvic acid**. During this glucose is split into two molecules of pyruvic acid and a small net amount of ATP is synthesised.

> ### Chapter Reference
> Digestion and the gastrointestinal tract are discussed in Chapter 9, 'Eating and Drinking' (see p. 241).

The **pyruvic acid (pyruvate)** formed in the reaction above can now go one of two ways:

1. If there is *no* oxygen available (**anaerobic respiration**) it can be reduced to **lactate** (lactic acid).
2. If there *is* oxygen available (**aerobic respiration**) it can be oxidised to **acetyl co-enzyme A** (acetyl Co-A) and enter into the mitochondria of the cell.

> ### Health Connection
>
> #### Lactic acid
> Athletes often talk about a wall. When muscle is used a lot in exercise there is a build up of lactic acid by anaerobic respiration. This causes pain and is part of the wall that the athletes reach, a pain barrier. They are in oxygen debt. Rest allows the oxygen debt to be paid back as aerobic respiration can compensate for the debt.

The Krebs (TCA) cycle

The mitochondria are the cell's powerhouse organelle. In the mitochondria the Acetyl Co-A enters a process called the Krebs cycle after its discoverer (also known as the TCA cycle – tricarboxylic acid cycle and the citric acid cycle). This cycle yields a further small amount of ATP and as a side product (waste product) carbon dioxide and water.

> ### Chapter Reference
> Waste is discussed in Chapter 10, 'Eliminating' (see p. 282).

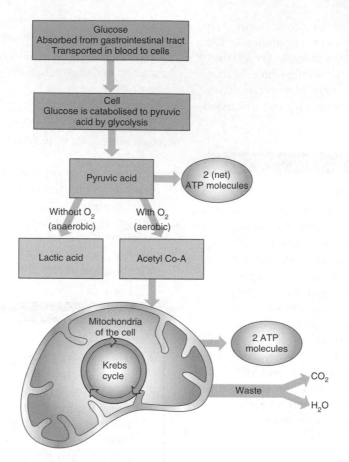

FIGURE 5.3 Metabolic pathways involved in cellular respiration

During both glycolysis and the Krebs cycle some ATP is used to fuel the reactions and some ATP is *synthesised* during the reactions. There is a *net gain* in the amount of ATP synthesised. Apart from glucose, fatty acids can also be digested, converted into Acetyl Co-A and enter the Krebs cycle. Fatty acids contain more calories than a similar mass of carbohydrates and therefore release more energy during catabolism.

At the end of the Krebs cycle only *four* molecules of ATP are synthesised. Most of the energy for fuelling the reactions of our bodies comes from molecules that are released during the Krebs cycles, but are used in the final process of oxidative phosphorylation.

Health Connection

Diets

Carbohydrates, fats and proteins all contain calories and can be used to generate energy and heat during their catabolism. As fats contain more calories than carbohydrates or proteins, removing them from the diet may help to encourage the use of stored fats in diets designed for weight reduction.

Redox reactions

The chemicals that are released from the Krebs cycle are in a **reduced** state. Reduced means that they have *hydrogen added* or *oxygen removed* to be in the reduced form.

Many reactions are oxidation:reduction reactions, also called **redox** reactions, for short. When glucose is broken down to carbon dioxide and water (with the production of ATP) this is an oxidation reaction, meaning oxygen is added or hydrogen is removed.

At the most fundamental level redox (oxidation reduction) reactions are:

- the removal of electrons or
- addition of protons.

Reduction

Oxidant + e⁻ ⟶ Product

(Electrons **gained**; oxidation number **decreases**)

Oxidation

Reductant ⟶ Product + e⁻

(Electrons **lost**; oxidation number **increases**)

For example:

$$2Mg + CO_2 \longrightarrow 2MgO + C$$

In this reaction the magnesium has become **oxidised** (gained electrons) and the carbon has become reduced (lost electrons). This is an example to demonstrate the importance of oxidation and reduction reactions. In metabolism glucose is gradually oxidised by the removal of hydrogen atoms. The hydrogen atoms join with the chemicals that are released from the Krebs cycle. These are **carrier molecules** and will be recycled back to the Krebs cycle. These molecules are **co-enzymes**.

The Krebs cycle may not generate much ATP, but the two other molecules it generates, the carrier molecules, can go on to do so. These are two co-enzymes:

1. **nicotinamide adenine dinucleotide (NAD+)** (derived from the vitamin niacin).
2. **flavin adenine dinucleotide (FAD+)** (derived from the vitamin B2 – riboflavin).

Both NAD+ and FAD+ can be reduced by the addition of hydrogen to NADH and FADH respectively. This is what occurs in the Krebs cycle. Once they are reduced they are released from the cycle with their hydrogen atoms (carried by them) to the inner part of the mitochondria where they will release the hydrogen atoms and become oxidised. They then return to the Krebs cycle and repeat the process. While they are carrying the hydrogen atoms they have high energy bonds and the energy is released through a series of reactions of oxidative phosphorylation linked to the **electron transport chain**.

Health Connection

Enzymes, genes and metabolic reactions

Most of the reactions described here are carried out by enzymes. Enzymes, which are specialised proteins, are made from genes. Many 'inborn errors of metabolism' are genetic disorders where the normal 'wild type' gene has undergone mutation. We have genes in our nucleus that code for many enzymes. However, we also have genes in our mitochondria that code for many of the genes involved in the formation of ATP and any lack of these genes can have serious consequences. Genes are discussed in Chapter 3, 'Growing and Developing'.

Electron transport chain and oxidative phosphorylation

NAD+ and FAD+ react with hydrogen ions to become NADH and FADH respectively. During this reaction they *gain* and *carry* electrons and are thus reduced. They can pass on their electrons and thus *lose* their electrons and become oxidised. The hydrogen atoms released are split into hydrogen proton and its electron. The electrons are passed along a chain and finally combine with the oxygen we breathe to form water. During the oxidation of NADH and FADH back to NAD+ and FAD+, energy is released and this generates ATP.

While the electron chain moves electrons along from donors to acceptors ending with water, oxidative phosphorylation allows phosphate molecules to join to ADP (ADP phosphorylation) in the oxidation (transfer of electrons) from reduced co-enzymes to oxygen (Figure 5.4).

Box 5.1 Summary – Glucose

- Glucose is oxidised to two molecules of pyruvate and then aerobically to co-enzyme A.
- These enter the Krebs cycle which produces some ATP and NADH and FADH. NADH and FADH enter the electron chain and the electrons are passed through a series of carrier molecules generating energy for oxidative phosphorylation, the addition of high energy phosphates to ADP so that it becomes ATP.
- The side products are carbon dioxide, from the Krebs cycle and water, from the electron chain.
- During this whole process 36 molecules of ATP are generated from one molecule of glucose during **aerobic (oxygenated) respiration.**

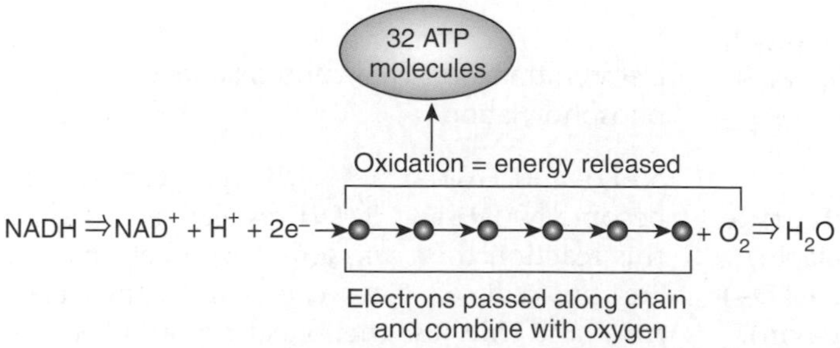

$$NADH \Rightarrow NAD^+ + H^+ + 2e^- \rightarrow \bullet \rightarrow \bullet \rightarrow \bullet \rightarrow \bullet \rightarrow \bullet \rightarrow \bullet + O_2 \Rightarrow H_2O$$

Oxidation = energy released

Electrons passed along chain and combine with oxygen

FIGURE 5.4 **Electron transport chain**

In the electron transport chain a series of proteins carry the electrons towards electron acceptors. Energy is formed during this process.

$$\text{Glucose} + O_2 \longrightarrow \text{ATP} + CO_2 + H_2O$$

As we said in Chapter 2, 'Working and Playing', 'there is no free lunch in the universe'. To be able to do work we must generate energy and generating energy takes energy and work!

Heat loss

Heat is generated or gained by our metabolism. It can be transferred around a body in the blood. When it reaches the skin it can be dissipated in blood vessels to cool the skin. At the same time it can cause evaporation of sweat, a liquid to a vapour. This helps to cool the skin.

Heat is lost to the environment from our surfaces via

- blood,
- skin and
- sweat glands.

Biology and homeostasis

Controlling body temperature

We continually lose heat from the surface of our bodies, the skin, via radiation and evaporation. Skin blood vessels and capillaries are filled with warm blood and it is this warmth that can be dissipated to the environment. We can cool ourselves down by evaporation of perspiration which takes the heat contained in the liquid with it as it evaporates into the surroundings. We need, therefore to control mechanisms for warming and cooling us so that we can keep a constant temperature.

As mentioned previously heat can be transferred in a variety of ways:

- **radiation** – emission of heat as electromagnetic energy;
- **conduction** – direct transfer of heat from molecule to molecule;

- **convection** – the transfer of heat from one by via the movement of air or water to another body;
- **evaporation** – loss of water from body surfaces as water changes from a liquid to a gas.

The body employs many of these ways to maintain our temperature.

There are various levels of controlling body temperature. At a behavioural level those that are able can carry out a number of *voluntary* actions that would affect body temperature:

- moving to a warmer or cooler place;
- removing or adding clothing;
- eating warm or cool foods;
- drinking warm or cool drinks;
- changing the temperature of the room by turning on heaters or coolers, opening or closing ventilation;
- moving or exercising to warm up, resting to cool down.

There are *involuntary* main mechanisms controlling body temperature. They are

- shivering;
- sweating and
- dilation or constriction of surface blood vessels.

These mechanisms occur in response to fluctuations of internal body temperature.

The body regulates body temperature through homeostatic mechanisms involving the **autonomic nervous system (ANS).**

Receptors that are specifically sensitive to temperature (temperature sensitive receptors or **thermoreceptors**) detect a change in temperature. This change is generally to stabilise internal temperature, but we also possess surface thermoreceptors that tell us about changes in temperature on our periphery so that we can detect hot or cold water and avoid burning ourselves. Some of these receptors detect an increase and some detect a decrease in temperature. When temperature fluctuates from an acceptable range (36–38°C) these receptors send signals to a control centre. In

this instance the control centre is the body's thermostat, the **hypothalamus** in the brain, which initiates heat-loss or heat-promoting mechanisms by sending signals via the ANS to **effectors.** The effectors carry out action that will alter the temperature back to within the acceptable range.

The effectors for this are

- sweat glands in the skin – controlled by autonomic nerves;
- blood vessels in the skin – controlled by autonomic nerves somatic nerves;
- involuntary movement of skeletal muscles (shivering) – controlled by a motor centre in the hypothalamus.

Chapter Reference

The nervous system is discussed in Chapter 4, 'Communicating' (see p. 102). Skin is discussed in Chapter 1, 'Maintaining a Safe Environment' (see p. 1) and Chapter 3, 'Growing and Developing' (see p. 64).

Sweating allows loss of body heat due to evaporation. A watery fluid from sweat glands located over the body secretes a dilute solution of sodium chloride. Adults have about 2.5 million sweat glands. Body heat is lost as the liquid takes up heat energy from our skin. This heat energy causes the liquid to evaporate as a gas from our skin. This is an active process requiring energy. Through this process we can lose up to 4 litres of liquid per hour.

Vasodilation (**vaso** – vessels; **dilation** – increase of diameter) of peripheral blood vessels also allows loss of heat. As the blood goes through these dilated vessels internal heat is taken to the surface of the skin where it is lost to the external environment through conduction and radiation.

Conversely, **vasoconstriction** (**constriction** is a reduction in diameter) of peripheral blood vessels reduces this heat loss by conduction and radiation. During vasoconstriction of blood vessels, blood is re-routed to deeper, more vital body organs to maintain them at constant heat, while the periphery of the body receives less blood.

We continually lose heat to the environment through fluid loss by diffusion of fluid through the skin which then evaporates. This is a passive loss which, together with fluid lost from the lungs during breathing, accounts for around 0.6 litres of liquid per day. This is called insensible water loss. Due to this loss and the loss of liquids through elimination we are in constant need of water balance – the amount lost must be replenished. This too is under homeostatic control and is discussed in Chapter 10, 'Eliminating'.

Chapter Reference

Muscles are discussed in Chapter 6, 'Moving' (see p. 163). Blood is discussed in Chapter 8, 'Transporting' (see p. 205).

Increasing body temperature, especially in cold climates, can be brought about by increasing metabolic rates and increasing muscle contraction. Muscular activity produces heat; however, muscular activity is usually accompanied by movement and movement uses energy. Making muscles move without using movement results in all the energy produced being taken up as heat. This can then be dissipated into the blood and circulated around the body. The blood thus transports heat. This type of muscular movement is *shivering* where there is a rhythmic contraction and relaxation of voluntary skeletal muscle at a rate of about 10–20 times per second producing heat. All the heat generated by shivering can be used to warm the body.

The homeostatic mechanism for controlling body temperature is an example of negative feedback where the variable is reversed or opposed. Whether the temperature is too high or too low both cause thermoreceptors to send messages to a control centre that coordinates an effect that is the reverse of the temperature. If we are too hot the effect is to cool us and if we are too cold the effect is to warm us. Positive feedback reinforces the variable and would result in us getting hotter if we were hot and colder if we were cold. Positive feedback, therefore, would not be effective in maintaining our body temperature within an acceptable range.

Temperature regulation in the newborn

Newborn babies and infants have a large surface area (body surface) to volume ratio compared to adults so they are more vulnerable to heat loss over this area. They cannot take voluntary actions to adjust their body temperature. Newborn babies are unable to shiver. They are able to utilise a special method of generating heat (**thermogenesis**) by using a specialised type of adipose tissue, **brown adipose tissue (BAT)**.

Chapter Reference

Tissues are discussed in Chapter 1, 'Maintaining a Safe Environment' (see p. 1).

Using up BAT does not result in the production of ATP. Instead all the energy released will be liberated as heat. BAT is available for the first six months of life.

Health Connection

Acclimatisation

We have the ability to live in various climates. At first we may be too hot or too cold when we move to a new climate. Gradually we 'get used to it' or acclimatise. During acclimatisation to heat, hormones, such as aldosterone, are released. This helps to re-absorb the secreted sodium chloride by the epithelial cells lining the sweat glands. As we sweat more in hot places, sodium chloride depletion becomes a problem and this mechanism helps us adjust. We also acclimatise to the cold, but the mechanisms for this are not understood.

Newborn babies lose heat through vasodilation. They possess fewer sweat glands than adults.

Hyperthermia

All forms of increase in body temperature are called **hyperthermia**. Most increases are temporary due to the homeostatic mechanisms discussed above. There are other forms that are more serious. These are

- fever;
- heat exhaustion and
- heat stroke.

During fever the normal range of body temperature of 36–38°C is re-set higher. This is usually caused as a result of an infection, but can be caused by trauma or stress. Factors from the immune system called **endogenous pyrogens** are released by defence cells of the immune system. These factors act on the hypothalamus. The ANS is then activated to conserve or generate heat by the mechanisms described above resulting in vasoconstriction and shivering and a feeling of being cold. When the pyrogen is removed the normal range of body temperature is re-set. This action may help to kill off an invading micro-organism, but it can also lead to damage to tissues.

Chapter Reference

The immune system and micro-organisms are discussed in Chapter 11, 'Cleansing and Dressing' (see p. 299).

Health Connection

Heat exhaustion

Heat exhaustion is caused when the thermoregulatory system cannot cope with demand. This can be due to excessive exercise, lack of water, excess sweating or salt deficiency.

Health Connection

Heat stroke

Heat stroke is usually caused by excessive activity in a hot climate and results in the thermoregulatory system failing. It can result in delirium, convulsion and unconsciousness and can be fatal if not treated.

Health Connection

Hypothermia

The body is hard to cool below 35.5°C. Once it cools below this level it is hard to warm it because shivering is not possible due to muscle weakness. Body temperature rapidly continues to drop in this situation to below 34°C. This results in confusion due to mental processes being affected. Between 32°C and 30°C there is loss of consciousness. Below 28°C the cardiovascular system is affected.

Control of cell numbers

Cells are continually made and lost. The numbers of cells that are made must meet the numbers that are lost. If there are too few cells we suffer from degenerative diseases. If there are too many cells made we suffer from tumour diseases such as cancer. Cell numbers must therefore be rigorously controlled.

Cell loss

Cells are lost due to wear and tear. They cease functioning properly and are able to commit suicide by a process called **apoptosis**. They are also lost through lack of nutrients, but this loss is not programmed and is the result of other processes in the body not functioning correctly.

Cell formation

Cell formation and growth are discussed in Chapter 3, 'Growing and Developing'.

During life we continually shed cells and replace with new cells. Sometimes we lose more cells than usual due to trauma. In the next section we are going to look at an example of controlling the repair of cell loss after trauma to demonstrate some of the homeostatic mechanisms involved. First we shall introduce the organ we are using as an example of repair and regeneration, the skin.

Health Connection

Tissue viability: Maintenance of the integrity of the skin

Wounding damages this integrity and brings many risk factors with it such as infections. Tissue viability specialists monitor any wounds and are responsible for wound care management, protection and treatment.

The skin as an example of control of repair and growth

In this part of the chapter we shall discuss the skin and its repair as an example of *cell growth* and *homeostasis* of cell growth.

The skin is part of the **integumentary system** comprising

- skin,
- nails and
- hair.

The skin is the largest organ of the body. In adults it covers and area of about 2 square metres and weighs 4–5 kg. It comprises about 16% of the total body weight. It ranges in thickness from 0.5 to 4 mm and consists of two main parts:

- epidermis – made of epithelial tissue;

- dermis – made of mainly connective tissues.

The structure of the skin

The type of epithelial cell skin is composed of is called keratinised stratified squamous epithelium. This is because it is composed of

- **keratin** – a tough fibrous protein. Keratin helps to protect the skin and underlying structures from heat, microbes and chemicals;
- **stratified** – because there are 4–5 strata (layers) of skin cells;
- **sqamous** – a squashy flat-shaped epithelial cell rather than cuboidal or columnar;
- the other cells in the epithelial layer are **melanocytes** which produce a pigment called melanin which gives colour to the skin. The more melanin we have, the darker our skin is.

The 4–5 strata of epidermis are composed of

- stratum basale,
- stratum spinosum,
- statum granulosum,
- stratum lucidum – this layer is only in areas exposed to friction and
- stratum corneum.

The layers of greatest interest are the **corneum** and the **basale**.

Corneum

This is the outermost layer of cells. It consists of 25–30 layers of flattened dead keratinocytes, cells containing keratin. These cells are disposable and are continuously shed and replaced by cells from the deeper layers. Our outside layer of skin is in constant contact with the external environment, all the chemicals and gases that it contains and all the damage it can do to us. To have a disposable, replaceable layer is, therefore, a very useful adaptation. The growing, healthy, new cells are kept away from the effects of the outside environment underneath this disposable layer.

Basale

The basale (base) layer is composed of a single row of columnar or cuboidal epithelia, rather than the squamous epithelia of the top layer. This layer is where the new cells are born from stem cells, so it is also known as the germinitive strata. The new cells gradually move up towards the surface corneum. As cells move up towards the corneum they become more keratinised (have more keratin in them) and they stop growing and dividing.

It takes about 4 weeks for a new cell to form in the stratum basale and rise to the surface, become keratinised and slough off in an epidermis 0.1 mm thick.

Melanocytes

These are the cells that produce melanin, a brown pigment that contributes to skin colour and absorbs damaging ultraviolet (UV) light. Melanin granules cluster to form a protective veil over the nucleus inside the keratinocytes, on the side facing the skin surface.

Health Connection

Vitiligo

This is the loss of normal pigmentation (melanin) from areas of skin resulting in white patches. It is most commonly seen on the face and hands. Usually the patches are distributed symmetrically on the body. The hair may also be white in the affected area. The disease occurs over months to years and the white patch area may continue to enlarge. It cannot be cured but 3 in 10 people regain their natural colour spontaneously.

The epithelial tissue provides a *disposable barrier* with the outermost layer sloughing off. It is due to this continual replenishment that we can use it as an example of the control of cell numbers.

Dermis

Underneath the epidermis of the skin is the dermis or dermal layer. This is composed of connective tissue containing collagen and elastic fibres. These are proteins secreted by cells in the connective tissue and the proteins give the skin its strength and ability to stretch and return to its original shape, its *elasticity*. The connective layer provides support and cushions the underlying muscle and bone. There are far fewer cells in the dermis than in the epidermis. Most of the layer is composed of these proteins and other structures such as follows:

- a few adipose cells, capillary loops, nerves, hair follicles, sebaceous (oil) glands and sweat glands are embedded in dermal tissue;
- blood capillaries from the cardiovascular system bringing nutrients and oxygen in the blood;
- nerve fibres and nerve endings are embedded in the dermis making it sensitive to touch giving rise to sensations of warmth, coolness, pain, tickling and itching;
- hair follicles help in insulation;
- nail beds, protecting the underlying skin;
- adipose cells (fat) allowing insulation and protection of the skin bruising against underlying bones.

This layer also has glands that secrete substances onto the skin. There are two types of glands in skin:

- sebaceous glands, secreting sebaceous oil;
- sweat glands, secreting sweat (Figure 5.5).

The outer epithelial cells have hairs and pores. The inner dermal layer has glands such as sebaceous glands secreting oil and sweat glands secreting sweat. There are also hairs and oil is secreted. There are fat cells at the bottom for insulation and capillaries for bringing nutrients to the skin and for heat regulation.

Health Connection

Stretch marks

While the dermis is able to stretch and return to its original shape due to the presence of elastin, extreme stretching may tear the dermis causing stretch marks. This is commonly seen in pregnancy.

Health Connection

Acne

Sebum normally drains into hair follicles and onto the skin. When the sebaceous glands produce excess sebum the follicles become blocked. The follicle can also become sealed by excess keratin. Bacteria multiply in the sebum causing inflammation of surrounding tissues. A rash due to blockage and inflammation of glands in the skin may occur. The most common form is acne vulgaris. It can be triggered by hormonal changes at puberty and is thought to be due to increased sensitivity to male sex hormone as it is most common in males and may have a genetic factor.

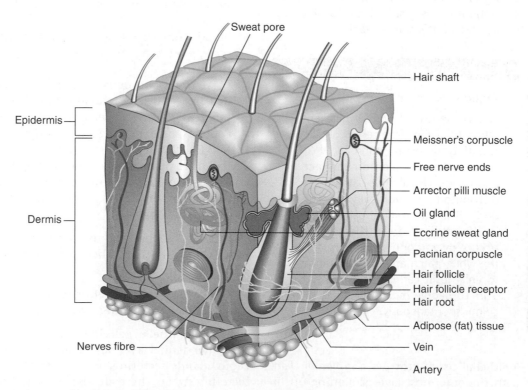

FIGURE 5.5 **Anatomy of the skin**

The function of the skin

The skin presents a barrier between our inner environment and the outer environment in which we live separating us from the world. It provides a number of functions including:

- protection,
- water resistance,
- sensation,
- excretion,
- absorption,
- heat regulation and
- synthesis of vitamin D.

Protection

- Keratin protects underlying tissues from abrasion, heat and chemicals and tightly interlocked keratinocytes resist microbes.
- The corneum forms multiple layers of dead cells to protect deeper layers from injury and microbial invasion.
- The corneum is in constant exposure to friction which stimulates the formation of a callus, an abnormal thickening of the stratum corneum.
- Lipids in the skin slow the evaporation of water protecting against dehydration and also slow the entry of water across our skin when swimming or showering.
- Sebum protects skin and hair from drying out and contains bactericidal chemicals that kill surface bacteria.
- Sweat is acidic and slows the growth of some microbes.
- Melanocytes contain the pigment melanin which shields the nuclear DNA from being damaged by UV light.
- With increased exposure to UV light the amount and darkness of melanin increases giving the skin a tanned appearance.
- The tan is lost when melanin-containing keratinocytes are shed from the stratum corneum.

UVB rays can damage DNA and produce genetic mutations in epidermal cells and can cause skin cancer.

Health Connection

Sunbathing

UVA rays from the sun can penetrate the dermis and produce oxygen free radicals (oxygen with free reactive electrons). These electrons can disrupt collagen and elastic fibres and disrupt their arrangement. This can result in severe wrinkling in those who spend a lot of time in the sun without protection

Water resistance

Our skin is also quite water resistant, it repels water. When we get in a bath the water stays in the bath rather than moving into us. This is due to lipids (fats) between the corneum cells that help to make the layer a water repellent barrier.

Health Connection

Burns

Damaged skin is able to regenerate. Extreme trauma, however, may challenge the skin too much. Burns may remove just the top layer, but deep burns may affect the growing layers leading to impairment in the skin's ability to grow new cells. Burns also remove the protective barrier layer of skin making the individual susceptible to infections. Infections are discussed in Chapter 11, 'Cleansing and Dressing'.

Sensation

There are a wide variety of nerve endings and receptors in the skin. These detect and send signals of sensation in the skin. These include

- tactile sensations – touch, pressure, vibration, tickling;

- thermal sensations – warmth and coolness;
- pain sensations – tissue damage.

Chapter Reference

Sensations and sensory information is discussed in Chapter 4, 'Communicating' (see p. 102).

Excretion

The skin is an excretory organ getting rid of waste material. About 600 ml of water containing waste is lost as sweat; more is lost if we are physically active. The waste contains small amounts of salts, carbon dioxide and urea and ammonia.

Chapter Reference

Excretion of waste is discussed in Chapter 10, 'Eliminating' (see p. 282).

Absorption

The skin can absorb chemicals through its layers.

- Lipid soluble materials do penetrate the skin; these include substances such as vitamins A, D, E and K, certain drugs (e.g. steroids), and gases oxygen and carbon dioxide.
- Some toxic materials can be absorbed, e.g. acetone, dry-cleaning fluid, heavy metals (lead, mercury and arsenic) and plant material such as poison ivy.

Health Connection

Nicotine patches

Nicotine contained in cigarettes is fat soluble. People wishing to stop smoking sometimes wear a nicotine patch on their skin to gradually reduce their addiction to the drug. Other drugs can also be absorbed through the skin.

Heat regulation

The skin is involved in many functions including maintaining body temperature. This is discussed above.

Synthesis of vitamin D

Synthesis of vitamin D requires UV light on the skin. The molecule is then modified in the liver and kidneys to form a hormone called calcitriol. This hormone aids the absorption of calcium from gastrointestinal tract into the blood.

Health Connection

Skin cancer

The skin is the barrier between us and the external environment. It is constantly being challenged by UV rays, chemicals and friction. The cells of the skin are sloughing off and new ones are being made. Because of the high turnover of cells in the basale, DNA replication is subject to error. Additionally, factors such as UV light can penetrate and damage the basale. The stem cells of the basale which form new skin cells are thus prone to growth errors such as cancer, uncontrolled replication of cell numbers.

Box 5.2 Summary – Skin

- The skin performs a number of functions.
- It is composed of two layers: Connective tissue – Dermis; and Epithelial tissue – Epidermis.
- The epidermis acts partly as a disposable barrier.
- The epidermis is continually sloughed off and new cells replace the lost cells.

Changes during lifespan and lifestyle

Controlling cell numbers: Repair and replacement of skin

Many tissues *degenerate* through wear and tear or through ageing. *Regeneration* is the replacement of tissue that has been destroyed. The regeneration is by similar tissue or cells. Not all tissues regenerate.

Tissues that regenerate easily are

- epithelial tissue and
- fibrous connective tissue and bone.

Tissues that regenerate poorly are

- skeletal muscle.

Tissues that are replaced largely with scar tissue are

- cardiac muscle and
- nervous tissue within the brain and spinal cord.

Health Connection

Replacing skin

As normal homeostasis skin is replaced by new cells in the **stratum basale**. When skin is damaged through **injury** or **trauma**, such as in **burns**, the rate of cell division in the stratum basale which will supply new cells must increase. New skin cannot regenerate if an injury destroys the stratum basale and its stem cells.

Because skin is constantly being lost it must be replaced. In cellular homeostasis, the rate of skin cell loss should match that of skin cell growth. Skin is constantly being replaced as the top, disposable layer is shedding. In fact, most of what you vacuum in your home is you – your skin and hair!

Destruction of skin leads to wound healing, which is a complex series of physiological events:

Health Connection

Forensic science and the integumentary system

As mentioned previously, at the scene of a crime forensic scientists collect and analyse biological material. The cells they collect contain DNA and each person's DNA is like a fingerprint with unique sequences that identifies the owner. As we shed hair and skin, these are the two main tissues analysed.

- inflammation,
- destruction,
- proliferation and
- maturation.

Skin trauma causes bleeding. During inflammation, which is the body's response to injury, the body is trying to prevent infection and stop bleeding, **haemostasis**. The stages of haemostasis are

- damaged blood vessel walls constrict to restrict supplies to the injured area;
- introduction of clotting proteins to start clotting process;
- fibrin mesh forms over wound trapping blood cells (dries to form a scab – temporary closure);
- initiation of prostaglandin and histamine release, dilation of blood vessels;
- fibrosis – repair by dense connective tissue (scar tissue).

During inflammation the capillaries become very permeable. These changes result in clinical signs such as redness, swelling, heat and pain.

Chapter Reference

Haemostasis and blood are discussed in Chapter 8, 'Transporting' (see p. 205).

During the **destructive phase** (days 1–6 post-trauma) there must be clearing of debris such as dead cells from the wound. This is done by the white blood cells (WBC), especially macrophage cells of the immune system which line the walls of the blood vessels and migrate into tissues to start phagocytosis of debris.

Health Connection

Apoptosis and necrosis

Sometimes cells must die because there are too many of them, and remodelling occurs. This process is called apoptosis, cell suicide. This helps a multicellular organism to work as a community of cells.

Sometimes cells die through lack of nutrients such as in **pressure sores**. This is called necrosis and can leave blackened, infected cells.

Health Connection

Psoriasis and cell over-production

There are several types of psoriasis (pronounced sor-I-A-sis).

In the affected skin new cells are produced at a much faster rate than dead cells are shed and excess skin accumulates to form thick patches. These patches of red, thickened, scaly skin often affect many areas of the body. The cause is unknown but it may be triggered by infection, injury or stress. A genetic factor is suggested as it does run in families. There is no cure, but treatment can relieve symptoms.

During the **proliferative phase** (days 2–24 post-trauma) there is active regeneration and construction of new tissue. Collagen protein from the dermis is formed from fibroblast connective tissue cells. This protein helps to repair and give structure to the skin. New capillaries grow into the wound margin, edge. There is formation of granulation tissue and regeneration of surface epithelium.

New skin cells are formed by stem cells in the lower, basale layers.

During the **maturation phase** (2 days to 2 years post-trauma) the finishing touches to wound healing occur. The wound edges move together through myofibroblast cells causing contraction. Epithelial cells from wound edges, hair follicles and sweat glands migrate over granulation tissue. Macrophages encourage remodelling and reorganisation of collagen. Some cells that are not needed die through the process of **apoptosis**, cell suicide.

Health Connection

Nutrition and wound healing

Vitamin C, iron and protein aid the proliferative phase of wound healing. Poor nutrition decrease wound healing or prolongs wound healing.

Health Connection

The environment and wound healing

Moist environments aid wound healing; hence dressings are chosen to allow moisture, but pressure must be avoided as pressure sores are more likely in moist environments.

Chapter Reference

Stem cells are discussed in Chapter 3, 'Growing and Developing' (see p. 64).

The new cells that are formed are from stem cells in the basale. Growth factors will help to stimulate growth of cells.

Chapter Reference

Growth factors are discussed in Chapter 3, 'Growing and Developing' (see p. 64) and in Chapter 4, 'Communicating' (see p. 102).

Health Connection

Pressure sores or ulcers

Pressure sores are areas of localised damage to the skin and underlying tissue, caused by pressure, sheer or friction. This type of damage is also known as pressure ulcers or bedsores.

When skin is subjected to long-term pressure, such as seen in immobile patients, sores or ulcers can develop. These can progress from affecting the epidermis (stages 1 and 2) to the dermis and to the underlying muscle and bone tissue (stages 3 and 4).

Chapter Reference

Other lifespan changes to our bodies are discussed in Chapter 13, 'Dying' (see p. 340).

Conclusion: Controlling and repairing

The external environment continually challenges us. We must be able to do two things:

- adapt to the external environment;

Health Connection

Bed making

While this may seem a simple act, learning to make a bed correctly for patients who are immobile is vital in reducing pressure sores and the **infections** that often follow on from them.

Health Connection

Leg ulcer

This is a persistent open sore usually on the lower part of the leg. It is more common in the elderly, those with reduced mobility or bedridden. An area of skin breaks down usually as a result of poor circulation and an open sore may then develop. Ulcers are slow to heal, painful and often reoccur. Nine out of ten leg ulcers are due to poor blood supply through the veins and often occur in people with varicose veins. Arterial ulcers develop due to poor blood flow through the arteries supplying the limbs.

- maintain our internal environment within strict ranges.

To do this requires homeostatic mechanisms and communication mechanisms. Our responses must be controlled and appropriate. We must respond to both changes in our internal environment and to any damage.

Chapter Summary

Body temperature

- We maintain our bodies around an optimum temperature of 37°C.
- This is by a homeostatic process called thermoregulation.
- This allows the metabolic processes, particularly enzyme reactions, to be carried out.
- We lose heat to our environment and must generate heat constantly.
- Heat is generated from metabolic reactions.
- Heat is taken from areas of metabolic reactions, cells to the blood and transported around the body.
- Metabolism and thermoregulation are, therefore, interlinked.
- To carry out any homeostatic mechanism requires energy.
- We not only make heat energy but also ATP energy.
- When healthy, feedback by thermoregulatory homeostatic mechanisms can adjust our temperatures and the amount of heat conserved or released during our various activities.
- Vasodilation and vasoconstriction help to regulate our body temperature.
- In extremes of cold temperature heat is sent as a priority to our vital organs.
- Too much heat requires us to cool down. If we don't we are at risk of causing damage to processes and molecules in our bodies. Our proteins, in particular, are damaged by heating.

Cell numbers

- Cells are destroyed and made constantly.
- Stem cells provide new cells through cell division.
- The skin is continually being remade.
- Traumas can increase the need for replacement and repair.

Moving

Chapter Outline

- Introduction: Moving as an activity of daily living
- The environment
- Pressure
- Mobility and movement
- The skeletal system: Bones and joints
- The muscle system
- Energy for movement
- Types of movement
- Changes during lifespan and lifestyle
- Conclusion: Moving
- Chapter summary

> *The great thing in the world is not so much where we stand, as in what direction we are moving.*
>
> **Oliver Wendell Holmes (1809–1894), American physician, professor, lecturer and author**

Introduction: Moving as an activity of daily living

Moving and mobility, the ability to get around, is one of the most essential of all the ADL. It gives us our independence and allows us to maintain our own lives. We are free to put our own food on our own tables, and not be reliant on others. If we lose our ability to move, say by having a broken leg, we can suffer feelings of acute disability; we are dependent on others and unable to carry out our normal activities. We start off in a dependent, immobile state as a baby. As our brains develop so do our muscles and the ability to coordinate our movements increase. Gradually we stand and move, we change from being supine to upright on two legs, *bipedal*, the mark of a human being.

The ability to move independently is one of the basic activities of life. The loss of this ability has severe effects on all the other ADLs. Feeding, washing, socialising, working and sleeping, for example, are all affected and this can have further effects on mental health and emotional well-being.

The environment

The external environment

The environment in which we live is thought of as enabling, it allows us to live. We talk of people who are disabled, unable to function in the environment. However, the environment which we create, our buildings, transport systems and furniture, may be disabling rather than the person being disabled.

Biological environment

We evolved in an environment which required that we find food and shelter. This may have required long treks through the terrain. We therefore relied on being *mobile* to find food and avoid being predated, ending up as something else's lunch.

About 3 million years ago bipedal animals evolved, those able to stand on their two hind limbs rather than on their hind limbs and fore limbs. As we bipedal animals (animals walking

163

on two legs rather than *quadripedal* animals on four legs) have survived there must be some advantages to walking upright. There are also some disadvantages.

Health Connection

The advantages and disadvantages of being bipedal

Advantages include

- the freeing up of the fore limbs as arms and hands to manipulate tools;
- the eyes are higher in a mobile skull allowing longer distance vision.

Disadvantages include

- the problems of getting blood to the brain, against gravity;
- bringing blood back from the lower body to the heart;
- uneven strain on the spinal bones due to uneven weight distribution compared to being on four limbs with an even weight distribution. The vertebrae become more compressed during the day;
- the need for extra muscles to hold organs in place;
- the development of an altered pelvis;
- higher wear and tear on joints due to increased stress and strain compared to distributing weight and movement on four limbs.

Health Connection

Immobility and oedema

When we are immobile our blood circulation is compromised. We especially find it a problem moving blood against gravity, upwards and back to our hearts for movement to our lungs for oxygenation and we find it problematic moving blood from our extremities, especially our legs. Poor circulation can result in oedema, the movement of fluids to tissues and their poor return back into the blood. This is seen as swelling around our feet which look 'puffy'.

Pressure

We increase *pressure* on our legs rather than distribute it on four limbs. Pressure is a measure of a force. We measure it using a scale of newtons (named after the physicist Sir Isaac Newton) applied to an area, in our case an area of our body, measured in metres.

Pressure is defined as force per unit area.

Pressure (Pa) = Force (Newtons)/Area (m^2)

To work out the amount of pressure of a patient lying in a bed we can take the weight of the patient and divide it by the area of the bed. That is because *weight* is, in fact, a force. It relies on our *mass*, measured in kilograms (kg) and the effect of *gravity* on that mass. Gravity is the force that pulls us towards the earth rather than letting us float off into space.

Weight = mass (kg) × gravity (ms^{-2})

We tend to use the term weight when we mean mass. Weight is a force dependent on mass and gravity. Gravity is measured as acceleration in metres per second, in this case, acceleration towards planet Earth, where gravity is 9.8 ms^{-2}. A person of 70 kg has a mass of 70 kg, but their weight is really their mass multiplied by gravity.

In this example weight = mass (70 kg) × gravity (9.8 ms^{-2})

Therefore weight = 686 newtons.

The force of this patient is 686 newtons.

An average bed is 2.0 metres long by 1.32 metres wide, so the surface area is these lengths multiplied together (2m × 1.32m = 2.64 m²).

Surface area = 2.64 m²

Pressure = Force (newtons)/Area (m²)

Here the Pressure is given by the Force (686 newtons) divided by the Area (2.64 m²)

686 newtons (force)/2.64 m²(area) = 260 newtons/m² (pressure)

Health Connection

Pressure sores

A patient lying on a well-constructed bed spreads the force of their body mass over a large area of bed. If the patient is standing up, the same force of body mass is now spread only through a small area, their feet. A badly constructed bed also means that their body mass may not be spread evenly across the bed and **pressure sores** arise.

Health Connection

Weightlessness and physiotherapy

People in weightless conditions, such as away from the Earth's gravity in space, do not put mass onto their legs. When returning from space trips it has been found that the amount of muscle and the strength of the bone are reduced. Both muscle and bone respond to use as part of homeostasis. Lack of use of muscle or bone by being immobilised, such as after a fracture, can lead to further muscle or bone wasting or weakness. Physiotherapy, therapeutic use of physical activity, can help to restore muscle and bone strength in these situations.

Mobility and movement

The three component systems that allow us to move are

1. **the skeleton** – which gives us support and is where muscles are anchored;
2. **the joints** – including ligaments, which allow the skeleton to have some flexibility;
3. **the muscles** – including tendons, which produce the mechanical movements.

The skeletal system: Bones and joints

The skeleton provides a strong, light moveable framework. There are 206 bones in the adult human skeleton. These are classified as either

- **appendicular** or
- **axial**.

The **appendicular** skeleton consists of 126 bones of the upper and lower limbs, the pelvic girdle (hip) and the pectoral girdle (shoulder). The 80 bones of the **axial** skeleton form the axis of the body consisting of the skull, ribcage and spine. Bones are not solid; if they were they would be very heavy to move. Instead they are a mix of materials that maximise strength and minimise weight.

Function of the skeleton

The skeleton is made of a hard substance, **bone**, and gives our basic shape and form. The main functions of the skeleton are to

- allow movement – bones act as levers to move the body. They in turn are moved by muscles;
- support the body – the skeleton provides a hard framework that allows attachment of muscles and organs;
- protect soft organs – e.g. the rib cage protects the organs of the thoracic cavity, the skull encloses the brain, the vertebrae surround the spinal cord;

- store minerals – calcium and phosphate in the matrix of the bone;
- produce blood cells – by a process called haematopoiesis from stem cells in red bone marrow within the cavities of spongy bone in long and flat bones;
- store fat – which acts as an energy reserve in the yellow bone marrow.

The two types of **bone tissue** are

- compact bone and
- cancellous bone.

Compact bone forms a dense outer layer of bone and looks as if it is solid. **Cancellous bone** is spongy and forms the inner layer of bone.

Bone is thus solid on the outside with a spongy interior. This gives the bone strength and lightness (Figure 6.1).

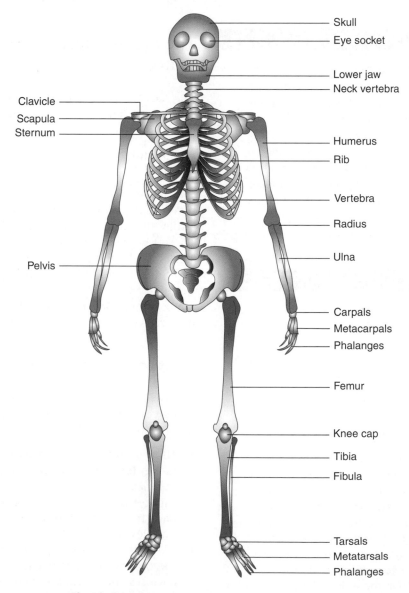

FIGURE 6.1 **The skeleton**

In adults the skeleton is composed of 206 bones arranged as axial or appendicular.

Types of bone

Bones are classified into four types according to their shape and function.

- long bones,
- short bones,
- flat bones and
- irregular bones.

Long bones have a long shaft and a head at each end. They are mostly made of compact bone tissue. The humerus of the arms and the femur of the legs are examples of long bones.

Short bones are roughly cube shaped and made of spongy cancellous bone tissue. Examples of these are the carpals of the wrists and ankles.

Flat bones have a flat shape and are mainly made of spongy cancellous bone tissue between two thin layers of compact bone. Examples of these are the parietal bone of the skull and the ribs.

Irregular bones have a complicated shape, such as that of a butterfly. Examples of these are the vertebrae (back bone) (Figure 6.2).

In a long bone, such as in the leg, the *shaft* of the bone, the long part of the bone, needs to be strong and hollow on the inside. They are made of compact bone tissues on the outside with less dense spongy bone at the ends.

Health Connection

Fractures

A fractured bone causes the severing of blood vessels around the break and the loss of blood. **Haemostasis**, the cessation of blood flow by blood clotting, begins. A clot forms, a fracture haematoma. Phagocytic cells of the immune system (discussed in Chapter 11, 'Cleansing and Dressing') and osteoclast bone cells remove cellular and bony debris. New blood vessels grow (**angiogenesis**) and the haematoma changes into **granulation** tissue. **Fibroblasts** (**connective tissue** cells) lay down collagen fibres across the fracture and **chondroblast** cells produce fibrous cartilage. The broken ends are connected together by this temporary fibrous tissue, **callus**. **Osteoblast** bone cells produce a spongy bone, which is gradually replaced with compact bone.

During the healing process *physiotherapy*, the physical movement of the patient, may be needed to prevent *atrophy*, the wasting and subsequent weakening of muscles.

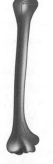 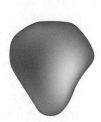 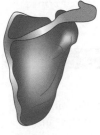 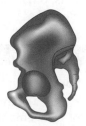

Long bone   Short bone   Flat bone   Irregular bone

FIGURE 6.2 **Types of bones**

The spaces inside the bone are often filled with red bone marrow. In adults this is the site of blood cell production, **haematopoiesis**. The long bones also contain a fatty yellow marrow, which is a store of fat for the body.

The joints

If the bones of the skeleton were fused together in solid joints it would have no flexibility. Instead, where one bone meets another, we have joints. Joints, therefore, allow the skeleton to move.

There are various types of joints that give different amounts of flexibility and therefore, different amounts of movement.

> ### Health Connection
>
> **Dislocation**
>
> A joint is dislocated when the bones are forced out of connection with each other. There may be damage to the ligaments and capsule.

Types of joints

There are three types of joints:

- **fibrous joints** found in the joints of the skull;
- **cartilaginous joints** found in the joints of the vertebrae and pubis;
- **synovial joints** found in the joints of the humerus, ulna, radius and carpal bones.

> ### Health Connection
>
> **Sprains**
> When a joint exceeds its ability of movement the muscles and ligaments over-stretch and the joint becomes damaged in a sprain.

Fibrous joints are joined by connective tissue and no movement is possible, they are fixed.

The ends of bones are **cartilaginous joints** are connected by cartilage. This allows a little movement.

The ends of bones at **synovial joints** are covered by **articular cartilage** (articular as in articulate, the ability to express something, here means the ability to move) which allows the joints to be freely movable (Figure 6.3).

Synovial joints, which are held together by **ligaments**, bundles of collagen protein fibre, are composed of a number of elements allowing movement between two bones:

- **articular cartilage** covers the ends of bones and allows smooth movement. It also acts as a shock absorber;
- **articular capsule** is an outer fibrous connective tissue that strengthens the joint and encloses an inner synovial membrane;
- **synovial fluid** is secreted by the synovial membrane to lubricate the joint. The knee joint contains 3–4 ml of synovial fluid;
- **joint cavity** which is a space containing the synovial fluid;
- **ligaments** which join bone to bone and reinforce the capsule for additional stability.

> ### Health Connection
>
> **Arthritis**
> There are many types of arthritis. In some forms of this disease the cartilage breaks down. This causes the bones to rub together which is painful and restricts movement at that joint.
> **Rheumatoid arthritis** is one form of arthritis. It is an autoimmune disease where the patient's own immune system attacks the joints. The symptoms begin with **bilateral** (both sides) inflammation of certain joints and can often lead to deformities.

Health Connection

Osteoarthritis

There are a variety of conditions called arthritis. Osteoarthritis is the most common form. Its symptoms are inflammation in the joints which results in pain. It is caused by the wearing away of the cartilage that covers the joint and acts as a cushion inside joints. The bone surfaces then become less well protected by cartilage and the patient experiences pain upon weight bearing, including walking and standing. Due to the pain this may result in the patient decreasing the amount of movement or exercise undertaken. Decreased movement can result in regional muscle atrophy, where the muscle reduces in size and loses its ability to function. Ligaments may become more lax.

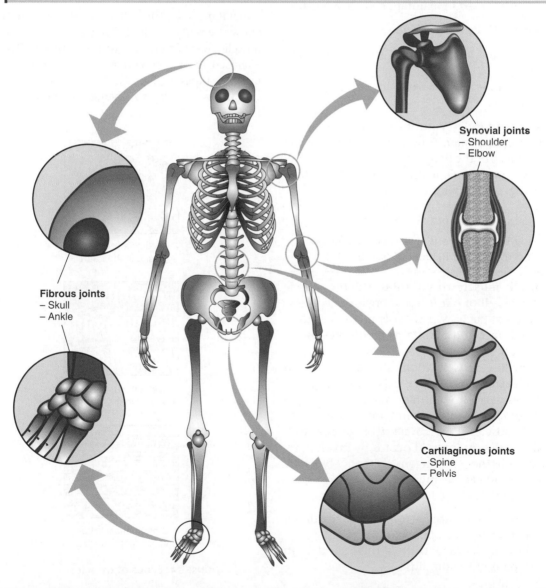

FIGURE 6.3 **Joints. Fibrous, cartilaginous and synovial joints have different properties and are found in different areas of the skeleton**

The muscle system

The main functions of muscles are listed below:

1. muscles contract or shorten causing movement;
2. skeletal muscles attach to bones by
   - tendons, allowing you to walk, leap, grasp, throw a ball or smile;
3. muscles help to maintain posture such as sitting or standing;
4. muscles produce heat during contraction which is used to maintain body temperature.

There are three types of muscle:

- **skeletal** – also known as striated or voluntary;
- **smooth** – also known as involuntary;
- **cardiac**.

Skeletal muscle (voluntary) has a variety of functions. Its main function is to produce the movement of the body and to maintain posture and stabilise joints. It also generates heat whilst moving, which helps to warm our bodies.

Chapter Reference

Body temperature is discussed in Chapter 5, 'Controlling and Repairing' (see p. 142).

Smooth muscle (involuntary) is the muscle that lines all of our internal organs and allows movement such as peristalsis in the gastrointestinal tract and maintains blood pressure in the arteries.

   Cardiac muscle looks similar to skeletal muscle which has stripes, called striations, but behaves as an involuntary muscle. It is a specialised muscle and is found only in the heart

   All muscles allow *movement* of bones in skeletal muscles, of internal organs by involuntary muscles or the pumping movement of blood by the heart in cardiac muscle.

   All muscles have four characteristics:

- they are **excitable** – responding to stimuli such as nervous innervation;
- they are **contractible** – they shorten in response to a stimulus;
- they are **stretchable** – they can lengthen without damage;
- they are **elastic** – they can return to their original shape after contraction or extension (Figure 6.4).

Both cardiac and skeletal muscles are *striated*, have stripes. Cardiac and smooth muscles are involuntary while skeletal muscle is voluntary.

Structure of skeletal muscle

Skeletal muscles, those attached to the skeleton, allow the body to move. They are composed of muscle cells which fuse to form muscle **fibres** enclosed by a connective tissue, **fascia**. Most muscles taper to form an extension of collagen fibres, similar to ligaments found across

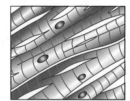

Cardiac muscle cell
(found in the heart)

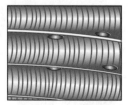

Skeletal muscle cell
(attached to the skeleton)

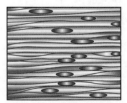

Smooth muscle cell
(found in major organs, such as stomach)

FIGURE 6.4 **Types of muscles**

bones. In muscles these fibres are called **tendons** and attach muscles to bone to produce movement. Skeletal muscles produce movement by crossing a joint, so that when *contraction* takes place one articulating bone is drawn towards another, providing *leverage*.

- the **origin** of a muscle is where it is attached via a tendon to a *stationary* bone;
- the **insertion** of a muscle is where the muscle is attached to a *movable* bone (Figure 6.5).

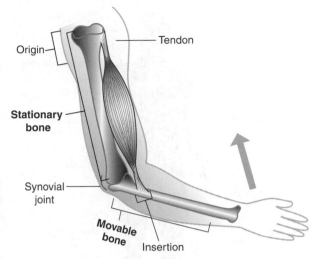

FIGURE 6.5 **Attachment of skeletal muscle to bone to allow movement of the skeleton**

Health Connection

Strains and sprains
- A **sprain** is when a **ligament** is over-extended (over-stretched).
- A **strain** is when a **muscle** is over-stretched.

Skeletal muscle cells fuse together to form muscle tissue which is then surrounded by a connective tissue fascia (meaning bandage) that protects and supports it. Inside the muscle tissue is a blood supply and a nervous supply. The cells of the muscles have many mitochondria as they have a high metabolic rate when contracting using ATP, synthesised in their mitochondria, to produce the energy needed for muscular contraction.

Chapter Reference

ATP is discussed in Chapter 2, 'Working and Playing' (see p. 35).

To make ATP requires oxygen and glucose which are transported in the blood to the muscles. Muscles, therefore, have a rich blood supply.

The muscle cells fuse together to form long **fibrils.** Along the length of the fibril are two types of protein molecules, **actin** and **myosin**. These two proteins are responsible for muscle *contraction*. Contraction is the *shortening* of muscle. This occurs when the actin and myosin molecules slide past each other, using ATP to do so (Figure 6.6).

Health Connection

Intramuscular injection
While intravenous injections get into the blood immediately, intramuscular injections get into the blood quickly due to the rich blood supply of muscles. This affects how fast a drug enters our bodies. Drugs are discussed in Chapter 12, 'Sleeping and Healing'.

There are two types of skeletal muscle fibre:

- extrafusal and
- intrafusal.

Extrafusal muscle fibres are the fibres that bring about *movement* through contraction. **Intrafusal muscle fibres** detect how much the muscle has been *stretched*. When the muscle is stretched intrafusal fibres are also stretched and send messages, electrical impulses, from sensory detectors on the fibres, to the brain. The sensory neuron wraps around the intrafusal muscle to form a **stretch receptor**. This allows feedback to the muscle to increase contraction if needed. This also helps us to know *where* our

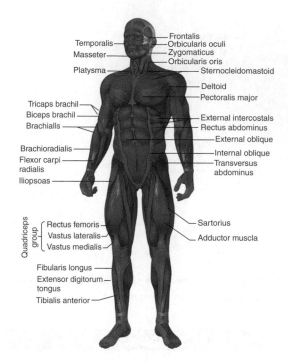
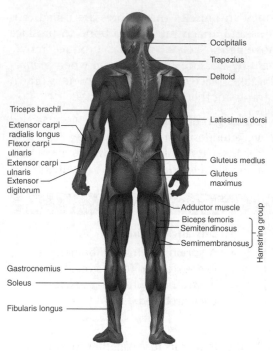
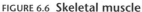

FIGURE 6.6 **Skeletal muscle**

Source: © Sebastian Kaulitzki 2010 / iStockphoto

limbs are in space, a sense called **proprioception.** In the tendon of a muscle is another sensory device, the **Golgi tendon organ** (*not the Golgi organelles found the cells!*), which relays information to the brain about how much stretch there is in a tendon.

> **Chapter Reference**
>
> Sensory and motor neurons are discussed in Chapter 4, 'Communicating' (see p. 102).

When muscles contract they generate heat, which helps to warm the body. If we do not have enough heat, muscles are made to contract without moving the body, *shivering*, to generate more heat.

> **Chapter Reference**
>
> Keeping the body warm is discussed in Chapter 5, 'Controlling and Repairing' (see p. 142).

Skeletal muscles also help blood return to the body, **venous return**, through the milking action they have when they move. Sedentary people have poor blood return to the heart.

> **Chapter Reference**
>
> Blood circulation is discussed in Chapter 8, 'Transporting' (see p. 205).

Skeletal muscles help in moving and in posture, as muscles, even when not contracting, maintain *tone* or firmness.

Muscle contraction

Muscles are excitable tissues. They are excited by action potentials, electrical impulses generated in neurons, cells of the nervous system. An action potential travels in a motor neuron, a neuron whose output is to a muscle; the motor neuron is said to *innervate* the muscle. When

fibres. The muscle fibres that a motor neuron excites are called a **motor unit** (Figure 6.8).

Health Connection

Duchene's muscular dystrophy

This is a genetic disorder (genes are discussed in Chapter 3, 'Growing and Developing'). It is a recessive disorder and is carried on the X chromosome so while females carry the faulty gene they do not suffer from the disorder, while some males receive the faulty maternal gene and tend to suffer from the disorder. It is a degenerative disorder where muscles 'waste' and this leads to loss of ambulatory ability (moving) and death. Symptoms of movement disorders appear in childhood and progress with muscle necrosis and paralysis of the voluntary skeletal muscles and eventually the involuntary muscles. Currently there are no effective treatments although drug trials, gene therapy (replacing the faulty gene) and stem cell therapies are all being trialled.

the electrical impulse in the motor neuron reaches the muscle there is a gap, a synapse, between the motor neuron and the muscle. This synaptic gap is called the neuromuscular junction. At this junction the neurotransmitter chemical **acetylcholine** (ACh) is released into the synapse. This travels to the muscle and binds to ACh receptors on the muscle. This causes excitement in the muscle. The excitement takes the form of a change in electric potential. This activates the muscle to contract, a *twitch* in the muscle fibres where the actin and myosin filaments slide over one another. The movement of the actin and myosin rely on ATP and calcium ions (Ca^{2+}). At the same time ACh is being broken down at the synapse to prevent constant excitation in the muscle, *tetanus* (Figure 6.7).

A muscle is made up of muscle fibres. Each motor neuron excites one or a number of muscle

Motor neurons

Motor neurons are the nervous tissue that takes messages from the brain to the skeletal muscles to innervate the muscles. There are two types of motor neurones:

- alpha motor neurons innervate extrafusal muscle fibres, those that contract to cause movement;
- gamma motor neurons innervate intrafusal muscle fibres, those that detect stretch.

Health Connection

Motor neuron disease

Muscle fibres are innervated, activated, by motor neurons bringing electrical activity to activate them and thus cause contraction diseases, such as motor neuron disease, that disable the motor neuron. This results in muscles not being able to contract.

Chapter Reference

Action potentials and neurotransmitters are discussed in Chapter 4, 'Communicating' (see p. 102).

When the muscle is excited by an action potential in a motor neuron, it contracts.

There are two ways a muscle can contract:

- **isotonic** and
- **isometric**.

In **isotonic** contraction the muscle length shortens while the tension in the muscle remains the same, as in bending your arm or leg.

In **isometric** contraction the muscle length stays the same, but the tension increases, as in adding weights to your arm. Isometric

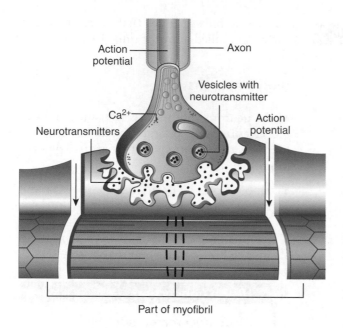

Action potential — Axon

Vesicles with neurotransmitter

Ca^{2+}

Neurotransmitters

Action potential

Part of myofibril

FIGURE 6.7 **Neuro-muscular junction**

contraction uses more energy than isotonic contraction. This is exploited in exercise regimes.

There are two ways to increase the strength of contraction:

- **recruitment** – this is where many motor units are activated in one muscle;
- **frequency** – this is where the frequency of action potentials in a motor unit is increased.

When a single action potential is released, a muscle fibre will twitch. To increase the amount of contraction in a fibre the fibre must be prevented from relaxing between twitches. This is done by increasing the frequency of electrical stimulation along a motor neuron. The muscle contractions are summed together forming a tetanus.

Energy for movement

Energy for muscle contractions

Energy for muscular contraction comes from the breaking of the chemical adenosine tri-phosphate, **ATP**, into adenine di-phosphate, **ADP**, and **phosphate**.

$$ATP \longleftrightarrow ADP + PO_4$$

During this reaction, energy is released and can be used by the body. We do not have a large store of ATP and muscles have only about 4–6 seconds' worth of ATP. Therefore more ATP must be synthesised from ADP and phosphate. There are a number of pathways for synthesising ATP in muscle:

- direct phosphorylation,
- aerobic respiration and
- anaerobic respiration.

Direct phosphorylation

Muscle cells contain another chemical with a high energy phosphate bone: creatine phosphate. Creatine phosphate can transfer its energy to ADP so that it can reform ATP. There are only about 20 seconds' worth of creatine phosphate stored in muscle and hence supplies are exhausted fast.

Aerobic respiration

In aerobic respiration a series of metabolic pathways occurs in the mitochondria where glucose sugar is broken down releasing energy that can be used to synthesise ATP from ADP. The by-products of this reaction are carbon dioxide and water. This is a slower reaction than direct phosphorylation and requires a continuous supply of oxygen.

Anaerobic glycolysis

In anaerobic respiration glucose is broken down to pyruvic acid and during this process energy is released, but without the need for oxygen. The pyruvic acid is then converted to lactic acid. This reaction is not as efficient as aerobic respiration because not as much energy is released, but it is fast. It requires huge amounts of glucose and the by-product, lactic acid, produces muscle fatigue.

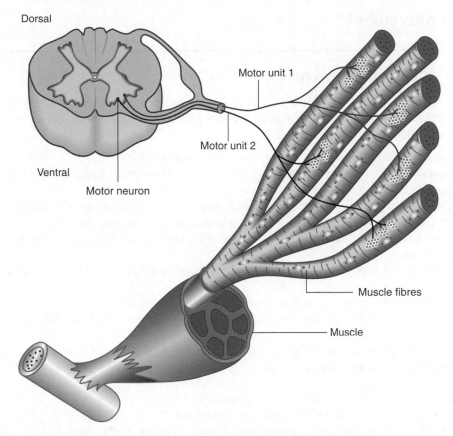

FIGURE 6.8 **Motor units. Each motor unit is composed of a motor neuron and the muscle fibre that it innervates**

Chapter Reference

ATP and metabolism are discussed in Chapter 2, 'Working and Playing' (see p. 35) and in Chapter 5, 'Controlling and Repairing' (see p. 142).

Muscle fatigue

When a muscle is fatigued, it is unable to contract. There are a number of reasons for muscle fatigue:

- oxygen debt,
- lactic acid increase and
- lack of ATP

In oxygen debt the oxygen used in aerobic respiration must be 'repaid' and more oxygen inhaled to remove the debt. Oxygen must be 'repaid' to tissue to remove oxygen debt.

Health Connection

Myasthenia Gravis

This disease is characterised by muscle fatigue. There are a number of possible causes including the possible abnormally high rate of breakdown of ACh or a failure of motor neurons to release sufficient ACh. In fact the main cause seems to be due to loss of ACh receptors on muscle.

Types of movement

Box 6.1 Directions of movement

Our bodies and various parts of it are capable of moving in many directions. These movement directions are brought about by the movement of joints, discussed above. The directions of movements include

- **flexion** – Bending movement that decreases the angle between two parts;
- **extension** – The opposite of flexion; a straightening movement that increases the angle between body parts;
- **hyperextension** – Movement of a body part beyond the normal range of motion;
- **abduction** – A motion that pulls a structure or part away from the midline of the body (or, in the case of fingers and toes, spreading the digits apart, away from the centre line of the hand or foot);
- **adduction** – A motion that pulls a structure or part towards the midline of the body or limb;
- **elevation** – Movement upwards, such as shrugging the shoulders;
- **depression** – Movement downwards, such as dropping the shoulders, the opposite of elevation;
- **pronation** – A rotation of the forearm that moves the palm so that it faces downwards;
- **supination** – The opposite of pronation, the rotation of the forearm so that the palm faces up;
- **dorsiflexion** – Flexion of the entire foot upwards;
- **plantarflexion** – Flexion of the entire foot downwards;
- **protrusion** – The anterior movement of an object. This term is often applied to the jaw;
- **retrusion** – The opposite of protrusion; moving a part backwards;
- **protraction** – Anterior movement of the arms at the shoulders;
- **retraction** – Posterior movement of the arms at the shoulders;
- **rotation** – A motion that occurs when a part turns on its axis. The head rotates on the neck, as in shaking the head to indicate 'no';
- **circumduction** – The circular movement of a body part, e.g. movement of the ball and socket joint by 'windmilling' the arms or rotating the hand from the wrist. Circumduction consists of a combination of flexion, extension, adduction and abduction;
- **opposition** – A motion involving a grasping motion of the thumb and fingers.

During anaerobic respiration lactic acid is a by-product. This increases the acidity of the tissue (the pH decreases). Changes in pH must be opposed by homeostatic mechanisms. Oxygen consumption helps restore the pH and remove the lactic acid. ATP is used up during muscle contraction and its use may outstrip its supply. A lack of ATP causes the muscle to contract less and become fatigued.

The arrangement of muscles

If a skeletal muscle contraction is strong the bone with which it is associated will move. Skeletal muscles are arranged in **antagonistic** pairs, where there is an associated muscle with the opposing effect. For example the biceps flexes the arm (decreasing the angle) while the triceps extends the arm (increasing the angle).

Muscles are attached to at least two points

- Origin – attachment to a movable bone and
- Insertion – attachment to an immovable bone.

Voluntary movement

When we decide to walk or dance, it is just that, a decision. These are made consciously, by our brains. Voluntary movement therefore starts in the brain. There are various areas of the brain that instigate movement. One of them, the **basal ganglia**, initiates action sending action potentials to the motor cortex.

Health Connection

Parkinson's disease

The basal ganglia initiate movement. If it is damaged or degenerates movement Parkinson's disease results. As the cells in the basal ganglia have died, they are not secreting enough of their neurotransmitter, dopamine. Synthetic dopamine, L-dopa that can cross the blood–brain barrier (discussed in Chapter 4 'Communicating'), can be administered to lessen the effects of the disease.

The motor cortex, in the forebrain, receives messages from the basal ganglia and sends electrical messages, action potentials, to specific muscles. It is organised with a representation of the body on it.

The motor cortex sends the action potentials to muscles via two possible routes:

- the brain stem or
- the cerebellum.

The messages are then carried to the spinal cord via pathways called the **cerebrospinal pathways**, where they exit at the appropriate level onto motor neurons that innervate skeletal muscle (Figure 6.9).

Interruption in any of these outputs or pathways will affect motor output and muscle contraction and therefore affect movement.

Reflex movement

Sometimes muscles are affected by a sudden change in environment such as an uneven pavement or a strong gust of wind. These changes alter the stretch in your muscles. We tend to be able to respond to these changes without thinking, a reflex action.

A reflex action can be initiated by a stretch, a stretch reflex. If a weight is added to a bag you are carrying, your arm lowers slightly and then instantly adjusts by using a corrective movement to restore it to its previous position. The additional weight has stretched your muscle. This stretch is detected by stretch receptors in the muscle. The stretch receptors have sensory neurons, neurons that take electrical information from the periphery of our bodies to the central nervous system, which is composed of the spinal cord and the brain. The sensory neuron takes a rapid action potential to the spinal cord. This action potential ends at a synapse. The synapse is directly passed onto a motor neuron, the motor neuron that will take an electrical impulse, action potential, back, in a *reflex arc*, to the muscle that has been stretched. This increases the activity in the motor unit of the motor neuron and the contraction increases, restoring the arm to its previous position. At the same time inhibition is increased in the antagonistic motor neuron and muscle so that it does not oppose the movement. If the stretch was in the biceps, the biceps will be made to contract a bit more, to flex, to counter the new stretch while the triceps will be inhibited from extension. These inputs (detecting the stretch) and outputs (contracting the arm) are organised locally by the spinal cord, without the involvement of the brain. They are thus reflex actions (Figure 6.10).

Reflex type actions are also responsible for rhythmic activities such as walking. Once the brain has decided to move, the actual movement of the limbs can be carried out at the

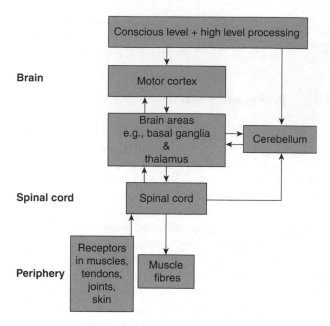

FIGURE 6.9 **Pathway of output of motor innervation**

Health Connection

Spinal injuries

As the motor neurons exit the spinal cord to innervate muscle, any damage to the spinal cord will affect skeletal muscle movement. The level at which the damage is done on the spinal cord will affect how many skeletal muscles are involved. The higher up towards the head that the damage is the less movement of the axial skeleton will be possible due to lack of signals to the muscles. This is due to the arrangement of the motor (and sensory, incoming), outgoing information on our bodies in regions called **dermatomes**, which are then arranged in a topographical order, preserving their place, in each vertebrae. This is discussed in Chapter 4, 'Communicating'.

---

level of the spinal cord without the brain having to 'think', be conscious about each movement. Just as you are not aware of the clothes on your body the whole time, you do not want to use high brain functions to carry out rhythmic activities. The spinal cord can act as a *pattern generator* controlling many *rhythmic* functions.

Nociceptive movements

As with the reflex action above, if we put our hands on a very hot dish we encounter an environment that can cause tissue damage in the form of burns. We have receptors that are tuned to extreme environments that can cause damage, called nociceptors that react to noxious stimuli. We move our hands away very fast in a reflex action. While this too can be thought of as a reflex action, the brain is informed of these changes and can inhibit them. If, for example, you stand on a very sharp rock, you may rush to remove your foot from it, but if you are on the edge of a cliff you may not be able to without falling off and dying! Your brain assesses the situation and stops the reflex action, moments after you reflexively start to lift your foot up. We take in information about our environment constantly, monitoring it and effecting actions that aid our survival. Just think of all the things you do before you cross a road and how when you have stepped off the pavement you can stop yourself if a car suddenly appears.

Posture and balance

Most of the time we maintain our posture without thinking about it. We have postural reflexes, similar to reflexes mentioned above that keep us in position. If we are standing on a train that suddenly moves we tilt backwards due to inertia, but then correct ourselves instantly. Our postural reflexes are constantly adjusting the tension in our muscles to maintain our position. It is aided by the *balance* mechanism in our ears discussed in Chapter 4, 'Communicating'.

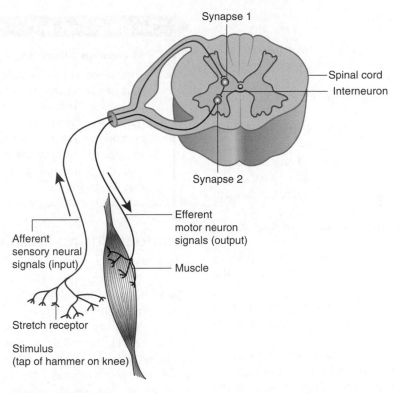

FIGURE 6.10 **Reflex arc**

Bad posture

Bad posture can be caused by

- poor sitting or standing habits,
- muscles that are weak due to lack of exercise,
- tight clothing,
- incorrect footwear and
- obesity and pregnancy– the extra weight pulls on the vertebral column and strains the back muscles

The consequences of bad posture can be:

- fatigue,
- backache,
- respiratory inefficiency,
- digestive problems,
- circulatory problems including varicose veins and
- lymphatic system inefficiency.

Moving forward

Putting all the processes together in voluntary movement relies on many complex interactions.

As an example, to move towards a place:

- one is already motivated to move towards this place;
- senses (sight) have detected the place and sent messages to the sensory parts of the brain detecting that the place is within range;
- the brain sends messages to the motor cortex;
- the motor cortex sends motor outputs to the spinal cord and to motor neurons in the legs;
- these motor outputs then synapse onto leg muscles causing them to contract and lift the leg up;
- a reflex action of balance and posture in other muscles and inhibitory messages to the other leg prevent falling over or lifting both legs at the same time;
- the leg is stretched out and the antagonistic muscles contract, by the same processes described, to bring the leg back down;
- stretch receptors feed back information that the leg has been stretched as part of the sense of proprioception and adjustments can be made if it is not appropriate;
- all of these actions are repeated in the other leg to move forward;
- messages are sent from the cerebellum controlling rhythmic movement and from the spinal cord for reflex actions and forward movement is generated until messages are sent to stop;
- all of this occurs so rapidly (and adjustments can be made for the slope of the terrain) that you are not aware of these processes. You are only aware of the processes when they do not occur!

> **Health Connection**
>
> **Movement disorders**
> This covers a wide range of disorders that can affect any part of the motor pathways, muscles and nervous tissue described here. Knowing how complex movement is may help us to understand how these pathways can be disrupted and cause an inability to move.

Changes during lifespan and lifestyle

The skeleton of an embryo is made mainly of cartilage, a connective tissue. This is a flexible tissue, but strong enough to cope with mechanical stress. The cartilage is gradually replaced by bone, a hard, connective tissue. The bone is formed by cells called osteoblasts. These cells secrete collagen protein which forms a fibrous framework. Into the gaps in the framework the mineral salts calcium and magnesium and phosphates are deposited. The salts make the bone hard (**calcification**) while the collagen makes bone able to bend slightly. The osteoblasts mature into osteoclasts which, although incapable of cell division, maintain compact bone by releasing calcium ions into the tissue. Rapid growth in height is due to increase in bone length by progressive calcification of cartilage. This cartilage is continually produced at the bone ends or joints, called **epiphyseal plates**. By the age of 16–20 humans cease growing taller as the epiphyseal plates become solid bone. All of the cartilage of the early skeleton is replaced with bone apart from where one bone moves against another, a **joint**. Cartilage remains in isolated areas such as the bridge of the nose and parts of rib. Bones are continually remodelled and lengthened until growth stops.

Growth hormone (GH)

If there is lack of growth in height **growth hormone**, produced normally from the pituitary gland (discussed in Chapter 4, 'Communicating'), may be administered to a child. This stimulates body tissues to divide and to absorb amino acids, used in protein formation. GH helps the breakdown of lipid stores in adipose tissue to provide cells with energy. The hormone appears to work by stimulating the liver to produce small protein molecules, insulin-like growth factors (IGF), which stimulate the growth of bone, cartilage and adipose tissue.

Fractures in the young and old

Fracture in the young may result in 'greenstick' fractures, like a young plant stem splitting. This is because the bones of children are not fully calcified and are quite soft. Healing is quite rapid in the young.

As we age, healing of bones slows down. This can be due to various reasons such as the reduced ability for repair of tissues or a poor blood supply.

Muscle degeneration

Muscles do not divide once they have grown. They can increase or decrease in size through activity (exercise). As we age we lose muscle mass. This can affect our strength, the ability to lift items for example. It also affects involuntary muscle and cardiac muscle, all of which weaken during ageing. Ageing will be discussed further in Chapter 13, 'Dying'.

During life, osteoblasts make new bone while osteoclasts engulf fragments of bone and break them down with the powerful **lysosomes** they contain in their cytoplasm. Bone, which is hard and rigid, is constantly worn down through life. Osteoclasts are responsible for the remodelling of bone, replacing old bone with new bone.

As we age there is a decrease in **muscle mass** and strength and a **demineralisation** (loss of mineral salts such as calcium and phosphate) from the bones. Our gait may become altered and thus our balance, posture and movement become impaired. We become susceptible to *falls*.

Hip replacement

Joints last a lifetime. If they break down, movement becomes restricted and painful. Artificial joints may be used to replace worn-out joints, such as hip replacements.

The amount of time we are mobile and the amount of time we are sedentary affects our muscle mass, the flexibility of our joints and the weight-bearing ability of our skeletons.

The consequences of immobility can include

- muscle weakness/wasting – *atrophy*,
- joint stiffness,
- chest infection,
- circulatory disorders,
- deep vein thrombosis and
- constipation.

Our circulatory system relies on our mobility to help 'milk' the blood in the veins between the skeletal muscles aiding the return of blood to the heart – venous return. Without this we can suffer from circulatory disorders and oedemas in the lower limbs (discussed in Chapter 7, 'Breathing').

While our gastrointestinal tract has smooth muscle aiding **peristalsis**, the muscular waves of contraction along the tract that help to move the food forward, the 'milking' action of our skeletal muscles in our abdomen, also helps. Sedentary people may suffer from constipation due to the lack of onward movement of faeces towards the rectum (discussed in Chapter 9, 'Eating and Drinking').

Health Connection

Obesity

With increasing body mass the force we put on our legs increases. If we have too great a force our legs cannot resist the force and can no longer hold us up. With increasing obesity the patient can end up immobilised. The lack of movement will further reduce the body's metabolic rate, so food will be stored as fat, increasing the body mass and further reducing mobility.

Health Connection

Manual handling

Manual handling is any activity involving the use of muscular force (or effort) to lift, move, push, pull, carry, hold or restrain any object, including a person or animal.

A number of activities can affect skeletal muscles, tendons and ligaments causing postural changes and pain, which can result in damage such as strains and sprains. Manual handling activities include

- repetitive activity seen in assembly work;
- sustained muscle exertion required to restrain or support a load;
- the effort needed to maintain the fixed postures that occur in the back and neck while typing.

When moving loads one needs to assess the

- *risk* that moving the load entails;
- *task* that needs to be done;
- *environment* in which the load and those that move it are in;
- *ability* of those that are required to move the load.

Increasingly the workplace is being designed to be **ergonomic**, applying scientific information concerning humans to the design of the environment and the objects in it.

Conclusion: Moving

Our skeletal bones provide support and protection for our internal organs and also provide anchorage, via tendons for muscles. It is muscles that allow us to be mobile and move ourselves around our external environment. Muscles, in turn, must be innervated by our nervous system. Our nervous system monitors our internal and external environments and sends messages to output effectors such as glands and muscles to change what we are doing or where we are. Muscles, therefore, are linked to homeostasis ensuring that our movements aid the maintenance of our internal environment (involuntary muscles) and move us around, as appropriate, our external environment (voluntary muscles) in response to signals from our nervous system. Damage to muscles or to our nervous system has an impact on our ability to move and this therefore has an impact on our health.

Chapter Summary

- The ability to move relies on many body systems including the muscular, skeletal and nervous systems.
- Skeletal muscle is under voluntary control and moves us in our external environment.
- Smooth muscle is under involuntary control and moves the muscles around our internal organs such as gastrointestinal tract and blood vessels and thus moves substances through these organs.
- Skeletal muscles are attached, via tendons, to bones of the skeleton.
- Bones are attached to each other via ligaments.
- Muscle movement requires energy, ATP, and produces heat as a by-product.

7 Breathing

CHAPTER

Then the Lord formed man of the dust of the ground and breathed life into his nostrils, the breath of life; and man became a living soul.

Torah, Bereshis (Genesis) II, 7

Chapter Outline

- Introduction: Breathing as an activity of daily living
- The environment
- The respiratory (pulmonary) system
- Changes during lifespan and lifestyle
- Conclusion: Breathing
- Chapter summary

Introduction: Breathing as an activity of daily living

From the first breath a baby takes, sometimes encouraged by a slap from the midwife, to our very last dying breath, the act of breathing defines for many of us the most basic aspect of being alive. The first question we ask in an acute situation is 'Are they breathing?'

We have all had the sensation of being 'out of breath' after exercise, finding it hard to 'catch our breath'. We may feel panicked by not being able to get enough air into our bodies. Sometimes we may *hyperventilate* (breath too much) leaving us feeling light-headed.

The environment

Our internal environment: Why we breathe

Every cell of our body requires energy to survive. Without energy all the complex processes occurring inside us cease and our chemical and physical structures unravel. It takes a lot of energy to keep us alive each day, around 2000 kilocalories.

We are composed of 10^{13} cells, each of which uses energy in the form of ATP in its

Chapter Reference

Calories are discussed in Chapter 9, 'Eating and Drinking' (see p. 241). Energy and ATP are discussed in Chapter 2, 'Working and Playing' (see p. 35).

daily metabolic processes. ATP is constantly being used; we have some 90 seconds' store of ATP in our body. Each cell therefore must constantly make ATP energy to replenish the ATP that it uses. Energy is made in the mitochondria of cells, small organelles often called the powerhouse of the cell. Energy is released by chemical reactions. In this case ATP energy is synthesised in the mitochondria by a chemical reaction that oxidises glucose. Oxidising glucose means that every cell requires a constant supply of both reagents, oxygen and glucose. The glucose is extracted from the food we eat and digest. The oxygen is extracted from air we breathe.

The glucose from food is extracted in our digestive tract. The oxygen from air is extracted in our lungs. Oxygen and glucose are collected into our blood and transported to every cell of our body. This transport relies on the cardiovascular system. Somehow, we have to

184

- get air to move from our surroundings into a collecting area inside of us, our lungs;
- extract the oxygen from the air collected in our lungs;
- transport the oxygen from our lungs into our blood;
- transport this oxygen in the blood to our cells;
- diffuse the oxygen from our blood into our cells;
- diffuse any waste gas from our cells into our blood;
- transport any waste gas in our blood back to our lungs;
- diffuse the waste gas from our blood into our lungs;
- expel any waste gases and air we do not need back into the external environment.

The act of breathing

Breathing, also known as *ventilation*, is the act of taking air into and out of our **lungs.** The process of getting air into our lungs is known as inhalation or inspiration. The process of expelling air out of our lungs into the external environment is known as exhalation or expiration.

Once the air is in the lungs it must diffuse into the blood and waste gases must diffuse out of the blood into the lungs. This process is called **gas exchange**, as one gas, that coming in, is exchanged for the gas going out. While ventilation, the movement of air in and out, occurs in the lungs, the whole act of breathing, ventilation and gas exchange, occurs in the **respiratory system**, comprising the passageways that the air travels in and out of the lungs, the lungs, the muscles that allow the lungs to expand and relax and the blood supply around the lungs.

The act of breathing is divided into two phases,

1. **external respiration** – getting gases from the lungs to the blood and waste gases from the blood to the lungs, getting air into and out of the lungs;

2. **internal respiration** – getting gases from the blood to the cells and waste from the cells to the blood.

In some more biochemical textbooks there is also a third respiration – **cellular respiration**. This is the enzymatic breakdown of glucose in the cytoplasm of the cell and the metabolism of the products of this with oxygen in the mitochondria of the cell. This is discussed further in Chapter 9, 'Eating and Drinking'.

What happens if breathing ceases

The cells of our body are continually using ATP as energy for movement, cell metabolism, growth, repair and transport. Without energy our cells cannot perform these basic functions that are part of living processes and they die. Without oxygen our cells cannot make ATP and death soon occurs. Our brains are very active, using 20% of the energy we synthesise. Our brains therefore require a constant supply of oxygen and glucose to make ATP. We can store surplus glucose as glycogen or fat. We cannot store oxygen so we must have a constant supply of it. This explains why cessation of breathing and therefore the supply of oxygen can very soon result in brain cells dying, brain death and, as the brain is the centre of homeostasis, the death of the entire person.

Chapter Reference

Chapter 2, 'Working and Playing' and Chapter 4, 'Communicating', explain the high energy needs of the brain maintaining the resting potential of neurons by means of the sodium-potassium pump (see pp. 35 and 102). Chapter 13, 'Dying', looks at various causes of death (see p. 340).

During the making of ATP in the cells waste products are also formed which must be eliminated from the cells and from the body. If they are not removed they build up to toxic concentrations. Some of the waste products are gases, that is carbon dioxide (CO_2) which is also transported away from the cells in the blood and back to the lungs where it is **exhaled** during breathing out. The other waste product is water (H_2O), which is transported away from cells by the blood to the kidneys for expulsion.

GLUCOSE (from food) + OXYGEN (from air) = ATP (energy) + CO_2 + H_2O (waste products)

To understand the importance of the activity of breathing and the effects of problems in breathing and delivering oxygen to cells, we must look at three interrelated systems:

- the respiratory system, consisting of lungs and airways;
- the transport system, consisting of the blood and lymph;
- the cardiovascular system, consisting of the heart and blood vessels.

In this chapter we shall consider the respiratory system. The blood, lymph and cardiovascular systems are discussed in Chapter 8, 'Transporting'.

The external environment in which we breathe

We humans live in a gaseous environment. There are various gases in the air that surround us. Nitrogen (N), usually in the form of a diatomic molecule, N_2, accounts for 80% of the gas in air. Other gases include oxygen (O) usually in the form of a diatomic molecule, O_2, argon (A), and carbon (C) which is found bound to oxygen as carbon dioxide (CO_2) and a small amount bound to oxygen as carbon monoxide (CO). The air that surrounds us also contains other elements in small amounts.

Chapter Reference

Molecules are discussed in Chapter 2, 'Working and Playing' (see p. 35).

While oxygen is one of the most abundant elements on this planet occurring usually in combination with other elements such as hydrogen in water, it accounts for only about 20% in air. It may seem strange therefore that oxygen is the substance in air that we require for our living processes rather than the more abundant gas, nitrogen. Oxygen has many chemical properties that make it ideal for how it is used in metabolic processes by living organisms and biology rests on the link between anatomy, what things are made of, and physiology, what things do. Some introduction and explanation of the properties of oxygen is given in Chapter 2, 'Working and Playing'. In water there is even more of a problem obtaining oxygen as it is in even lower concentration than in air. This is partly why we cannot breathe under water; we cannot extract the breathable oxygen at the concentration it exists dissolved in water. Obviously fish can live at this lower concentration of oxygen and this demonstrates how organisms are adapted to the environment in which they live. High concentrations of oxygen for prolonged periods are dangerous. While it may be needed medically to administer oxygen when our respiratory system is compromised, this tends to be a temporary solution.

As we have said above, air, and the gas we need from it, oxygen, exists in our gaseous surroundings and is affected by events in the external environment. These events include pressure, climate and pollution.

Pressure

We may not be able to see the molecules of gases in the air but we can feel them as *air pressure*, the resistance to our movement.

Pressure is something that many people find hard to imagine. If you push your right hand onto your left arm you are exerting pressure on your arm. Because you can feel it you may find it easier to understand. On this planet the atmosphere, composed of air, is pressing against you. We are not very sensitive to it, but it holds us back at sea level when we are running, but at high altitude, where the air is 'thinner', the pressure is less and as we run our bodies meet less resistance from air pressure. At high altitude there is less air and less air pressure on us reducing resistance. Conversely, there is less available oxygen making breathing more laboured.

Pressure, measured in a unit called a Pascal (Pa), is the force, measured in units called newtons, per unit area, measured in metres squared:

Pressure (Pa) = Force (newtons)/Area (m²)

Forces are influences that move free bodies such as air or you. They are usually perceived as pushing or pulling a body.

Chapter Reference

Force and Pressure and its measurement are discussed in Chapter 6, 'Moving' (see p. 163). Pressure and its measurement in blood vessels, blood pressure, is discussed in Chapter 8, 'Transporting' (see p. 205).

Our bodies are subject to a constant pressure, called atmospheric pressure. This pressure is measured in Standard International units (**SI**) called kilo Pascal or in older units on a barometer using a scale of millimetres that mercury travels up a *tube*. Atmospheric pressure on our bodies is about 100 kPa in SI units or 760 mmHg in old units. This is due to the weight of air above any point on the surface of the Earth. As one goes higher (increase of altitude) there is less weight of air above us or less atmospheric pressure above us. Atmospheric pressure varies with weather conditions and can be measured by a barometer. Water vapour can contribute to atmospheric pressure. Dry air has little water pressure adding to the total atmospheric pressure. Each gas in dry air contributes pressure according to its partial pressure. This is important in medical settings where air or oxygen may be delivered as a dry gas and need to have moisture added to it.

Partial pressure is a measure of the concentration of a gas in a mixture of gases. It is measured in millimetres (mm) of mercury (Hg) in an apparatus similar to that which measures blood pressure, a barometer (Table 7.1).

Health Connection

Pressure

Various types of pressure measurements are made in clinical settings. Blood pressure is one example and is discussed in Chapter 8, 'Transporting'. A barometer with a scale in millimetres is used as a standard to compare.

Chapter Reference

The variation in oxygen levels may be exploited in sports training. This is discussed in later in Lifestyle (see p. 201).

Table 7.1 Partial pressures and constituents' of gases in air

Gas	Partial pressure of air	%
CO_2	0.3 mmHg	1%
O_2	159 mmHg	21%
N_2	593 mmHg	78%
Total	760 mmHg	0%

Climate

While our body temperature is maintained at 37°C, air temperature varies. Air frequently needs warming before being transported in the blood.

Air is usually quite dry and may need to have moisture added to allow diffusion from the lungs to the blood to occur.

Health Connection

Oxygen

Oxygen is delivered to hospitals in canisters. The pressure of the oxygen delivered to the patient must be carefully monitored to avoid having such high pressure that it damages the lungs. The oxygen is also moistened.

How warming and moistening of air is done is discussed below.

Dust and other pollutants in air

Air may be polluted with small particles and need *filtering* to remove debris and micro-organisms before entering the blood. We have various points of entry and the nose and mouth are lined with cells are at the interface between our internal environment and the external world. These cells have special properties which help to filter debris from the atmosphere and will be discussed in the respiratory section below.

Health Connection

Caution: Oxygen

Oxygen, while vital for the process of making energy in cells, is also a very **reactive chemical** and can cause **damage** to cells and the environment. Oxygen is needed in certain concentrations in the body, but too much oxygen is also dangerous. The use of oxygen by health professionals must be monitored carefully.

Oxygen is a colourless, odourless gas. Oxygen does not burn, but it can support **combustion**. When this occurs oxygen combines to make oxides and heat, light (flame) and other products such as carbon dioxide are released.

Oxygen can be toxic to cells in high concentrations for prolonged periods or at high pressure. Oxygen tanks can release oxygen under high pressure and this must be avoided when delivering oxygen to patients.

Oxygen delivery can also cause damage by drying the moist mucosal membranes (see below) and the oxygen supply may need to be moistened.

Chapter Reference

Micro-organisms are discussed in Chapter 11, 'Cleansing and Dressing' (see p. 299).

Box 7.1 Summary – Breathing

- Breathing brings gases, air, to the lungs for respiration.
- Respiration is the exchange of gases between the environment and the lungs, the lungs and the blood and the blood and the tissues.
- Oxygen is extracted from air in the lungs and transported to the cells to combine with glucose to make energy, ATP.
- Waste products, carbon dioxide and water are also formed in this metabolic process by each cell and must be removed.
- Breathing thus combines the respiratory, transport and circulatory systems to supply cells with a constant source of oxygen and to remove waste products.

The respiratory (pulmonary) system

Each day, we inhale and exhale some 20,000 times taking in 10,000 litres of air. The air we inhale must be filtered from pollutants, warmed to body temperature and moistened for gaseous diffusion; the oxygen is extracted and diffused into our blood while the waste must be removed and exhaled. The movement of oxygen from the air to the body requires the respiratory, blood and cardiovascular systems. In this chapter the respiratory system is discussed. The respiratory system is part of the **pulmonary system** of the cardiovascular system discussed in Chapter 8, 'Transporting'.

The constituents of the respiratory system

The constituents of the respiratory system are

- the upper respiratory tract or **conducting zone** – the areas or passageways through which air passes on its way to the respiratory zone;
- The lungs or **respiratory zone** – a collecting and diffusing area for **gas exchange** (Figure 7.1).

The upper respiratory tract or collecting zone

The passage of air from the environment to our lungs

Air passes from the external environment into our **lungs** through a series of **tubes** or **tract**. This tract starts in our head and continues into our **thoracic cavity** where our lungs are situated.

The tract consists of

- **nasal passage (nose) or mouth,**
- **conchae,**
- **pharynx,**
- **larynx,**
- **epiglottis,**
- **trachea,**
- **bronchi,**
- **bronchioles,**
- **lungs** and
- **alveoli.**

Air passes through our nasal passage, past our conchae into the pharynx, which is shared with the food passageway into the gastrointestinal (GI) tract. The passageways then separate and the air enters the larynx, past the vocal cords, into the trachea. After this the air enters the

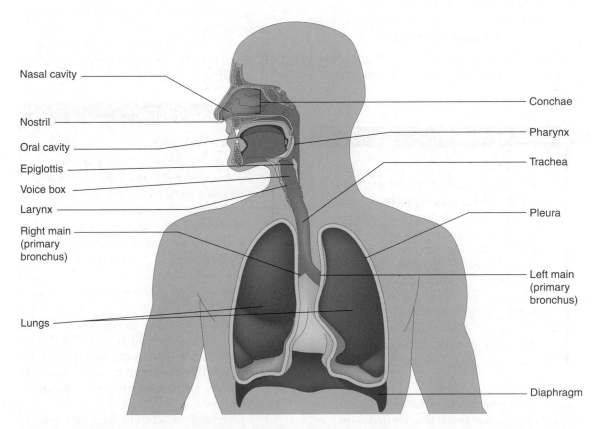

Nasal cavity

Nostril

Oral cavity

Epiglottis

Voice box

Larynx

Right main (primary bronchus)

Lungs

Conchae

Pharynx

Trachea

Pleura

Left main (primary bronchus)

Diaphragm

FIGURE 7.1 **The organs of the respiratory system**

lower tract, the right and left bronchi for the right and left lungs.

The nose is the only visible part of the respiratory system. It is composed of nostrils, which consists of a nasal cavity divided in two by a **septum**. The roof of the cavity is bony; the floor of the cavity is shared with the roof of the mouth and has hard palate in front and soft palate behind.

The nasal cavity is lined with **ciliated columnar epithelium**, a tissue type that forms linings and secretary glands to many cavities. The cilia are small hairs on the epithelial cells. Mucus is a sticky watery substance. The layer of epithelium in the nasal cavity forms a mucous membrane containing mucus-secreting cells (**goblet cells**). These are exocrine glands formed from one type of secretary tissue. There are also hairs in the anterior (front) end of the nasal cavity. There are also sinuses, cavities in the bone containing air, also lined with mucous membrane.

Chapter Reference

Epithelial cells and glands are discussed in Chapter 1, 'Maintaining a Safe Environment' (see p. 1).

Health Connection

Sinusitis

The sinuses lighten the skull. They are air filled spaces within the bones of the skull. The sinuses are joined to the nasal cavity via small orifices called ostia. These become blocked relatively easily by allergic inflammation, or by swelling in the nasal lining which occurs with a cold. If this happens, normal drainage of mucus within the sinuses is disrupted, and sinusitis may occur.

The mucosal layer is very moist. It is also sticky. Inside the nose are projections called **conchae**, which increase the *surface area* of the nasal

cavity and increase turbulence of the inhaled air. This allows a greater deflection of air, and thus any polluting particles to be caught on the sticky mucous.

The nasal cavity is very *vascular* (it has many fine blood vessels). Blood carries heat from the muscles of the body. The fine blood vessels in the nose can thus warm the air.

The nose is also lined with sense receptors that detect odorous chemicals giving us our sense of smell.

Chapter Reference

Senses are discussed in Chapter 4, 'Communicating' (see p. 102).

The anatomy of the nose and the whole upper respiratory tract prepares air for its entry into lungs. It does this in three ways:

1. warms air by the blood supply around the nose and tract;
2. moistens air by the mucus secretions;
3. filters air by the mucous membranes and cilia that trap debris.

Health Connection

Smell and colds

When we have a cold our sense of smell is diminished by the thick covering of mucous over our sense receptors. The mucous increases in the first line of defence of the immune response discussed further in Chapter 11, 'Cleansing and Dressing'.

Once the air has passed through the nostrils it reaches an area at the back of our throats consisting of a tube called the **pharynx**. From there it passes into the **larynx**. The tubes of the pharynx and larynx are shared with the digestive system.

The pharynx is 12–14 cm long and consists of three areas:

- the **nasopharynx**, closest to the nasal cavity;
- the **oropharynx**, closest to the oral cavity;
- the **laryngopharynx**, closest to the larynx.

In the nasopharynx are openings, **auditory tubes**, into the middle ear. On the posterior wall there are **pharyngeal tonsils** at the back of the nasopharynx. Tonsils are part of the immune system being composed of lymphoid tissue, a type of tissue in the immune system discussed in Chapter 11, 'Cleansing and Dressing'.

Chapter Reference

The pharynx, larynx and swallowing food are discussed in Chapter 9, 'Eating and Drinking' (see p. 241).

The oropharynx lies behind the mouth and contains the **palatine tonsils**, also part of the immune system. The nasopharynx and oropharynx are separated by the **soft palate** and **uvula**.

The laryngopharynx continues into the larynx.

At the larynx the tube separates. One tube goes into the **oesophagus**, which passes food into the gastrointestinal tract. The other tube goes into the **trachea** (windpipe) which allows air to enter the respiratory system. There is a flap, the **epiglottis**, that covers the trachea when food is swallowed. This is to prevent food entering the trachea blocking the trachea and preventing air passing along it. During swallowing, the larynx moves upwards and the epiglottis closes over it. The only passage left open is then the oesophagus that leads into the stomach. The epiglottis is a leaf-shaped cartilage covered with stratified epithelium and acts as a lid over the larynx preventing food entering the trachea.

The pharynx has a mucosal lining as well as fibrous tissue and muscle tissue which help in swallowing by moistening food.

The tubes of the larynx consist of cartilage, ligaments and membranes connecting the cartilaginous tissue to the hyoid bone. The larynx contains the **voice-box** and is, therefore, involved in the production of sound. Sound is produced by the movement of air over vocal cords contained in the voice-box. The vocal cords are two folds of mucous membrane with free cord-like structures. Muscles around the cord can constrict or relax altering the length of the cord and changing the pitch and volume of the sound made.

Health Connection

Caution: Blockage – food going down the wrong way

We have all had food go 'down the wrong way' which it literally does, by going down into the trachea instead of the oesophagus. Coughing is a **reflex action** that helps to bring the food particles back up to the larynx for swallowing into the oesophagus and thus freeing up the trachea for the passage of air. Occasionally coughing does not free the food. The Heimlich manoeuvre, where a jolt to the diaphragm helps to increase pressure and free the food, may be needed.

The **trachea** is a tube of about 10 cm in length and about 1.8 cm in diameter. It is made of connective tissue and smooth, involuntary muscle. Unlike the oesophagus which is pushed open as food passes down, the usual movement of air will not open the trachea which must, therefore, be held open by 16–20 C-shaped rings of hyaline cartilage. The trachea is lined with ciliated epithelium. The **cilia** (little hairs) help to transport mucous and trapped particles upwards to the epiglottis for swallowing.

Once air has passed into the trachea it then separates into two tubes:

- a **left bronchi** which takes air into the left lung;
- a **right bronchi** which takes the air into the right lung.

The two lungs are sac-like structures covered in membranes called **pleura**. The two bronchi pass into the lungs where they gradually become narrower and branch out into multiple, **bronchioles** – little bronchi, dispersing the air into finer and finer tubes.

The **bronchi** consist of the same tissue as the trachea and, like the trachea, are lined with ciliated epithelium. Each bronchus divides into two smaller tubes which each divide a further 15 times into increasingly smaller tubes.

The bronchi and bronchioles are part of the **conducting zone**, the zone or area that moves air from the external environment, through the passageways to the lungs.

Terminal bronchi divide seven times into **respiratory bronchioles**. The tubes end in the **functional** part of the lungs, the **alveoli**, small sacs.

Air, which has been warmed, moistened and filtered in the conducting zone, passes from the trachea into the bronchi and then into a series of finer tubes, the bronchioles. The air then enters the respiratory zone and into the alveoli for gas exchange. The alveoli (plural; alveolus – singular) are very thin sacs of epithelia surrounded by pulmonary capillaries (Figure 7.2).

The respiratory zone

Gas exchange occurs in the **respiratory zone**, which consists of

- respiratory bronchioles,
- alveolar ducts and
- alveoli.

The walls of the bronchioles become thinner losing their muscular and fibrous walls as they divide into smaller and smaller tubes ending in tiny sac-like alveoli. The **alveoli** are very thin sacs formed of **epithelial tissue** with no muscle or fibrous tissue and are surrounded by blood vessels called **pulmonary capillaries** which are also very fine. The area of the alveoli and the pulmonary capillary is called the **respiratory membrane**. The alveoli are kept moist to allow gas exchange by *diffusion* (Figure 7.3).

The alveoli are composed of epithelial cells. They are surrounded by pulmonary capillaries, which are also composed of epithelial cells. Between these epithelial cells is basement membrane sticking the thin epithelial layers together. Due to the thinness gases can exchange from and to the blood and from and to the alveoli. Gas exchange is discussed below.

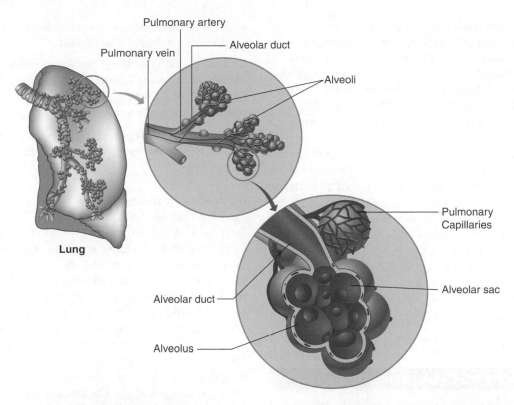

FIGURE 7.2 **The respiratory zone**

Chronic obstructive pulmonary disorder (COPD)

The respiratory system is part of the pulmonary system. Chronic obstructive pulmonary disorder – COPD – is exemplified by two major conditions:

- **chronic bronchitis** – affecting the bronchioles (discussed above);
- **emphysema** – affecting the alveoli (discussed below).

With both conditions breathing becomes more difficult, laboured (**dyspnea**) and becomes progressively more severe with retention of carbon dioxide in the blood. This leads to hypoxia and respiratory acidosis – discussed below.

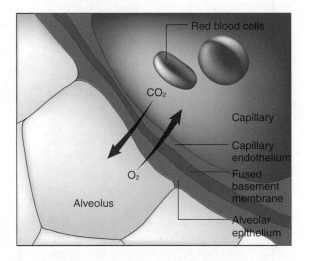

FIGURE 7.3 **The respiratory membrane**

How we get air into our lungs

The lungs are contained in the **thoracic cavity** (chest) consisting of the chest wall, ribcage and **sternum** (breastbone). The thoracic cavity is separated from the abdominal cavity by a large dome-shaped muscle, the **diaphragm.** The lungs and chest wall consist of **elastic tissue.**

Around the outside of our lungs are membranes, **pleural membranes**, with **pleural fluid** between them. There are two membranes, the visceral membrane lining the outside of our lungs and the parietal membrane lining the chest wall. These two membranes are held together by surface tension formed by the pleural fluid in the same way that two sheets of glass can be held together by a film of water between them. The pleura protect the lungs, allow them to glide with reduced friction when moving and hold the lungs to the muscular chest wall allowing the lungs to be increased and decreased in volume by the movement of the muscles surrounding the lungs.

- Pulmonary ventilation – moving air in and out of the lungs.

Health Connection

Pneumonia

Pneumonia is an inflammation of the lung and the fluid from the inflammation may be present in the alveoli. The inflamed alveoli fill with white blood cells and secretions. This would impair gas exchange and leave patients 'hungry' for air as oxygen cannot diffuse across the walls of the alveoli into the bloodstream as easily resulting in laboured breathing. It usually only affects part of a lung but can affect both lungs and be life-threatening.

It is caused by infections such as by bacteria, viruses, protozoa, and fungi. It can also be caused by inhaling vomit or chemicals. Complications include pleurisy, pleural effusion and septicaemia. It is often treated with antibiotics, but results in about 27,000 deaths each year in the UK.

- External respiration – gas exchange between pulmonary blood and alveoli.

Getting air into our lungs requires maintaining *pressure* differences between our lungs and the environment in which we live, the atmosphere (see 'Pressure' section above).

- The **parietal pleura** line the *thoracic cavity.*
- The **visceral pleura** form the *outer layer of the lungs.*

Both pleura are made of serous connective tissue. They have serous fluid between them. The serous fluid sticks the parietal to the visceral pleura. When the parietal pleura covering the muscles of the thoracic cavity move, the visceral pleura move (are pulled by the parietal pleura) too. As the visceral pleura are on the lung, when they move (expand or contract) the lung expands or contracts. The confusion for some people is the word contract – to become smaller. Muscles contract – shorten – when they are in tension. The diaphragm muscle contracts (downwards) and pulls the lungs with it. The lungs thus expand. When the diaphragm muscle relaxes it recoils into a dome shape and the lungs reduce (contract) in size. So the lungs expand when the muscles contract and the lungs contract when the muscles relax (Figure 7.4).

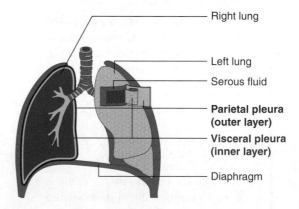

Right lung

Left lung

Serous fluid

Parietal pleura (outer layer)

Visceral pleura (inner layer)

Diaphragm

FIGURE 7.4 **Pleura of lungs**

The mechanism of breathing

Our lungs are composed of elastic tissue and are capable of being expanded and then recoiling back to their original shape. Muscles are needed to act on the elastic tissue to move it as elastic tissue does not move itself.

> **Chapter Reference**
> Movement by muscles is discussed in Chapter 6, 'Moving' (see p. 163).

Our lungs are surrounded by muscles. Between our ribs are **intercostal muscles (external and internal)**. Dividing the thoracic cavity and the abdominal cavity is the **diaphragm**. These muscles can contract and relax. If the intercostal muscles contract they pull the rib cage up and out. If the diaphragm contracts it moves downwards. Both of these sets of muscles contracting serve to increase the volume of the thoracic cavity. By doing this the lungs expand. If these muscles merely contracted and relaxed the thoracic cavity would expand and contract in volume, but little else would happen. Due to the pleura the muscles are attached to the lungs so that when the muscles contract they pull the lungs with them, increasing the volume of the lungs. When the muscles relax, the lungs, due to their elasticity, recoil back. As mentioned above, the parietal pleura cover the lining of the rib cage and the visceral pleura cover the lungs. Between the two pleura is serous fluid. When the muscles contract they take their covering of parietal pleura with them. Due to the serous fluid, the visceral pleura around the lungs are held close to the parietal pleura by surface tension. When the parietal pleura are moved by being attached to muscles, they pull the visceral pleura with them. The visceral pleura are closely attached to the lungs so when they move the lungs are moved. Thus, by contracting muscles which are not directly attached to the lungs the lungs expand and contract. As the lungs expand the alveoli expand.

As the lungs expand their volume increases, but there is nothing more inside them so air rushes in to 'fill the void'. In other words, as the volume increases, the pressure decreases so air is sucked in to equalise the internal (lung) pressure with the external atmospheric pressure. When the lungs decrease in volume the pressure inside the lungs increases so air is pushed out to reduce the pressure and equalise it again with the atmospheric pressure.

Health Connection

Asthma
Asthma affects many children and adults. It is caused when the muscles in the airways go into spasm causing them to constrict (get narrower). It may occur as a reaction to pollutants in the air including cigarette smoke.

Health Connection

Pleural fluids
Serous fluid holds the two pleural membranes together by surface tension thus aiding breathing. In pneumothorax, air enters the pleural cavity. In haemothorax, blood enters the pleural cavity. In pleural effusion there is excess fluid in the pleural cavity.

All of these conditions will compromise the ability of the lungs to expand and recoil (inflate and deflate) by affecting the surface tension between the two pleural membranes.

Inhalation is an *active process*, active because muscle contraction is involved and actively uses ATP energy (calories are used). Exhalation is a *passive process*.

The amount the muscles contract affects the amount the lungs expand and relax (contract) and thus the air flow:

- during inhalation and shallow breathing the diaphragm muscle contracts and moves down about 1.5 cm;

- during deep inhalation the diaphragm moves about 7 cm;
- during normal shallow breathing the increase in thoracic volume is brought about by the diaphragm moving down (inhalation) and up (exhalation) and the external intercostal muscles moving upwards and outwards (inhalation);
- During deep breathing the internal intercostal muscles as well as muscles in the neck shoulders and abdomen are involved.

Box 7.2 Summary – Inhalation and exhalation

During inhalation or inspiration our thoracic cavity *expands* and thus increases in volume and in consequence our lungs are pulled open with the thoracic cavity and are expanded and inflate. During exhalation or expiration, our thoracic cavity *contracts* or decreases in volume and our lungs therefore deflate.

- **Inhalation** – muscles constrict, chest expands, volume increases, pressure decreases, lungs inflate.
- **Exhalation** – muscles relax, chest contracts, volume decreases, pressure increases, lungs deflate (Figure 7.5).

How our lungs maintain a pressure difference

Creating changes in volume creates changes in pressure. As the volume of the thoracic cavity and the lungs increases during inhalation, a pressure difference is formed where there is a higher pressure outside the lungs (atmospheric pressure) than inside the lungs. The lungs have a negative pressure relative to the outside. This means that the space inside the lungs has expanded, but there is little to fill that space. The alveoli are kept open by the presence of a fluid surfactant. Air rushes in to equalise the pressure outside and inside and the alveoli are filled with this air. The air is drawn in through the nose and upper tract so it is filtered of debris, warmed and moistened.

How often we normally breathe

Our lungs act like a bellows with air entering and leaving in a cycle of respiration and can be measured as the **respiratory rate** (RR). This cycle occurs 12 to 15 times per minute in adults during normal quiet breathing. It consists of three phases

- inhalation,
- exhalation and
- Pause.

The rates change during our lifespan and during different activities.

How much air we breathe in and out

The volume of air breathed in and out with each normal quiet breath, the **tidal volume**, is around 0.5 litres. Deep breathing allows extra air volume, **inspiratory reserve volume**, to be inhaled. Breathing out hard allows extra volume, **expiratory reserve volume**, to be exhaled. There is always a small amount of air, the **residual volume**, remaining in the lungs. Our **vital capacity** is the maximum volume of

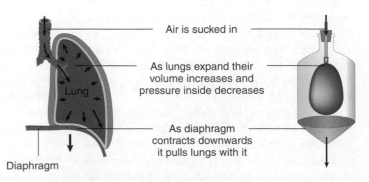

Diaphragm

Air is sucked in

As lungs expand their volume increases and pressure inside decreases

As diaphragm contracts downwards it pulls lungs with it

Lung

FIGURE 7.5 **Mechanism of breathing**

air that can be moved in and out of the lungs (Table 7.2).

Table 7.2 Average lung volumes in litres. Males and females are assumed to differ due to size and height differences

	Males	Females
Tidal volume	0.5	0.5
Inspiratory reserve volume	3.3	1.9
Expiratory reserve volume	1.0	0.7
Residual volume	1.2	1.1
Total lung capacity	6.0	4.2

Vital Capacity = Tidal Volume + Inspiratory Reserve Volume + Expiratory Reserve Volume

Gas exchange

External respiration: The movement of air from the external environment to the internal environment

Ventilation is the process by which we move gases into and out of our lungs and is the first stage of **respiration**. This is covered in the mechanism of breathing above.

Once in the lungs oxygen from the air must now pass to our blood for delivery to tissues. In exchange, carbon dioxide, a waste product of cell metabolism, must flow from our tissues to our blood and out of our lungs back into the atmosphere. These are all parts of gas exchange, exchanging one blood gas for another. It occurs due to the mechanism of diffusion discussed in Chapter 1, 'Maintaining a Safe Environment'. Substances diffuse (passively move) from an area of high concentration to an area of low concentration down a concentration gradient.

For gases to diffuse across areas of the body they must be 'dissolved' in liquids, hence the need to moisten air either during the passage though the upper respiratory tract, or artificially when administering oxygen. The alveoli are kept moist to allow gas diffusion to occur. The moisture can, however, act to hold the alveoli together, preventing them from expanding. The presence of a substance called **surfactant** reduces the surface tension of the moisture in each alveolus and allows them to expand while also being moist.

External respiration relies on the different concentrations of gases in the lungs and in the **blood:**

- if oxygen concentration is high in the alveoli of the lungs and low in the blood it will diffuse into the blood;
- if carbon dioxide is high in the blood and low in the alveoli of the lungs it will diffuse into the lungs.

They are thus exchanged.

The concentrations of gases in inhaled and exhaled air (Table 7.3) show the percentages of O_2, Co_2 and N_2. The remainder of the concentration is made up of other compounds.

In external respiration the oxygen diffuses from the alveoli into the **pulmonary capillaries** surrounding each alveolus while carbon dioxide in the pulmonary capillaries diffuses into the alveoli.

During inhalation the alveoli fill with air. The pulmonary capillaries bring de-oxygenated blood from the tissues full of carbon dioxide to the lungs. In Figure 7.6 carbon dioxide is expelled from the blood into the alveoli and exhaled while oxygen diffuses into the blood and is taken to the body tissues.

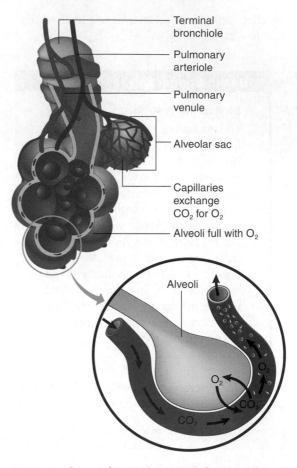

Terminal bronchiole

Pulmonary arteriole

Pulmonary venule

Alveolar sac

Capillaries exchange CO_2 for O_2

Alveoli full with O_2

Alveoli

O_2

O_2

CO_2

CO_2

FIGURE 7.6 **Gas exchange in external respiration**

Chapter Reference

Diffusion is discussed in Chapter 1, 'Maintaining a Safe Environment' (see p. 1).

Internal respiration is the movement of oxygen from our blood to our cells and carbon dioxide from our cells to our blood. Internal respiration relies on the different concentrations of gases in the tissues and in the **blood** (Figure 7.7):

Table 7.3 Partial pressures and constitution of inhaled and exhaled air

Gas	Concentration of gases in inhaled air	Concentration of gases in exhaled air
H_2O	Variable	Variable
CO_2	0.04%	4%
O_2	20%	16%
N_2	79%	79%

- if oxygen concentration is high in the blood and low in the tissue it will diffuse into the tissue;
- ff carbon dioxide is high in the tissue and low in the blood it will diffuse into the blood.

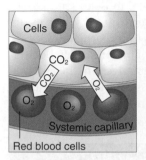 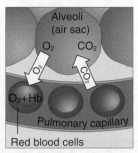

FIGURE 7.7 **Internal and external respiration and gas exchange**

Oxygen is constantly used to form ATP. During the synthesis of ATP, carbon dioxide is formed in the cells and diffuses into the blood to be carried to the lungs where it will diffuse into the alveoli and be expelled during exhalation.

The use of oxygen to produce ATP and the production of waste carbon dioxide occurs at the cellular level in mitochondria as part of cellular metabolism. It is also known as **cellular respiration.**

Chapter Reference

Cellular respiration is discussed in Chapter 1, 'Maintaining a Safe Environment' (see p. 1) and in Chapter 9, 'Eating and Drinking' (see p. 241).

How we control our rates of breathing: Homeostasis

Respiratory centres in the brain composed of nerve cells (neurons) control the rate and depth of our breathing. The centres are found in the **brainstem**, an area at the base of the brain near

Box 7.3 Summary – Internal and external respiration

In both cases oxygen and carbon dioxide are the gases that are exchanged.
Oxygen

- in external respiration oxygen is diffused into the blood;
- in internal respiration oxygen diffuses from the blood to the cells.

Carbon dioxide

- in external respiration carbon dioxide diffuses from the blood to the alveoli;
- in internal respiration carbon dioxide diffuses from the cells into the blood.

Health Connection

Emphysema

Emphysema is a disease affecting the alveoli. The alveoli enlarge as adjacent chambers break through and the airways collapse during exhalation. Patients use a large amount of energy to exhale. Patients can suffer from cyanosis – turning blue at the extremities due to lack of oxygen in the blood and tissues. Over-inflation of the lungs leads to a permanently expanded barrel chest.

the spinal cord, especially in an area called the medulla oblongata and the pons. Motor signals exit through the **phrenic** and **thoracic nerves**.

Chapter Reference

Nerve conduction and brain areas are discussed in Chapter 4, 'Communicating' (see p. 102). Muscle contraction is discussed in Chapter 6, 'Moving' (see p. 163).

To inhale and exhale the respiratory muscles must be **innervated** (stimulated) by the nervous system. **Innervation** means the stimulation of the muscle to contract and is initiated by the conduction of **electricity** to the muscle from nerves. The diaphragm is *innervated* by the **phrenic** nerve and the intercostal muscles by the **thoracic** nerves.

Our breathing in and out in a regular pattern is controlled by signals from the medulla region of the brain, a control centre for ventilation acting as a **respiratory pacemaker**. Two types of signals are sent to the phrenic and thoracic nerves. One type fires during inspiration, and the other type fires during expiration. The inspiratory firing inhibits the expiratory firing and vice versa.

During inhalation the medulla sends signals to the inspiratory nerves to stimulate contraction of the diaphragm and intercostal muscles. Stretch receptors in the intercostal muscles send signals back to stop firing. The expiratory nerves are then free to send signals to relax the muscles.

This regular pattern of breathing can be over-ridden in response to changes in the internal environment. If we are being active and using more ATP, more oxygen is required and more carbon dioxide is produced.

Health Connection

Respiratory acidosis

Decreased respiration (hypoventilation) causes increased blood carbon dioxide and decreased pH. This causes the blood to become acidic.

Acute respiratory acidosis occurs when an abrupt failure of ventilation occurs. This may be due to

- depression of the central respiratory centre due to a disease in the control centre of the brain;
- a neuromuscular disease reducing the ability to ventilate adequately (e.g. myasthenia gravis, amyotrophic lateral sclerosis, Guillain-Barré syndrome, muscular dystrophy);
- airway obstruction related to **asthma** or chronic obstructive pulmonary disease **(COPD)** exacerbation.

Chronic respiratory acidosis may be seen as a secondary symptom brought on by other disorders, including COPD.

Chapter Reference

As discussed in Chapter 1, 'Maintaining a Safe Environment' (see p. 1), control of homeostasis involves receiving information by receptors, sending the information to a control centre and the control centre integrating and sending a response to motor outputs.

Receptors, specifically **chemoreceptors**, monitor changes in gas levels in the blood. These receptors are located either

- centrally, in the brain;
- peripherally, in the arch of the aorta and the carotid arteries.

The **central chemoreceptors** measure the levels of H+ ions in the cerebrospinal fluid. Hydrogen ions will increase in extracellular fluid if there is an increase in the partial pressure of carbon dioxide in the plasma. This is because the **carbon dioxide** in the plasma will react with water and form hydrogen carbonate ions and hydrogen ions.

$$CO_2 + H_2O \leftrightarrow H_2CO_3 \leftrightarrow H^+ + HCO_3^-$$

An increase in hydrogen ions decreases pH and increases acidity. Changes in acidity are tightly regulated. Cells can withstand changes in many conditions for various periods of time, but changes in pH are poorly tolerated.

> **Chapter Reference**
>
> pH and ions are introduced in Chapter 1, 'Maintaining a Safe Environment' (see p. 1).

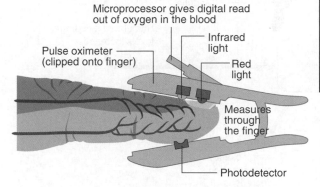

FIGURE 7.8 **A pulse oximeter allows the amount of oxygen in the blood to be determined**

The **peripheral chemoreceptors** are sensitive to decreases in the concentration of **oxygen** in the blood and send signals to the respiratory centres in the brain to increase ventilation (Figure 7.9).

> **Chapter Reference**
>
> Transport of gases in blood is discussed in Chapter 8, 'Transporting' (see p. 205).

Electrical messages innervate muscles to contract and relax in response to the amount of carbon dioxide and hydrogen ions in the blood (centrally) or the amount of oxygen in the blood (peripherally).

Many factors can alter the rate of breathing including

- compliance,
- airway resistance and
- surface tension of alveolar fluid.

Compliance is a measure of the stiffness of the lung. A stiffer lung is less compliant. It is a

> **Health Connection**
>
> **Cot death**
>
> Sudden infant death syndrome (SIDS) also known as cot death is a form of sleep **apnoea** (stoppage of breathing). The cause could be due to the malfunction of chemoreceptors, reflex changes which are subconscious. There are various theories about this syndrome, its causes and factors that exacerbate the chances of this happening.

static measure of lung and chest recoil and is expressed as a change in lung volume per unit change in airway pressure. Compliance decreases with certain diseases and increases with emphysema and with age, perhaps due to the reduction in elastic tissue.

Airway resistance is the opposition to flow. Airway resistance decreases as lung volume increases because the airways distend as the lungs inflate, and wider airways have lower resistance. Resistance to flow can be effected by friction caused by pollution and diseased tissue.

Surface tension of alveolar fluid: During development the alveoli secrete a fluid surfactant that allows the alveoli to expand during inhalation while remaining moist for gas exchange.

Changes during lifespan and lifestyle

In the foetus the lungs are filled with fluid and are not fully inflated with air until two weeks after birth. Surfactant that lowers alveolar surface tension is not present until late in foetal development and may not be present in premature babies.

Respiratory rates change during lifespan:

- newborns – 30–40 respirations per minute;
- infants – 30 respirations per minute;
- age 5–adult – 25 respirations per minute;
- adults – 12 to 18 respirations per minute.

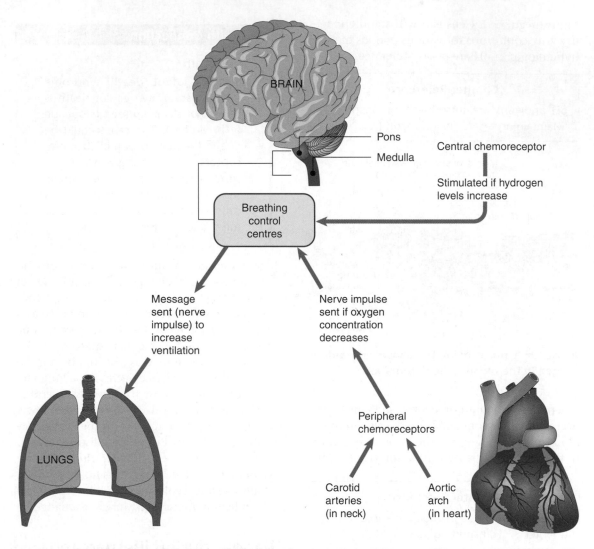

FIGURE 7.9 **Control of breathing (ventilation) by the nervous system**

Health Connection

**Surfactant and premature/
pre-term babies**

Babies born before the 34th week of gestation have difficulties expanding their lungs. This is due to the lack of production of surfactant. Surfactant coats the inside of the alveoli and reduces surface tension allowing the alveolar to expand during inhalation.

Health Connection

Cystic fibrosis

This is a genetically inherited disease (see Chapter 3, 'Growing and Developing'). It results in poor ion and osmotic exchange in the lungs leading to over-secretion of thick mucus clogs in the respiratory system.

The rate often increases somewhat with old age to compensate for poor compliance and hypoxia (decreased oxygen levels).

Sleep

Respiratory rates are not as tightly regulated while asleep as while awake. Sometimes during sleep we stop breathing – sleep apnoea. This can be due to a decrease in sensitivity of chemoreceptors to the partial pressure of carbon dioxide. Another reason for this occurrence during sleep is the failure of contraction of the muscles which hold the tongue in place. The tongue can then drop back and block the airways.

Chapter Reference

Chapter 12, 'Sleeping and Healing', discusses further events during sleep (see p. 324).

Exercise

When we exercise we are using our muscles more than when we are at rest. Our muscles are mechanical devices that aid movement. To be mechanical they need energy. This energy comes in the form of ATP. At rest we use ATP in transporting substances across membranes and in maintaining our electrical potentials in the brain. During exercise we use additional ATP.

This has two effects. More ATP must be made and more waste products removed.

To make more ATP in the cells of the muscles, blood must flow faster to the muscles to supply the muscle cells with oxygen from the lungs and glucose or its stored version from the liver. The heart must, therefore, pump blood faster and to do this the heart rate must increase. Blood pressure increase also helps to speed the flow of blood to the muscles. While blood is transporting oxygen to the muscles, more oxygen is needed so the respiratory rate must increase.

At the same time more waste products, carbon dioxide and water, are being made in the muscles. These must be transported away in the blood. Carbon dioxide is transported in the blood to the lungs and expelled. Water is transported in the blood to the kidneys and sweat glands.

Making ATP through combining oxygen with glucose is called aerobic respiration. There is also a pathway that uses anaerobic respiration, respiration without using oxygen. This is a pathway using glucose and converting it to pyruvate. The waste product is lactic acid. Our muscles use this pathway during prolonged exercise when there is a lack of oxygen, but eventually lactic acid must be disposed of and this requires oxygen.

The result of this exercise is that we breathe faster to get oxygen in and carbon dioxide out of our bodies and our heart beats faster to pump blood to our muscles.

Health Connection

Lung cancer

The surfaces of the lungs are in constant contact with factors from the external environment, hence the need to filter air entering the lungs. Epithelial cells turn over (are renewed). Each time a cell is replaced with a new cell through replication there is a chance of mutation, especially of factors that control growth such as hormone receptors. Lung cancer is an abnormal growth of lung cells. There are three common types:

- squamous cell carcinoma,
- adenocarcinoma and
- small cell carcinoma.

Lung cancer accounts for one third of all cancer deaths in the United States and there appears to be increased incidence associated with smoking.

Chapter Reference

Heart rate and blood pressure are discussed in Chapter 8, 'Transporting' (see p. 205). Kidneys are discussed in Chapter 10, 'Eliminating' (see p. 282).

Conclusion: Breathing

Breathing is the most obvious of the ADLs associated with the living processes of biology.

It provides the basis for all the metabolic processes in the body which require energy from ATP which must constantly be made using oxygen gained from the air. We cannot store oxygen and so we need a constant supply. Any interruption to that – blockages of the airways, lack of ventilation – severely compromise our health and well-being and if not corrected immediately can lead to death.

Chapter Summary

- Oxygen is needed by every cell in the body to synthesise ATP.
- Carbon dioxide is a waste product of this synthesis and must be removed.
- The lungs supply the blood with oxygen and remove carbon dioxide.
- Ventilation – inhalation and exhalation – allows the movement of gases.
- Ventilation is brought about by the movement of muscles which are attached via pleura and serous fluids to the lungs.
- The gases are filtered, warmed and moistened on their passageway to the alveoli.
- The alveoli are the site of gas exchange. They are thin walled and are surrounded by pulmonary capillaries.
- Gas exchange is by diffusion.
- Gas exchange requires a moist environment.
- The alveoli are kept moist by secretions.
- The alveoli also need surfactant to reduce the surface tension of the moisture that would otherwise hold the walls of the alveoli together and reduce the area for gas exchange.
- The rate and depth of breathing are controlled by innervation of the intercostal and diaphragm muscles by the phrenic and thoracic nerves, respectively.
- These nerves are under the control of a respiratory pacemaker in the brain.
- The requirements for oxygen and removal of carbon dioxide vary during wakefulness and sleep, and during activities.
- Chemoreceptors monitor the levels of hydrogen ions (formed as a result of build up of carbon dioxide in plasma) centrally or oxygen molecules peripherally and send signals to the respiratory centres in the brain to change the rate or depth of breathing. This is an example of homeostasis, maintaining a safe internal environment for our cells.

Transporting

Every perfect traveller always creates the country where he travels.

Nikos Kazantzakis (1883, Kandiye, Crete, Ottoman Empire – 1957, Freiburg, Germany), Greek writer and philosopher

Introduction: Transporting as an activity of daily living

Substances that we take into or make in our bodies do not just get to where they are needed, they must be *transported* there. To do this we need a number of systems:

- a *medium* – in this case a liquid in which they can be transported, **blood** and **lymph**;
- some *routes* – in this case vessels along which they can be transported, the **vascular system**;
- a *mechanism* – in this case a *pump* which is a way of moving the liquid through the vessels, the **heart**.

If any of these systems are not working effectively, the substances do not reach their targets; homeostasis is disrupted and ill health ensues.

The environment

The external environment

In the external environment things move via a number of mechanisms. They may be moved by outside forces such as oceans, currents, wind, air or they may move themselves such as in the locomotion of an ant. In the former the object is being passively moved. In the latter the ant is moving itself, actively.

We are multicellular and all our cells need a constant supply of substances, many of which are in the external environment. We must move or collect these external substances, gather them into our bodies and then distribute them around to all our cells. As we need to move substances around our bodies, so we need a transport system and modes of moving substances into cells.

The internal environment

In Chapter 1, 'Maintaining a Safe Environment', different methods of transport of substances were mentioned:

- diffusion,
- facilitated diffusion,
- osmosis,
- active transport and
- engulfment.

All of these are employed at the cellular level. At the organ and organism level, because we are such large, multicellular organisms, we need an entire system devoted to moving substances around the internal environment.

The blood system

Blood is a medium for transporting substances, a bit like a car carrying people and luggage. Many of the terms associated with blood contain the root 'haem', for example haematology, haemoglobin, haemophilia.

There are three main functions of blood:

- **transport** of substance such as
  - nutrients, gases, waste, hormones and heat;
- **regulation** of variables such as
  - temperature, pH by blood buffers, osmotic water content of cells;
- **protection** of which there are two types:
  - **Haemostasis** – stoppage of blood flow clotting broken blood vessels
  - **Immune surveillance** and destruction of pathogens by white blood cells.

Blood carries out a number of physiological functions due to its composition, what it is made of, and due to what it contains.

Blood composition

Blood is a liquid formed from **connective tissue**. Most connective tissue is solid such as that found in cartilage and bone. Blood is formed from cells found inside a special part of some bones, the red marrow. This liquid blood

- flows and
- carries substances.

The small molecular substances that blood can carry are called **solutes**. The larger ones are cells. The substance carrying these solutes and cells, the liquid, is called a **solvent**.

Blood is composed of **two phases**:

- a liquid phase (solvent) and
- a cellular phase.

Usually these two phases cannot be distinguished as the cells float in the liquid phase. If a sample of blood is removed and **centrifuged** (spun under centrifugal gravitational forces) the two phases can be separated and seen. The upper yellow liquid is called **plasma.** The lower red phase is composed of red blood cells. Between these two boundaries is a small cellular phase composed of white blood cells (Figure 8.1).

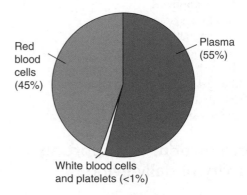

Red blood cells (45%)

Plasma (55%)

White blood cells and platelets (<1%)

FIGURE 8.1 **Composition of blood after centrifugation**

Plasma makes up about 55% of the volume while the cells make up the rest. Plasma is composed mainly of water (98%) with dissolved solutes and small molecules dispersed in it. The cells of our bodies cannot be placed in pure water due to the **osmotic pressure**. If the cells were placed in pure water, the water would move into the cells by osmosis (diffusion of water). This would cause the cells to swell up and burst.

Chapter Reference

Osmosis and ions are discussed in Chapter 1, 'Maintaining a Safe Environment' (see p. 1).

Plasma contains

1. **water;**
2. **solutes**
   - **electrolytes** – ions that are dissolved in a solvent;

3. **plasma proteins**
   - some of which help to maintain osmotic balance
   - involved in haemostasis.

The **cellular phase** of blood contains three types of cells:

- **red blood cells,**
- **white blood cells** and
- **megakaryocytes (platelet forming cells).**

The most abundant of the cell types are the red blood cells. White blood cells are involved in the immune system. Platelets are fragments of megakaryocytes.

Chapter Reference

White blood cells are discussed in Chapter 11, 'Cleansing and Dressing' (see p. 299).

The amount of each cell type is an indication of health.

Health Connection

Blood counts

Blood **samples** can be taken and the amount and type of cells counted in a **haematology** laboratory. Per cubic millimetre of blood in healthy adults there are

- platelets = 150,000–400,000;
- white blood cells (WBC) = 5.000–10,000;
- red blood cells (RBC) = 4.8–5.4 million.

Plasma, the watery fluid part of the blood, is a medium of transport. It transports

- cells, such as red blood cells, white blood cells and platelets;
- nutrients, such as glucose;
- gases, such as oxygen and carbon dioxide;
- electrolytes, such as sodium and potassium ions, involved in osmotic balance;

- ions, such as hydrogen ions and bicarbonate ions, involved in pH balance;
- hormones (message chemicals), such as insulin, to their target cells;
- waste products of metabolism, such as urea, uric acid and creatinine, to the kidneys and liver for elimination;
- plasma proteins, such as albumin involved in osmotic balance, lipid and steroid hormones, immunoglobulins involved in immune surveillance and defence of the body, and the inactive versions of clotting factors, such as fibrinogen.

Health Connection

Serum and plasma

Serum is plasma without the **clotting factors**. Synthetic versions can be made for clinical use.

There are three main types of **blood cells**:

1. red blood cells, also called **erythrocytes**, are involved in the transport of oxygen;
2. megakarytocytes and the cells derived from them, **platelets**, are involved in **haemostasis**, blood clotting, stopping blood flowing out from wounds to the blood vessels (discussed below);
3. white blood cells (WBC) are involved in the **immune system**, that is, the defence of the body from invading micro-organisms. This system is discussed in Chapter 11, 'Cleansing and Dressing'.
   WBC come in various types:
   - **Agranulocytes (lymphocytes, monocytes/macrophages);**
   - **Granulocytes (eosinophils, neutrophils, basophils).**

Chapter Reference

Development and differentiation are discussed in Chapter 3, 'Growing and Developing' (see p. 64).

Formation of blood cells

Blood cells in the early embryo are formed in the yolk sac. As the embryo develops, the site of formation moves to the liver. In adults blood cells are formed in the bone marrow of the sternum and iliac crest. In the bone marrow are **haematopoietic stem cells (HSC)**. These are the cells that form all the cells of the blood. Stem cells are cells that, on dividing, replace themselves with one of the newly formed cells and produce offspring with the other newly formed cell. This offspring cell will divide many times to form blood cells through a process called **differentiation**.

Health Connection

Leukaemia

Leukaemia is the **cancer** of the **blood** or **bone marrow** characterised by an abnormal proliferation of blood cells, usually white blood cells (leukocytes). It is part of the broad group of diseases called haematological **neoplasms**. Damage to the bone marrow, by way of displacing the normal marrow cells with increasing numbers of malignant cells, results in a lack of blood platelets, which are important in the blood clotting process. This means people with leukaemia may become bruised, bleed excessively or develop pin-prick bleeds (petechiae).

White blood cells, which are involved in fighting pathogens, may be suppressed or dysfunctional, putting the patient at the risk of developing infections. Red blood cell deficiency leads to anaemia, which may cause dyspnea. All symptoms may also be attributable to other diseases; for diagnosis, blood tests and a bone marrow biopsy are required.

Blood cells are formed from haematopoietic stem cells (HSC) in the bone marrow. These proliferate to form many descendant cells. The descendant cells differentiate to form the different types of cells of the blood (Figure 8.2).

Rate of blood cell production

Only about one in every 100,000 cells in the bone marrow is an HSC, but their production rates are very prolific.

Stem cells in the bone marrow produce about 10 trillion blood cells daily. If the body needs emergency replacements, the process speeds up.

Approximately a quarter of the cells in the human body are red blood cells.

Red blood cells, the most numerous cells in the blood, are *formed* at a rate of about 2 million each second to meet the loss or turnover of these cells. Red blood cells are *destroyed* mainly in the **spleen**.

White blood cells and platelets make up only about 1% of the blood and are produced at a slower rate.

Red blood cells

Red blood cells are part of the haematopoietic lineage made in the bone marrow in adults from haematopoietic stem cells. They circulate in the blood vessels and have a lifespan of 120 days. This means that new blood cells are constantly being made in the bone marrow. Destruction of red blood cells starts in the spleen.

Red blood cells do not have a nucleus. This means that they can have more space for cytoplasm. The cytoplasm of the red blood cell is full of a transport protein, haemoglobin. The advantage for the red blood cell is the ability to have more haemoglobin inside the cell than if a nucleus had been there. The disadvantage is that as the proteins wear out they cannot be replaced because the instruction machinery of how to make proteins, the genetic material DNA, is not there because DNA resides in the nucleus. So the red blood cell has a limited lifespan.

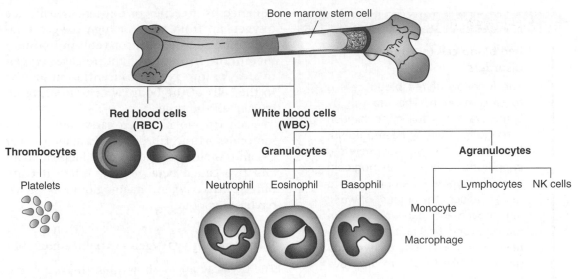

FIGURE 8.2 **Blood cell formation and types**

Chapter Reference

DNA and cell growth are discussed in Chapter 3, 'Growing and Developing' (see p. 64).

within the cell. The function of the red blood cell (RBC) is to carry oxygen. As the RBC must pick up oxygen quickly in its transit through the **pulmonary capillary** by the **respiratory membrane**, having most of its content on the surface allows the rapid diffusion of oxygen into the cell.

Chapter Reference

The pulmonary capillary and the respiratory membrane with the alveoli of the lung are discussed in Chapter 7, 'Breathing' (see p. 184).

Red blood cells have a particular structure called a **biconcave disc** as both sides cave in. This allows the cell to have most of its content on the surface of the cell rather than deep

The membrane is also very flexible, which, together with the lack of a **nucleus**, allows the RBC to squeeze through narrow capillaries.

The red blood cell and oxygen

The RBC is a highly specialised cell. Not only is the *shape* of the cell adapted to its *function*, but the *content* of the cell is also highly adapted. The RBC is full of a **protein** called **haemoglobin** (Hb). This protein is exquisitely designed as a carrier of oxygen. It will take **oxygen** up from areas of high oxygen concentration such as in the **alveoli-pulmonary membrane** in the **lung** and **release oxygen** in areas of low oxygen concentration such as in the cells of the body, which are using up oxygen all the time.

Each Hb molecule can carry four oxygen molecules as the Hb protein is made of four globin protein chains (two called alpha globin and two called beta globin). When it combines with oxygen, haemoglobin is called oxyhaemoglobin.

$$\text{Hb} + 4\,O_2 \leftrightarrow \text{Hb}(O_2)_4$$
$$\text{Haemoglobin} + \text{Oxygen} \leftrightarrow \text{Oxyhaemoglobin}$$

The two-way arrow shows that this is a *reversible* reaction.

The association of oxygen with haemoglobin is affected by:

- pH,
- temperature and
- a molecular substance called 2,3-diphosphoglycerate (2,3-DP.).

An increase in **acidity** (**decreased pH**) will dissociate oxygen from oxyhaemoglobin. The reaction above will move to the left. This is useful in, for example, exercise. During muscular movement lactic acid builds up. This will lower the pH in the muscle. As muscles use up oxygen to make ATP for use in movement, a muscle with lactic acid will need more oxygen. At this lower pH, oxyhaemoglobin will release the oxygen to the muscle more readily.

Likewise with temperature, an increase in muscular activity increases temperature. At increased temperature oxyhaemoglobin dissociates to oxygen and haemoglobin, i.e. again the oxyhaemoglobin releases the oxygen to the muscle.

2,3-DP is a product that is made during the formation of **ATP** from glucose. An increase in **metabolism**, such as in exercising muscle, will increase the amount of 2,3-DP. This increase will encourage the release of oxygen from oxyhaemoglobin.

How carbon dioxide is carried in blood

Carbon dioxide is formed as a **waste product** during cellular metabolism. It is removed by the blood. The carbon dioxide dissolves in the blood plasma as carbonic acid and bicarbonate, or hydrogen carbonate:

$$CO_2 + H_2O \leftrightarrow H_2CO_3 \leftrightarrow HCO^- + H^+$$
Carbon dioxide + Water ↔ Carbonic acid ↔ bicarbonate + hydrogen ion

About 7% of carbon dioxide is carried this way, **dissolved in plasma.** The effect on the plasma is to **lower the blood pH.** The red blood cell carries 70% of the carbon dioxide due to the presence of an enzyme in RBC, **carbonic anhydrase**, which allows rapid combination of carbon dioxide with water. This allows the rapid uptake of carbon dioxide from the body tissues. This uptake also helps to regulate blood pH so that carbon dioxide does not accumulate and lower the blood pH.

Haemostasis and serum proteins

There is a balance to be struck between blood *flowing around* the body inside the blood vessels and blood *flowing out* of the body after damage to a blood vessel.

Blood clotting which *stops* the flow of blood and therefore the loss of blood from the body occurs in response to damage of blood vessels. When a blood vessel is damaged, **haemostasis**, a stoppage of blood flow, occurs by clotting.

This stoppage of blood flow uses the **constituents** of blood to carry out its function.

As discussed above, blood is composed of a cellular fraction and a liquid fraction.

In the **cellular fraction** there are cells called **thrombocytes**, also called **platelets**, that help with blood clotting.

In the **liquid fraction** there are various protein molecules, including the **clotting proteins**.

To stop loss of blood and promote healing, a number of mechanisms occur.

1. **Platelet plug formation**. After tissue damage to the endothelium of blood vessels, platelets break down and become sticky. This breakdown is due to the protein thromboplastin. The platelets clump and attract more platelets, which stick to vessel wall forming a plug (positive feedback).
2. **Vasoconstriction** (vascular spasm). Platelets become sticky and adhere to the damaged vessel wall and release serotonin which constricts the vessels (vascular spasms), reducing blood flow.
3. **Coagulation**. Clotting factors (proteins) work to eventually form a clot (coagulation) and stop blood flow, haemostasis. This involves a positive feedback of various factors in a cascade reaction. It also involves the activation of proteins in the liquid phase of the blood.
4. **Fibrinolysis**, finally, results in the removal of the clot and healing of the blood vessel.

Prothrombin and **fibrinogen** are **proteins** normally found in blood.

- prothrombin is the *inactive* form of **thrombin**;
- fibrinogen is the *inactive* form of **fibrin**.

You do not want these proteins to be activated to thrombin and fibrin and start a clotting cascade unless there is tissue damage. If this happened when there was no damage, you would have blood clotting all the time and prevention of blood flow and transport. If this doesn't happen when there is tissue damage you will bleed continuously (Figure 8.3).

During the cascade reaction:

- **thromboplastin** from the platelet plug causes the protein prothrombin to become the protein thrombin;
- thrombin causes the protein fibrinogen to become fibrin;
- fibrin forms a clot over the damaged endothelium of the blood vessel preventing blood leaking out into the body cavities.

The clot formed is an insoluble mesh of fibrin which traps blood cells and is stronger than the platelet plug.

In the final stages the plasminogen activator acts on the plasma protein prothrombin.

Control of coagulation

Coagulation is an example of a self-perpetuating or positive feedback system; once it has started blood clotting continues.

It is prevented from starting and forming unnecessary clots by

- smooth blood vessels with no damage;
- presence of anticoagulants, e.g. heparin;
- inactivation of thrombin by thrombin receptor.

Haemostasis (the stoppage of blood flow) is kept under strict **homeostatic** (the maintenance of a suitable internal environment) control.

Health Connection

Haemorrhage

Haemorrhage means particularly severe bleeding space. Loss of 10–15% of total blood volume can be endured in a healthy person. The complete loss of blood is referred to as exsanguination. Haemorrhage generally becomes dangerous, or even fatal, when it causes hypovolemia (low blood volume) or hypotension (low blood pressure). If either of these occur there are various mechanisms to maintain the body's homeostasis. Death from haemorrhage can occur quickly. This is because of 'positive feedback'. An example of this is 'cardiac repression', when poor heart contraction depletes blood flow to the heart, causing even poorer heart contraction. This kind of effect causes death to occur more quickly than expected. Blood transfusion (see below) can replace lost blood.

Health Connection

Haemophilia – Disorders of blood clotting

Haemostasis stops blood flow after damage. Some people are unable to stop the blood flow, generally due to a genetic mutation causing the condition haemophilia. There are various types of haemophilia affecting different parts of the clotting mechanism due to mutations in different genes, which cause different clotting proteins to be affected. Haemophiliacs, people with haemophilia, are given the normal protein factor that they lack to allow blood clotting to occur when needed.

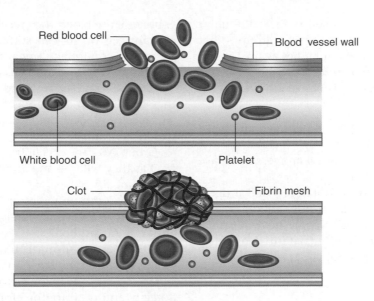

FIGURE 8.3 **Clotting at a site of injury**

Blood groups

There are many blood groups, but the main ones of concern in health are the **ABO** blood groups and the **Rhesus (Rh)** blood group.

Blood is a mixture of **plasma**, a liquid, and **cells**, either red cells that carry oxygen or white cells that protect us against pathogens. For the ABO and Rh blood groups it is the red blood cells that are of interest.

On the surface of every cell of our bodies are 'markers' made of proteins with sugars attached called **glycoproteins**. These markers are called **antigens**. Each one of us has individual protein antigens that mark us out from each other. However, there are common ones such as the ABO group. These glycoproteins are found on red blood cells. As they are a type of marker they can be classified as an antigen. Our immune system can make other proteins, antibodies which recognise and attach to antigen. When this happens an immune reaction is activated, somewhat like a clotting cascade. Our immune system can make **antibodies** that bind to antigens. These antibodies are also protein molecules which can be released into our plasma and bind antigens such as the ABO antigens. We do not want to bind antibodies to our own antigens, but we do want to bind antibodies to antigens that we detect in out bodies as not our own. These latter antigens, 'foreign antigens', may be on viruses or bacteria for example. Binding antibodies against them prevents the spread of an infection.

> ### Chapter Reference
>
> The immune system is discussed in Chapter 11, 'Cleansing and Dressing' (see p. 299).

On the surface of our red cells we can have either type A antigen or type B antigen, both A and B type antigen or we can have no antigen (O). Those with either A or B antigen are said to belong to Group A or Group B. The individuals without A or B antigens on their cell surface and are said to be Group O. Some individuals have both A and B on their surfaces and are said to be Group AB.

If we have an antigen on our cell surface, we don't want to make antibodies to it otherwise our own immune system would attack our own cells. So if we belong to Group A, we have

A type antigen on our cell surface. We don't want to make antibodies against group A, but we do want to make antibodies against group B, which is a foreign group to us.

To summarise blood antigen groups and the antibodies made,

- those in Group A have A antigen and make anti-B antibodies;
- those in Group B have B antigen and make anti-A antibodies;
- those in Group O do not have A or B antigen, but make anti-A and anti-B antibodies;
- those in Group AB people have A and B antigen so they don't make anti-A or anti-B antibodies (Figure 8.4).

Transfusion

The human body generates blood at a rate of about **2 litres per week.** This allows people to be blood donors, donating up to half a litre every six months. Donated blood is checked for infections and, most importantly, to categorise it into a blood group.

The antigen on our cell surface is the important factor in deciding which blood we can accept and to whom we can donate blood because it is the cell antigens that cause antibodies to be made or not. That is why blood in transfusions must be *matched* for blood groups.

Group A people can receive blood in a transfusion from other A donors as they will not see the donated blood with its A antigen as foreign. They can also receive blood from Group

O because the blood they receive will not have any antigen on its cell surface (O). Group A recipients won't make any antibodies to group O as group O has no antigens.

Group B can receive blood from Group B as they won't see B antigen as foreign. They can also receive blood from Group O for the same reason as Group A.

Group AB can receive from group AB, A, B or O as they will see any antigens as similar to their own.

Group O can only receive from Group O as they see A, B and AB as foreign and will make anti A, B, AB antibodies.

Group O can **donate** blood to all blood groups because they have no antigens on their surface so no other blood group sees them as 'foreign' and they are therefore known as **universal donors.** However, Group O are limited receivers of blood. They make antibodies to A and B antigens so they cannot receive blood from A, B or AB blood groups. The antibodies that are transferred with their blood (in this case antibodies to A and B) do not matter so much as they are protein molecules with limited lifespans. It is the antigens on the cell surface that must be matched.

AB people are the reverse to O group. They can **receive** blood from all blood types (**universal recipient**) as they don't make anti-A or anti-B antibodies, but they can donate only to AB people, i.e. people who do not make antibodies as they possess both antigens on their own cells. Group AB has both A antigen and B antigen on their cell surface; so if we give

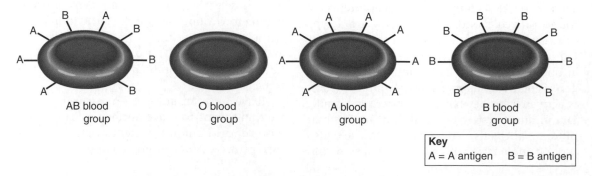

AB blood group   O blood group   A blood group   B blood group

Key
A = A antigen   B = B antigen

FIGURE 8.4 **Antigens on RBC**

AB blood to a Group O person, the AB markers will be antigenic and cause the Group O to make antibodies to A and B antigens. If we gave AB blood to a Group A person, they would make antibodies to B marker. If we gave AB to a Group B person, they would make antibodies to A marker.

Box 8.1 Summary – Blood donation

- Group A can donate blood to group A and AB and receive blood from A or O.
- Group B can donate blood to group B and AB and receive blood from B or O.
- Group AB can only donated blood to AB, but can receive blood from A, B, AB or O.
- Group O can donate blood to group A, B, AB or O, but can receive blood only from O.

Health Connection

Transfusion reactions

If the wrong blood group is transfused, a reaction by the recipient against the donor blood can occur (host versus graft reaction) and a reaction by the donor blood to the recipient can occur (graft versus host reaction).

Reactions include clumping of donor cells by host antibodies affecting flow of blood in blood vessels and blockages of small blood vessels.

Lifespan

During development our haemoglobin changes because the amount of oxygen (the pressure of

Health Connection

High altitude

People in **high altitudes** have adapted to the **lower partial pressure** of oxygen by increasing the number of red blood cells they have per mm^2 of blood, thus increasing the amount of haemoglobin they have to carry the sparser amounts of oxygen available. Athletes sometimes train at high altitude to increase their red blood cell count.

---

oxygen) changes. In the womb we encounter less oxygen, as the level gets depleted by the time it reaches the placenta, than when we are in the external environment. We have a different type of haemoglobin which can take oxygen at lower concentrations. There are three main types of haemoglobin:

- **embryonic Hb**,
- **foetal Hb** and
- **adult Hb**.

Reactions can also occur in the womb due to blood type differences. Apart from the ABO blood group there are various other ones. One of these is Rhesus (Rh). Like the ABO group, Rh is an antigen on the cell surface. Most of us are Rhesus positive (Rh+) which means we have the Rh antigen on our cell surface. Some of us, who have blood group O, do not have the Rhesus antigen – we are Rhesus negative (Rh–). If you are Rh+ you do not make antibodies to Rh. If you are Rh– you make antibodies to the Rh antigen.

If a mother is Rhesus negative (does not possess the Rhesus antigen) she will make anti-rhesus antibodies in her plasma. These may react with the developing infant, especially if she has already given birth to a Rhesus positive child before because she is already 'primed' against that antigen. This is discussed further in Chapter 11, 'Cleansing and Dressing'.

The lymphatic system

Apart from oxygen, which is carried by red blood cells, other constituents of blood such as nutrients, hormones and electrolytes are carried in the plasma. These constituents must be transferred from the plasma to the cells. The exchange is, in fact, between the plasma and the **interstitial fluid**, the plasma-like fluid that surrounds each cell. From the interstitial fluid the substances needed by the cell are transported into the cell across the cell membrane. Substances also pass from the cell into the interstitial fluid. This is then removed as lymph before rejoining the circulatory system in the plasma.

Chapter Reference

Cell transport is discussed in Chapter 1, 'Maintaining a Safe Environment' (see p. 1).

The lymphatic system: Anatomy

The lymphatic system consists of

- a network of lymph vessels;
- lymph fluid;
- lymph tissue consisting of lymph nodes and nodules.

The lymph fluid is contained in the lymph vessels similar to plasma contained in blood vessels. The larger lymphatic vessels are similar to veins having an endothelial lining supported by fibrous connective tissue between which are muscle fibres. There are also valves to prevent the backflow of fluid.

The larger lymph vessels feed into smaller lymphatic capillaries, which, in turn, feed back to large vessels or veins called **lymphatics**.

The lymphatics empty into the lymph nodes. The **lymph nodes** allow the lymphatic fluid from the vessels to be filtered and pathogens are trapped and inactivated by cells of the immune system.

Our blood may deliver substances to and collect substances from our cells, but these substances must move from the blood vessels to the cells and back across membranes. This movement occurs through various transport mechanisms such as diffusion or active transport. **Solutes** are substances that are carried in, dissolve in or are transported in a **solvent**. Usually the solutes are solids such as salts and nutrients. The solvent is a liquid such as water. Each cell is surrounded by interstitial fluid, a solvent. The fluid is formed by exclusion from the blood. The blood is continually losing fluid through the capillaries into the interstitial space and thus forming interstitial fluid called **lymph**.

What the lymphatic system does: Physiology

There are three main roles of the lymphatic system:

- to circulate plasma that leaks from the blood vessels into the interstitial spaces back to the blood;
- to defend the body against pathogens by cleansing the leaked plasma and lymph of bacteria and other micro-organisms;
- to absorb lipid, fats, from the gastrointestinal tract.

Chapter Reference

Inactivation of pathogen is discussed in Chapter 11, 'Cleansing and Dressing' (see p. 299). Transport of lipids, fats, is discussed in Chapter 9, 'Eating and Drinking' (see p. 241).

Lymph

Lymph is a fluid that is very similar to **plasma** but without the plasma proteins. It consists, therefore, mainly of water, electrolytes and gases. It is composed of the same substances as intercellular (also called interstitial) fluid.

Lymph formation

Lymph is formed from the movement of fluid from the capillaries into the interstitial space. Small molecules diffuse out from the capillaries into the interstitial space. Additionally blood pressure, **hydrostatic pressure**, also pushes the fluid out. Large molecules such as proteins remain inside the capillaries. This creates a difference in osmotic pressure between the inside and outside of the capillary called **colloidal osmotic pressure**. Water is drawn into the capillary to try to balance the pressure. The two pressures, hydrostatic pressure and colloidal osmotic pressure, are in opposite directions (they oppose each other). If hydrostatic pressure is greater, water is forced out. If colloidal osmotic pressure is greater, water is forced into the capillary.

The hydrostatic pressure varies along a capillary from 40 mm Hg at the arterial end to 15 mm Hg at the venous end. The colloidal pressure remains at 25 mm Hg overall. At the arterial end there is a net outflow of liquid and at the venous end a net inflow of liquid. However, the outflow is greater than the inflow. If this remained so, there would be a build up of interstitial fluid around cells and there would be a lack of fluid in the blood. The lymphatic system works as a drainage system for about 10% of the interstitial fluid, returning it to the blood via the lymph vessels and the subclavian veins. The walls of the lymph vessels consist of endothelial cells that overlap each other. When interstitial fluid enters the lymph vessel to become lymph fluid, it cannot go back as the cells act as one-way traps. This one-way trap is similar to the valves in the heart vessels.

Chapter Reference

Osmosis is discussed in Chapter 1, 'Maintaining a Safe Environment' (see p. 1). Hydrostatic pressure is discussed again in Chapter 10, 'Eliminating' (see p. 282). Heart valves are discussed below.

Health Connection

Oedema

This is a build up of interstitial fluid, usually found in the ankles and feet due to an increase in the secretion of fluid or decrease in removal. Many people who have sedentary lifestyles have oedema and this affects venous return.

The lymph passes along several lymph **nodes** which act as filters, removing foreign material. The nodes contain cells of the immune system such as macrophages that help engulf and destroy micro-organisms. This helps prevent the spread of infections. The nodes also contain cells called lymphocytes which are also part of the immune system. Lymphocytes monitor the lymph and can attack foreign antigens. Apart from the nodes there are other organs associated with the lymph: the spleen, tonsils and Peyer's patches, all of which act as nodes (Figure 8.5).

Chapter Reference

Fluid balance is discussed in Chapter 9, 'Eating and Drinking' (see p. 241) and in Chapter 10, 'Eliminating' (see p. 282).

The cardiovascular system

Introduction

The beating heart is a symbol of life and of emotions such as love in many cultures. We express this in phrases such as 'our heart beat quickened' or that a person causes your heart to 'skip a beat'. It has been seen as the organ of love and the organ of the soul. The biology of the heart is altogether more mundane!

Cardio means heart and **vascular** means vessels, so the cardiovascular system includes the heart and blood vessels, the long, tube-like containers in which liquid is contained.

Box 8.2 Summary – Blood and lymph

- Blood is a liquid, connective tissue.
- Blood is composed of two fractions or phases, cells and plasma.
- Plasma is the main transport medium.
- Plasma transports cells, gases, proteins, nutrients, waste, hormones and ions.
- The cells of the blood are red (erythrocytes), white (leucocytes) and platelets.
- Leucocytes are involved in the immune system.
- Platelets are involved in clotting.
- Erythrocytes contain haemoglobin, which binds and releases oxygen.
- Oxygen is transported mainly bound to haemoglobin.
- Carbon dioxide is transported mainly bound to bicarbonate ions.
- Oxygen and carbon dioxide enter and leave the blood by diffusion across thin membranes.
- Oxygen diffuses into the blood from the lungs during external respiration.
- Carbon dioxide diffuses from the blood into the lungs during external respiration.
- Oxygen diffuses from the blood into cells during internal respiration.
- Carbon dioxide diffuses from the cells into the blood during internal respiration.
- The normal composition of the blood is maintained during health.
- Changes to the normal composition of blood are an indication of malfunction.
- Changes to the composition of blood can include
  - changes in blood gas levels and
  - changes in relative cell numbers.
- Changes in blood composition can be due to factors such as anaemia.
- The lymphatic system contains a fluid that is similar to plasma, but does not contain plasma proteins.
- The composition of the lymphatic fluid is identical to interstitial fluid.
- The lymphatics allow the exchange of nutrients and waste between blood and cells via interstitial fluid.
- Interstitial fluid returns to either the blood or the lymph.
- Interstitial fluid also functions to absorb lipids, fats, from the digestive system.

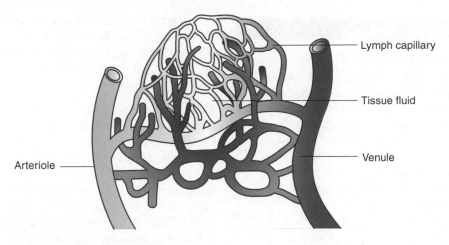

FIGURE 8.5 **Lymph circulation**

The function of cardiovascular system: Physiology

Blood, the liquid transport medium discussed above, flows through the body held in or restricted in vessels. As it is a liquid it would tend to settle under gravity. The heart provides a **pump** to push this liquid blood through the blood vessels. As blood carries so many vital substances to and from cells, any interruption in its flow causes severe problems.

The constituents of our circulatory system

Both the heart and the blood vessels are made of similar structures. They both consist, as do many organs, of three layers:

- **an inner epithelial tissue layer;**
- **a middle muscular tissue layer** and
- **an outer connective tissue layer.**

Innervating the muscular (**myo**) layer are nerves conducting electrical impulses to stimulate the muscle to contract.

The heart is a continuation of the blood vessels developing from them during **embryogenesis**, the development of the embryo. The heart is, therefore, a specialised area of the vascular tissues.

The heart: Anatomy

The three layers in the heart are called

- **endocardium – consisting of epithelial tissue;**
- **myocardium – consisting of cardiac muscle;**
- **pericardium – consisting of fibrous connective tissue.**

The inner endocardium consisting of tightly joined epithelial tissue called **endothelium** forms a watertight surface to contain blood and provide a *smooth* surface for blood to flow through the heart.

The myocardium makes up the bulk of the heart, the muscular pump. Cardiac muscle is one of the three types of muscle tissue. It has the appearance of voluntary skeletal muscle, but behaves like involuntary, smooth muscle. Because it is a mechanical pump, the heart muscle uses up energy, ATP, to contract. The heart muscle must, therefore, have a good supply of oxygen and glucose to maintain its ability to synthesise ATP. Glucose and oxygen are brought to the heart muscle in the cardiac circulation.

Chapter Reference

Movement of muscle is discussed in Chapter 6, 'Moving' (see p. 163).

Health Connection

Myocardial infarction
The heart receives its own blood supply in the **cardiac circulation**. Interruption of this blood flow to heart muscle reduces the ability of the heart muscle to synthesise ATP and therefore to pump. This stoppage of blood supply to cardiac muscle can be caused by a number of factors.

The pericardium is composed of two sacs:

- **outer sac – consisting of fibrous tissue** and
- **inner sac – consisting of two layers of serous tissue.**

The outer sac adheres to the **diaphragm** and the **tunica externa** (adventitia) of the large blood vessels to hold the heart in place and prevent over-expansion.

The inner sac has two layers of serous membranes:

- **parietal pericardium** and
- **visceral pericardium or epicardium.**

The parietal pericardium lines the fibrous sac; the visceral pericardium lines the heart muscle. Between the two layers is serous fluid.

The pericardium

- anchors the heart to the chest wall;
- allows the heart muscle to expand and contract;
- provides a friction-free environment for the heart muscle to expand and contract (Figure 8.6).

The heart is often described as a four-chambered organ: The heart is divided into a **right** and **left** side by the **septum**.

Each side is divided into an

- upper **atrium** on each side (right and left) = two atria and
- lower **ventricle** on each side (right and left) = two ventricles.

These **atria** (plural) and **ventricles** are the four chambers of the heart, each one lined with endocardium and contracted by myocardium.

Valves of the heart

Between the atria and the ventricles are valves called **atrioventricular valves**. These allow blood to flow from the atria to the ventricles, but prevent blood flowing from the ventricle to the atria. There are also valves where the ventricle meets blood vessels exiting the heart. The valve in the right ventricle is the **pulmonary valve**. The valve in the left ventricle is the **aortic valve**. Valves are discussed below.

The four valves of the heart are thus

- **the right atrioventricular valve (also called tricuspid);**
- **the left atrioventricular valve (also called bicuspid or mitral);**
- **the aortic semi-lunar valve;**
- **the pulmonary semi-lunar valve.**

For convenience it is easier to colour the heart. The colours used here are

- **right side** of the heart – **black** and
- **left side** of the heart – **red**.

This reflects the functions of the right and left side of the heart.

Coming to and leaving from each side are **blood vessels:**

- blood vessels called **veins** bring blood *towards* the heart;
- blood vessels called **arteries** take blood *away* from the heart.

When you look at a diagram of the heart (see Figure 8.7) it is divided into right and left by a septum – the patient's right and left, not the reader's! There are two upper chambers, right atria and left atria, and two lower chambers, right ventricle and left ventricle. The upper chambers (atria) receive blood and the lower chambers pump blood. There are valves between the atria and ventricles to stop the backflow of blood during ventricular pumping and valves between the vessels leaving the heart (arteries)

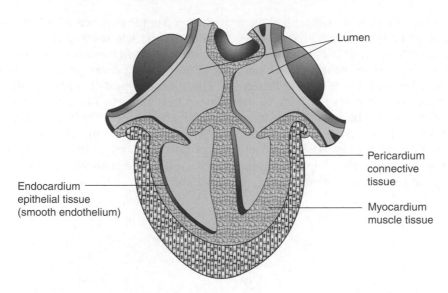

FIGURE 8.6 **Layers of the heart**

and the ventricles to stop the backflow of blood when the ventricles relax.

What the heart does: Physiology

The heart carries out two main functions:

- it pumps blood to all the tissues of the body – **the systemic system**;
- it pumps blood to the respiratory system – **the pulmonary system**.

The systemic system allows blood to deliver and collect substances to and from all the cells of the body, including the heart itself.

The pulmonary system allows blood that has become **deoxygenated**, that is the blood has given up its oxygen in its journey around the systemic system, to become re-oxygenated in the **lungs**.

This is why the heart has **two sides**:

- the left side is involved with **delivering oxygenated** blood through the systemic system;
- the right side is involved with **collecting deoxygenated** blood from the systemic system and pumping it to the pulmonary system.

Chapter Reference

The pulmonary circulation is also discussed in Chapter 7, 'Breathing' (see p. 184).

The two halves must be kept separate to stop the blood from each side mingling.

Health Connection

Hole in the heart

Some children are born with a congenital disorder (birth defect, but not genetic) where the septum of the heart is not fully formed and there is a hole in it. This allows deoxygenated blood and oxygenated blood to mix. This results in the systemic system taking both types of blood around the body and not enough oxygen reaching the tissues. The symptoms are thus fatigue, lethargy and breathlessness.

The systemic circulation takes blood from the heart to the tissues where the oxygen in the blood diffuses to the cells for use with glucose to synthesise **ATP.** Waste from that process, including carbon dioxide, diffuses from the cells into the blood by gas exchange. This blood, now deoxygenated and full of carbon dioxide, comes from the systemic system back to the heart. The deoxygenated blood is then pumped by the heart to the lungs where carbon dioxide diffuses from the capillaries into the alveoli and oxygen diffuses from the alveoli into the capillaries. The blood is thus re-oxygenated and the carbon dioxide removed. This is the **pulmonary circulation.** The re-oxygenated blood returns to the heart and is ready to be pumped around the body by the systemic circulation once more. The cycle is repeated continuously with every heart beat and inhalation of oxygen.

The two sides of the heart receive and pump different oxygen compositions of blood, deoxygenated (shown in black in Figures 8.7 and 8.8) and oxygenated (shown in red in Figures 8.7 and 8.8).

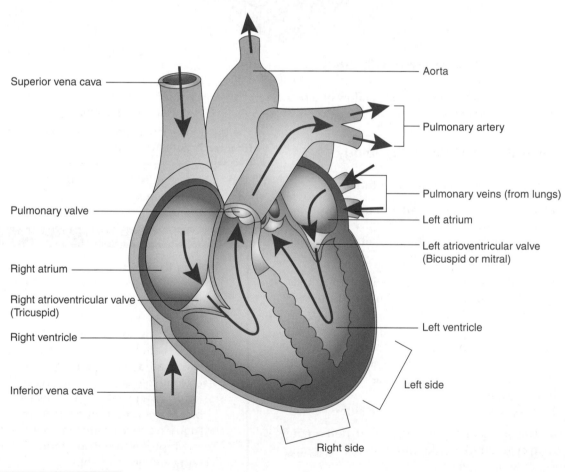

Key
→ Deoxygenated blood
→ Oxygenated blood

FIGURE 8.7 **Diagram of the heart**

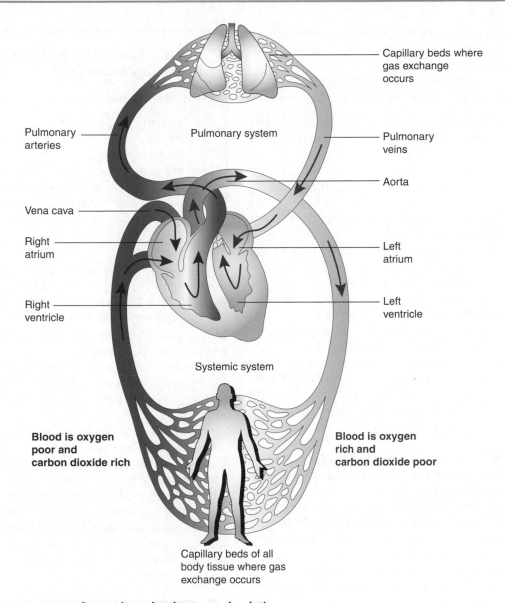

FIGURE 8.8 **Systemic and pulmonary circulation**

How the heart pumps blood to the systemic and pulmonary systems

Each side of the heart, left and right, acts as a pump.

The upper chambers of the heart, the left and right atria, are *receiving* chambers. Each atria receives blood.

- the left atria receives oxygenated blood from the pulmonary system;

- the right atria receives deoxygenated blood from the systemic system.

The lower chambers of the heart, the left and right ventricles, are *pumping* chambers.

- the left ventricle pumps oxygenated blood to the systemic system;
- The right ventricle pumps deoxygenated blood to the pulmonary system.

So while each side, left and right, contains only oxygenated or deoxygenated blood, respectively, each side receives blood and pumps blood from and to the pulmonary and systemic system.

If we follow the circulation of blood in a general description the following happens.

- oxygenated blood is pumped out of the **left ventricle** via an artery (**the aorta**) to the systemic system;
- the blood travels through the arteries to capillaries where oxygen, nutrients, hormones and electrolytes diffuse to cells and waste including carbon dioxide diffuses from cells to blood;
- the deoxygenated blood travel back to the heart in veins;
- the deoxygenated blood enters the **right atrium** from the main collecting veins, the **inferior and superior vena cava**;
- the blood collects in the **right atrium** and then flows into the **right ventricle**;
- blood is pumped during contraction of the heart muscle from the right ventricle into an artery, the **pulmonary artery**, taking the blood to the lungs. The pulmonary artery is the only artery to carry deoxygenated blood;
- blood loses its carbon dioxide and gains oxygen passing through the **pulmonary capillaries**;
- oxygenated blood is taken from the lungs in the pulmonary veins towards the heart. The pulmonary veins are the only veins to carry oxygenated blood;
- oxygenated blood enters the **left atrium** and then flows into the **left ventricle**;
- oxygenated blood is pumped from the **left ventricle** during muscular contraction of the myocardium into the **aorta** to be delivered, once again, to the systemic system.

Valves

Blood flows one way through the heart due to heart **valves**.

When the ventricles contract the liquid blood is pushed around the contracting ventricles. It tries to find an exit and will go out any

---

Box 8.3 Summary – Systemic and pulmonary blood flow

The flow of blood is thus:

- **systemic**: Left ventricle, aorta, arteries, capillaries, tissues, veins, vena cavae, right atria;
- **pulmonary**: Right atria, right ventricle, pulmonary arteries, lungs, pulmonary veins, pulmonary capillaries (lungs) pulmonary arteries, left atria.

---

way it can. It would flow back into the atria if the valves were not there. The valves allow blood to flow from the atria to the ventricles, but not the other way. They are like a one-way door flap allowing one-way movement of traffic. When the blood tries to flow back into the atria the pressure of the blood pushes the valves closed. The only exit open to the blood is therefore the arteries, either the pulmonary or aorta.

There are also valves in the pulmonary artery and aorta. After the ventricles have contracted and pushed the blood into these arteries, the heart relaxes allowing blood to flow into the atria and ventricle ready for another contraction. When the heart relaxes, the blood in these arteries could flow back into the ventricles. To stop this, the valves in the pulmonary artery and the aorta prevent the backflow of blood into the ventricles.

Health Connection

Damaged valves

In some cardiac conditions the heart valves fail to function properly. There are various effects depending on which valve fails. Generally circulation of blood is compromised causing fatigue and lethargy. Heart valves can now be replaced, surgically.

Heart beat

A heart beat is a cycle, a **cardiac cycle**, of events lasting about 0.8 seconds which, being a cycle, can be started at any point. It is a cycle of contraction and relaxation of cardiac muscle fibres. The contraction pumps blood through chambers and vessels. The relaxation allows the chambers to re-fill and the cycle to repeat itself. When the ventricles, the main pumping area of the heart, are contracted they are said to be in **systole**. When they are relaxed they are said to be in **diastole**. The beating sound is caused by the movement of liquid blood through chambers and past valves into arteries. In other words, it is the sound of the heart pumping blood.

Health Connection

Heart sounds

The cardiac cycle can be monitored through a **stethoscope**. Contraction pushes liquid blood around chambers and vessels and the movement of the fluid can be heard through a stethoscope. The main sounds are a low pitch, quiet 'lubb' sound that lasts a while and corresponds to the closing of the two AV valves by the contraction of the ventricles. This contraction causes the blood in the ventricle to swirl. A higher pitched louder and sharper 'dupp' sound lasting a shorter time is then heard corresponding to the closing of the semi-lunar valves in the arteries.

How the heart pumps blood

Basically, the heart is a muscle with four chambers. It has an ability to beat by itself, intrinsically, if it has a supply of nutrients and oxygen. Within the heart are some specialised muscle cells within the wall of the right atrium near to where the superior vena cava meets the right atrium. This area of muscle is called the **sinoatrial node (SAN)** and the SAN functions as the heart's **pacemaker.** It contracts at 80 beats per minute and sets the pace for the other muscle fibres. Because initiation of muscle activity requires movement of ions and ions have electrical charges, a wave of electrical activity is established by the SAN each time the SAN contracts. This is transmitted through the right and left atrium as the muscle fibres of the heart are connected to each other. This leads to contraction of the atrial fibres. As this wave of activity reached down the atria towards the ventricles, another group of specialised muscle fibres, the **atrioventricular node (AVN)**, is excited to contract.

Here the impulse is slowed down allowing time for the atria to fully contract forcing blood into the ventricles, before the ventricles themselves contract. The AVN sends impulses to the **Purkinje bundle fibres**, or **atrioventricular bundle** (also known as the **bundle of His**) between the ventricles. The conduction then reaches the rest of the Purkinje fibres and spreads out to the other ventricular muscle fibres which commence contraction. The contraction begins at the base of the heart spreading upwards through the ventricles forcing blood from the ventricles into the arteries.

Chapter Reference

Nerve conduction is discussed in Chapter 4, 'Communicating' (see p. 102). Muscle contraction is discussed in Chapter 6, 'Moving' (see p. 163).

In summary, a wave of contraction emanating from the SAN passes over the atria to the AVN which slows the speed of conduction of the electrical activity. The activity then passes into the Purkinje fibres which form a bundle, the atrioventricular bundle or the bundle of His. The conduction is sped up and the impulse continues into all the Purkinje fibres and then into all the ventricular fibres which then contract. The base of the heart contracts first.

This heart beat or cardiac cycle allows blood to fill the atria, then the ventricles and then be pushed up into the arteries, before relaxing and starting to fill the atria once more (Figure 8.9).

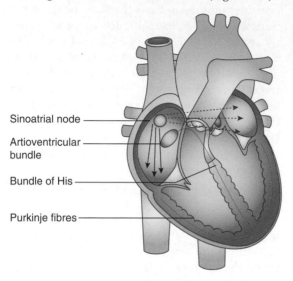

Sinoatrial node

Artioventricular bundle

Bundle of His

Purkinje fibres

FIGURE 8.9 **The electrical conduction of the heart**

The electrical conduction of the heart commences at the sinoatrial node (pacemaker) and

Health Connection

Pacemakers

The sinoatrial node contains cells that are the pacemaker for electrical stimulation and coordination of the heart. If they do not work properly the heart can start beating too fast, tachycardia, or too slowly, bradycardia or irregularly, arrythmically. A synthetic pacemaker can be implanted, surgically, to reset and maintain a regular heart beat. The pacemaker has detectors to adjust the rate as needed.

continues to the atrioventricular node and on to the bundle of His and Purkinje fibres.

The electrical stimulation is thus rapidly dispersed over the entire myocardium to enlist a full contraction of the muscle tissue for maximum force and blood output.

Health Connection

ECG

Muscles are innervated by electrical activity before they contract. The electrical activity of the heart can be monitored by **ECG** (electrocardiogram).
The ECG can tell the nurse about:

- cardiac electrical conduction;
- cardiac muscle (myocardium) contraction.

The normal ECG is composed of

- a 'P wave', corresponding to depolarisation of the atria, before atrial contraction;
- a 'QRS complex', corresponding to depolarisation of the ventricles before ventricular contraction;
- a 'T wave', corresponding to re-polarisation of the ventricles, as the ventricles relax.

The SAN innervates this pattern of electrical activity which is called **sinus rhythm**. Sinus rhythm is usually 60–80 beats per minute. Faster heart rate is called **tachycardia**. Slower heart rate is called **bradycardia**.

In practice: Why was a particular patient's ECG taken? What signs had they shown that an ECG should be taken? What had caused the changes in their ECG? (Figure 8.10)

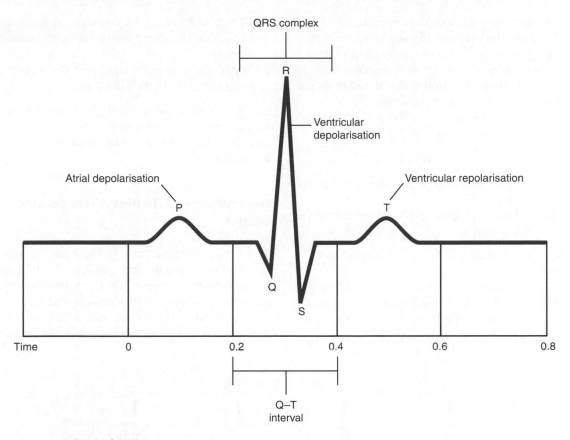

FIGURE 8.10 Typical ECG

Figure 8.11 shows, in milliseconds, the electrical conduction over the atria and into the ventricles. This activity is caused by the movement of ions, depolarisation and the ions are then re-polarised by active transport of ions against their concentration gradients. This is discussed further in Chapter 4, 'Communicating'.

How much blood the heart pumps

With each cardiac cycle or heart beat, a volume of blood is pumped into arteries. The amount, the volume, of blood that is pumped out into arteries by the ventricles in one minute is called the **cardiac output**. Obviously, it is expressed as a volume in millilitres or litres per minute. The amount depends on two factors:

- the **heart rate** measured in beats per minute;

- the **stroke volume** measured in millilitres or litres.

Thus **Cardiac Output (CO) = Stroke Volume (SV) × Heart Rate (HR)**

Heart rate is the number of beats per minute and can be measured by listening or taking a **pulse**. At rest the heart beats some **70** times per minute in adults. In the newborn the heart beats some 120 times per minute. By three years the rate has reduced to about 90 beats per minute.

Chapter Reference
Pulse is discussed below (see p. 235).

Stroke volume is the amount of blood pushed out of the ventricles each time the ventricles contract. This contraction is called a stroke, similar to the stroke of the engine of a car. Each time the engine strokes, an amount of fuel is ejected and burnt to release energy to move the car. The **stroke volume** is calculated from cardiac output and at rest it averages 70 ml.

If the stroke volume is 70 ml and the heart rate is 70 beats per minute then

$$CO = SV \times HR$$

If SV = 70 ml and heart rate = 70 beats per minute (bpm)

CO = 70 ml × 70 bpm = 4900 ml per minute = 4.9 L/min

So CO is almost 5 litres per minute in an adult at rest.

The electrical innervation and the strength of muscle all help to have a large, coordinated force to squeeze the liquid blood out into the arteries to circulate around the body.

- When the ventricles contract and pump blood out the blood into arteries it is called **systole**.
- When the ventricles relax and the atria fill with blood it is called **diastole**.

While it is hard to measure the heart directly we can measure the amount of pressure of systole and diastole as part of blood pressure in the blood vessels.

How different activities affect cardiac output

The cardiac output can be altered through homeostatic mechanisms according to changes in conditions or needs. This can be done by altering the stroke volume or the heart rate.

In general we do not alter our stroke volume. Athletes have stronger muscles, including heart

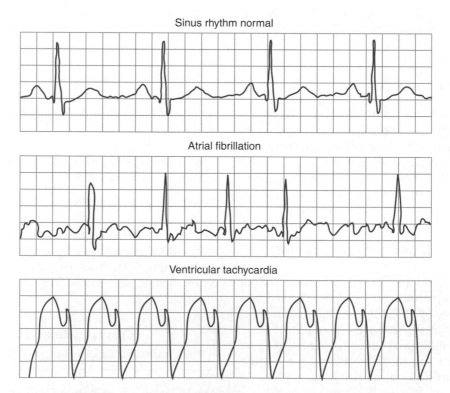

FIGURE 8.11 **Some examples of ECG when either the atria of ventricles become arrythmic**

muscle. Their stroke volume is larger and hence to have a cardiac output of 5 L/min they do not need to have such a high heart rate. For example, if their stroke volume is 100 ml/beat and their heart rate is also 70 bpm then:

CO = 100 ml × 70 bpm = 7000 ml/min = 7 L/min

rather than the 5 L/min of non-athletes.

For most of us we maintain a stroke volume of 70 ml and alter our heart rate for the conditions needed, for example:

CO = 70 ml × 100 bpm = 7000 ml/min = 7 L/min

The same amount as the athlete, but with a faster heart rate.

Changing conditions can lead to demands for changes in the supply of nutrients and oxygen to provide more or less fuel to make ATP. Cardiac output, especially **heart rate**, is one part that can be changed to accommodate these needs.

Health Connection

Heart rate

The heart rate is measured at rest. This is to see what the background rate is rather than the rate during physical activity. In adults it should be in the range 60–80 bpm. Alterations in this range are indicative of vascular problems such as atherosclerosis (discussed below) or haemorrhage.

Our cardiac output, especially heart rate, however, is not the only control that we have on how blood is delivered to the organs of our body to suit our activities during the day or during our lifespan. The vascular system is also involved.

The vascular system: Blood vessels

While our heart pumps out fluid blood carrying nutrients and gases, this blood must be carried in a series of vessels, the **vascular system**, to all the parts of our body and collected again from our body in vessels back to the heart.

Blood must be contained in these vessels rather than being allowed to leak all over the body which would be hard to control in terms of delivery and collection. If the heart is the pumping powerhouse and the blood a transport system, the vascular system is like a network of highways allowing the transport system to flow, bypassing, re-directing, putting speed limits and increasing traffic flow as is needed. Blood flows not just in a circuit from the heart to the body or lungs, but at the same time to many organs simultaneously as needed (Figure 8.12).

Constituents of the vascular system

The vascular system is made of a series of tubes, blood vessels. As discussed above these vessels are similar in structure to the heart. The vessels have a general structure that consists of three layers:

- an **outer** connective tissue layer – **tunica externa or adventitia**;
- a **middle** muscle tissue layer – **tunica media**;
- an **inner** endothelial tissue layer – **tunica interna**.

The muscle layer, like that of the heart, is **smooth muscle**, an involuntary muscle that is innervated, stimulated, by the sympathetic and parasympathetic autonomic nervous system.

Chapter Reference

The nervous system is discussed in Chapter 4, 'Communicating' (see p. 102).

The muscles of the tubes can **contract** and **relax**, just as the heart does, and therefore, help to pump the liquid blood around the body.

The blood exits from the heart in vessels called **arteries**. Arteries always carry blood away from the heart and usually contain oxygenated blood except for the pulmonary artery. Arteries carry blood under high pressure and are thick-walled with large middle layers, tunica media, of muscle. The largest artery, the aorta, has walls that are about 2 mm thick and a diameter of some 2.5 cm. Other arteries are about 1 mm thick and about 0.4 cm in diameter.

Arteries branch into smaller **arterioles**, which are about 30 μm thick almost all of

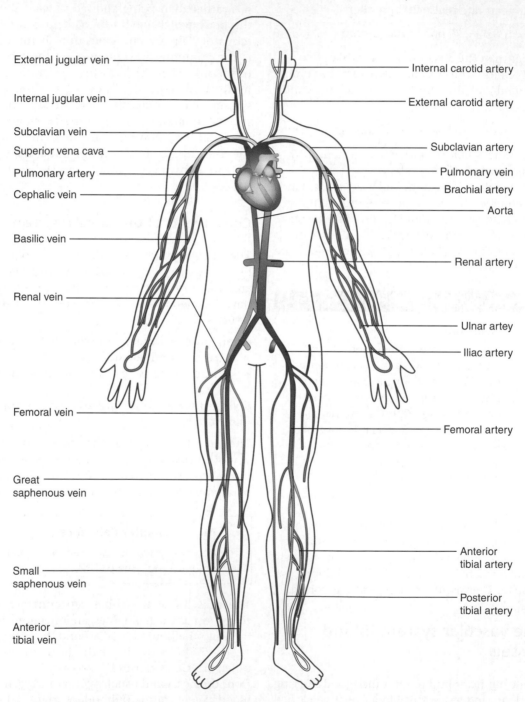

FIGURE 8.12 **Circulatory systems of the body**

which is smooth muscle. Their inner lumen is about 20 μm thick. Because of their muscle wall and small lumens arterioles' constriction of the muscle would further decrease the size of the lumen and cause an increase in **peripheral resistance.** Arterioles are involved in maintaining **blood pressure.**

Chapter Reference

Peripheral resistance and blood pressure are discussed below (see p. 236).

The network of tubes gets smaller and smaller as it branches away from the heart until it reaches fine tubes consisting of just one layer, the inner endothelium. These thin tubes are the **capillaries,** the functional end point of the network of blood vessels, similar in size and function to alveoli. These thin tubes are about 1 μm thick and about 5 μm in diameter where movement of solutes occurs. There are many fine capillaries just as there are many alveoli. Some 5% of the total blood volume is contained in the capillaries.

Venules, small veins, collect blood from the capillaries taking it back to the veins. **Veins** take blood back towards the heart via the vena cavae, the largest veins. Veins usually contain deoxygenated blood, apart from the pulmonary vein coming from the lung. Veins tend to be thinner-walled than arteries, lacking thick muscular walls. Instead of pumping blood towards the heart, veins depend on the milking action of skeletal muscle. As the skeletal muscle moves, it squeezes the veins pushing the blood along. Veins have valves to prevent the backflow of blood. There is some smooth muscle in the walls of the veins that can be contracted and relaxed to help move blood towards the heart. Veins have large lumens (Figure 8.13).

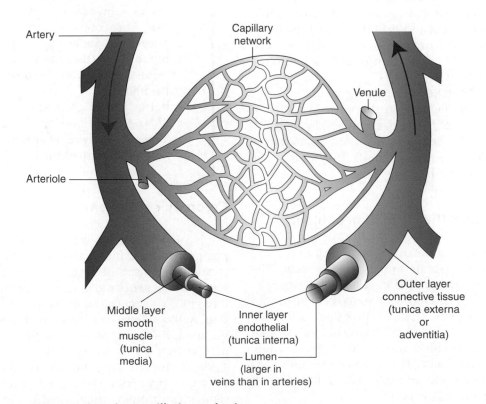

FIGURE 8.13 **Arteries, capillaries and veins**

What the vessels do: Physiology

The vessels transport blood around the body.

- the arteries take blood under high pressure away from the heart to the arterioles;
- the arterioles pump blood to the all the parts of the body via the capillaries;
- both arteries and arterioles are part of a large delivery network. They start at the ventricles of the heart;
- the **capillaries** allow for transport of substance, solutes and solvent into the interstitial spaces and into the cells of the body. Substances from cells enter the interstitial space and can be transported back into the blood;
- the capillaries feed into the venules;
- the venules join to the veins, which take blood back to the heart under low pressure;
- both the venules and veins are part of a large collection network. They end at the atria or the heart.

Perfusion: The circulation of blood

In the section on the heart the systemic and pulmonary circulations were discussed. The systemic (or somatic) circulation, the circulation serving the body or soma, is divided into various regions. These are now discussed.

When the blood leaves the left ventricle of the heart it enters the aorta, the main artery leaving the heart. This then divides into various arteries and arterioles taking blood to all the organs on the body.

Coronary circulation

While blood passes through the heart and is pumped into the pulmonary and systemic circulations the heart itself is an organ and needs a supply of nutrients and gases to maintain itself. It has its own circulation, the **coronary circulation**. As blood leaves the left ventricle and enters the aorta, the aorta has two branches, the coronary arteries taking blood to the heart. About 4–5% of blood leaving the left ventricle enters the coronary arteries. These arteries branch into capillaries through which oxygen can diffuse into the heart muscle. These then drain into coronary veins and into the coronary sinus which drains directly into the right atrium.

Cerebral circulation and the blood–brain barrier

The brain of humans has about 100 billion cells. As the brain is the central control region of the body including controlling homeostasis, brain cells need a constant supply of nutrients and oxygen. The brain takes about 15% of the total cardiac output. Blood is delivered by four arteries, two **carotid arteries** which branch to form the internal and external branches and two **vertebral arteries** which join to form the basilar arteries. The basilar artery branches and joins with the carotid arteries to form the Circle of Willis. As there are branches entering and forming the Circle of Willis, any blockage in one branch can be compensated by the other branches to ensure a blood supply to the brain. The supply to the brain barely changes even during exercise when the muscles are using up more oxygen and demanding a greater blood supply.

Blood drains from the brain into the jugular veins and returns to the heart via the superior vena cava.

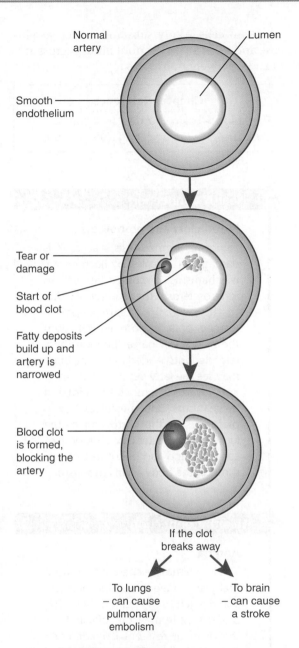

FIGURE 8.14 **Atherosclerosis**

Health Connection

Stroke

Atherosclerosis can block the arteries to the brain and neck. Narrowing of the carotid arteries can lead to brain **ischaemia** and **stroke** (Figure 8.14).

Apart from the constant need for nutrients and oxygen, the brain uses about 20% of all the oxygen entering the body, and the brain is exquisitely sensitive to chemical imbalances. The capillaries of the brain are specially adapted to allow oxygen and some chemicals such as steroid hormones to diffuse across into the brain cells, but they prevent many other substances crossing to the brain cells, forming a **blood–brain barrier**. The endothelial cells of the capillaries are joined by tight junctions and surrounded by 'foot-processes' from a type of cell of the brain called glial cells. The foot-processes store chemicals from metabolism and transfer them from the capillaries to the brain cells. Many substances, such as glucose and amino acids, cannot diffuse across and must be actively transported.

Chapter Reference

The blood–brain barrier is discussed in Chapter 4, 'Communicating' (see p. 102).

Health Connection

Blood clots and embolisms

In normal homeostasis if a vessel is damaged it is sealed by haemostatic mechanisms discussed above. In atherosclerosis the damage is due to the build up of fatty deposits. Instead of a smooth endothelium the blood now passes through these fatty deposits. Added to this the body may see the fatty deposits as damage and start haemostatic clotting mechanisms. Both processes end in blockages or the narrowing of the lumen. In the latter case a **blood clot** can form and can break off to travel through the body as an **embolism.**

Health Connection

Angina

This is a cramp-like chest pain brought on by an inadequate supply of blood and oxygen to the heart muscle. The blood supply may be sufficient for the heart at rest but is inadequate during exertion. The main cause of angina is atherosclerosis, but can be caused by a temporary spasm of the coronary arteries.

An embolism can move from where it is formed to another part of the body. If it moves to the lungs it causes pulmonary embolism. If it moves to the brain it can cause a stroke.

Health Connection

Myocardial infarction

This is the death of part of the heart **muscle** due to a blockage in a **coronary artery** and loss of blood supply. Its main causes include **atherosclerosis**, thrombosis, embolism and ventricular fibrillation. Depending on the extent of the damaged muscle, complications may occur, such as an arrythmias, heart failure, damage to the heart valves, pericarditis or cardiac arrest.

Circulation to the skin

The skin accounts for about 8% of cardiac output, but can increase the circulation 150 fold. This is done by **shunts**, which are special channels connecting arterioles to venules without the blood passing through capillaries. These shunts are found in extremities such as fingers, toes, palms and ear lobes. When body temperature rises, vasodilation occurs particularly in the shunts. Heat loss is thus increased.

Chapter Reference

Body temperature is discussed in Chapter 5, 'Controlling and Repairing' (see p. 142).

Circulation to the muscles

Skeletal muscle receives 15% of cardiac output at rest. During exercise this can increase to 90%, with oxygen consumption increasing from 20 to 90%. This is brought about by vasodilation in the capillary beds in the skeletal muscle.

Venous return

While the heart pumps out blood at high pressure into the arteries the problem for blood circulation is getting the blood back to the heart, **venous return**. The blood returning to the heart in veins is under low pressure. Getting blood back to the heart is aided by

- gravity – blood from the head goes back under gravity, but blood from the parts of the body lower than the heart does not;
- skeletal muscles and the diaphragm – veins travel through muscles and so the movement of the muscles helps to squeeze the veins and their contents, blood, back towards the heart;
- valves – veins have valves which help prevent the backflow of blood.

The pulse

In healthy individuals every time our heart beats our pulse beats too indicating that heart beat and pulse are related.

When the ventricles of the heart contract they push out a volume of blood, about 70 ml, called the stroke volume. This 70 ml of blood goes into the aorta, one of the major blood vessels. The volume of blood stretches the aorta, a bit like air going into a balloon. The walls of the aorta and of many arteries, vessels that carry blood away from the heart, have thick middle layers, tunica media, made up of smooth muscle and elastic tissue. As the walls distend and stretch, the elastic tissue makes the walls recoil and spring back to their former shape. When this happens the liquid inside the walls, the blood, is forced along the aorta. By this method blood is pushed around the arteries and arterioles into the capillaries were exchange of nutrients and oxygen from the blood to the surrounding cells can occur.

The stretching and recoil of the arteries can be felt over superficial arteries and is called a pulse. So each time blood is ejected from the ventricles of the heart, a pulse should be felt in the vascular system of arteries.

Health Connection

Sites to measure a pulse

As blood is pumped out of the left ventricle into the aortic artery the thick wall of the aorta expands. Due to the elastic nature of the wall it then recoils back, like the stretch and recoil of an elastic band. This expansion and recoil occurs in many arteries as blood is pumped into them. This expansion and contraction is a **pulse**. A pulse can be taken at various sites on the body, wherever an artery is near a skin surface. The common sites are illustrated in Figure 8.15. They are

- radial artery – inside of wrist,
- brachial artery – inside of elbow,
- carotid artery – sides of neck,
- temporal artery – sides of forehead,
- femoral artery – groin,
- popliteal artery – inside of knee,
- tibial artery – inside of ankle and
- dorsalis pedis artery – top of foot.

The pulse should be the same as the heart rate. A pulse can tell the nurse many points about the heart including:

- heart rate,
- heart beat regularity and
- heart beat strength.

Health Connection

The pulse

If the pulse is slower than the heart it is indicative of either

- narrowing or blocking of peripheral arteries, for example in atherosclerosis or angina,
- failing heart and
- haemorrhage.

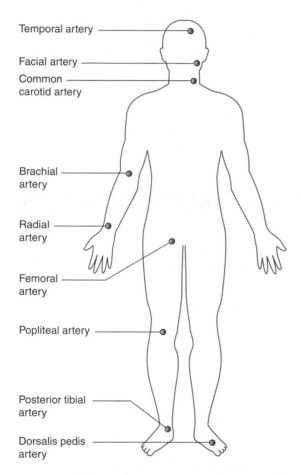

Temporal artery

Facial artery

Common carotid artery

Brachial artery

Radial artery

Femoral artery

Popliteal artery

Posterior tibial artery

Dorsalis pedis artery

FIGURE 8.15 **Pulse points**

Measuring the pulse, which is about **70 beats per minute** at rest in an **adult**, tells us that the vascular system is working and can be compared to the sounds of the heart beat.

If the pulse varies from the heart beat – they should both be about 70 beats per minute at rest – something is wrong. If pulse is less than heart rate either the arteries have narrowed or blocked or the heart is diseased or failing or the blood is not flowing due to blood loss.

How different amounts of blood are delivered according to needs

Blood pressure and peripheral resistance

Blood needs to be transported around the entire body to provide nutrients and gases and to remove waste from cells. Blood, a liquid medium, is contained in blood vessels, which can vary in size from large arteries to small capillaries.

Organs of the body have different requirements for nutrients and oxygen according to their metabolic rates. The brain has a high need; the skeleton a lower need. When muscle is being used a little it has a low need, but during exercise, for example, the need of the muscle for nutrients and oxygen to provide energy in the form of ATP increases. The body must adjust the flow of these nutrients and oxygen, and therefore the flow of blood, to suit the needs of the organs. *Different percentages of blood are delivered to different organs depending on their metabolic rates at rest and when exercising.* This is part of a homeostatic mechanism.

There are various ways to adjust blood flow. Either the heart can pump faster (**tachycardia**) or slower (**bradycardia**). If the heart rate changes this will alter the cardiac output (the amount of blood the heart pumps out per minute) as discussed above. Altering cardiac output (CO) alters the flow of blood generally, rather than specifically to a particular area or organ. The other way to alter amount of blood reaching various organs is for the blood to be pushed through the vessels at greater or lesser force altering the rate of flow, faster or slower. The force with which blood flows affects blood pressure. **Blood pressure (BP)** depends on force or pressure of blood on blood vessel walls. The pressure of blood inside an artery vessel comes up against two forces:

1. the pressure of the liquid pushing against the wall and
2. the pressure of the walls pushing against the liquid.

For example if you had a plastic bag and filled it with water, the water would push against the walls and fill the bag and the bag would push against the water. You could increase the pressure in the bag by either filling in more water or by making the bag smaller, squeezing on the sides of the bag. Blood pressure (BP) works the same way.

There are two components to BP, **Cardiac Output (CO)** and **Peripheral Resistance (PR)**

$$BP = CO \times PR$$

As discussed above, **cardiac output** is the amount of blood ejected each time the ventricles contract (stroke volume) in litres/min. In adults the stroke volume is about 70 ml/beat. How often the heart ejects blood in a minute is determined by the heart rate, which is about 72 beats/min. If CO = SV × HR then the cardiac output is 5 litres/min. This can be altered by speeding up or slowing down the heart rate.

Peripheral resistance (PR) is the resistance to blood flow in the peripheral blood vessels.

A few things that alter peripheral resistance are

1. the viscosity of the blood, how fluid or how thick it is;
2. the diameter of the blood vessels;
3. the length of the blood vessels.

To have an effect on blood pressure we could alter peripheral resistance by

1. altering the viscosity of the blood: We can add factors to dilute blood such as drinking fluids when dehydrated (or medically adding saline or plasma) or to thicken the blood such as when we make more red blood cells or clotting factors as needed;
2. altering the diameter of our blood vessels, which is the most usual way, we control our blood pressure, by altering our peripheral resistance in our arteries (and altering our heart rate) as required during different activities such as sleeping or running; we cannot, however, alter the length of the blood vessels once they have reached their full length in adulthood.

If we have a garden-hose that is attached to a tap we can alter the amount of water flowing through the hose in two ways.

- firstly, we can turn the tap more or less on. This is the same as the **cardiac output**, the *central* control of the amount flowing out of the source;
- secondly, we can *squeeze* the hose, and reduce its diameter (constrict it), the **peripheral** part of the system. This will make the water spurt out. This is the same as peripheral resistance.

Peripheral resistance can be altered by the *constriction* and *dilation* of arteries and arterioles. These vessels have a thick middle layer of tissue, the tunica media, composed of smooth muscle and elastic fibre. Smooth muscle is innervated (served by) the autonomic nervous system (ANS). The ANS, has two branches, the sympathetic, which tends to increase activity in a system, and the parasympathetic, which tends to decrease activity in a system. If the smooth muscle around an artery is activated by the sympathetic ANS, the muscle will contract. When it contracts it makes the lumen, the inner space of the artery, smaller. It constricts it. This will increase the pressure inside the artery. If the parasympathetic ANS sends signals to the smooth muscle, the muscle does not contract, the lumen increases in size and the artery dilates. The pressure inside the artery will decrease. Peripheral resistance, the resistance or opposition of blood flow around the body affects thus blood pressure.

Chapter Reference

The Autonomic Nervous System (ANS) is discussed in Chapter 4, 'Communicating' (see p. 102).

Box 8.4 Summary – CO, BP, PR

Once blood has left the heart it must flow in vessels to all parts of the body.

The **rate of blood flow** is affected by many factors:

1. **Cardiac output** (CO) which is influenced by heart rate and stroke volume.
2. **Blood pressure** (BP) is affected in turn by
   (a) cardiac output and
   (b) peripheral resistance.
3. **Peripheral Resistance** (PR) is in turn affected by
   (a) blood viscosity,
   (b) length of the blood vessel through which the blood is flowing and
   (c) diameter of the blood vessel.

Thus to maintain the flow of blood at the correct rate to serve all the organs and tissues of the body, the heart (cardio) and vessels (vascular) systems can be controlled. The heart can alter blood flow by altering the amount of blood pumped out of the heart (stroke volume) or the rate of pumping blood out of the heart (heart rate, corresponding usually to pulse rate). The vascular system can alter blood flow by altering blood pressure. Blood pressure is affected by peripheral resistance and heart rate. The principal method of altering peripheral blood flow is by altering the diameter of arterioles thereby altering resistance to flow and thus altering blood pressure.

Health Connection

Measuring BP

We can measure the pressure inside vessels by measuring what pressure it takes to stop the blood flowing and at what pressure the blood starts flowing again. The first pressure corresponds to the systolic pressure from the heart, the push of blood out of the ventricles into the aorta. The second pressure corresponds to the relaxation of the heart.

Blood pressure (BP) is measured in mm HG and expressed as systolic on the top and diastolic on the bottom (Figure 8.16). The measurement of blood pressure thus consists of two components:

- **systolic pressure** which occurs during discharge of blood from ventricles and is about 120 mm Hg in adults;
- **diastolic pressure** which occurs when heart is resting after ventricular contraction and is about 80 mm Hg in adults.

Adult blood pressure BP is thus around 120/80 mm.

Health Connection

Atherosclerosis

Arteries and arterioles have endothelium in their inner surface so that blood can flow smoothly. If arteries and arterioles get damaged blood flow is interrupted. In atherosclerosis plaques build up on the inner endothelium altering blood flow and peripheral resistance and thus blood pressure.

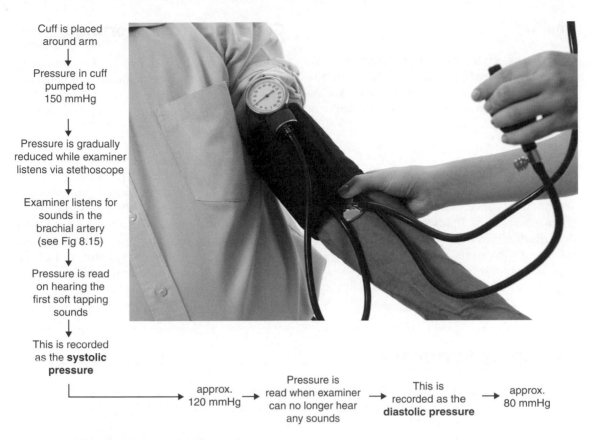

Cuff is placed around arm
↓
Pressure in cuff pumped to 150 mmHg
↓
Pressure is gradually reduced while examiner listens via stethoscope
↓
Examiner listens for sounds in the brachial artery (see Fig 8.15)
↓
Pressure is read on hearing the first soft tapping sounds
↓
This is recorded as the **systolic pressure**
→ approx. 120 mmHg → Pressure is read when examiner can no longer hear any sounds → This is recorded as the **diastolic pressure** → approx. 80 mmHg

FIGURE 8.16 **Blood pressure measurement**
Source: © trismile 2011 / iStockphoto

When the left ventricle ejects blood into a full aorta, systolic pressure, this causes distension and recoil in arterial system. This relies on elasticity of artery walls. This distension and recoil can be felt as a **pulse**, discussed above. During cardiac diastole the elastic recoil of arteries maintains diastolic pressure.

Changes during lifespan and lifestyle

Heart rate in newborns is 100–160 beats per minute and 70–120 beats per minute in children aged 1–10 years old. In adults the resting heart rate should be around 60–80 beats per minute. The pulse should be the same as the heart rate.

Blood pressure in newborns is 73/55 mmHg. By six months the BP is 90/53 mmHg, by 9 years it is 100/61 mmHg and by 15 years BP is 114/65.

Adults have BPs around 120/60 mmHg.

Elasticity in the arteries and heart reduces with age. This will affect peripheral resistance and cardiac output and thus blood flow in turn is affected.

Smoking

One of the major factors in atherosclerosis is smoking which increases damage to the endothelium of the blood vessels causing ischaemia or severe damage such as stroke or MI.

Diet

Saturated fats also seem to play a large part in atherosclerosis, as lipids can be deposited on the endothelium of blood vessels causing narrowing of the vessels, reducing blood flow and increasing blood pressure.

Conclusion: Transporting

Substances must be transported to and from all parts of our body to maintain homeostasis. Any interruption in the flow of substances has serious consequences for the organ involved. The heart is the main pump for the transport system, but can itself be affected by blood flow, or lack of it. Without a transport system our cells do not receive the nutrients and gases they need to continue their metabolic processes, nor rid themselves of waste. Blood is the liquid medium that allows all the substances to travel. Any interruption in its flow, volume or contents affects our transport systems and affects out abilities to carry out our daily lives.

Chapter Summary

- The function of the heart is to keep blood flowing to and from the tissues of the body and to send deoxygenated blood to the lungs for re-oxygenation.
- The function of the vessels is to contain the blood, to deliver and collect blood to and from the tissues.
- The heart pumps blood at the rate required by the tissues of the body.
- This rate is maintained through homeostatic mechanisms.
- There are control centres in the brain.
- Alterations in heart rate alter the delivery rate of blood and its constituents such as oxygen and glucose.
- The rate of blood delivery can also be altered by changing the pressure of blood in the vessels.

Eating and Drinking

> *All flesh is grass*
> Tanach (Bible) Isaiah, 40:6–8

Introduction: Eating and drinking as an activity of daily living

From the newborn baby taking its first feed to our last supper, eating and drinking play an important part in our lives. One of the main signs of independence is the ability to feed oneself, the ability to put one's own food on one's own table. One of the signs of adulthood is to earn a salary, from the word *sal* meaning salt, with which to feed oneself. Centurions in ancient Rome were paid in salt, hence the word salary. Not being able to feed oneself physically due to illness or disability removes feelings of independence and makes us feel infantilised. Not being able to earn a salary to put food on the table makes us feel diminished.

Food seems to fill so many functions. We use food biologically for growth and development and for our survival, to maintain our biological integrity, our homeostatic balance. We use food psychologically as a comfort. We use food sociologically to bind us together in groups. More and more people from biochemists and food scientists to nutritionists and dieticians have something to say about the food we eat and the food we should eat. For many people food has become an enemy. Diets, fads and allergies blamed on food have become a major source of income for many so-called experts. Public health and health promotion tell us daily what is good for us to eat only to recant the advice the next day. What constitutes a healthy diet seems more a matter of opinion than of fact. For many centuries people have managed to eat and thrive without all the advice and mixed messages we currently get. What constitutes a balanced, nutritious diet and what constitutes a desirable diet are often at odds. There has always been hunger and shamefully there still is in many parts of the world and for many people while others have surplus. How much we need and how much we have are seldom matched. While food plays so many roles in our lives there may always be a conflict between what we need biologically and what we need psychologically and sociologically. Food, at its very basis, sustains life and it is its biological function that will be the main focus of this chapter.

In Chapter 2, 'Working and Playing', we discussed the formation of *energy* from *food* and how material chemicals can be altered into different forms. When this process occurs energy is released. This fuels us and our living processes to allow us to carry out activities of daily living. This chapter investigates food and our ability to use food to re-structure our bodies and fuel our physical processes.

> ### Health Connection
>
> **Energy intake and metabolic output**
>
> There is a close link between our energy intake, in the form of calories in our food, and our ability to maintain and repair our bodies and carry out tasks requiring energy such as active transport and movement.

The environment

As discussed in Chapter 2, 'Working and Playing', 'there is no free lunch in the universe'. For us to maintain ourselves, to be alive, there is a cost in terms of energy. We expend energy every time we move a muscle or move a molecule by active transport.

> ### Chapter Reference
>
> ATP is discussed in Chapter 2, 'Working and Playing' (see p. 35). The movement of air is discussed in Chapter 7, 'Breathing' (see p. 184).

For us to maintain ourselves, our internal environment, energy in the form of ATP is used. As mentioned previously to use ATP we must make in the first place. We cannot really store ATP, we have about 90 seconds' worth of ATP stored in our bodies, and so we are constantly synthesising and using it. To make ATP requires the **oxidation** of **glucose**. We obtain the oxygen from the external environment, air, via our lungs. We obtain the glucose (sugar) from the external environment via our mouths. We then extract what is needed, oxygen from air,

and glucose from the mixed food we intake. Oxygen extraction is discussed in Chapter 7, 'Breathing'. Glucose extraction is discussed in this chapter.

As discussed in Chapter 2, 'Working and Playing', everything in the external environment is composed of matter and all matter is composed of chemicals. We too are composed of the same material as the external environment, chemicals, and use substances in the external environment, such as food, to maintain our internal environment as part of homeostasis and health. You are what you eat!

Food and nutrients

Food, the chemicals we imbibe or **ingest**, whether it is 'organic' or processed, is a material substance composed of chemicals. The branch of chemistry called organic chemistry investigates the chemistry of carbon. We eat other life forms such as plants and animals and their products. These, like us, are carbon based. The main chemical food types we need are carbohydrates, fats and proteins. These constitute our main **nutrients**, the group of chemicals that are nutritious to us. These particular chemicals are not inherently nutritious or special; they are nutritious to us because they are similar to us and can be converted into material such as cells or energy such as ATP that we can use. In other words nutrients are merely useful chemicals to us. Carbohydrates, proteins and fats contain **carbon**, because we are a carbon-based life form and we need to take in carbon to maintain ourselves. Additional chemicals in food include chemicals such as hydrogen, oxygen and nitrogen.

> ### Chapter Reference
>
> Chemicals and macromolecules such as carbohydrates are discussed in Chapter 2, 'Working and Playing' (see p. 35).

The main **nutrients** and the **foods** in which they are found that we need to sustain our cells are listed in Table 9.1. The foods that we consume are called our **diet**. Most of the foods we consume are large macromolecules which need to be broken down, **digested**, into smaller constituent parts that can enter the blood and body cells. The macromolecules are broken down in the **digestive tract** discussed later in this chapter.

Carbohydrates

Carbohydrates, consisting of carbon, hydrogen and oxygen, are the major source of energy in animal, including human, diets. There are various types of dietary carbohydrate. One way that carbohydrates are classified is by size:

- Monosaccharides – are simple sugars consisting of one basic unit.
- Disaccharides – are simple sugars consisting of two basic units.
- Polysaccharides – are long chains of linked simple sugar units, polymers; the chains can sometimes be branching.

Polysaccharides are large **polymers** – molecules formed from joining basic structures together, in this case polymers of **monosaccharides**, also known as **sugars**, and including **starch** and **cellulose** from plants and **glycogen**, a stored form of glucose, from animals. Disaccharides include **sucrose** and **lactose**. Monosaccharides include **glucose** and **fructose**. One other source of polysaccharide is **cellulose**, a plant material also called **fibre** or **roughage**. It is a non-starch

Table 9.1 Major nutrients needed in our diets, the constituent part and the foods in which they are found

Major nutrients	Constituent (unit) part	Foods in which they are found
Carbohydrate (polysaccharides)	A complex arrangement of sugars (monosaccharides) – molecules linked together to form a polysaccharide.	Plants. Starch from grains, legumes, root vegetables. Sugar and cane sugar from fruits. Lactose sugar from milk. Glycogen from meat.
Lipids (fats)	Large polymer of fatty acid and glycerol.	Saturated fats from animal products. Unsaturated fats from seeds, nuts, vegetable oils. Cholesterol from egg yolks, meat, milk.
Proteins (polypeptides)	A complex arrangement of amino acids.	Eggs, milk, meat, nuts, legumes, cereals.
Vitamins	Organic molecules that form co-enzymes.	Many fruits and vegetables.
Minerals	Mineral salts or ions (also called electrolytes) such as sodium, potassium, chlorine, magnesium, calcium.	Many foods such as fruits, meats, dairy.
Water	A liquid solvent composed of hydrogen and oxygen in which ionic or polar substrates dissolve.	All normal foods i.e. not dessicated or dehydrated foods.
Nucleic acids (e.g. DNA and RNA)	Composed of nucleic acids such as adenine, thymine.	All living organisms (viruses, bacteria, plants and animals).

polysaccharide which cannot be digested by humans. It is discussed later (Figure 9.1).

Monomer sugar units (such as glucose) can join together to form a two-sugar entity, a disaccharide, or join many monosaccharides together to form a polymer, a polysaccharide such as starch or cellulose as discussed in Chapter 2, 'Working and Playing'.

Lipids

Fats and **lipids** are found in both plants and animals. They are mainly formed from carbon and hydrogen with some oxygen. Because they are formed from covalent carbon and hydrogen units they are insoluble in water (hydrophobic).

There are three main types of lipids in humans:

1. **Triglycerides**
   - Contain three units (tri-).
   - Composed of fatty acids and glycerol.
   - Act as the main lipid stored in humans as fat, usually just below the skin, as a source of energy.
   - They can be saturated (no double bonds between the carbon atoms) or unsaturated (double bonds between the carbon atoms).
   - Saturated fats can line up together and form weak interactions which allow many to be solid at room temperature (such as butter).
   - Unsaturated fats are not as linear due to 'kinks' in the bonding and tend to be liquid at room temperature, such as oil.
2. **Phospholipids**
   - Contain lipids (hydrophobic) joined to a hydrophilic phosphate (PO_3) tail.
   - Allow the lipid to be fat soluble at one end and water soluble at the other end.
   - Form the lipid bilayer of the plasma membrane around cells.
3. **Steroids**
   - As the name suggests these fats include **cholesterol**, some **steroid** hormones, bile salts and vitamin D.

Health Connection

Fats

There is a lot of debate about plant fats being **unsaturated** and better for us than animal **saturated** fats. We are capable of synthesising fats ourselves. Surplus carbohydrates can be converted to fats and we need to synthesise cholesterol, a vital constituent of cell membranes and the basis of all the steroid (cholesterol) hormones.

Proteins

Proteins, or **polypeptides**, are a complex chain of **amino acids** joined together into peptide chains. There are numerous types of amino acids, but only approximately **20** found in living organisms. Of the 20 we can synthesise some from basic materials, but eight of them are *essential* in our diet as we cannot synthesise

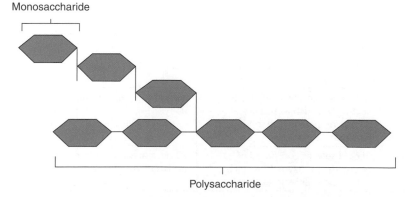

Monosaccharide

Polysaccharide

FIGURE 9.1 **Monosaccharides, disaccharides and polysaccharides**

them. The amino acids are classified according to the behaviour of their side chains, part of their molecular structure which affects aspects of their behaviour such as whether they are acidic, basic, polar or non-polar at a neutral pH. Amino acids are composed of carbon, hydrogen, oxygen, nitrogen and sometimes sulphur. Their name derives from their having an **amine** group (similar to **ammonia**, NH_3, in chemical form) and an **acid** group.

Proteins make up over half of the body's organic matter. They are used to

- provide the structure of body tissues;
- act in physiological processes in the cell;
- act as enzymes, hormones and antibodies.

> **Chapter Reference**
>
> The chemical nature of carbohydrate, fats, proteins and amino acids are discussed in Chapter 2, 'Working and Playing' (see p. 35).

Vitamins

Vitamins are a chemically diverse group of organic molecules found in many foods. Vitamins are often divided into water soluble and fat soluble types. Water soluble vitamins are excreted in the urine. They have a variety of functions in the body and many are precursors of **co-enzymes**, non-protein molecules that are associated with enzymes and play a crucial role in their catalytic activity. Some enzymes are part of signalling pathways inside cells, helping gene expression and thus protein synthesis.

Health Connection

Storage of vitamins

Fat soluble vitamins are more prone to storage in our body fats and *overdose* is therefore more possible while the water soluble vitamins are more easily eliminated from the body.

Some vitamins are **antioxidants**, helping to limit the harmful effect of **free radicals**, atoms with an unpaired electron that are extremely reactive and can cause tissue damage. While many advocate vitamin supplements, over-consumption of vitamins is as bad as under-consumption (Table 9.2).

Health Connection

Excess vitamins

Excess vitamin B6, a water soluble vitamin, can damage the peripheral nervous system. Excess fat soluble vitamin A can cause liver and bone damage, hair loss, double vision, vomiting and headaches. Overdose of this in pregnant women can lead to birth defects in the unborn child.

Minerals

These are 'inorganic' molecules, not based on carbon. Minerals are, really, mineral salts. They are made of **ions** which, in water, become **electrolytes**, conducting electricity. They have a variety of functions in the body including structural components of cells and tissues, intercellular communication, components of molecules, components of enzymes as co-enzymes and osmotic balance (Table 9.3).

Health Connection

Amount of vitamins and minerals in a diet

For both vitamins and minerals there are consequences if there is either too little or too much. People on restricted diets or those taking surplus vitamin or mineral tablets may, therefore, be liable to changes in homeostasis and health.

Nucleic acids

Nucleic acids are composed of rings of carbon with nitrogen, oxygen and hydrogen as the main other constituents. They can polymerise with other nutrients to large molecules such as the genetic material of life, DNA.

Chapter Reference

Nucleic acids and DNA are discussed in Chapter 3, 'Growing and Developing' (see p. 64).

The other important **nucleotide** containing molecule is **adenosine triphosphate (ATP)**. It provides the chemical energy used by all cells. Energy is released by breaking high energy phosphate bonds in the ATP which then becomes **adenosine diphosphate (ADP)** – in other words the three (tri-) phosphates have been become two (di-) phosphates. ATP is replenished from ADP by oxidation of food fuels (Figure 9.2).

We use ATP for all the work processes of our body by breaking it from being a **tri**phosphate (ATP) to a **di**phosphate (ADP) and releasing the energy stored in the bond which can then do work:

$$ATP \leftrightarrow ADP + energy$$

To make ATP again from ADP, glucose is oxidised and energy is put in. The energy released from ATP is exactly the same amount required to make ATP from ADP. It is a **reversible** reaction as discussed in Chapter 2, 'Working and Playing'.

Metabolism and calorie requirements

Why we need to eat

Food provides nutrients, chemicals that can be used in the body for a variety of functions. For example, carbohydrates provide sugars that can be used for energy production. Fats can also be converted into energy. They can also be used for insulation and as a store for future use as an energy supply. Proteins provide amino acids, which can be recombined to make new proteins such as enzymes, hormones and transport proteins such as haemoglobin. Nucleic acids are used in the synthesis of the genetic material, the instruction code, of each cell in the body. Vitamins help in the function of many proteins and processes in the body. Minerals are involved in many processes such as water balance, nerve conduction and muscle contraction. Food, therefore, provides the body with the necessary chemicals that can be used for a variety of functions including building blocks for new proteins and cell growth.

Fibre does not have any nutritious value. In other words, it does not release compounds that can be used by the body. Fibre is required in the diet for the proper functioning of the digestive system.

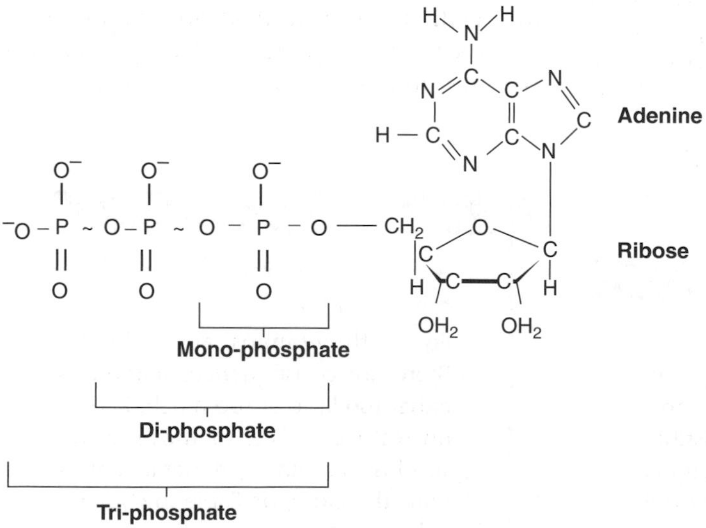

FIGURE 9.2 **ATP**

It aids transport of foods, nutrients and waste through the digestive system.

Glucose, for example, is a very important constituent of our diets. It is made by plants by a process called photosynthesis. We cannot synthesise it so we must imbibe external sources of it. We then need to extract the glucose from all the foods we have eaten. Once glucose has been extracted it is oxidised in the cells in the body to produce ATP. The glucose acts as an energy source to fuel the processes of the cells and hence of the entire body. This is in a manner similar to releasing energy from petrol in a car. The petrol, which is chemically very similar to glucose, is burnt in oxygen. We 'burn' glucose in oxygen at a much lower temperature due to the presence of specialised proteins called enzymes that lower the energy required to activate a reaction so that it can proceed in our bodies at 37°C. Higher temperatures would affect our proteins, including our enzymes, which would no longer function.

The process of making ATP is part of metabolism; the energy used and synthesised by cells. Metabolism can be **catabolic**, breaking down substances such as glucose, or **anabolic**, synthesising substances such as proteins.

ATP is both synthesised from ADP in an anabolic process which requires the *input* of energy in the form of glucose and broken down to ADP to release energy as an *output* in a catabolic process (see Figure 9.2).

Why we need to drink

Water is the major **solvent** of the body. Many chemical substances can be transported in it or dissolved in it. Cells are kept under a narrow range of osmotic pressure which relies on the movement of water into and out of the cell. This movement also allows the transport of some substances.

Chapter Reference

Water balance and drinking is discussed later in the chapter (see p. 278).

How much food we need

As discussed, we need food for the nutrients it contains. Different foods contain different nutrients, in other words different foods contain different chemicals that the body needs. The amount of each type of nutrient needed varies with the activities of the body. For instance, blood cells have a limited lifespan. New blood cells are made daily. If more were required due to infection or more were lost than the usual daily turnover due to an injury new blood cells would be needed in larger amounts than normal. Cell growth and multiplication depend on the presence of many chemicals such as amino acids to make new protein, nucleic acids to make new genes for new cells and vitamins to help in the process. Foods containing these chemicals would be needed in greater amount than usual.

Health Connection

Diet and wound healing

Wound healing is discussed in Chapter 3, 'Growing and Developing' (see p. 64), may be enhanced by a balanced diet and impaired by a poor diet.

Protein-rich food such as meats (including fish, which is an animal and is, therefore, considered to be meat) and pulses can be digested to release the amino acids that the proteins contain. Food labelling may list the amino acids that are contained in the proteins and it may state the amount, in grams, of protein in the food.

Foods that contain energy-rich foods, polysaccharides and lipids that can be digested to release their constituent monosaccharides or fats, will generally be labelled with the amount of kilocalories or kilojoules they contain.

Chapter Reference

ATP is discussed in Chapter 1, 'Maintaining a Safe Environment' (see p. 1) and in Chapter 7, 'Breathing' (see p. 184).

Table 9.2 Vitamins. The common name and the chemical name of the vitamin are given. Vitamins are either water soluble or fat soluble. The dosages per day are listed as well as what diseases one can suffer from if there is too little or too much of a vitamin in our diet.

Vitamin (and its solubility)	Food Source	Function	Deficiency disease	Overdose (toxicity)
Vitamin A Retinol (fat soluble)	Cod liver oil, carrots, egg yolks	Eyesight, growth, repair	Night-blindness	Fat soluble so can be stored in body for a long time
Vitamin B1 Thiamine (water soluble)	Cereal, yeast, red meat, nuts, wheatgerm	Nervous system, digestion, muscles	Beriberi, tingling in fingers and toes. Weakness	Drowsiness or muscle relaxation with large doses
Vitamin B$_2$ Riboflavin (water soluble)	Meat, fish, eggs	Skin, nails, hair, lips, eyesight, digestion	Itchy mucous membranes, cracked lips	
Vitamin B$_3$ Niacin, niacinamide (water soluble)	Meat, eggs, grain	Digestion, nervous system, skin and mucous membranes	Pellagra	Liver damage (doses > 2g/day)
Vitamin B$_5$ Pantothenic acid (water soluble)	Meat, whole grain	Synthesis of coenzyme A Synthesis and metabolism of proteins, fats and carbohydrates	Fatigue, weakness	Diarrhoea; possibly nausea and heartburn
Vitamin B$_6$ Pyridoxine (water soluble)	Meat, fish, bananas, dairy products	Skin and nerves, absorption of nutrients	Skin inflammation, anaemia peripheral neuropathy	Impairment of proprioception, nerve damage (doses > 100 mg/day)
Vitamin B$_7$ Biotin (water soluble)	Meat, dairy, eggs	Cell growth, fatty acid metabolism	Dermatitis, enteritis	Not known
Vitamin B$_9$ Folic acid (water soluble)	Leafy green vegetables, pumpkin, avocados, beans	Red blood cell	Tiredness In pregnancy, lack can lead to birth defects, such as neural tube defects	May mask symptoms of vitamin B$_{12}$ deficiency.

Vitamin	Sources	Function	Deficiency	Toxicity
Vitamin B$_{12}$ Cobalamin (water soluble)	Liver, poultry, milk, eggs	Red blood cells, Nerve formation	Tiredness, tingling in hands and feet. Megaloblastic anaemia	No known toxicity
Vitamin C Ascorbic acid (water soluble)	Most citrus fruits, potatoes, peppers	Immune system Wound healing	Tiredness, slow wound healing, scurvy	Diarrhoea and nausea
Vitamin D Calciferol (fat soluble)	Cod liver oil, sunlight	Bones and teeth	Rickets and osteomalacia, unhealthy teeth	Fat soluble, so can be stored in the body
Vitamin E Tocopherols, tocotrienols (fat soluble)	Vegetable oil, nuts, soyabeans	Antioxidant	Deficiency is very rare; weak muscles, mild haemolytic anaemia in newborn infants	Not known
Vitamin K Quinone (fat soluble)	Leafy green vegetables	Assists blood clotting	Bleeding	Increases coagulation in patients taking warfarin

Table 9.3 Major minerals. Minerals, also known as salts, are formed from metals as discussed in Chapter 1, 'Maintaining a Safe Environment'. They form positive cations in ionic bonds. When they dissolve in water they are called electrolytes.

Mineral	Functions	Food sources	Deficiency disease	Overdose (toxicity)
Calcium (Ca)	Bones and teeth. Blood clotting. Nerve and muscle function.	Milk, cheese, yoghurt and canned fish, green leafy vegetables, white and brown flour and bread, fortified soya products and nuts.	Bone weakening – rickets and osteomalacia.	Rare in healthy people.
Sodium (Na)	Regulation of body water content. Nerve impulses.	Salt.	Fatigue, nausea, cramps. Thirst is experienced.	Linked to hypertension.
Potassium (K)	Constituent of body fluids. Functioning of cells. Nerve conduction.	Widely distributed in fruits, vegetables, milk, meat.	Weakness, mental confusion and heart failure.	Excess can be harmful especially if the kidneys are not functioning properly.
Magnesium	Bone, body fluids, involved in energy transfer in the cell, in enzyme activity and in nerve and muscle functioning.	Wholegrain cereals, nuts and green leafy vegetables, milk, potatoes.	Cardiovascular contractions, (heart attack) Neurological problems (depression, irritability, fits, tiredness).	Not known.
Phosphorus	Bones and teeth. Essential component of all cells, energy storage as ATP.	Milk, cheese, meat, fish, eggs, cereals.	Dietary deficiency unknown.	Not known.

Calories

Calories are a measure of the amount of energy that can be released from a material substance, food. Releasing energy from food (catabolism) is the reverse of synthesising food from energy, the process plants carry out called photosynthesis, discussed above.

Calories are calculated by releasing the *maximum* amount of energy a food can contain. Each calorie is the amount of energy released that can heat one gram of water by one degree Celsius. Generally calories are expressed as kilocalories, thousands of calories, or the amount of energy released that can heat 1000 g or water by 1°C.

Foods are labelled as containing a number of kilocalories (kcal). The modern SI unit, the joule, is also sometimes used.

Calories are a very misunderstood concept in most diets. They are an attempt to relate the amount of a material (food) to the amount of energy it contains. It assumes the amount contained in the food is the same as the amount released in all circumstances. As there are variations between people and our ability to digest foods may also vary, we may not all release the same amount of energy from the same foods as other people. We each have variations in our metabolic rates. Calories, as used in diets, are an attempt to link the amount consumed to the amount expended; the amount eaten to the amount used.

Different nutrients yield different amounts of energy, as measured by calories or joules, for the same amount of food. Each gram of a nutrient contains different amounts of energy in the form of calories or joules. Fats contain more energy than carbohydrates or proteins (Table 9.4).

Health Connection

Diets and weight

Different daily nutrient requirements – diets – suit different people. This may reflect the amount of energy each person uses during the day. It may reflect our different metabolisms or our different abilities to digest foods. This may account for our varying calorie needs and that some people lose weight on a diet that others do not. With sedentary patients, calorie needs change yet again, but not all sedentary patients have the same needs – one size may not fit all. As a rule of thumb the amount of calories you eat should match the amount you use. If you consume more than you use you will store the excess as fat, you put on weight. If you use up more than you consume you will use your fat stores up and you will lose weight. It is another example of the balance of homeostatic mechanisms as discussed in Chapter 1, 'Maintaining a Safe Environment'.

Metabolism and metabolic rate

Metabolism is the process of chemical reactions that occur within the cells of the body. There are many chemical reactions in cells. The main ones of interest in health are those that are catabolic, breaking down molecules into constituent parts, and those that are anabolic, forming molecules into new arrangements

Table 9.4 The energy yield of different nutrients

Nutrient	Available energy/kcal per gram	Available energy/kjoule per gram	Daily intake %
Carbohydrate	4	15–17	50
Fat	9	37	35
Protein	4	16	15

as needed by the body. Catabolic reactions often release energy which can be converted into ATP for use by the cells of the body. Anabolic reactions often use up ATP energy. Catabolic and anabolic reactions are often linked in terms of energy output and energy consumption.

Not all the potential energy contained in food is converted into usable energy. Some of it is released as heat. This heat can be used to maintain body temperature.

Energy generated = energy used + heat released

The **basic metabolic rate** (BMR) is measured in an individual who has not eaten for 12 hours, is at rest and at a comfortable temperature. It is the minimum calories you would need to sustain your life without much activity, e.g. when lying in bed all day. It uses your weight, height, age and gender to calculate your BMR.

The formula for calculating your BMR in metric is:

Women: BMR = 655 + (9.6 × weight in kilos) + (1.8 × height in cm) – (4.7 × age in years).
Men: BMR = 66 + (13.7 × weight in kilos) + (5 × height in cm) – (6.8 × age in years).

Chapter Reference

Blood cells are discussed in Chapter 7, 'Breathing' (see p. 184). Cell growth is discussed in Chapter 3, 'Growing and Developing' (see p. 64) and Chapter 1, 'Maintaining a Safe Environment' (see p. 1).

A balanced diet

A balanced diet depends on our individual needs, but generally suggests that we need a selection of different foods as each food contains different nutrients. As we require protein-rich foods for cell growth and repair, energy-rich foods for metabolism and muscle contraction, fats for maintaining the cell membrane, mineral salts for muscle contraction, nerve impulse and water balance, and nutrients such as vitamins to help enzyme function a balanced diet needs to include all the nutrient sources, foods, containing this mix. How much and in what mix we need foods depends on our daily activities and the stage we are at in our lives. Typical values are shown in Table 9.5.

People vary, as discussed above, in terms of their activities, metabolic rates and digestive abilities so their dietary needs vary. Table 9.5 shows the average daily nutritional needs for adults.

Health Connection

Exercise and ATP

An athlete uses up energy in their sport. Running causes the muscles, especially in the legs, to contract rapidly and for prolonged periods of time. Muscle contraction is an active process using ATP. ATP must be synthesised from oxygen and glucose in every cell of the body. Those people who are very active therefore use more ATP and require more energy-rich foods, foods containing monosaccharides and lipids (fats).

Health Connection

Pregnancy

During pregnancy women often claim they need to 'eat for two', themselves and the embryo. In fact no more calories are needed until the last couple of months and then only about 200 more calories a day are sufficient. During breast feeding an extra 400 calories a day may be needed.

There is also a food we consume that has no nutritious value, but is needed in our diet, **roughage** also known as fibre.

Table 9.5 Average nutrient requirements in adult life

Nutrition	Men over 24 years	Women 25–50 years	Women over 50 years
Calories	2900	2200	1900 maximum
Fat	96 g maximum	73 g maximum	63 g maximum
Saturated fat	32 g maximum	24 g maximum	21 g maximum
Cholesterol	300 mg maximum	300 mg maximum	300 mg maximum
Protein	63 g	50 g	50 g maximum
Carbohydrates	446 g	335 g	283 g
Fibre	20–30 g	20–30 g	20–30 g
Sodium	2400 mg maximum	2400 mg maximum	2400 mg maximum

Roughage or fibre

This substance contains a plant polysaccharide called cellulose. It has no nutritional value as we do not have the enzyme to digest cellulose and release the monosaccharide sugars it contains, so we cannot get energy from cellulose. Cellulose remains in its large chewed form in our digestive system and never enters our blood to be carried as a nutrient to cells.

Why we need roughage

Because we cannot digest, break down and release, the nutrients in cellulose it remains in our intestines and is excreted in our faeces. Roughage adds bulk to our food intake and helps to move food particles through our intestines. It helps eliminate undigested food particles and waste. Without sufficient roughage food particles and waste remain in our intestine where bacteria in the gut start to break down these particles and can cause illness. It may come as a shock that our waste is the meal of another species and the bacteria in our gut use our 'waste' as their food. In return they release, as their waste, some vitamins such as **vitamin K** which we cannot make for ourselves. These bacteria are called **'commensals'** from the Latin 'mensa', meaning table. They *share* the table with us and are beneficial to us and we are useful to them; the 'cost–benefit' balances with each side benefiting. However, too much fibre in the diet may *prevent* vitamin absorption in the large intestine or bowel.

Chapter Reference

Bacteria are discussed in Chapter 11, 'Cleansing and Dressing' (see p. 299).

Health Connection

Constipation and bowel movement

Humans on an average healthy diet (food intake) should be excreting waste faeces at least once a day. Less than that indicates a very slow transit through the gastrointestinal tract and may indicate constipation where faecal stools are very hard. This can be due to low roughage in the diet, with low bulk making it hard to move matter through the tract, but allowing time for water to be absorbed. Passing faecal matter may then become painful. There are many over-the-counter remedies to aid the movement and expulsion of waste from the tract. Health professionals often ask patients about their 'bowel movement', when and how often they have expelled faecal waste. Not expelling waste regularly also has other health implications – all waste attracts microbes such as bacteria and can result in infections. Immobile or inactive people have poorer frequency of bowel movements as mobility helps to push waste through the tract.

What happens if there is a lack of nutrients in the diet

A lack of nutrients in the diet can lead, over the long term, to **malnutrition**. For most people malnutrition is a lack of food and therefore a lack of nutrients such as sugars, water and mineral salts. This would lead to severe lack of energy production. Stored fats can be converted to energy producing food. Once the fats have been used proteins from areas such as muscles can also be converted to energy producing food. The reduction in stored fat reduces insulation and more energy is required to maintain a stable temperature. The reduction of muscle leads to weakness.

For some people, malnutrition is not due to lack of food, but to a poor diet.

Health Connection

Fluid intake

While drinking will be discussed later in this chapter, the amount of fluids and the types of fluids we consume may also affect the calories we consume. Alcohol and sugary drinks have a high calorie load and must be taken into account when assessing how many calories have been consumed when trying to maintain a healthy weight.

Box 9.1 Health promotion and diet

Much is written about a 'balanced diet'. There are many theories about what constitutes a good diet for humans, but there are many humans with different needs. Scientific research will eventually be able to ascertain a generally healthy diet, but until then there will be many fads and opinions.

Increasingly obesity and its consequences diabetes, heart disease and stroke, are affecting parts of the western world, particularly the USA and UK. If obesity is seen in particular countries epidemiologists are interested in its causes. As obesity is seen across the populations of the USA and the UK it is likely that there is an environmental cause rather than a genetic cause as both populations are quite heterogeneous, quite diverse. It appears that our diets may be to blame rather than our genes. When experts working in health promotion look at other countries and their diets and diseases Japan is often cited as a country where the people eat a healthy diet and have low obesity associated diseases. The Japanese diet is very low in dairy products and quite low in red meat, both of which contain saturated fats, although they do eat fats from fish. As a result, we are told that the Japanese diet is the one to follow. The Swedish diet is very high in dairy products, but the Swedish people do not have an obesity problem or obesity related diseases. Both Japan and Sweden have very high life expectancy. Both of these countries are quite homogeneous in their populations so genes and environments may work together. But it is more complicated than we think and simple solutions or one style of diet may not work for all people.

Our foods contain increasing amounts of preservatives and hormones, such as oestrogen and growth hormone. These aid rapid growth of the food source, plants or animals. This means that a plant or animal can be fed the hormone and grow faster and be harvested for consumption sooner. These chemicals can have deleterious effects on us and on the planet. The food packaging may also have effects on the food and therefore on us. When we consume the food we consume all the chemicals in the food. Eating foods that are not grown locally, eating out of season, not having regional foods and not eating enough fresh foods may be the source of the problem.

Genetically Modified (GM) foods, however, should not need additional chemical additives and may be a way forward for both us as a species and the planet. With increasing populations an increase in food production is needed, but the method of this larger production (chemicals or genes) may affect our health.

Food charts and monitoring food intake

People who are not able to feed themselves, for instance due to being immobilised, need to have their nutritional status evaluated, how much and what sort of food they require. Food charts and monitoring food intake helps to ensure that the appropriate foods and amounts have been consumed. Poor nutritional status may prevent or prolong healing as vital nutrients for use by the cells of the body may not have been consumed.

Box 9.2 Summary – Food

Food in the external environment is a source of nutrient chemicals that our internal environment needs to replenish cells and produce energy for living processes. Food contains many different nutrients which we require in varying amounts for a healthy **diet**.

Eating

Digestion and nutrient absorption

Once we have found the food we need in the external environment we must ingest it and convert it into a form that the body can use. **Eating** is the first part of the process – ingesting food. The food comes as large molecules which must be broken down into small molecules for **absorption**, transport from the tract into the blood and transport to all the cells of the body. The breakdown of large food molecules into small molecules for absorption is done by the **digestive system**.

The constituents of the digestive system

The digestive system is separated into two parts: the **gastrointestinal tract (GI tract)** also called the **alimentary canal (AI)** and the **accessory organs**. In this chapter we shall refer to the tract as the gastrointestinal or **GI** tract. The GI tract runs from the mouth to the anus and is some 4.5 metres long. The tract contains food which is ingested into the mouth before passing down the tract for digestion. Undigested food is eliminated, or excreted, from the anus.

Chapter Reference

Hormones and the nervous system are discussed in Chapter 4, 'Communicating' (see p. 102).

The **accessory organs** include the **salivary glands**, the **pancreas** and the **liver** which aid digestion in the tract. As with all systems, it is under hormonal and nervous system control.

The digestive system is composed of a group of structures running from the head region, through the thorax, with most of the system in the abdominal cavity ending in the pelvic cavity. It consists of:

- **mouth** or **oral cavity** containing:
  - teeth
  - tongue
  - salivary glands;
- **pharynx;**
- **larynx;**
- **epiglottis;**
- **oesophagus;**
- **stomach;**
- **small intestine** or small bowel or small colon containing
  - duodenum
  - jejunum
  - ileum;
- **large intestine** or large bowel or **large colon** containing
  - ascending colon
  - transverse colon

- descending colon
- sigmoid colon;
- **rectum**
  - anus.

The gastrointestinal tract runs from the mouth into the oesophagus, stomach and then into the small intestine and large intestine. The small intestine is longer than the large intestine, but narrower (Figure 9.3).

The general structure of the GI tract

The GI tract is a series of coiled, hollow, muscular **tubes** or **lumen** of varying diameter and shape. These tubes pass from the mouth through the thoracic cavity to the abdominal cavity and end in the pelvic cavity. The lumen is where the food travels through.

Many systems of the body are made of *three* layers of tissues. In all these body systems usually

- the outer layer is connective tissue;
- the middle layer is muscle tissue;
- the internal layer is epithelial tissue.

Chapter Reference

Cavities and tissues are discussed in Chapter 1, 'Maintaining a Safe Environment' (see p. 1).

The digestive system or tract follows this arrangement, but has an additional connective

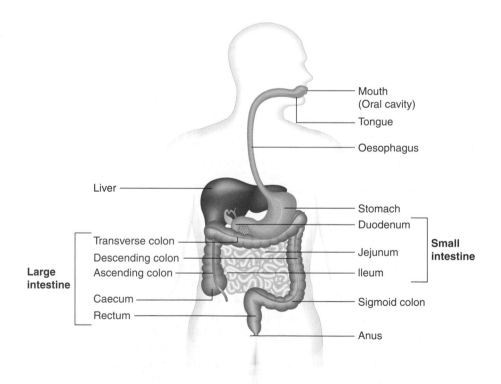

FIGURE 9.3 **Gastrointestinal tract and accessory organs**

tissue layer protecting the innermost **mucosal epithelium**.

The **four** layers of the tract are

- the innermost epithelial layer of **mucosal** cells;
- a connective tissue layer of submucosa;
- a muscle layer of outer longitudinal and inner circular muscle;
- a connective outer double layer of serosa or adventia tissue called peritoneum with visceral peritoneum lining the tract and parietal peritoneum lining the body cavities.

When the epithelial tissue is internal it is called endothelium. The endothelium of the gastrointestinal tract is associated with glands that secrete mucus (also known as mucous). This watery-salty mucus protects the tract from food particles, enzymes and other chemicals secreted into the tract to aid digestion. Even so there is a rapid turnover of epithelial cells in the tract. In the small intestine 17 billion epithelial cells are shed into the lumen and replaced every day. The cells are formed from other cells called **stem** cells.

Chapter Reference
Lifespans of cells are discussed in Chapter 1, 'Maintaining a Safe Environment' (see p. 1).

The mucosa also has a rich blood supply. Absorbed nutrients from the tract (discussed below) are transported in a blood vessel called the hepatic portal vein or in the lymphatic system to the liver.

The submucosa contains blood vessels, nerves and lymphoid tissue involved in protection of the tract from infection. The neurons are part of the enteric nervous system which controls the release of neurotransmitters that influence the production of digestive secretions and the peristalsis in the tract.

Chapter Reference
Lymphoid tissue is discussed in Chapter 7, 'Breathing' (see p. 184). Protection from infection is discussed in Chapter 11, 'Cleansing and Dressing' (see p. 299) and nervous tissue in Chapter 4, 'Communicating' (see p. 102).

Health Connection

Cancers of the tract

Dividing cells are more susceptible to mutation than non-dividing cells. The epithelial cells of the tract have a high turnover and can form epithelial cancers called **carcinomas**. Cancers of connective tissues are called **sarcomas**. Cells that are dividing are sensitive to agents that kill dividing cells. Because of the continual cell turnover the epithelial cells of the tract are also very sensitive to agents that inhibit cell division such as ionising radiation and chemotherapeutic drugs used in the treatment of cancer. This means that even when treating another cancer in a different part of the body non-cancerous epithelial cells of the tract can be killed by therapeutic treatments.

The muscles of the tract are involuntary, under unconscious control. They are there to propel food along the tract. This propulsion is called **peristalsis** (discussed below). Food is pushed, by peristalsis, through the lumen. The lumen is lined with mucosal cells that moisten the food and protect the tract (Figure 9.4).

Chapter Reference
The nervous system is discussed in Chapter 4, 'Communicating' (see p. 102).

The outer connective tissue, **serosa**, supports the tract and, due to the double serous layer with serous fluid between the layers allows friction free movement.

Chapter Reference
Tissue types and glands are discussed in Chapter 1, 'Maintaining a Safe Environment' (see p. 1).

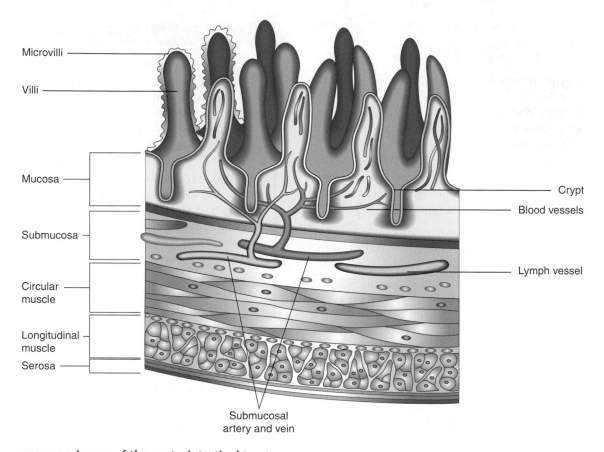

FIGURE 9.4 **Layers of the gastrointestinal tract**

Other adaptive features of the tract will be discussed as we travel along the tract from mouth to anus.

The physiological function of the tract

The digestive system is the system that *divides* or breaks food into small, molecular chemical particles, nutrients. These chemicals are then able to cross from the tract into the blood to be distributed around the body to provide nutrient chemicals to all the cells.

Chapter Reference

The transport by the blood is discussed in Chapter 7, 'Breathing' (see p. 184).

The gastrointestinal tract carries out four main processes:

- **digestion** – dividing, changing large complex food molecules into smaller chemical nutrients;
- **motility** – movement of food through the tract from mouth to anus by muscular peristalsis;
- **absorption** – chemical nutrients released by digestion are absorbed from the tract to the blood for distribution to all the tissues of the body;
- **elimination** – removal of undigested food from the tract.

How the tract digests food

A number of steps must be taken for food to be digested fully to release the chemical nutrients that it contains and that the cells of our bodies require for proper functioning.

Ingestion

Before food can be digested it must first be **ingested**. Ingestion is the process of putting food in the mouth. It is usually a voluntary, independent action. Babies have the ability to ingest food by a suckling activity the moment they are born.

Once ingested into the mouth the process of digestion begins.

Mechanical digestion

Mechanical digestion occurs throughout the tract. It uses mechanical movement and force to digest food. It includes

- biting by teeth,
- chewing by teeth,
- mixing of food by tongue,
- churning by muscles in the stomach and
- segmentation in the small intestine.

How the mouth aids digestion

The mouth, or oral cavity, is lined with mucus membrane which helps to protect the mouth and moisten food. The mouth contains teeth which aid digestion by biting food into a manageable size for entry into the tract. The teeth also help to grind the food into a pulp by chewing or mastication, increasing the surface area and making the food easier to break down. All of these actions are a form of mechanical digestion.

The mouth allows the

- mastication (chewing) of food,
- mixing masticated food with saliva,
- initiation of swallowing by the tongue and
- allowing for the sense of taste.

The hard teeth allow the grinding action needed to mechanically digest (break)

Health Connection

Chewing

Many people do not chew or 'masticate' their food sufficiently. Chewing helps to digest food and to make the food particles moist and small for passing through the tract. If large food particles are swallowed they must be moved through by peristalsis. If the food blocks the tract the muscular movements in peristalsis may be disturbed and food may be sent back up the tract, regurgitation, rather than proceeding down the tract.

food into pieces that are small enough to pass by swallowing into the throat. The tongue secretes saliva which helps to moisten food and aids in taste. The saliva also has chemicals in it which aid digestion, chemical digestion (Figure 9.5).

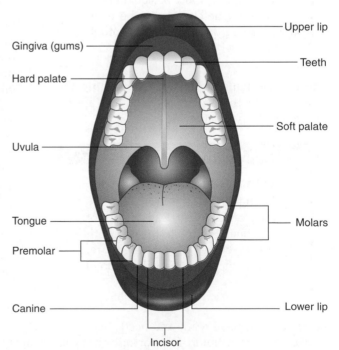

FIGURE 9.5 **The mouth and teeth**

In the mouth the teeth masticate (chew) food. Humans have two sets of teeth:

1. **deciduous** – baby or milk teeth
   - 20 teeth are fully formed by age 2;
2. **permanent teeth**
   - Replace deciduous teeth beginning between the ages of 6 to 12;
   - A full set is 32 teeth, but some people do not have wisdom teeth.

Health Connection

Naso-gastric tubes

Sometimes a person is not able to feed themselves through the mouth (they could be unconscious or have chewing or swallowing problems, for example). A naso-gastric tube can be inserted through the nose and into the food passage at the back of the throat avoiding the mouth. If this is done, the food that is fed into the tube must be moist as it will not be moistened in the mouth and it must be liquidised as it will not be chewed by the teeth into a **size** that would pass through the tract.

The tongue helps the teeth by presenting the food to the teeth, moving the food into appropriate positions for chewing.

Health Connection

Tooth loss and digestion

The health of the teeth can be compromised and lead to loss of individual teeth. Each lost tooth impairs chewing and, therefore, reduces the mechanical digestion in the mouth.

Babies do not have teeth and need their food intake to be in a liquid form or one that can become liquid by the addition of saliva.

Swallowing

Once the food has been bitten, ingested, chewed and moistened it is formed into a **bolus,** a small compact lump, and ready to enter the tract. The food is moved by the **tongue** towards the back of the mouth. This is a voluntary action. It is then swallowed, **deglutination**, and the process of moving food particle through the tract begins.

At the back of the mouth is the throat consisting of the **pharynx** and **larynx.** Both air for breathing and food for digestion enter the throat. The two systems then have separate tubes. The air tube, **trachea**, is held open by cartilage and is at the front of the neck. You can feel it if you put your fingers on the front of your throat and press lightly. The resistance to pressure is due to the cartilage in the trachea.

The tube for food runs behind the trachea. It is important that **food** does not enter the trachea. To prevent this from happening during swallowing a flap called the **epiglottis** covers the larynx and prevents food from entering the trachea.

The phases of swallowing are

1. **buccal phase**. This is *voluntary*, and occurs in mouth where the bolus is forced into the pharynx by the tongue;
2. **pharyngeal-oesophageal phase**. This is the *involuntary* transport of the bolus by peristalsis towards the stomach. All passageways except to the stomach are blocked
   (a) the tongue blocks off the mouth.
   (b) the soft palate (uvula) blocks the nasopharynx.
   (c) the epiglottis blocks the larynx.

Chapter Reference

The epiglottis and blockage of the trachea by food is discussed in Chapter 7, 'Breathing' (see p. 184).

Once food has been swallowed it is propelled past the throat into the first part of the tract, the oesophagus, a tube 15 cm long which links the mouth to the stomach. Food must enter the oesophagus and not the trachea. The oesopha-gus travels through the **thoracic cavity** and links the mouth to the stomach to transport food. The stomach is located in the **abdominal cavity** under a muscle called the **diaphragm.** The thoracic cavity is filled with the lungs and heart so food must be moved from the mouth to the abdominal cavity where the GI tract is.

Health Connection

Tongue

In some mouth cancers the tongue or part of it may be surgically removed. Not only will speaking, discussed in Chapter 4, 'Communi-cating', be compromised, but eating will also be compromised as the tongue cannot aid in the presenta-tion of food to the teeth for chewing or moving the bolus towards the back of the mouth for swallowing.

The oesophagus enters the stomach through the **cardiac sphincter** or **cardio-oesophageal.** The sphincter is a flap to prevent the backflow of food. While food is in the oesophagus there is little or no digestion, merely transport by peristalsis past the thoracic cavity which is full with the cardiac and respiratory system and on into the abdomen where most of the tract is contained. The cardiac sphincter is opened when food presses against it.

Health Connection

Vomiting, food hygiene service

Food may contain toxic substances. We have reflexes that avoid damage from hazardous substances. Vomiting is a response triggered by a number of different stimuli such as the distension of the stomach and small intestine and activation of chemore-ceptors that respond to noxious chemicals or toxins in the gut.

Mechanical digestion in the stomach

The stomach is a J-shaped sac with an **inner curvature** and an **outer curvature.** The stom-ach can vary in **volume** from 0.05 litres to 1.5 litres. This variation is due to the stomach being folded up when empty. The inner mucosal epi-thelium layer of the stomach lies in folds called

---

Health Connection

Gastric bands

Obesity is an increasing problem in many countries where food intake exceeds the use of energy. As more food is put into the stomach the rugae unfold and the volume of the stomach increases. Normal food portions and meal sizes should not stretch the stomach to its full volume. Repeated large meals repeatedly stretch the stomach so that it stops folding back to a smaller volume and is extended to a larger volume. The amount of stretch in stomach tells us how full we are. There are 'stretch receptors' in the walls of the stomach that feed back to the control centre in our brain. Effectors then tell us we are full and should stop eating. This is part of the homeostatic mechanism discussed in Chapter 1, 'Maintaining a Safe Environment'. If the stomach is continually over-stretched our bodies never tell us we are full and it takes increasing amounts of food to fill our stomach. Gastric bands, similar to elastic bands, can be bound, surgically, around our stomachs to decrease the size. This decreases the capacity of the stomach making it almost impossible to put too much in and makes us feel the stretch so that we feel full with less food. It is one treatment for obesity.

rugae when the stomach is empty. These can expand and smooth out when the stomach is full. As food enters the stomach the rugae unfold and the volume of the stomach increases.

There are three main regions of the stomach: the **fundus**, the **body** and the **pylorus.** Food enters from the oesophagus via the cardiac sphincter into the fundus, then the body and then the pylorus before emptying into the duodenum of the small intestine via the pyloric sphincter (Figure 9.6).

The oesophagus enters the stomach by the cardiac (near the heart) sphincter. Food enters and is then mechanically churned to chime. After about three hours the food is released at the pyloric sphincter into the duodenum, the first part of the small intestine.

The inner layer of mucosal epithelial cells is columnar in shape with millions of deep gastric pits which lead into gastric glands. The gastric glands contain cells that secrete gastric juices.

These juices contain digestive enzymes and hydrochloric acid (HCl). The mucus cells in the upper part of the gland produce sticky mucus to protect the stomach wall from acid pH and enzymes.

The stomach has three layers of **smooth, involuntary muscle:**

- outer longitudinal muscle fibres;
- middle circular folds of muscles fibres;
- inner oblique muscle fibres.

These muscles help to churn, pummel and mix the food into a watery mix and aid mechanical digestion. For the muscles of the tract to contract nerve fibres must innervate them, so there are projections from nerves cells, neurons, to the muscles of the tract.

Chapter Reference

Nerves are discussed in Chapter 4, 'Communicating' (see p. 102). Muscles are discussed in Chapter 6, 'Moving' (see p. 163).

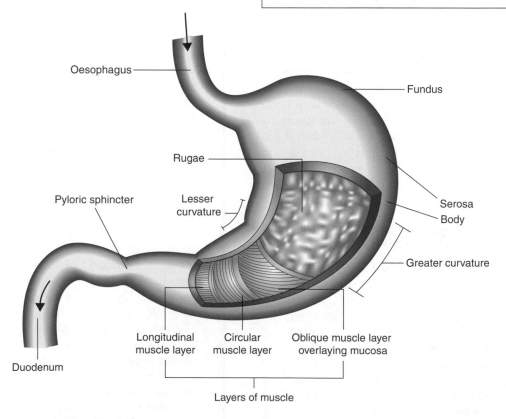

Oesophagus
Fundus
Rugae
Pyloric sphincter
Lesser curvature
Serosa
Body
Greater curvature
Longitudinal muscle layer
Circular muscle layer
Oblique muscle layer overlaying mucosa
Duodenum
Layers of muscle

FIGURE 9.6 **The stomach**

Peristalsis and segmentation

Food is moved through the tract by an action called **peristalsis** which propels the food along. It does this by the contraction and relaxation of the muscles in the walls of the tract in a coordinated wave-like pattern which is under involuntary control. Food is detected in the tract, the messages relayed back to the brain and the effector messages sent to the smooth muscle of the tract to start waves of contraction. This is **motility**.

In the small intestine there is both peristalsis to push food along the tract and segmentation which moves food back and forth to aid mixing of the food with the chemical secretions into the small intestine (Figures 9.7 and 9.8).

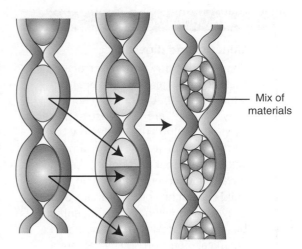

FIGURE 9.8 **Segmentation – moving materials back and forth to aid in mixing in the small intestine**

Chemical digestion

While the start of digestion is carried out by mechanical digestion, this only allows the foods

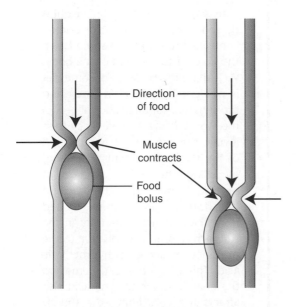

FIGURE 9.7 **Peristalsis – food is pushed through the tract by the muscular layer contracting and relaxing and thereby squeezing the food through. This should be in one direction only, from mouth towards anus**

to be broken down to a certain extent into a chyme. Finer digestion into molecular units requires the equivalent of a finer pair of scissors to cut the food up. This is done by chemical digestion. Chemical digestion is the breaking down of foods by chemical actions, usually by enzymes. As discussed in Chapter 2, 'Working and Playing', enzymes are catalytic proteins that speed up the rate of a reaction without themselves being changed. Enzymes specifically break the bonds between the polymers of foods releasing the monomers. Each food type is broken by its own enzymes. Polymers of sugars, polysaccharide, have different enzymes to polymers of amino acids, polypeptides or proteins. Cellulose, a polysaccharides can be digested by many animals, but humans do not have the specific enzyme to break the bonds between the cellulose monomers. Cellulose, therefore, remains as a polymer and cannot pass from the tract to the blood.

Polymer + enzyme → Monomer + enzyme

Each major food group uses *different* enzymes in chemical digestion to break down food molecules into their building blocks.

- carbohydrates are broken to simple sugars;
- proteins are broken to amino acids;
- fats are broken to fatty acids and alcohols.

Genetics and digestion

There are many inborn errors of metabolism where children are born with a gene that is not functioning fully. Genes are the instruction manual telling the cell how to synthesise proteins from amino acids. If the malfunctioning gene is for a particular enzyme protein, the child will not be able to produce that enzyme and will not, consequently, be able to break certain bonds in chemical digestion. Phenylketonuria (PKU) is one such error. Children with this disorder cannot digest an amino acid, phenylalanine, and must be kept on a phenylalanine-free diet.

Chemical digestion in the mouth

The mouth contains **salivary glands** that secrete **saliva.** Saliva contains water which helps to moisten the food which, combined with the chewing action of the teeth, helps to make the food into a **bolus** that is easy to swallow and move through the tract. Saliva also contains an enzyme, salivary **amylase.** This enzyme chemically digests carbohydrates. It also contains **lysozyme**, which breaks down the walls of bacteria and antibodies which help to kill bacteria. The tongue also contains taste receptors.

There are three **saliva-producing glands** in the mouth:

- parotid glands – located anterior to ears;
- submandibular glands;
- sublingual glands.

These glands produce fluids which aid the chemical digestion of food. The fluids are:

- a mixture of mucus and serous fluids;
- helps to form a food bolus;
- contain an enzyme, salivary amylase, to begin **starch** digestion;
- dissolve chemicals so they can be tasted.

Glands in the mouth and throat produce saliva and mucus. The saliva moistens food, as does mucus, and contains enzymes which start the digestion of carbohydrates (Figure 9.9).

Chemical digestion in the stomach

The stomach continues digestion of food. It does this in a number of ways:

- by secretion of 1.5–2 litres per day of gastric juice, discussed below;
- mechanically because the stomach is a muscular bag that can churn food;
- chemically because the gastric juice contains pepsin which helps to digest protein.

Gastric juice contains water which moistens food allowing the food to become, once mechanically churned around by the muscular walls of the stomach, a soupy mix called **chyme.**

Bulimia

One way of not putting on weight is by reducing the amount of calorie-containing food being absorbed from the GI tract to the cells of the body. We can do this by diet. For some diet is not enough. Food is eaten and the sensation of taste and fullness in the stomach is achieved. They then invoke the process of regurgitation of the stomach contents, vomiting, by using the reflux reaction of putting fingers into the back of their throat. Food is then vomited from the stomach. The food in the stomach is at an acid pH due to the presence of secreted hydrochloric acid. This affects the teeth removing the enamel covering. The acid also affects the cells lining the throat. This way of controlling weight often has psychological components. The condition of controlling weight in this extreme fashion is called bulimia.

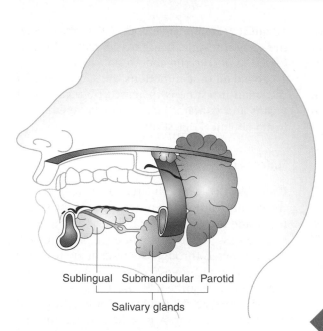

Sublingual   Submandibular   Parotid

Salivary glands

FIGURE 9.9 **Saliva and glands**

The stomach also protects us from harmful bacteria that enter on food. The gastric juice contains **hydrochloric acid**, a strong acid of pH 2 which helps to kill bacteria and other microorganisms.

Health Connection

Vomiting

Toxic substances can be ingested with food. Vomiting is a reflex action that, like swallowing, requires the coordination of a number of muscles controlled by a vomiting centre in the brainstem. It can be initiated by extension of the stomach or small intestine or by signals from the tract to the vomiting centre such as increased pressure in the skull from concussion, chemical stimuli in the brain such as in response to drugs or sensory information during movement as in travel sickness.

There is some chemical digestion in the stomach. Hydrochloric acid secreted from the mucosal

cells not only helps kill bacteria but it also helps in the activation of the enzyme **pepsin** from its inactive form **pepsinogen** secreted from specialised cells in the glands. Pepsin works best at this low, **acidic pH**. Pepsin is an enzyme that chemically breaks the bonds of **polypeptide proteins** releasing monomers of **amino acids**. Hydrochloric acid also helps break down food as it is a strong acid. The hydrogen ions react with ionic or polar molecules in the food, particularly in proteins to disrupt their bonds so that they de-nature and break up their physical structure.

Renin enzyme is also active in the stomach helping to break down milk. Some people are **lactose intolerant** (discussed below).

Health Connection

Ulcers

Ulcers are formed by the erosion of the epithelium of the tract. It was thought that this was due to the presence of HCl, but it is now thought that it may be due to bacteria, *Heliobacter pylori*, that produce substances toxic to epithelial cells. Antibacterial therapy has proved very successful in treating ulcers.

Amylase, the enzyme found in saliva, cannot work at acid pH and is *inactivated* in the stomach. The stomach, therefore, does not chemically digest carbohydrates although it helps in their mechanical digestions.

Thus the stomach helps in the chemical enzymatic digestion of proteins but not in the chemical digestion of carbohydrates or fats.

The cells in the mucosal also secrete a hormone, **gastrin**, and a protein, **intrinsic factor**, which is needed for vitamin B12 absorption.

The stomach also acts as a **temporary storage tank** storing food until it can pass further down the tract. The stomach empties completely in 4–6 hours.

There is very limited absorption of nutrients from the stomach into the blood or lymph. Some water, drugs and alcohol can be absorbed.

After 1–3 hours of mechanical and chemical digestion **chyme** is released from the stomach through the **pyloric sphincter** into the **small intestines** or small bowel.

- simple columnar epithelium
  - mucous neck cells – produce a sticky alkaline mucus
  - gastric glands – secrete gastric juice
  - chief cells – produce protein-digesting enzymes (pepsinogens)
  - parietal cells – produce hydrochloric acid
  - endocrine cells – produce gastrin;
- gastric pits formed by folded mucosa;
- glands and specialised cells are in the gastric gland region.

Chemical digestion in the small intestine

The small intestine has various functions, but its two main functions are

- chemical digestion of food into nutrients using enzymes secreted into the small intestine from the pancreas, liver and intestinal epithelium;
- absorption of nutrients into the blood and lymph for transport to all the cells of the body.

The small intestine and accessory organs

The small intestine is a series of tubes 3 metres long and about 4 cm wide. The small intestine is longer than the large intestine. It is called the small intestine due to its narrow width. The tube is divided into three areas:

- the **duodenum**, 25 cm long;
- the **jejunum**, 1 metres long;
- the **ileum**, 2 metres long.

As adult humans are about 1.8 metres long, the small intestine, being over 3 metres long, is folded to fit into the abdominal cavity.

To aid all of its functions the surface area of the small intestine is increased by a variety of means and contains cells that secrete enzymes to aid chemical digestion.

Surface area

If an object is a smooth circle the surface area is the circumference, the outer edge, of the circle. If you add lots of projections onto the circle the surface area, the area at the edge, is increased. As food travels through the tract enzymes must act on it to aid digestion into small particles that can be absorbed. If the food travels too quickly through the tract it is not fully digested and absorption is not possible. Increasing the surface area increase the chances of having enough area to secretes enzymes and absorb nutrients. Again this illustrates how the structure of an organ or tissue helps its function; the anatomy aids the physiology.

The small intestine increases its surface area in a number of ways (Figure 9.10):

- **plicae** or circular folds: these are permanent folds in the mucosa and submucosa that increases the surface area;
- **villi**: finger-like projections (0.5–1 mm) which contain blood capillaries and lymph vessels (lacteals) increase the surface area;
- **microvilli** (or brush border): contain microscopic projections of the columnar epithelial cell walls. Microvilli contain enzymes, which complete chemical digestion.

Intestinal **glands** are situated between the villi; these secrete mucus and enzymes.

Lymphoid tissue is found in the submucosa towards the end of the small bowel to help protect against bacterial infection.

There are also two ducts (small tubes) into the duodenum. These ducts allow secretions from two organs to enter the lumen of the small intestine. The two organs that have digestive secretions into the small intestine are the pancreas and the liver.

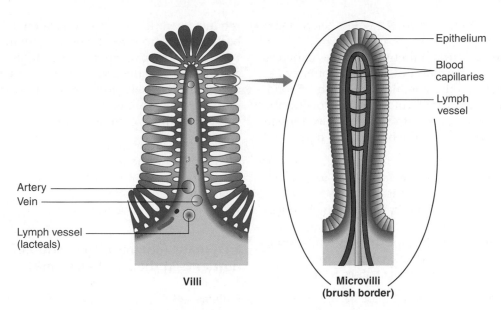

FIGURE 9.10 Surface area in the small intestine is increased by folding of surfaces or projections from cells (villi, microvilli)

There are various enzymes that are secreted into the small intestine to aid chemical digestion. In turn, these enzymes are manufactured in various locations. The main areas that enzymes of the GI tract are made are

- intestinal cells of the small intestine (brush borders);
- pancreas.

As well as these enzymes **bile**, made by the liver, enters the small intestine from the gall bladder. Bile aids the digestion of lipids.

The small intestine and its enzyme

The lining of the small intestine secrete many digestive enzymes into the lumen aiding chemical digestion as seen in Table 9.6.

The pancreas

The pancreas is a long gland that has *endocrine functions* as it secretes hormones into the blood. The pancreas secretes the hormones insulin and glucagon into the blood which control blood

Table 9.6 Enzymatic secretions of the small intestine

Enzyme	Digests
Aminopeptidase	Proteins and peptides
Dextrinase	Dextrins into glucose
Lactase	Lactose (milk sugar) into glucose and galactose
Sucrase	Sucrose (sugar) into glucose and fructose
Maltase	Maltose (dissacharide from starch) into glucose

glucose levels. It also has an *exocrine function*, secreting fluid into **ducts**.

> **Chapter Reference**
>
> Glands are discussed in Chapter 1, 'Maintaining a Safe Environment' (see p. 1).

The secretions from the pancreas pass into ducts in the pancreas that then, together with secretions from the liver, pass into the duodenum via a sphincter called the sphincter of Oddi (Figure 9.11).

The exocrine functions of the pancreas include the secretion of a number of enzymes that help in the chemical digestion of food, breaking small molecular bonds allowing the food to be digested into particles small enough to be absorbed into the blood and lymph.

- pancreatic enzymes play digestive function:
  - help complete digestion of starch (pancreatic amylase);
  - carry out about half of all protein digestion (trypsin, etc.);
  - are responsible for fat digestion (lipase);
  - digest nucleic acids (nucleases);
  - alkaline content neutralizes acidic chyme.

Pancreatic enzymes are part of the exocrine function of the pancreas and are secreted into ducts that empty in the small intestine and break the chyme into subunits of various monomers (Table 9.7).

The pancreas also produces bicarbonate ions HCO_3^-. This helps to alter the very **acidic** chyme entering the duodenum into a more **alkali** chyme in which the pancreatic enzymes can function.

The liver

The liver performs a number of functions in metabolism. One of these functions is to produce an exocrine secretion called **bile.** Bile is a mixture of bicarbonate ions, phospholipids, a fatty substance called cholesterol and its derivative called bile salts. There are also waste products in bile from the breakdown of the haemoglobin from red blood cells (bilirubin). Bile leaves the liver in the hepatic duct and can be stored in the gall bladder. It enters the duodenum and helps in the emulsification and breakdown of fats (Figure 9.12).

Roles of the liver in digestion:

- detoxifies drugs and alcohol;
- degrades hormones;
- produces cholesterol, blood proteins (albumin and clotting proteins);
- plays a central role in metabolism.

Enzymatic (chemical) digestion of nutrients in the small intestine

Proteins

The enzymes trypsin and chymotrypsin break down proteins entering the small intestine. These are then broken down further by two enzymes:

- **carboxypeptidase** (affect the carboxy-acid part of amino acids) from the pancreas;
- **aminopeptidase** (affects the amino group of amino acids) from the brush border interstitial cells of the small intestine.

This results in the peptides being broken down into amino acids.

Carbohydrates

Carbohydrate digestion begins in the mouth with salivary amylase. It then ceases in the acid

Table 9.7 The pancreatic enzymes

Enzyme	Digests
Trypsin, chymotrypsin, elastase	Proteins into amino acids
Carboxypeptidase	Proteins and peptides (polypeptides)
Amylase	Polysaccharides into disaccharides and glucose
Lipase	Triacylglycerol into fatty acids
Ribonuclease, deoxyribonuclease	Nucleic acids (RNA, DNA) into nucleotides

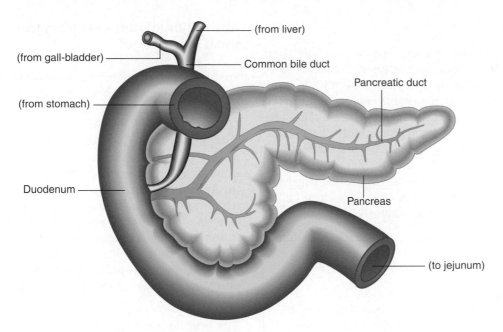

FIGURE 9.11 **The pancreatic and bile duct**

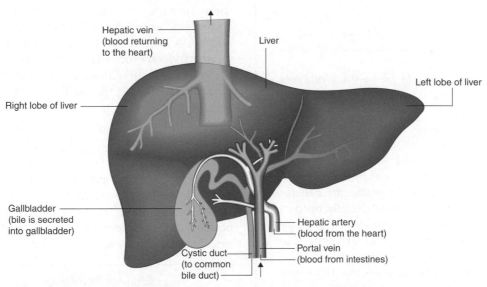

FIGURE 9.12 **The liver**

environment of the stomach. The small intestine has more alkali and carbohydrate chemical digestion is completed here. Pancreatic amylase converts polysaccharides into disaccharides.

There are two fates for the disaccharides: the enzyme **maltase**, from the brush borders of the small intestine, converts disaccharides into monosaccharides or short chains of glucose (dextrins). These dextrins are then broken down into glucose by the enzyme **dextrinase** from the small intestine.

Fats and lipids

Most dietary lipids are consumed as fats. These are insoluble in aqueous (watery) solutions – they are hydrophobic. To digest fats both bile, from the liver, and pancreatic **lipase** are needed. The chyme entering the small intestine contains large fat droplets. Bile, which consists of bile salts, cholesterol and phospholipids, disperses the large fat droplets into smaller drops. This process is called **emulsification** and results in a much larger surface area for the enzyme lipase to cleave the fats (triacylglycerols) into smaller units.

Box 9.3 Summary – Chemical digestion

- The chemical digestion of nutrients is completed as the food travels along the small intestine from the duodenum via the jejunum to the ileum.
- During this passage, proteins, carbohydrates and fats are digested to their constituent parts by the action of secreted enzymes shown in Tables 9.6 and 9.7.
- Bile emulsifies fat to small droplets allowing lipase to convert fats to fatty acids.
- Proteins are digested into amino acids.
- Carbohydrates are digested into sugars.
- Once chemical digestion by pancreatic and intestinal 'brush border' enzymes is complete the large surface area of the small intestine allows absorption to occur.
- The small intestine is also the major site of absorption of nutrients due to its large surface area as discussed above.
- Any nutrients remaining in the lumen are moved on, by peristalsis, to the large intestine via the ileocaecal valve.

Absorption of nutrients from the small intestine

The absorption of nutrients consists of the transport of nutrients from the small intestine into the blood or lymph for transport to the cells of the body to provide nutrients for growth, repair and energy. Nutrients must cross from the lumen into the blood or lymph. The small intestine has a number of villi, finger-like protrusions into the lumen of the small intestine, which increase the surface area of the small intestine and thus aid absorption of nutrients from the lumen across into the blood.

Sugars, amino acids and nucleic acids are absorbed into the capillary blood and are transported to the liver via the hepatic portal vein.

Fats, acids and monoglycerides

These are hydrophobic and can diffuse from the lumen and enter the interstitial cells. They then combine with other substances such as cholesterol and fat soluble vitamins such as vitamin A and vitamin D into small droplets called **chylomicrons**. These are extruded into the lacteals of the villi and transported to the systemic circulation via the lymph in the thoracic duct.

Amino acids and monosaccharides

Both amino acids and monosaccharides are polar and hydrophilic. They cannot, therefore, diffuse across, but must be transported by specialised proteins in the cell membrane of the small intestine (facilitated diffusion or active transport).

Chapter Reference

Diffusion is discussed in Chapter 1, 'Maintaining a Safe Environment' (see p. 1).

Minerals, vitamins and water

Water is absorbed along the length of the small intestine. It is transported across by osmosis.

We ingest about 2 litres of water per day in our food and drink. Our GI tract secretes 7 litres of water into the lumen.

Crypt cells in the small intestine also secrete a watery fluid, similar to extracellular fluid mentioned below. This fluid aids absorption of water soluble nutrients.

Salts are mainly absorbed by active transport.

The digested substances once absorbed into the blood and lymph are then transported to the liver by the hepatic portal vein or lymph.

Box 9.4 Summary – The functions of the small intestine

- **Peristalsis**. Food must be moved through the tract.
- **Secretion**. 1.5 litres of intestinal juice, similar to gastric juice, is secreted per day. This juice contains water, mucus, mineral salts and enzymes.
- **Chemical digestion**. Chemical catalysts, enzymes, secreted in the intestinal juice make the food particles into their smaller constituent molecules and atoms.
- **Absorption**. Nutrients must be moved from the tract of the small intestine into the blood and lymph.
- **Hormones**. Hormones involved in homeostasis of the tract are secreted into the tract.

Fate of amino acid, fats and carbohydrates absorbed from the small intestine

Once food has been digested to its constituent parts, monomers, it can be absorbed from the small intestine into the blood or lymph.

Most **amino acids** are used by cells for synthesis of new proteins. Surplus amino acids can be converted to keto acids by the removal of their amino molecular groups. Keto acids can then be used to synthesise fatty acids or can be used in the TCA cycle. Amino groups combine with hydrogen to form ammonia which is highly toxic. It is converted in the liver to urea and excreted by the kidney.

Fats are absorbed into the lymph. They enter the lymph as **chylomicrons** and then pass into the bloodstream. They are transported by lipoproteins (lipid–protein complexes).

- low-density lipoproteins (LDLs) are transported to body cells;
- high-density lipoproteins (HDLs) are transported from body cells to the liver.

Those that are used in the formation of energy must first be broken down into acetic acid. In the mitochondria the acetic acid is completely oxidised to produce ATP, water and carbon dioxide.

Fats in the liver are used to

- synthesise lipoproteins;
- synthesise thromboplastin, a blood clotting chemical;
- synthesise cholesterol;
- broken down into simpler compounds and released into the blood.

Those released into the blood are used by the body cells' fat together with cholesterol to build membranes and steroid hormones.

The functions of cholesterol as follows:

- it serves as a structural basis of steroid hormones and vitamin D;
- it is a major building block of plasma membranes;
- most cholesterol is produced in the liver and is not from diet;
- cholesterol and fatty acids cannot freely circulate in the bloodstream.

Glucose, the most important sugar in human diets, is controlled by two hormones, **insulin** and **glucagon**. If there is a lot of sugar in the blood after a meal, insulin is released by the β **(beta) endocrine cells** of the **pancreas**. This causes glucose to be taken up by cells and used in metabolism. If there is surplus glucose it is converted to **glycogen** and triacylglycerol fats and stored in the liver and other tissues. When stored glycogen is needed by cells for metabolism it is converted to glucose by the hormone **glucagon** made by the α (alpha) endocrine cells of the **pancreas**. Glucose is used to fuel the TCA cycle discussed in controlling body temperature in Chapter 5, 'Controlling and Repairing'.

Glucose is stored or used for the following:

- Glycogenesis:
  - glucose molecules are converted to glycogen;
  - glycogen molecules are stored in the liver.
- Glycogenolysis:
  - glucose is released from the liver after conversion from glycogen.
- Gluconeogenesis:
  - glucose is produced from fats and proteins.

Box 9.5 Summary – Small intestine

- Most digestion and absorption occurs in the long, narrow, small intestine. Chyme takes 4–6 hours to pass through the small intestine.
- Chyme enters the large intestine at the **ileocaecal** sphincter or valve which prevents the backflow of chyme from the large intestine into the small intestine.

Health Connection

Diabetes

Pancreatic enzymes together with those of the small intestine are secreted to aid chemical digestion. Pancreatic enzymes are also involved in the fate of nutrients. Insulin and glucagon, discussed above, maintain the correct glucose levels in the blood. The glucose is transported in the blood to all the cells of the body. There it is used to synthesise energy, ATP.

The glucose released from food after digestion and absorption enters the blood and remains in the blood unless insulin is released. This hormone helps in the absorption of glucose from the blood to body cells. A lack of production of insulin in β (beta) endocrine cells of the pancreas prevents glucose in the blood being absorbed into the cells of the body. It remains in the blood while the body cells are gradually starved of glucose. The body cells must then use stored fats and even amino acids for the production of ATP. The lack of insulin causes a disease called diabetes. Its treatment is by changes in diet (type 2 diabetes) or by the provision of injected insulin (type 1 diabetes).

Chapter Reference

The further fate of glucose and fat metabolism, energy and heat generation are discussed in Chapter 5, 'Controlling and Repairing' (see p. 142).

The large intestine

The large intestine is about 1.5 metres long, much shorter than the small intestine, but its width is about 6 cm. It is divided into three parts, the **caecum**, the **colon** and the **rectum**.

As the chyme enters the large intestine it is termed **faeces** (Figure 9.13).

The large intestine is wider than the small intestine, but shorter. It meets the small intestine at the ileum at the bottom of the small intestine and, to fit into the body, must be wound upwards and around. Muscular action, peristalsis, must then move the contents against the force of gravity around the large intestine.

The large intestine has the same structure as the rest of the tract. The inner mucosal layer contains many goblet cells secreting mucus. The mucus lubricates faecal contents. Longitudinal

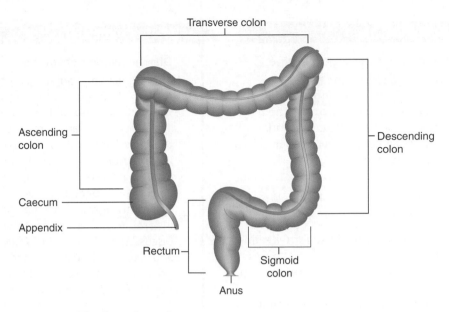

FIGURE 9.13 **The large intestine**

muscle in bands tends to pucker the wall of the large intestine which can expand as faeces enter the bowel.

This wider, shorter part of the tract, the large intestine, colon or bowel, is involved with the

- removal of waste;
- absorption of water and salts.

Only about 4% of digested material is absorbed in the large intestine.

About 1.5 litres of chyme enters the **caecum** of the large intestine from the ileum through the **ileocaecal** valve, a sphincter between the ileum of the small intestine and the caecum of the large intestine. It takes about 12–14 hours to transit the large intestine.

The chyme of the large intestine contains mainly:

- secretions from the small intestine;
- waste from the liver;
- undigested material such as fibre.

As mentioned earlier, the large intestine is heavily colonised with bacteria called **commensal** that off our waste or undigested food and in return synthesise vitamin B12, vitamin K, vitamin B1 (thiamine) and vitamin B2 (riboflavin) which the large intestine can absorb. There is also some lymphoid tissue, the appendix, associated with the large intestine. Lymphoid tissue is part of the immune system, discussed in Chapter 11, 'Cleansing and Dressing'.

> **Health Connection**
>
> ### Appendicitis
> The appendix can become inflamed and if so it can be surgically removed without affecting the digestion of food or absorption of nutrients. It appears not to have a function in humans and is redundant.

Undigested polysaccharides are broken down in the large intestine by bacteria and 0.4–0.7 litres of gas are produced daily. The gases produced in the large bowel are mainly nitrogen and carbon dioxide, but include hydrogen, methane and hydrogen sulphide.

Health Connection

Antibiotics and the large intestine

Antibiotics – discussed in Chapter 11, 'Cleansing and Dressing' – kill bacteria. They can also kill the commensal or useful bacteria and upset the balance of vitamin production and absorption.

Health Connection

Diarrhoea and dehydration

If the remaining contents (waste) of the large intestine transit too quickly water is not absorbed fast enough. The faeces that are eliminated are therefore very watery. This occurs in **diarrhoea**. Diarrhoea is usually due to bacterial infection not by commensal bacteria, but instead by a **pathogenic** bacteria causing illness. Pathogenic bacteria are discussed in Chapter 11, 'Cleansing and Dressing'. With diarrhoeas the greatest health risk is **dehydration** due to loss of water with the waste.

The large intestine therefore has *three* main functions:

- absorption of water and salts to form a semi-solid waste;
- production of vitamins by commensal bacteria;
- the onward movement of waste or residue.

Digestive enzymes are not produced in the large intestine so no further enzymatic cleavage of food polymers can occur. There are resident bacteria (commensal bacteria) that digest the remaining nutrients that have not been fully digested or absorbed in the small intestine. These bacteria use what would be waste as their nutrient source. In return these bacteria produce as their waste vitamins that we need, vitamins K and B, and release gases, also as waste, which we eliminate.

Water and vitamins K and B are absorbed in the large intestine. All remaining materials are eliminated as waste via faeces. There is slow movement through the large intestine by sluggish peristalsis. This allows time for water to be absorbed and as a result the faeces to become more solid waste.

Excretion from the large intestine

Waste products of digestion and undigested food must be eliminated from the tract. To move the waste through the colon a *sluggish peristalsis* occurs, as discussed above, allowing water to be re-absorbed. Mass movements occur, which as slow powerful movements of waste three to four times per day move the waste towards the

rectum. Bulk or fibre in the diet increases the strength of colon contractions and softens the **stools**, the bolus of waste material. As the waste products pass along the large intestine by peristalsis, water is absorbed to make a semi-solid waste called **faeces**.

The rectum is normally empty. As faeces enter the rectum the walls of the rectum stretch which initiates a reflex action contracting the walls of the sigmoid colon and rectum. In the final part of the large intestine is the opening to the external environment. There are two sphincters in the anus, an internal sphincter under involuntary control and an external sphincter under voluntary control. The internal anal sphincter relaxes and the faeces pass along towards the external anal sphincter. This is under voluntary control and delays defecation until convenient. Defecation occurs with the relaxation of the external, voluntary anal sphincter.

Chapter Reference

Elimination from the large bowel is discussed again in Chapter 10, 'Eliminating' (see p. 282).

Faeces

The faeces consist of undigested residue (fibre) water, some minerals, shed epithelial cells, mucus and bacteria in the following proportions:

- 75% water
- 25% solid waste:
  - bacteria (33%)
  - undigested fats and protein (33%)
  - cellulose (33%)

The colour of faeces is due to bile pigments and breakdown of **red blood cells (bilirubin)**. Their odour is due to the bacterial action in intestine releasing gases such as nitrogen products and hydrogen sulphide.

Health Connection

Colonic stomas and bags

Problems such as colonic cancers and degenerative diseases may result in some of the large intestine being removed or non-functional. A tube can be inserted into the colon and attached externally to a bag for the collection of waste. Where the tube is inserted will affect the consistency of the waste collected. If the tube is near where the small intestine enters the colon the material will be very fluid. If the tube is near the rectum the material will be more solid as water will have been absorbed along the colonic tract. The bag will need emptying as needed (Figure 9.14).

Homeostasis, appetite and control of eating

We need to obtain material from the external environment, food for the chemicals and energy inside it. We need to eat a variety and the right amount to maintain our internal

Health Connection

Ulcers

Ulcers are formed by the wearing away of the lining of the gut, the epithelial cells. In more severe cases the erosion can extend into deeper layers of the tract. The acidic environment plays a part in this erosion. However, the bacteria *Heliobacter pyloris* is found in 67% of patients with ulcers and is now thought to be the causative agent of ulcers. Antibiotics (discussed in Chapter 11, 'Cleansing and Dressing') are given to treat this condition.

environment, our bodies. How do we know when to eat (**hunger**) and when to stop eating (**satiety**)? How is our **appetite**, the amount of food we want, controlled?

There are three phases of gastrointestinal control:

- cephalic,
- gastric and
- intestinal.

The **sensory detection** (detection by our sense organs) of food by its smell, taste and sight as well as by chewing stimulates nerve cells (neurons) in the brain which act to increase peristalsis and secretions. This is called the cephalic phase.

Food entering the stomach causes the stomach to distend, decreases stomach acidity and releases peptides. All of these act to cause the hormone **gastrin** to be released. This stimulates acid to be released. This is part of the gastric phase.

The distension and acidity in the small intestine cause hormones to be released that stimulate **bicarbonate** to be released. This is part of the intestinal phase. The bicarbonate raises the pH of the chyme so that pancreatic enzymes are able to work. Pancreatic secretions of enzymes are controlled by the presence of food in the tract and by bicarbonate secretions.

How much we need and how much we have, as stated above, are seldom balanced. How much we need and how much we want also are often not balanced. Our **appetite**, the amount of food we want, does not always match the amount of food we need.

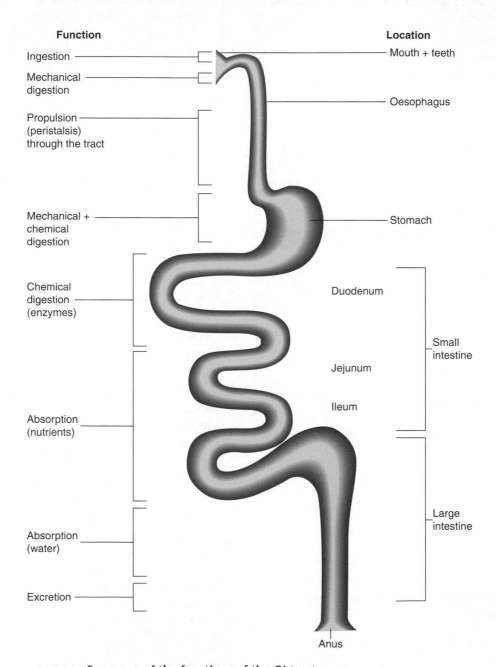

FIGURE 9.14 **Summary of the functions of the GI tract**

Box 9.6 Summary – Eating

- Food, discussed in the first part of this chapter, from the external environment is brought into our internal environment via the mouth.
- Food is ingested and the process of digestion, the division and breaking down of food into its constituent parts, nutrients, begins.
- Mechanically food is sheared by teeth.
- It is moistened by saliva.
- It is chemically digested by enzymes in the saliva.
- It is then swallowed moving past the throat into the oesophagus (the epiglottis prevents food entering the trachea and lungs).
- The food enters the stomach and is churned into chyme mechanically.
- There is some chemical digestion in the stomach.
- The food is then moved into the small intestine and through this by peristalsis.
- The small intestine secretes enzymes that digest the food further.
- The food is now digested into its constituent chemicals, nutrients.
- These nutrients are absorbed into the blood and lymph.
- Non-absorbed and non-digested material is moved through into the large intestine for excretion as faeces.
- The large intestine absorbs water from the waste before it is excreted.

Drinking

Drinking and fluid balance

Water is a solvent in which many substances or solutes will dissolve.

Solutes include electrolytes such as

- sodium (Na^+),
- potassium (K^+),
- chloride (Cl^-),
- calcium (Ca^{2+}) and
- magnesium (Mg^{2+}).

Water forms the main solvent of the body and all chemical reactions take place in a watery milieu. In Chapter 7, 'Breathing', it was seen that even inhaled air must be moistened in the upper respiratory tract before it enters the lungs and oxygen diffuses into that watery transport medium, the blood. Our cells are bathed in fluids and the interior of our cells, the cytoplasm and nucleus, are full of watery fluids where all the metabolic reactions of the cells occur.

We live on land, rather than in the sea, so our main problem and the problem for all land animals, is dehydration. Our bodies are made up of about 50% water and we must maintain this amount so that reactions and transport can occur. As our blood is watery, any loss of water will affect blood volume and thus affect blood pressure. This in turn will affect the amount of blood reaching vital organs.

Chapter Reference

Blood pressure is discussed in Chapter 7, 'Breathing' (see p. 184).

From the Chapter 7 it may be seen that all pressure relies on the fluid pressing on the container and the container pressing on the fluid. This means that the greater the volume of liquid the more the fluid presses on the container or the smaller the container the more it presses on the liquid. Likewise, blood pressure relies on the volume of blood in the vascular tubes and the dimensions of the tubes. Maintaining the correct blood pressure during homeostasis thus relies not only on altering the constriction of blood vessels through the autonomic nervous system sending signals to the smooth, involuntary muscles in the artery and arteriole walls, but also on the volume of the blood. Blood is composed of a watery plasma with proteins and cells floating in it. The watery plasma volume can alter during the day and this can be controlled to affect blood pressure.

How much water do we contain

The total volume of water found in our bodies is 40 litres. This is contained in various compartments of the body:

- intracellular (inside cells): 25 litres;
- extracellular (outside cells): 15 litres
  - interstitial (between cells): 12 litres
  - plasma (in blood): 3 litres.

While our blood volume is approximately 5 litres, 3 litres of it is plasma. The majority of our 40 litres is contained in the 10^{13} (10 trillion) cells of which we are made.

- changes in electrolyte balance cause water to move from one compartment to another which
  - alters blood volume and blood pressure
  - can impair the activity of cells.

Water balance

Because we live on land water evaporates from us all the time. We lose it in sweat when we are hot and in urine and faeces when we eliminate waste.

We lose 2500 ml (2.5 litres) of water each day through various routes:

Chapter Reference

Temperature regulation is discussed in Chapter 5, 'Controlling and Repairing (see p. 142). Elimination of waste is discussed in Chapter 10, 'Eliminating' (see p. 282).

- Urine: 1500 ml
- Insensible loss (skin/lungs):   700 ml
- Sweat: 200 ml
- Faeces: 100 ml
- TOTAL OUTPUT: 2500 ml

To balance this we must take in 2500 ml of water each day. We do this through various routes:

- Drink: 1500 ml
- Food: 750 ml
- Metabolism: 250 ml
- TOTAL INPUT: 2500 ml

If we lose more than we put in we dehydrate. If we gain more than we lose we over-hydrate or hyper-hydrate.

Health Connection

Measuring water input and output

Water output through the urine is often measured by collection and measurement of urine volume. It is equally important to measure the amount of liquid taken in through drinking.

Negative fluid balance is where there is more **output** than **input** leading to dehydration. It can occur through two routes; either there is an excessive loss of fluid or there is an inadequate intake of fluid.

Negative fluid balance – lack of fluid – can result from excessive loss or inadequate intake.

Excessive loss of fluid can occur for a number of reasons:

- haemorrhage (loss of blood);
- vomiting – losing gastric juice (chyme);

- diarrhoea – where water has not been absorbed from the large intestine;
- high temperature and excessive sweating (febrile) usually due to an infectious disease;
- burns where the protective layer of epithelium is removed and water can easily evaporate from the body surface.

Inadequate intake of fluids can occur for a number of reasons. It is a risk for the very young and very old as well as those unable to drink, such as due to a physical disability and those not knowing they should drink such as those with learning difficulties, unconscious or depressed. It is also a problem for patients who cannot control their water intake or those 'nil by mouth' pre- or post-operative patients.

Excessive fluid loss or lack of intake leads to a disturbance of electrolyte balance and blood pressure. Some of the signs of dehydration include:

- low blood pressure,
- dry mouth,
- furred tongue,
- inelastic skin,
- thirst,
- lethargy,
- concentrated urine and
- delirium.

It is possible that some patients who are deemed to be confused are in fact dehydrated due to inadequate water intake. It is important therefore to chart output *and* input, particularly in those at risk.

Regulation of water balance

Regulation is primarily by hormones being released in response to changes in blood pressure. This will be discussed further in Chapter 10, 'Eliminating'. In general water balance can be achieved by altering the amount of water lost in the urine or by altering the amount of salts lost in the urine. When salts are lost, water is also lost to balance osmosis.

Health Connection

Water and osmotic balance in patients

The main route for water intake is orally, by drinking it. If a patient is incapable of drinking, the water can be delivered by a naso-gastric tube along with food which needs to be moistened, or intravenously. If the intravenous route is used it is not water that is introduced into the vein as that would have a deleterious effect on the osmotic balance of the plasma, interstitial fluid and intracellular fluid. Saline, water with electrolytes in the same proportion as plasma and interstitial fluids, is used instead.

Two hormones are responsible for water balance:

- antidiuretic hormone (ADH) prevents excessive water loss in urine;
- aldosterone regulates sodium ion content of extracellular fluid:
  - triggered by the rennin-angiotensin mechanism (discussed in Chapter 10, 'Eliminating').

Cells in the kidneys and hypothalamus of the brain are active monitors of this.

Chapter Reference

Hormones are discussed in Chapter 4, 'Communicating' (see p. 102).

Changes during lifespan and lifestyle

Our dietary needs alter with our development from newborn to adolescent to adult and on into old age. Growth and movement both contribute to our energy needs.

Diet

The estimated average requirements (EAR) for energy vary during lifespan and due to gender. Males usually require more than females.

Babies up to 6 months require about 500–600 calories per day. From 7 months to 1 year the requirements increase up to 1000 calories in a day. Gradually through childhood and adolescence the requirement increases up to 2000–2800 per day and then decrease for adults to 1900–2400 per day. During pregnancy there is only a need for about an extra 200 calories per day – no need to eat for two! Lactation, however, requires about an extra 450 calories per day.

Digestive tract

The newborn GI tract is not fully formed. All the layers are present, but the villi are not finger shaped but leaf shaped. Up until the age of 10–15 the villi are not fully developed. The digestive enzymes in a newborn also vary. Intact proteins can cross the wall of the tract. The tract is shorter than in an adult and must continue to grow in length until maturity.

Other changes in digestion include the ability to digest lactose, the sugar found in milk. Newborns have an enzyme, lactase, that can digest lactose. Indeed, milk lactose is the sole source of sugar for the newborn. During adolescence this enzyme is no longer made by the brush borders of the small intestine, causing **alactasia**. In Northern Europeans this does not occur and they can continue digesting lactose as adults.

There are different metabolic requirements for a newborn, youth, adult and older person due to their different needs. While a baby is small and not physically active it is growing and needs nutrients to aid growth. A child and youth are physically active and growing and have a need for nutrients for growth and

---

Health Connection

Lactose intolerance

Those who cannot digest lactose can become lactose intolerant. The enzyme, lactase, is not synthesised and the lactose remains as a disaccharide in the lumen. It is too large to be absorbed. Bacteria that use lactose as a food source grow and affect the person resulting in watery diarrhoea and abdominal pain. This reaction can result from even a small ingestion of milk, but does not occur when lactose is converted into lactic acid in yoghurt.

---

movements. Older people may become more sedentary and their metabolic needs diminish which is reflected in their reduced need for calorific foods.

Water

The water content of the body varies during lifespan. In babies the water content is about 70–75% of the body. It gradually decreases in age with the adult water content making up 50–60% of the body, while in the elderly it is about 45% of the body.

Conclusion: Eating and drinking

We obtain food and water from the external environment. Obtaining these nutrients is the basis of our concept of work. We use these nutrients to do further work in the body, making energy, growing and repairing tissues. Our ability to do internal work rests on finding the correct nutrients in the correct amount.

Chapter Summary

- The food we eat is called our diet.
- It consists of a variety of chemical nutrients that aid growth, repair and energy formation.
- Metabolism can be catabolic, breaking substances down and releasing energy, or anabolic, building substances up and requiring energy.
- Energy is contained in food matter, particularly fats and carbohydrates.
- The energy we need is measured in calories or joules.
- The gastrointestinal tract is responsible for ingestion, propulsion, mechanical digestion, chemical digestion, absorption of nutrients and the elimination of waste.
- These activities occur along the route of the tract.
- The small intestine is responsible for most of the chemical digestion and absorption.
- The large intestine is responsible for most of the absorption of water and the elimination of waste.
- Different amounts of nutrients are required through life.
- The tract is not fully developed in the newborn and alters through life.
- Water is one of the most important 'nutrients' of our bodies as all the chemical reactions of metabolism and our transport system occur in a watery solution.
- Water and electrolytes are balanced for osmosis.
- Water output per day is 2500 ml, so we need 2500 ml of water input per day. Some of this, 1500 ml, is through drinking.
- Negative water balance leads to dehydration and eventually death.
- We can survive some time without food, but only a few days without water.

Eliminating

Chapter Outline

Introduction: Eliminating as an activity of daily living

Not only do we eliminate waste, but we also produce our own waste in the first place. The production and elimination of waste occurs throughout life; even the developing foetus must eliminate waste material. While a healthy human at any stage of development eliminates, there are social boundaries on this activity. When we are infants, always producing waste, we are trained to eliminate it in an appropriate place. Eliminating waste appropriately is seen as a right of passage of child development and brings increasing independence to the infant. The elderly or the immobile may not be able to eliminate waste independently causing them embarrassment and distress with a feeling of dependency and infantilism. Our ability to carry out the final stages of elimination, the ridding of urine (**micturation**) and the ridding of faeces (**defecation**), as an enormous impact on our health. While the internal elements of forming waste may still be carried out, our ability to control its output may vary.

Just as accumulation of waste material in our kitchens and bathrooms affects the cleanliness and functioning of our homes, so the build up of waste in our bodies affects their functioning.

Should our ability to produce or eliminate waste cease, our health can be severely compromised.

The environment

Our waste products

There are two main types of waste found or manufactured in the body:

● undigested food and
● metabolic waste.

Undigested food is food that has entered the gastrointestinal (GI) tract and passed through the stomach and small intestines without being mechanically or chemically digested. It is therefore too large to be absorbed through the villi in the small intestine into the blood for transport as a nutrient to the cells of the body. Instead, it remains in the small intestine and then passes into the large intestine for passage out of the body by elimination through the rectum and anus.

Undigested food can consist of nutrients that passed through too quickly to be digested or absorbed due to an infection causing rapid transit resulting in a condition called **diarrhoea**. Alternatively, undigested food can be food for which we do no possess enzymes to break it down to release the nutrients it contains. Roughage, a type of carbohydrate for which we do not possess the appropriate enzymes, remains unabsorbed in our intestines and is eliminated as undigested material. It helps to push other undigested food through the tract.

Chapter Reference

Digestion is discussed in Chapter 9, 'Eating and Drinking' (see p. 241). Infections are discussed in Chapter 11, 'Cleansing and Dressing' (see p. 299).

◆ Health Connection

Diarrhoea

Diarrhoea can be caused by microbes in our food. The result is rapid transit of foods through the GI tract without full absorption. This can result in malnutrition and, due to the high water content of the faecal material, dehydration.

Metabolic waste comes from the metabolic activities of the cell including

- **anabolism**, synthesising ATP, proteins, other molecules, cells and tissues;
- **catabolism**, breaking down molecules such as ATP to release energy, proteins and cells during repair and maintenance.

Each activity of the cell can produce wanted substances for cell growth, repair and survival, but it can also produce side products or waste products that need to be eliminated.

Each type of waste is dealt with in different ways by the body.

Chapter Reference

Metabolism is discussed in Chapter 9, 'Eating and Drinking' (see p. 241) and in Chapter 1, 'Maintaining a Safe Environment' (see p. 1).

The need for elimination of waste from our environment

Undigested food in the bowel, *waste*, still contains matter that can be a rich source of

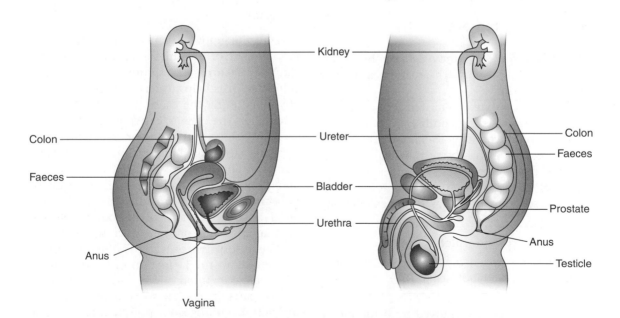

FIGURE 10.1 **Female and male large colon and bladder positions in the pelvic cavity**

nutrients for other organisms and, micro-organisms such as bacteria and must, therefore, be eliminated from the body. It can provide a source of nutrients for unwanted, opportunistic micro-organisms and can, therefore, lead to infections.

A build up of undigested material in the bowel can also cause obstructions to the normal functioning, including water absorption and commensal bacteria activity such as the synthesis of some vitamins.

Metabolic waste from the breakdown of molecules including drugs can release molecules that affect the pH, osmotic pressure and chemical environment of cells. It must be eliminated from the body before it alters the internal environment of the cell that produced it by altering the conditions of the cell beyond its tolerance range and cause cell death. **Necrosis**, large numbers of cell deaths in areas of tissue, can lead to the cessation of function of the tissue and, ultimately, the death of the organism.

Chapter Reference

Micro-organisms are discussed in Chapter 11, 'Cleansing and Dressing' (see p. 299).

How waste is removed

Undigested food is removed from the bowel by elimination though the rectum and anus into the exterior.

Metabolic waste is removed in a variety of ways. The waste is transported away from the cells that produced it by the blood. The blood must then have the waste it is transporting removed from it.

Gases such as carbon dioxide are removed from the blood by the lungs during exhalation.

Chapter Reference

Removal of carbon dioxide is discussed in Chapter 7, 'Breathing' (see p. 184).

Other substances are removed from the blood by filtering them through the **kidneys** which then passes the waste to the **bladder** in the form of **urine**, ready for elimination to the exterior.

Elimination from the bowel

The final part of the digestive tract, the **large bowel**, also known as the **colon** or the **large intestine** (Figure 10.2), is also the site of elimination of unabsorbed material. As discussed in Chapter 9, 'Eating and Drinking', some ingested food does not cross from the **gastrointestinal (GI)** tract into the bloodstream for use by the body. This food remains in the tract. It may do so because it cannot be digested. Food containing cellulose is one such food. This constitutes roughage and helps provide bulk and push food through the tract. When this unabsorbed food reaches the large bowel it is too late for it to be digested or absorbed. The large bowel is an area of the GI tract involved in elimination.

This part of the GI tract, the large intestine, is a tube of about 1.5m long and is wider than the small intestine having a diameter of about 6cm. It consists of three areas:

- caecum,
- colon and
- rectum.

Chyme, the soupy substance in the GI tract, exits the last part of the small intestine, the **ileum**, into the **caecum** past a sphincter, the ileocaecal sphincter. This helps to regulate the amount of chyme entering the caecum so that about 1.5 litres enters the caecum in about 12–24 hours.

As discussed in Chapter 9, 'Eating and Drinking', the large intestine absorbs water and salts and about 4% of digested material. The absorption of water and salts is highly regulated under homeostatic control to suit the needs of the water–electrolyte balance of the body as well as in maintaining blood pressure (discussed below).

The absorption of water in the large intestine results in the formation of faeces (**stools**) which are composed of one part solid material to two parts water. The solid material consists of bacteria, undigested polysaccharides, bile pigments, cholesterol and protein.

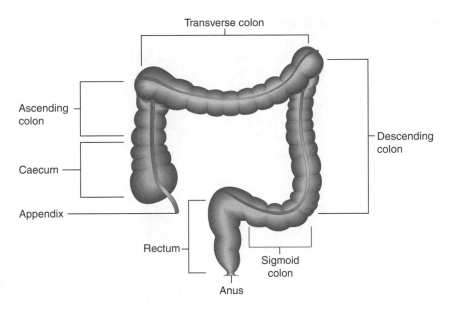

FIGURE 10.2 **The large intestine**

The removal of faeces from the GI tract: Defecation

The colon is subject to slow waves of contraction moving faeces through the bowel. There is a reflex pathway – the **gastrocolic reflex** – where extrinsic nerves of the GI tract are activated by **stomach distension**. After a large meal the stomach distends and a wave of contraction passes along the large intestine propelling faeces present in the large intestine into the rectum. This distends the rectum and initiates a **defecation reflex** action of the internal anal sphincter. This sphincter is normally closed, but now opens. The faeces pass into the anal canal. The external anal sphincter is under voluntary control and faeces are passed out of the anus at a convenient time and place. This voluntary action is learnt during childhood, but it can be lost during illness and age.

Health Connection

Roughage

Carbohydrates that cannot be digested increase the rate of movement of faeces in the large intestine due to distension of the gut. This distension is a stimulus for the activation of the smooth muscle surrounding the gut wall to act in peristaltic movement. This undigested carbohydrate can be broken down by bacteria and produces gases (see Chapter 9, 'Eating and Drinking') or it remains in the large intestine as roughage. Health promotion has looked at the epidemiology of diseases such as colon cancer, heart disease and diabetes. Those with diets high in roughage, or fibre, tend to have lower incidences of these diseases. The movement of faeces along the bowel may help to reduce constipation and haemorrhoids (piles). If faeces remain in the bowel longer there is a build up of toxic wastes. Fibre may also bind to these toxins aiding their elimination from the GI tract. However, high fibre diets may result in a lowering of vitamin absorption as fibre can also bind vitamins and prevent them from crossing the GI tract into the blood.

Elimination from the kidneys

Metabolic waste is collected from cells and transported in the blood to the **kidneys**. There it must be removed from the blood and eliminated from the body. The kidneys, the organs that remove waste from the blood, form part of the **renal system**, one of the **excretory systems** of the body.

The constituents of the renal system

The excretory system consists of

- two kidneys,
- two ureters, one from each kidney,
- one bladder and
- one urethra.

The kidneys work by filtering waste from the blood which is then transported via the **ureters** to a temporary storage area, the **bladder**, which, when quite full will release its contents, **urine**, down the **urethra** to be voided from the body (Figure 10.3).

There are two kidneys situated at the back of the body behind the digestive organs in the abdominal cavity. The bladder is in the pelvic cavity with the ureters connecting the kidneys to the bladder.

The kidneys are bean shaped, dark red to brown in colour and approximately 12cm × 6cm × 3cm in size. Each kidney is surrounded by an outer connective tissue layer, the renal capsule. The inner part of the kidney is in three layers (Figure 10.4):

- outer layer or renal cortex,
- middle layer or renal medulla and
- inner layer or renal pelvis.

The inner renal pelvis connects with the ureters to transport the urine formed by the kidneys to the bladder.

Each kidney contains approximately one million **nephrons**. The nephrons are the functional part of the kidney; each one acting as an independent filtering unit. Each nephron receives blood to be filtered of waste. The

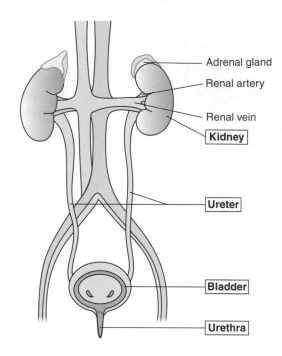

FIGURE 10.3 **The renal system**

filtered blood re-enters the blood circulatory system. The waste enters the rest of the nephron to be treated and excreted.

Chapter Reference

Diffusion and osmosis are discussed in Chapter 1, 'Maintaining a Safe Environment' (see p. 1).

How waste is moved from the blood to the kidneys

Blood containing metabolic waste enters the kidneys in the renal arteries and is removed in the renal veins. The blood entering the kidneys come from the liver where **metabolites**, products of metabolism, have accumulated, along with waste products from cell metabolism. Between entering and leaving the kidneys the blood is cleared of waste metabolites. The waste from the blood is passed into a watery fluid, **urine**, ready for excretion into the outside by **micturation** (voiding). The blood with the waste removed re-enters the general circulation into veins and the vena cava.

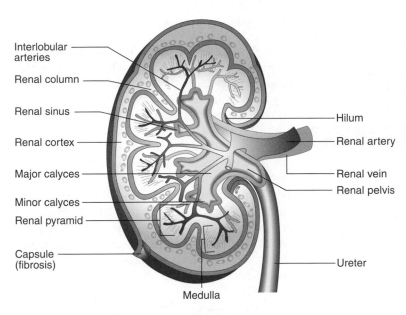

Interlobular arteries

Renal column

Renal sinus

Renal cortex

Major calyces

Minor calyces

Renal pyramid

Capsule (fibrosis)

Medulla

Hilum

Renal artery

Renal vein

Renal pelvis

Ureter

FIGURE 10.4 The kidney in cross-section

The blood is brought to the kidneys in blood vessels called **renal arteries** which break into smaller blood vessels. These bring blood to the individual nephrons in **afferent** (towards) **tubules** or blood vessels called **arterioles**. The arterioles enter the nephron at a region called the **glomerulus**, which is a network of very fine blood vessels called **capillaries**. Here the blood is filtered.

The filtered blood is removed from the nephron in **efferent** (away from) **tubules** back into the general blood circulatory system via the renal vein.

The **filtrate** (waste from the blood) enters the nephron tubule in an area called the **Bowman's capsule** which surrounds the glomerular arteriole. The filtrate then passes through a long tube consisting of three parts:

- the distal convoluted tubule,
- the loop of Henlé and
- the proximal convoluted tubule.

The **proximal** (close or in close proximity, near) convoluted tube is lined with epithelial cells which contain many **microvilli** (membrane projections) which increase the surface area of the cells allowing for **absorption**. The proximal tubule enters the loop of Henlé where

the epithelial cells have no microvilli and are very thin. This area allows passive diffusion of substances such as water and ions. As the tubule ascends into the distal tubule the epithelia become thicker. This is a site of ion absorption. Around the proximal and distal tubule are a series of capillaries, the **peritubular capillary system**, into which absorbed solutes are transported. The tubule then enters a collecting tubule which together with other collecting tubules enters the renal pelvis to connect with the ureters and bladder. The bladder acts as a temporary storage unit until the filtrate, now called urine, enters the urethra for voiding to the exterior.

Urine is formed in the tube of the **nephron** starting at the Bowman's capsule and continuing along the tubule to the collecting ducts. It then passes out of the kidney via the **renal pelvis** into the **ureters**. There are three stages to urine formation:

- glomerular filtration,
- tubular re-absorption and
- tubular secretion.

Glomerular filtration

The blood entering the kidneys in the renal arteries is under system blood pressure. The arteries branch into very small diameter afferent arterioles which decrease in width but still have the same volume of blood. This causes an increase in blood pressure. The arterioles then branch into capillaries around the nephrons. These capillaries are called the **glomerulus**. Blood pressure is affected by blood volume and the diameter of the vessel. As just mentioned the vessels of the glomerulus now have a small diameter with the same blood volume in them as before, so the pressure increases. This high **hydrostatic**

blood pressure in the glomerulus forces water and solutes across the glomerular capillary walls and through pores in their walls as filtrate. The filtrate is forced out of the glomerular arteriole blood vessels into the first part of the kidney nephron called the **Bowman's capsule.**

Health Connection

Kidney stones

The stones found in the kidney in this condition are crystal deposits of varying sizes. Most are made of calcium salts which may be due to a diet rich in calcium or oxalic acid. Small stones may dislodge from the kidney and move through the urinary tract eventually passing out of the body in the urine. If the stones are larger they may cause excruciating pain, frequent, painful passing of urine, nausea and vomiting and blood in the urine. If a stone lodges in the ureter the build up of urine can result in swelling of the kidney (hydronephrosis).

Kidney stones may be caused by inadequate fluid intake and low blood pressure and urine output as well as long-standing urinary tract infections. Some drugs can cause stone formation.

The filtrate consists of water and small molecules, for example glucose, vitamins, amino acids, urea and other waste and electrolytes. Larger molecules (plasma proteins) and blood cells do *not* enter the Bowman's capsule as the pores in the walls of the capillaries are too small for them to exit the glomerulus and enter the Bowman's capsule. Large molecules therefore remain in the blood capillary.

Chapter Reference

Blood pressure is discussed in Chapter 7, 'Breathing' (see p. 184).

Tubular re-absorption

The filtrate, in the nephrons, water and small molecules, has now been filtered from the blood. It passes along from the Bowman's capsule into the first part of the tubule, the proximal convoluted tubule. In this part of the tubule 99% of the filtrate is re-absorbed into the blood. Water and some substances such as glucose and amino acids are completely re-absorbed. Some substances are poorly re-absorbed such as urea, uric acid and creatinine, which are breakdown products of amino acids and form the main solutes of urine. They remain in the tubule. Some substances are partially re-absorbed according to need such as water and electrolytes.

Tubular secretion

As the filtrate passes along the tubule into the distal convoluted tubule substances are secreted from the blood into the filtrate. These substances move out of the peritubular capillaries through the tubule cells into the filtrate. They include substances such as

- hydrogen H^+,
- potassium K^+,
- creatinine,
- drugs.

Health Connection

Chronic renal failure

Chronic conditions are long term. Chronic renal failure can be caused by hypertension, diabetes mellitus, sickle-cell disease or polycystic kidney disease.

The symptoms are weakness, loss of appetite, shortness of breath, muscle twitching, cramps in the legs, pins and needles, persistent hiccoughs, nausea and vomiting, pale, itchy and easily bruised skin.

Health Connection

Acute renal failure

This occurs when there is a loss of the function of both kidneys. Waste products and excess water build up in the body disrupting the normal chemical balance of the blood.

Acute failure could be due to shock and hypotension or sudden blockage causing hydronephrosis or toxic chemicals or drugs.

The symptoms are very little urine produced, nausea and vomiting, drowsiness and headache and back pain (Figure 10.5).

Health Connection

Polycystic kidney disease

This is an inherited (genetic) disorder in which multiple fluid-filled cysts gradually replace the tissue in both kidneys. The kidneys become larger and progressively less able to function until they eventually fail. If the kidney is further damaged high blood pressure may result. Blood in the urine and vague discomfort or episodes of severe abdominal and lower back pain, but as seen in other Health Connections these symptoms can occur in other kidney and urinary diseases.

The role of the kidney

The kidney has various roles due to its action on blood:

- It forms urine by the removal of waste products from blood.
- It regulates water and electrolyte balance due to the regulation of partially re-absorbed substances such as water and salts.
- It regulates blood pressure due to its altering blood volume by the removal of water from the blood during filtration and the addition of water to the blood during re-absorption – depending on needs.
- It regulates blood pH due to the secretion of H+ ions into the urine in the distal convoluted tubule.
- It also has an endocrine function secreting a hormone – erythropoietin – which is responsible for the formation of red blood cells.

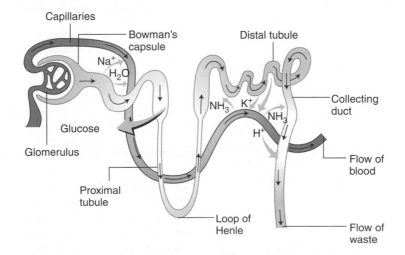

FIGURE 10.5 **The parts and functions of a kidney nephron**

The regulation of all these functions by the kidney is under hormonal control.

> **Chapter Reference**
>
> Hormones and the endocrine system are discussed in Chapter 4, 'Communicating' (see p. 102).

Renal clearance

The renal clearance of a substance is the volume of plasma from which the substance is completely cleared from the kidney in a unit of time. The amount of a substance that is excreted relies on how much is filtered, re-absorbed and secreted into the urine. If a substance is not secreted or re-absorbed the **glomerular filtration rate** (GFR), the filtering of substance in the glomerulus into the tubule, defines how much of the substance is cleared from the blood. However, all naturally occurring substances in the body are re-absorbed or secreted. Creatinine is not re-absorbed and very slightly secreted so it is used as a standard for GFR. To measure the amount of removal of a substance from the blood the amount present in the blood and the amount excreted in the urine in a set time must be measured.

Glomerular filtration rate

The glomerular filtration rate (GFR) is the volume of fluid filtered by the kidneys over a set time. For a 70 kg adult it is about 180 litres per day (125 ml/minute). From Chapter 7, 'Breathing', you may remember that there are 5 litres of blood in the adult body of which 3 litres are plasma. Other capillaries in the body have a flow of about 4 litres per day. The kidneys thus filter at a very high rate. In fact 25% of the blood ejected from the left ventricle (cardiac output) is received by the kidneys.

The rate of filtration by the kidneys is dependent on three factors:

- Blood pressure in the afferent and efferent arterioles of each nephron.

- The permeability of the wall of the glomerulus and Bowman's capsule.
- The osmotic pressure in the glomerular capillaries and Bowmans' capsule.

> **Chapter Reference**
>
> Blood pressure and cardiac output are discussed in Chapter 7, 'Breathing' (see p. 184).

Regulation of kidney function

Glomerular filtration rate is controlled at the junction between the loop of Henlé and the arterioles, the peritubular capillary system (discussed above). This is because the tubule passes very close to the glomerulus just after the loop of Henlé, between the afferent and efferent arterioles. This junction is called the **juxtaglomerular apparatus**. The epithelial cells at this part of the tube are specialised cells, **macula densa cells**. The epithelial cells of the arterioles are the **juxtaglomerular cells**. These produce an enzyme called **renin**. The hormone renin decreases the diameter of blood vessels, thus increasing blood pressure in the arterioles. This in turn affects the filtrate which is then detected by the macula densa cells. The macula densa cells can respond by releasing factors that effect renin production and release.

Re-absorption in the tubules relies on two mechanisms:

- Changes in permeability of the membranes of the tubules to water and ions.
- Passive osmosis along the tube due to the varying concentrations of solutes in the filtrate and surrounding fluids.

Homeostatic regulation of water

In Chapter 9, 'Eating and Drinking', the importance of water balance is discussed and some basic mechanisms for controlling water levels are introduced. Here we discuss how the kidneys regulate water and electrolyte balance for the body fluids.

Water and sodium are filtered and re-absorbed by the kidneys. Normally water and sodium intake matches output (Table 10.1).

The actual amount of water and salt that we take in our diets varies from day to day. Our output of water can also vary from 0.4 litres to 25 litres per day, depending on the amount ingested. Also, as discussed in Chapter 9, 'Eating and Drinking', bouts of vomiting or diarrhoea can effect water and salt loss, as can sweating in hot weather during thermoregulation, discussed in Chapter 5, 'Controlling and Repairing'.

We have 40 litres of water in our body. It is held in two body compartments:

- **intracellular** (inside cells): 25 litres,
- **extracellular** (outside cells): 15 litres,
  - interstitial (between cells): 12 litres,
  - plasma (in blood): 3 litres.

Water passes between these sites as part of its role in transport and changes in water levels are monitored by **osmoreceptors** in the hypothalamus of the brain.

Chapter Reference
The brain is discussed in Chapter 4, 'Communicating' (see p. 102).

When the water content of the body decreases the body fluids become more concentrated (increased osmolarity). When this occurs the brain releases **antidiuretic hormone** (ADH). This hormone changes the membranes of the epithelial cells of the collecting ducts to increase their permeability to water which will allow more water to be absorbed from the tubules back into the concentrated blood arterioles surrounding the tubule.

ADH can also be released in response to the detection of the amount of stretch in the vascular system caused by changes in blood volume. A drop in blood volume will encourage the release of ADH. This will result in water being re-absorbed from the tubules, the urine being more concentrated and the blood gaining water and thus increasing volume and pressure.

Health Connection

Alcohol
Alcohol inhibits the release of ADH. As alcohol is consumed, urination increases while dehydration increases.

Health Connection

Diabetes insipidus
In this condition the ability to synthesise ADH is decreased, often due to damage to the hypothalamus. Copious urine is thus produced. It is treated by the administration of ADH.

Homeostatic regulation of sodium and potassium levels

The regulation of sodium levels relies on two factors:

- filtration in the glomerulus and
- re-absorption in the tubules.

Table 10.1 Water and sodium chloride input and output

	Water	Sodium chloride
Drink	1500ml	
Food	750ml	10.5g
Metabolism	250ml	
TOTAL INPUT	2500ml	10.5g
Urine	1500ml	10.0g
Insensible loss (skin/lungs)	700ml	
Sweat	200ml	0.25g
Faeces	100ml	0.25g
TOTAL OUTPUT	2500ml	10.5g

Filtration rates in the glomerulus rely on blood pressure in the glomerular arterioles. The macula densa cells (discussed above) detect changes in filtration and secrete a hormone **renin**. Renin can also act on a small polypeptide protein produced by the liver, **angiotensinogen**. Renin causes it to be cleaved to **angiotensin I**, which is then converted to **angiotensin II** by another enzyme, **angiotensin converting enzyme**, located in the capillary endothelial cells. Angiotensin II is a hormone that acts to change the GFR by causing the constriction of blood vessels and thus increasing blood pressure.

Re-absorption of sodium from the kidney tubules is effected by a steroid hormone, **aldosterone**, which is produced by the adrenal glands which are situated on the top of the kidneys.

> **Chapter Reference**
> Hormones are discussed in Chapter 4, 'Communicating' (see p. 102).

Aldosterone alters the numbers of sodium transport proteins in the epithelial cells which increase sodium re-absorption. Angiotensin II stimulates aldosterone production.

If there is too much sodium in the blood **atrial natriuretic factor** (ANF) is released which inhibits sodium re-absorption and increases GFR to accelerate sodium filtration and excretion.

Potassium ions are very important in active transport. Potassium can be secreted in the distal tubule under the control of aldosterone.

Regulation of pH: Buffers

The pH of most body fluids is slightly alkaline at pH 7.4. The pH is affected by levels of hydrogen ions (H+). Too many hydrogen ions lead to acidosis; too few to alkalosis. Hydrogen ions accumulate due to the production of carbon dioxide during respiration.

Within blood, in the plasma liquid phase, are many chemicals. One of them is a chemical that acts as a **buffer**: it mops up hydrogen

> **Chapter Reference**
> Respiration is discussed in Chapter 7, 'Breathing' (see p. 184). ATP and CO_2 production are discussed in Chapter 2, 'Working and Playing' (see p. 35).

ions and it mops up hydroxyl ions depending on which are most present, concentrated, in the blood. This chemical is called **bicarbonate**, H_2CO_3.

When carbon dioxide is formed it combines with water to form carbonic acid (H_2CO_3) which dissociates, separates, to form hydrogen ions and bicarbonate ions (HCO_3^-)

$$CO_2 + H_2O \leftrightarrow H_2CO \leftrightarrow HCO_3^- + H^+$$

The symbol $\leftrightarrow$ means that the reaction can go either way. The reactions with this $\leftrightarrow$ symbol are *reversible*. They can be driven to the right if there are lots of CO_2 molecules and they can be driven to the left if there are lots of H+ ions. The bicarbonate molecule thus acts as a buffer, buffering CO_2 or H+ as needed.

This reversible binding of hydrogen ions acts to buffer the numbers of hydrogen ions in the blood. Excess hydrogen ions are excreted by the kidneys. Bicarbonate ions are filtered in the kidneys. Hydrogen ions are secreted and bind to the filtered bicarbonate ions and other ions in the filtrate.

Health Connection

Diabetic kidney disease
Long-term diabetes mellitus damages the blood vessels in the glomeruli. This causes protein to leak into the urine and reduces the kidneys' ability to remove wastes and excess water from the body.

When the kidney damage is severe the symptoms of chronic renal failure appear: vomiting, drowsiness, shortness of breath and high blood pressure.

Chapter Reference

Hormones are discussed in Chapter 4, 'Communicating' (see p. 102).

The kidney also acts as an **endocrine gland** secreting the hormone erythropoietin which increases red blood cell production.

Health Connection

Dialysis

If the kidneys fail, toxic waste products and ions build up in the blood. A treatment for this is dialysis. Blood from an artery is connected to a semi-permeable tube that allows the passage of water, salts (ions) and small molecules into fluid surrounding the tube (dialysis fluid) by diffusion. These small molecules are either removed, if waste, or re-introduced if needed. The filtered blood is then passed back into a vein (Figure 10.6).

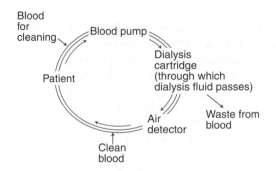

FIGURE 10.6 **Dialysis mechanism**

How waste is removed from the bladder

Once urine has been formed in the nephrons it is conveyed to the calyxes and into the renal pelvis, joining the urine from all the nephrons of each kidney. The urine then enters the **ureter**, one

from each kidney, tubes that convey the urine from the kidneys to the bladder. The ureters convey urine from renal pelvis to the posterior of the bladder a distance of about 25–30 cm. They have an oblique entry into the bladder (Figure 10.7).

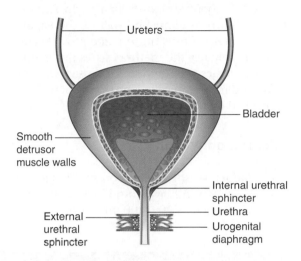

FIGURE 10.7 **The bladder**

The bladder

The bladder is located in pelvis, behind the symphysis pubis. It is a collapsible hollow muscular sac. The walls are thick and folded in the empty bladder. The bladder can expand significantly. It has three layers of smooth detrusor muscle walls that aid **peristalsis**, the muscular contractions that move substances along vessels. It has an inner lining of transitional epithelium tissue. There are three openings (**trigone**) in the bladder: two are inputs, ureters, bringing urine from the kidney. The output is into a thin-walled tube, the **urethra** that carries urine from the bladder to the outside of the body by peristalsis.

The urethra

The urethra conveys urine to the exterior. It contains two **sphincters** (muscles): an internal urethral sphincter at the junction of the bladder and urethra which is under involuntary control and an external urethral sphincter at the pelvic floor which is under voluntary control by an early age. In males the prostrate gland surrounds urethra where it leaves the bladder. In females the urethra is about 3–4 cm (1 inch) while in males it is about 20 cm (8 inches). In females the urethra runs along the wall of the vagina while in males it runs through the prostate and penis. In females the urethra carries urine only while in males the urethra is a passageway for urine and for sperm cells. The release of urine is controlled by the two sphincters.

Micturation: Voiding

The bladder is only a temporary storage for urine. It slowly fills with urine from the ureters. When there is 200–300 ml of urine in the bladder, the bladder becomes stretched. This activates stretch receptors in the wall of the bladder. The reflex travels to the sacral spinal cord and then back to the bladder via the splanchnic nerves. It causes the internal sphincter to relax. Urine then passes out of the bladder via the internal sphincter into the urethra.

Both sphincter muscles must open to allow voiding of urine from the bladder to the urethra. The external urethral sphincter must be voluntarily relaxed. The stages of micturation are

- reflex contraction of bladder wall;
- urine forced past internal sphincter (urge);
- contraction stops – reflex again as bladder fills more;
- voluntary relaxation of external sphincter results in micturation.

Health Connection

Urinary incontinence

Being unable to control micturation is a very debilitating condition. Urinary incontinence is where there is complete or partial loss of voluntary control over bladder function. There are different types of incontinence:

- Stress incontinence: small amounts of urine are expelled involuntarily during coughing, exertion or sneezing. This is usually due to weakness of the pelvic floor muscles.
- Urge incontinence: repeated episodes of involuntary loss of urine preceded by a sudden, urgent need to empty the bladder. This can be due to an infection such as cystitis, to having a weak pelvic floor or disorders of the nervous system, e.g. stroke.
- Overflow incontinence: this may be due to an obstruction to the flow of urine, e.g. enlarged prostate, and this causes an intermittent dribble.
- Total incontinence: no bladder control usually caused by a nervous system disorder, e.g. spinal cord injury.

Health Connection

Bladder stones

Stones can form in the bladder if waste products in the urine crystallise. Most stones consist of salts of **calcium**. They can occur if the urine stagnates in the bladder due to incomplete emptying or due to recurrent cystitis.

Urinary retention

As opposed to incontinence, retention is the inability to empty the bladder completely or at all. It can be caused by anything that exerts pressure on the urethra such as an enlarged prostate, urethral stricture, pregnancy or constipation. The bladder neck may be obstructed by bladder stones or tumours or there may be nerve damage. Urinary retention can cause kidney damage if the urine cannot drain from the kidneys.

Acute retention: abdominal pain, a distressing painful urge to pass urine but the inability to do so.

Chronic retention: a frequent urge to pass urine, swelling of the abdomen, difficulty in passing urine, a weak flow of urine that ends in a dribble.

Urine

Urine is an amber coloured, clear aromatic liquid if fresh with a pH of about six which can vary depending on what is being excreted. It has a specific gravity (SG) of 1.010–1.035, which means it is a little denser that water due to the presence of solutes. It is composed of 96% water with added solutes. These solutes include

- products of amino acid breakdown including
  - urea,
  - uric acid,
  - creatinine and
  - ammonia.
- electrolytes including
  - sodium,
  - potassium,
  - chlorides,
  - phosphates and
  - bicarbonates.

Abnormal constituents of urine

Urine contains the waste of metabolic processes. It should not contain

- blood proteins,
- white blood cells,
- red blood cells,
- ketones,
- glucose and
- micro-organisms.

The presence of glucose, for example, is an indication of diabetes mellitus where there is too much glucose in the blood and not enough in the cells of the body. The excess glucose in the blood has to be excreted via the kidneys. The presence of micro-organisms shows a potential infection as urine should be sterile (no living cells or organisms in it) when it is first voided. The presence of immunoglobulin proteins from the blood is indicative of disease. This is why urine is *collected* and *tested.* The presence of abnormal constituents is *diagnostic* of various disease processes.

Urinary tract infections (UTIs)

Infections are discussed in Chapter 11, 'Cleansing and Dressing'. In UTI a bacteria, E coli, which is a normal constituent of the GI tract and in faeces, colonises the genito-urinary tract. This usually occurs due to poor toilet hygiene where the faeces are wiped towards the urethra. Children should be taught to wipe from front to back, from the urethral area towards the anus. Because toilet hygiene is one of the main causes of UTI it is more common in women than in men due to their shorter urethra. In UTI the E coli bind to the surface of the tract and multiply. They can then move back and colonise the bladder. They are usually eliminated by a treatment with antibiotics. If untreated they can move back and colonise the kidney causing severe diseases in the nephron. The main signs and symptoms are a burning sensation when passing urine. Drinking water, and some say cranberry juice, helps the flow of urine and helps to flush out the E coli.

Changes during lifespan and lifestyle

Small imbalances in water salts or waste have a very severe effect on babies as small changes have a large effect due to the smaller volumes of fluids in babies. Not all the glomeruli are functional at birth. Blood flow to the kidneys is low. However, urine production is high. At birth the filtration rate falls and sodium excretion falls. It gradually rises during the first week after birth. Adult rates are reached at about 2–3 years of age.

As we age our kidneys shrink in size and have a 50% reduction in blood flow and therefore in filtered blood. Our sensation of thirst diminishes with age; therefore older individuals are susceptible to dehydration. There is also an increase in **urinary tract infections** and an increase in urination, urinary **retention** (due to blockages), **incontinence** (due to muscle tone), **nocturia** (needing to urinate during normal sleep time) and **dysuria** (painful urination).

Alcohol

One of the main alterations in our water balance and kidney output is due to alcohol consumption. While drinking many pints of beer

Cystitis

Cystitis is one of the most common urinary tract infections (UTIs). The lining of the bladder becomes inflamed. The symptoms are burning when passing urine (due to the inflamed bladder), frequent urge to urinate with little urine passed, a feeling of incomplete emptying of the bladder, pain in the lower abdomen or lower back, fever and chills.

It is mostly caused by a bacterial infection from the vagina or bowel entering the urethra and the bladder.

The risk of contracting cystitis is increased if diabetic or if the bladder cannot be emptied fully due to an enlarged prostate or urethral structure.

would be thought to act as a hydrator, in fact the alcohol in the beer dehydrates as it interferes with ADH. This results in more urine being excreted than the volume of alcohol consumed (Figure 10.8).

Catheters

Catheters are tubes that can be inserted into a vessel or duct in the body. They can then be used to drain fluids. A common catheter is a urinary one inserted into the urethra and up into the bladder to drain urine. This is done when there is a blockage or when a person is unable to control micturation (incontinence) due to illness or in situations such as anaesthesia or hospitalisation (Figure 10.8).

Body image

Some changes to our bodies through development such as puberty, through trauma, such as the loss of a limb, or through illness, such as urinary tract surgery may leave us with altered bodies. With some diseases we may need a permanent in-dwelling catheter, for example. This has a profound effect on our body image, how we see ourselves and how comfortable we are in our bodies. It can also have profound effects on our social and personal lives and leave us isolated and lonely, affecting our mental well-being.

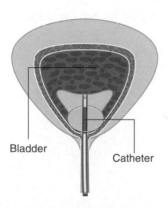

Bladder

Catheter

FIGURE 10.8 Catheter inserted through the urethra into the bladder. The external end is then connected to a bag to collect the urine

Conclusion: Eliminating

We cannot stop the production of waste as the activities in the body produce waste as a by-product. The waste we produce can become toxic if it is not removed. The ADL of elimination is one which most of us are keen to be able to maintain independently throughout our lives. Inability to eliminate waste has major impacts on our health. Inappropriate elimination of waste (incontinence) has major impacts on our feelings and our ability to participate in other activities.

Chapter Summary

- Excretion is necessary to rid the body of waste products.
- Waste from ingestion is excreted via the large colon and rectum.
- Waste from metabolism is excreted via the kidneys.
- The kidneys regulate water, salts (ions), hydrogen ion (pH) and waste levels in the blood and thus also affect blood pressure via blood volume.
- Waste is filtered into kidney tubules with water and forms urine.
- Regulation of urine content and amount is under hormonal and enzymatic control.
- Urine is excreted from the kidneys via ureters into the bladder.
- The bladder acts as a temporary storage tank.
- When the bladder has 250–300 ml of urine the stretch in the walls of the bladder causes a reflex action.
- Urine passes into the urethra past the involuntary sphincter.
- When convenient, urine passes the voluntary sphincter for excretion from the body.
- Urine mainly contains water, salts, urea, uric acid and creatinine.
- The analysis of the amount of water produced and the contents of urine can help in the diagnosis of various diseases.

Cleansing and Dressing

Chapter Outline

- Introduction: Cleansing and dressing as activities of daily living
- The environment
- Pathogens
- The immune system
- Detection and prevention of infection
- The innate immune system and response
- The adaptive immune system and response
- Changes during lifespan and lifestyle
- Conclusion: Cleansing and dressing
- Chapter summary

Introduction: Cleansing and dressing as activities of daily living

There can be few greater pleasures than bathing in clean, warm water. The feeling of being relaxed and refreshed revitalises. They say that 'Cleanliness is next to Godliness'. Even babies and children have an affinity for splashing in water. We all know the consequences of dirty, contaminated water and the resultant diseases such as **cholera**.

It is estimated that more people have died of **infections** than all the wars put together. Infections are caused by what we tend to call 'germs', organisms so small that we need a **microscope** to view them, hence their name **micro-organisms**. Washing our bodies and clothing and having anything we imbibe (take into our bodies) clean and free of 'germs' are attempts to cleanse ourselves and our environment of these threats. Dressing also protects us from the environment.

In the arena of health care, the study of **microbes** and their impact on our health has large consequences. Infections due to micro-organisms are the reason for many visits to general practitioners and hospitals. Clean water and the disposal of waste have reduced the spread of infection in many areas and reduced the illness and death rate (**morbidity** and **mortality**) due to infectious disorders. **Nosocomial** infections, infections acquired while in hospital, cost the health services large sums in money and time. Much work to reduce these infections is recommended as a health priority. One of the most effective ways of preventing infection is basic hygiene: the simple act of washing before handling foods and between patients can reduce the spread of infectious disorders. When cleanliness through washing and using clean dressings is not maintained infections can spread. In this chapter we will discuss infections and protection from infections.

The environment

We do not have sole dominion on the planet. Nor is the planet populated with other species merely for our dining table. We share the planet with many other species and we are quite recent arrivals having only been here some one million years. This may sound as if we have an ancient ancestry, but the first species on this planet arose four hundred million years ago and their descendants are still here. We are the new boys and girls on the block! The planet and other species, therefore, existed before us and could exist without our presence on it.

It is often said that we humans are at the top of the 'food chain'. This is a very inaccurate description of our place on the planet. We might possess the highest levels of consciousness of any species on the planet currently, but we are certainly not at the top of the food chain. We are *in* the food chain. Just as we look to other species for food, the source of our nutrients, other species look to us as their lunch. This includes not only large animals such as crocodiles and tigers, if we happen to stray into their path, but also very small species such as **bacteria** and **viruses**. In fact, if any organisms are at the top of the food chain it is these minute, microbes or micro-organisms (microscopic organisms), organisms that are so minute they can only been seen with a microscope, which have found so many food sources including us.

We live in a *permissive* (it allows us to be here), but *indifferent* (it won't miss us if we are not here) environment. In health we must maintain ourselves, the integrity of our body, by homeostatic mechanisms. However, we are constantly confronted by other organisms trying to maintain themselves – to survive and thrive. We must protect our own bodies, our cells, from being used as a source of energy and nutrients by other organisms.

Micro-organisms (microbes) are all around us. When we breathe in, inhale, millions of micro-organisms enter our air passages. We have many cilia, hair-like projections that help to filter the air we breathe in to clear these microbes.

Chapter Reference

Filtering air during inhalation is discussed in Chapter 7, 'Breathing' (see p. 184).

Most of these microbes are harmless to us. They exist in the environment but are not looking to us for a food source. This is just as well as there are far more species of microbes than of large organisms! When they find a suitable food source, one which provides the nutrients they need in a manner they can absorb them, they can grow and reproduce, multiply, in minutes so they are capable of outgrowing us.

Health Connection

Microbes and breathing
In Chapter 7, 'Breathing', we talked about the upper respiratory tract being covered in mucus and cilia as part of the **filtering** function that needs to be carried out to clean the air as it enters our internal environment. The mucus and cilia trap dust and **microbes** in the external environment.

Types of microbes

It is estimated that there are five million, trillion, trillion microbes on the planet. That is the number 5 followed by 30 zeroes. Microbes are the largest group of organisms. They are a very successful group as they can evolve very quickly though mutation, due to their rapid reproductive rates. Humans have a very low reproductive rate. It takes us about 12 years to reach reproductive potential and then each offspring takes 9 months to develop in the uterus followed by 12 years to reach sexual maturity. Microbes, with an appropriate food source for energy and growth, can reproduce in about 20 minutes and form offspring that can also reproduce in about 20 minutes. In a short while one microbe can form millions of offspring.

Apart from the microbes that exist in the environment independent of us, there are some microbes that do use us as food and home. These microbes come in two types:

- **commensals** and
- **pathogens.**

Commensal means to share a table and these microbes share the table with us. They live on us, but do us no harm. Many of them do us good helping to digest food and produce vitamins in the large bowel. They also, by living on our skin, hair and body entrances such as the upper respiratory tract, provide a barrier to the more menacing microbes which cannot get a foothold as they are outnumbered by the commensals. While we are made of 10^{13} cells there are some 10^{12} microbes living on or in us. Approximately 1 kg of our weight is attributable to these commensals.

Pathogens

Pathogens are a subgroup of microbes. They are the microbes that cause disease through infection. In other words they cause a **pathology**. As with all microbes they come in a variety of types including

- bacteria,
  - rickettsia,
  - mycoplasma,
- viruses,
- protozoa,
- fungi,
- parasitic worms.

Bacteria

There are two main groups: the bacteria and the cyanobacteria. Bacteria include all of the commonly known species such as Escherichia coli (E. coli bacteria), Salmonella bacteria, Staphylococci, Listeria and the Clostridia. Cyanobacteria form a separate type of bacteria that are able to photosynthesise – they can also be called blue-green algae.

They are the commonest cause of infections. They come in various forms such as **cocci**, which are spherical, **bacilli**, which are rod shaped, **NS spirochaetes**, which are corkscrew-shaped bacteria, some of which cause syphilis (Treponema bacteria) and Lyme disease (Borrelia bacteria).

Cocci or bacilli type bacteria that have thick cell walls are termed **gram positive** because of

the way they take up the Gram stain. Those with thin cell walls are termed **gram negative.**

> ### Health Connection
>
> #### Gram staining
> Gram staining is a way of differentiating between different bacteria. It is a stain that some bacteria take up and are then dyed purple while others are not. It is useful in pathology laboratories to diagnose what type of bacteria has invaded us and what type of treatment is most appropriate.

Rickettsia and Chlamydia

These are bacteria which can only live and survive inside other living cells. They are often carried by ticks, fleas and lice. One type causes the disease **typhus.**

Mycoplasmas

These are bacteria, but with no cell wall. They have no fixed shape, but are capable of independent metabolic activity. These can infect humans and cause pneumonia. Their main areas of infection are surface linings such as found in the gastrointestinal tract, the respiratory tract and the genitourinary tract. *Mycoplasma pneumoniae* is one of the commoner causes of atypical pneumonia, an infection of the lungs.

> ### Health Connection
>
> #### Antibiotics
> Bacterial cells can be killed or prevented from growing by a range of antibiotic drugs such as penicillin. These drugs *do not* act against viruses or **fungi**. They mainly work by interfering with the **bacterial cell wall** and thus altering the osmotic pressure of the bacterial cell, usually ending in **lysis**. Some interfere with the replicative machinery of the cell.

Viruses

These are at the other extreme from bacteria. They are not independent and cannot feed or reproduce themselves. They are comprised of just genetic material in a protective protein coat. To reproduce they attach themselves to a 'host' cell wall, inject their genetic material into the host and get the host to replicate the viral genetic material, make the protein coat, wrap the genetic material in the protein coat and export the new viral particle(s) to infect other cells, often killing the host cell at the same time. Viral infections are discussed in the T lymphocytes section.

Chapter Reference

Replication of genetic material and reproduction are discussed in Chapter 3, 'Growing and Developing' (see p. 64).

Protozoa

These are single-celled organisms such as amoeba that cause diseases such as amoebic dysentery, trichomonosis and malaria.

Fungi

These are plant-like organisms such as moulds and yeast found in air, soil and water. They can cause diseases such as athlete's foot if found on the surface or **histoplasmosis** if found in the systemic system.

Parasitic worms

Parasitic worms such as roundworm, pinworm and tapeworm cause these infections.

Health Connection

Nosocomial infections

Methicillin-resistant staphylococcal infection (MRSA)

Hospitals face a very large problem of diseases that are acquired in hospitals (nosocomial infections). The health care worker or the visitor may not be susceptible to certain diseases, but once a barrier such as the skin is broken in an operation or drugs are given that may reduce the immune response, patients may be susceptible to the 'germs' carried by worker or visitors. Coupled to this is the over-use of antibacterials and antibiotics. These do not distinguish between commensals and pathogens. If you eliminate the commensals you leave room for the opportunistic pathogen. MRSA is one such opportunistic bacteria. It is a staphylococcal type bacteria present in many of us, usually in our noses. It is opportunistic because it can, if it gets the chance, infect other parts of our bodies. This chance is provided by moving it inappropriately to a site it would not normally invade, such as skin. If it invades a new site it is no longer commensal and it can cause disease. This can occur if healthy people with the bacteria inappropriately infect vulnerable patients.

The best defence is hygiene.

Infections

Infections are the presence in the body of a pathogen that can multiply and cause disease in the host by damaging the host.

There are various ways, routes, a pathogen can enter our bodies:

- inhalation;
- ingestion: e.g. cholera, salmonella and polio;
- sexual contact: e.g. herpes, gonorrhoea and HIV;
- inoculation: via the skin and mucus membranes by accidental injury;
- puncture of skin by bites or injections: e.g.

rabies, malaria, clostridium tetani, HIV, hepatitis B;

- via the placenta: e.g. rubella.

An infection has four stages:

- **Incubation period** – the time between the organism entering the host and the onset of symptoms.
- **Prodromal period** – the time from the onset of non-specific signs and symptoms to the specific symptoms of the infection.
- **Full stage of illness period** – with a general feeling of illness.
- **Convalescent period** – with a recovery from the infection occurring.

How *many* microbes infect you, the *dose*, has an outcome on how *severe* an infection is as well as other factors such as *infectivity*, how able the organism is to invade and multiply and how pathogenic it is in its ability to produce disease. Killing us, the *host*, eliminates the microbe's food source so many microbes are commensal rather than pathogenic.

Health Connection

Burns and trauma

The skin is a waterproof lining and a protective barrier against microbes. Burns and traumas that damage large areas of skin remove this barrier and put the patient at risk not only of dehydration, but also of infection from microbes in the atmosphere.

Patients with broken skin or traumas are very susceptible to infection. When this infection occurs there is often an inflammatory response (discussed below). In an inflammatory response our temperature increases. This is why patients with burns or traumas have their temperature measured frequently to see if they are having an inflammatory response which is a sign of infection.

Health Connection

Surgery, infection and latex gloves

Most surgery involves cutting the skin. While the operating theatre may provide a **sterile** environment – an environment free from microbes – once out from the theatre the patient is susceptible to infection. One sign of infection is a rise in temperature due to an inflammatory response or fever (discussed below). Post-operative patients are, therefore, monitored regularly for changes in temperature which may be indicative of an infection.

The health care worker and any visitor need to be vigilant not to bring microbes that are usually harmless to themselves into contact with open wounds where the skin barrier is no longer able to prevent infection. Hygiene such as hand washing before touching each patient would help to reduce contamination. The use of latex gloves can mask the problem. Using them can lead the health care worker to think that the gloves are to protect the health care worker from infection. In fact, the gloves are worn to protect the vulnerable patient from the source of infection, the health care worker. They therefore need changing between patients and if the carer touches surfaces on which there may be microbes. Wearing a pair of gloves to go to reception or answer the phone and then wearing the same pair to attend to a patient happens when the carer thinks the gloves are to protect the carer. In these instances the patient is under severe threat and danger from the carer. As the quote at the top of the chapter says 'Soap and education are not as sudden as a massacre, but they are more deadly in the long run.'

First encounters with pathogens

For a pathogen to infect us it must first get onto us or into our internal environment. We have natural barriers to infections. Our skin is one of our most effective barriers, preventing microbes entering our body cavities and cells.

First line defences

There are various **barriers** and general defence mechanisms that prevent microbes, including pathogenic microbes, from entering in the first instance. Together these barriers are often referred to as **first line defence**.

First line defences are **non-specific** and are not part of the immune system itself, but are general barriers against infection. Imagine a pile of barbed wire and rocks on a beach. These would provide a barrier to anyone landing on the beach from the sea. First line defences are similar. They provide a natural barrier: rather than attacking the invader, they prevent the invader entering. They come in various types:

- physical,
- chemical,
- mechanical and
- biological.

Physical barriers are barriers such as

- skin,
- mucous and intact membranes,
- intact skin and
- hairs in epithelial and respiratory tracts that trap foreign material.

Chapter Reference

Skin is discussed in Chapter 5, 'Controlling and Repairing' (see p. 142).

While they are undamaged and continuous the membranes present a fairly impermeable membrane.

Chemical barriers are substances such as

- **hydrochloric acid** in the stomach;
- **lysozyme**, enzymatic **chemicals**, in mucous, tears and saliva which have an antibacterial action (not to be muddled with **lysosomes** found in cells);
- **acid** in sweat;
- **antibacterial proteins** and **zinc** in semen;
- **mucous** secretions in tracts.

Some of these alter the pH and effect cell growth and cell metabolism; some are specifically targeted against bacterial proteins; and some prevent bacteria adhering to target (host) cells.

Mechanical barriers are the effect of movement. While fluids are moving, a microbe in the fluid has less time to gain a foothold on a cell and attach and infect the cell; it is moved by the liquid. Mechanical barriers include the

- flow of tears preventing infections of the eyes;
- flow of urine preventing infections in the genitourinary tract.

Biological barriers include the natural, **commensal** microbes found on and in us that prevent pathogenic microbes having space to grow. They are found in the gastrointestinal and genital tract. These commensal bacteria grow in many areas that are open to infection. Their presence in these areas prevents other 'opportunistic' bacteria being able to adhere and infect us.

If these general barriers are breached; for instance if the skin is broken or a microbe enters that can survive the acidic pH of the stomach, an infection can occur. When this happens a system of the body is activated which has the sole responsibility for ridding us of pathogens and maintaining the balance of our cells and commensals in the body in homeostasis. This system is called the **immune system**.

Health Connection

Wound healing

When we encounter a noxious stimulus such as a mechanical pressure or an extreme temperature we have a rapid reflex response by the nervous system to remove ourselves from the stimulus. This is generated due to pain pathways and is to avoid tissue damage. The skin has receptors that monitor pain (discussed in Chapter 12, 'Sleeping and Healing', and in Chapter 4, 'Communicating'). Once the skin has been damaged a temporary recovery is instigated. To avoid blood loss haemostasis (cessation of blood flow to the area) is initiated through a positive feedback homeostatic pathway. Proteins in the plasma are converted to clotting agents to seal up the wound and prevent blood loss and pressure reduction (discussed in Chapter 7, 'Breathing'). Inflammatory pathways are also enlisted (discussed below). A fibrin clot is formed over the wound by the haemostatic mechanisms. It provides a scab while wound healing takes place. Platelets release a growth factor that stimulates cell division in the epidermal and dermal layers of the skin and enlist white blood cells to remove debris. Fibroblast cells migrate to the wound area and produce collagen and actin proteins that form a ring around the wound. These proteins and cells can contract to bring the edges of the wound together. Epidermal cells secrete material into the dermal ring and form new cells around the wound. The healing tissue is vulnerable and must be kept clean and not broken again for healing to proceed. Gradually the skin reconstitutes itself and within 2–4 weeks a tough impermeable elastic skin is restored.

The anatomy of the skin and wound healing is discussed in Chapter 5, 'Controlling and Repairing'.

Box 11.1 Summary – Barriers to pathogens

- We have a number of barriers to prevent the entry of harmful pathogens entering our bodies.
- These barriers act in a day-to-day manner.
- There are physical barriers such as skin.
- There are biological barriers such as commensal bacteria.
- There are chemical barriers such as HCl in the stomach.
- There are mechanical barriers such as the flow of urine.

Health Connection

Asepsis, sterile and infection control

The barriers of our bodies are trying to prevent harmful microbes from entering our internal environment. The intention is that our internal environment is sterile, having no micro-organisms. In infection control we try to keep the environment sterile by aseptic techniques using sterile gloves, instruments that have been sterilised and sterilised fluids. These are all measures to prevent contamination by microbes and the spread of microbial infections.

The immune system

The immune system is a network of **cells** that, unlike a solid organ, are **mobile** and can travel through the body. They are transported in the main transport systems of the body, the blood and lymph, and are thus known as types of blood cells and cells of the lymph: **white blood cells** – or **leucocytes** (where **cytes** means cells and **leuco** means white). The main component, thus, of the immune system is white blood cells (WBC) which consist of a number of different types of white blood cells and there are subdivisions of those types:

- **granulocytes** (granules or grainy cells)
  - neutrophils,
  - basophils,
  - eosinophils.
- **phagocytes**
  - monocyte/macrophages
- **antigen presenting cells**
  - macrophages.
- **natural killer cells**
- **lymphocytes**
  - T lymphocytes (T cells)
    - T killer,
    - T helper,
    - T suppressor,
    - T memory.
  - B lymphocytes
    - B plasma cells,
    - B memory,
    - B suppressor.

The immune system also consists of a number of **chemicals** including

- **antibodies (Ab)**,
- **complement**,
- **cytokines**,
- **interferon**,
- **chemicals of the inflammatory response.**

Where is the immune system?

The immune system is comprised of a number of different cell types that circulate in the blood and lymph tissues. Some of the cells are quite mobile moving through these transport systems. Other cells, such as macrophages, burrow into tissue and can remain there.

The lymph tissue is composed of lymph vessels and lymph nodes. The lymphoid system is the main area in which the adaptive immune system (discussed below) responds. The immune system is also found in the tonsils, spleen and thymus (Figure 11.1).

> **Chapter Reference**
> The lymph is discussed in Chapter 7, 'Breathing' (see p. 184).

Origins of the immune system

All the cells of the immune system are synthesised on bone marrow. This is an area inside particular bones and is also called the red bone marrow (Figure 11.2).

> **Chapter Reference**
> Bones are discussed in Chapter 6, 'Moving' (see p. 163).

Haemocytoblast stem cells give rise to all the other cells that eventually are found in the blood and lymph.

All organs contain cells called stem cells that are capable of forming all the cells of the organ. The bone marrow contains cells called **haemocytoblast stem cells**. These haemocytoblast stem cells, like all stem cells, are immortal and undifferentiated but can divide to form two daughter cells. One replaces the original stem cell and the other goes on to divide many times forming many offspring cells. These offspring, progenitor, cells then differentiate to form the terminal (non-dividing) functional end cells – the cells that carry out the physiological functions of the organ. In this case they form the functional cells of the blood such as the red blood cells and platelets (discussed in Chapter 7, 'Breathing') and the white blood cells discussed here.

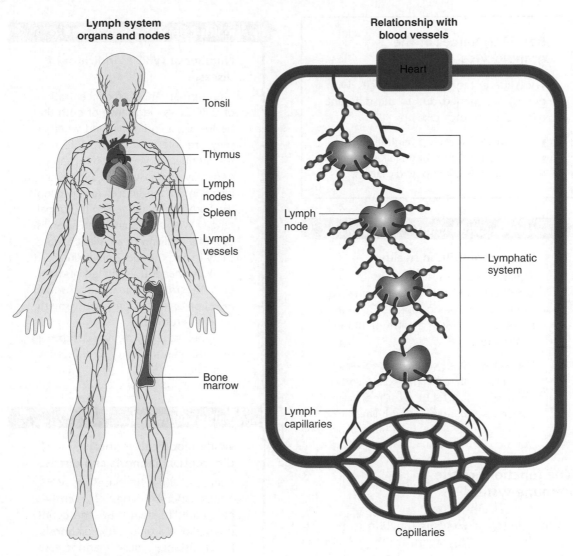

FIGURE 11.1 **Lymphoid system**

There are seven main types of white blood cells (WBC) or leucocytes:

1. neutrophils,
2. basophils,
3. eosinophils
4. monocyte/macrophages,
5. natural killer cells,
6. T cells and
7. B cells.

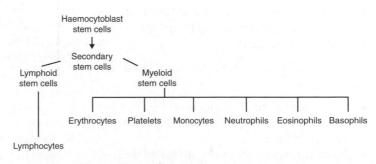

FIGURE 11.2 **Cells of the bone marrow**

Box 11.2 Names of the granulocytes

The different granulocytes (cells with grains) are named due to the different types of stains they take up:

- Neutrophils take up neutral stains.
- Basophils take up basic (alkali) stains.
- Eosinophils take up acidic stains.

Health Connection

Number of WBC in health

The numbers of each type of white blood cell can be indicative of what type of infection is being fought. The normal numbers of WBC per litre of blood in health are

Neutrophils	$2–7.5 \times 10^9$ cells/litre of blood
Eosinophils	$0.04–0.4 \times 10^9$ cells/litre of blood
Basophils	$< 0.1 \times 10^9$ cells/litre of blood
Monocytes	$0.2–0.8 \times 10^9$ cells/litre of blood
Lymphocytes	$1.5–4.0 \times 10^9$ cells/litre of blood

The functions of the immune system

To be able to carry out its function in protecting us from invading organisms the cells of the immune system perform a variety of functions:

- patrolling the body;
- recognising pathogens;
- activating cells of the immune system;
- inactivating or destroying pathogens;
- clearing pathogens.

Each type of white blood cell has a particular *target*:

- Neutrophils and monocytes protect the body against bacteria and small particles of foreign matter.
- Basophils take part in the allergic response.
- Eosinophils kill parasites and are involved in the allergic response.

Health Connection

Number of WBC as indicator of disease

The normal range of concentration of WBC is also indicative of both the health of the individual and whether they are infected. During infection the numbers of WBC should change, generally increase, to counter the infection. At the end of an infection the numbers should return to normal ranges. WBC counts are often taken as part of a profiling of a patient in care to try to find the cause of an illness.

A permanently elevated number of WBC may indicate a chronic infection or an inappropriate growth of cells, a tumour.

A permanently depleted number of WBC may indicate a deficiency disorder.

Health Connection

White blood cell counts, differential diagnosis and disease

Because different types of WBC attack different types of microbes being able to stain WBC and count them allows a differential diagnosis. If, for instance, there is an increase in eosinophils it would indicate a parasitic disease and treatment against parasites could begin. If there is an increase in basophils there may be an allergic reaction and treatment such as antihistamines may be given.

- Natural killer cells can attack virus infected cells.
- Lymphocytes are part of the adaptive or specific immunity. The B cells produce antibodies against foreign organisms and the T cells protect against viruses.

Many of the cells of the immune system are thus **cytotoxic** (cyto means cells and toxic means lethal).

Detection and prevention of infections

How do we detect other organisms while not attacking our own cells? There are two remarkable facets to the immune system that allow it to detect foreign invaders and protect us from repeated infections:

- self and non-self,
- memory.

Self and non-self

The immune system does a remarkable feat. It can distinguish self (that is ourself) from non-self (other organisms). Each one of us has a molecule on the surface of their cell called the MHC (Major Histocompatibility Complex), which is different, either slightly or very, from anybody else's MHC. It is like a personal signature on each of our cells. Our immune system will attack any infecting organisms without our signature on it. Our immune system, particularly the T lymphocytes of our immune system, is trained to **not** attack any cell containing our own MHC. If we did attack our own cells it would cause an **autoimmune disease**.

Health Connection

Types of grafts

Different types of graft or transplants have different prognoses (outcomes). Some are more likely to be accepted by the host than others. In transplant clinics the 'best match' or closest fit is preferred where the graft or transplant tissue is from a donor that has a close genetic or antigenic match to the recipient to avoid host versus graft reactions where the recipient host mounts an attack on the donor graft. The graft tissue can also mount an attack on the host (Graft versus Host – GvH). Both Host v Graft and Graft v Host are called rejection reactions. The main types of grafts are

Autografts – tissue is transplanted from one site to another on the same person, such as in skin grafts after a burn. These are ideal as there is no rejection reaction.

Isografts – tissue grafts from an identical person (identical twin). This graft also has very low probability of a rejection reaction.

Allografts – tissue taken from an unrelated person. This is quite common, but requires a close 'tissue match' to avoid rejection.

Xenografts – tissue taken from a different animal species. These are not successful without immense manipulation of the graft and immune suppression of the host.

The ability of the immune system to recognise non-self can present problems for clinical transplantation.

Memory

The other remarkable feat of the immune system apart from being able to distinguish self from non-self is that it has a *memory*. This means that we seldom become infected with the same pathogen twice. If you have been infected by a particular microbe, the immune system can remember having seen that *particular* microbe before and mounts a quicker and, therefore, more lethal attack on the invader.

As with all memories, it can only remember what it has known. Just like remembering a person, you can only do that if you have already met them or learnt about them. The immune system can learn and remember. The ability to have a memory is exploited in the clinic in a form called vaccination, which will be discussed later.

Health Connection

Transplants

In transplant operations donor tissues (tissue from a donor) are transplanted (grafted) into a recipient whose own tissue or organ is defective. For instance, a kidney donor can donate one of their kidneys to a recipient. The recipient is the host to the donor tissue. The host can see the donated graft as 'foreign', i.e. not of the owner's or host's body, because of the differences between the host's MHC and the MHC of the graft. Rejection can occur where the host's immune cells attack the foreign graft. Immunosuppressive drugs are given to the host to reduce the functioning of the host's immune cells to reduce their ability to attack the graft. Unfortunately, the side effect of the drugs is to make the host more susceptible to infections.

Antigens

What is it that our immune system sees as 'foreign' and non-self and can remember if it encounters it again? The characteristics that elicit these responses from the immune system are called **antigens**. An antigen is any substance (cells, toxin, tissue, protein) that triggers an immune response.

The immune system is trying to prevent the invasion of substances that may cause us harm. Antigens include

- **micro-organisms,**
- **foreign proteins,**
- **nucleic acids,**
- **large carbohydrates,**
- **some lipids,**
- **pollen grains.**

All the cells of our bodies have many surface proteins and proteins combined with sugars or fats. These are our own antigens. We see them as part of our repertoire. If they were put into another person they would be seen as foreign and that person's immune system would attack them. This is the problem in transplants. Antigens, often on the cell surface of other organisms, that are different from ours are seen as foreign and we mount an immune response to them. Our immune system should protect us from foreign invading organisms. It should not attack our own antigens and cause us harm. If it attacks our own antigens we have an autoimmune disease.

Health Connection

Autoimmune diseases

In these diseases the cells of the immune system attack the cells of the body rather than pathogenic microbes. There are a variety of these diseases such as

- **Multiple sclerosis** – the white matter of brain and spinal cord are destroyed.
- **Myasthenia gravis** – where communication between nerves and skeletal muscles is impaired.
- **Juvenile diabetes** – pancreatic beta cells that produce insulin are destroyed.
- **Rheumatoid arthritis** – destroys joints.
- **Systemic lupus erythematosus (SLE)** – affects kidney, heart, lung and skin.
- **Glomerulonephritis** – impairment of renal function.

Immunosuppressive drugs may be given to reduce the effects of the immune system. However, reducing the action of the immune system can result in increased vulnerability to disease.

How do the cells of the immune system recognise and destroy pathogens?

The cells of the immune system recognise the cells of the host as host cells and all other cells as foreign. This is an **innate** ability, a characteristic that does not need to be learnt. There are also cells of the immune system that not only recognise host cells as host, but recognise each type of unique foreign pathogen once they have encountered it. This is an **adaptive** response, an ability that is learnt. Different types of cells of the immune system behave in either an innate or adaptive way and are termed part of the innate or adaptive immune system. It should be remembered, however, that these are merely terms that are used to describe events and that the immune system behaves, ultimately, as one system.

The innate system is also called the second line of defence. The adaptive system is also called the third line of defence.

To understand the difference between the innate and adaptive system imagine entering a country such as the UK or any other country (here the country behaves like your body) with passport control acting as the immune system. Anybody carrying a UK passport is allowed in (i.e. is seen as self or part of your body). All other passports are seen as non-UK (non-self) and are not allowed entry. This is equivalent to the innate system. It sees you and your cells as self and all other cells as non-self. The adaptive system is more sophisticated in its recognition. If it were at passport control it would recognise all UK passports as self, just like the innate system, but it would be able to distinguish each foreign passport, not just see them as non-UK, but, for example, distinguish Peru from Argentina, Mozambique from Zaire, Norway from Iceland. It recognises each individual rather than just as a non-self group. Your innate system sees you as self and all other cells as non-self. Your adaptive system sees all your cells as self and recognises each non-self cell in its own right. Basically, your body is xenophobic!

The innate immune system and response

The innate immune system is responsible for a rapid immune response and helps in the activation of the entire immune system. The innate system recognises all cells that are not host cells as foreign, non-self, and destroys them in a variety of ways. The arsenal of tools that the innate system has at its disposal includes

- phagocytic cells: monocytes and macrophages;
- the inflammatory response: activation of the immune system and destruction of pathogen;
- fever;
- contact mediated cytotoxic cells: granulocytes;
- natural killer cells;
- complement: a series of proteins;
- interferon: a protein.

Phagocytosis

Phagocytosis means **cells** (**cytes**) that **engulf** another cell or particle. In the case of the immune system phagocytic cells engulf and destroy pathogens. The main phagocytic cells are **macrophages**, large cells derived from monocytes, that are large enough to engulf and destroy bacteria. Other phagocytic cells include **neutrophils** and **monocytes**. These two types of cells can roam freely in the blood and lymph to areas of **inflammation**, while macrophages are less mobile lodging themselves in organs and tissues throughout the body.

During phagocytosis the phagocytic cell adheres to the pathogen and then engulfs it. Once ingested the pathogen is digested; i.e. it is broken down in a similar fashion to that of the gastrointestinal tract. This digestion is carried out by the action of enzymes and chemicals contained in the **lysosomes** of the phagocytic cells. These chemicals include powerful oxidants such as hydrogen peroxide (Figure 11.3).

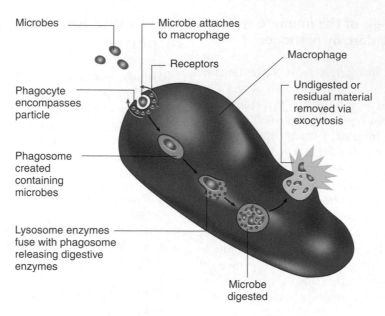

FIGURE 11.3 **Phagocytosis. Here a large cell (macrophage) engulfs and digests a microbe**

Chapter Reference

The GI tract and the digestion of food are discussed in Chapter 9, 'Eating and Drinking' (see p. 241).

Inflammation

We have all suffered the results of inflammation to a part of our body. The signs of inflammation include

- redness,
- swelling,
- heat,
- pain and
- loss of function.

Inflammation is caused in response to tissue injury. When tissue is injured by trauma, extreme temperature leading to hot or cold burns, infection by micro-organisms or chemical damage inflammation may occur. Inflammation, which we may think of as a bad thing, is in fact the immune system at work. Inflammation helps to

- localise the damage,
- stop the spread of any infection to other parts of the body,
- remove the cause of the damage and
- aid wound healing.

It also helps to inform the rest of the immune system of tissue damage and recruit help to prevent infection.

Tissue damage elicits an **inflammatory response** (Figure 11.4) in an attempt to localise the damage and destroy any incoming material. When tissue is damaged chemicals from the damaged tissue leak out into the surrounding tissues and blood. These chemicals include **prostaglandins** that can cause pain. Prostaglandins are chemicals that are released from damaged cells. They help to attract the immune system to the area of damage. White blood cells, particularly basophils and monocytes, are then attracted to the area of damage. Basophils release inflammatory chemicals such as **histamine** that leads to **vasodilation** (increased diameter) of blood vessels and increased blood flow to the area. This results in the redness and heat associated with inflammation. The chemicals allow the blood vessels to

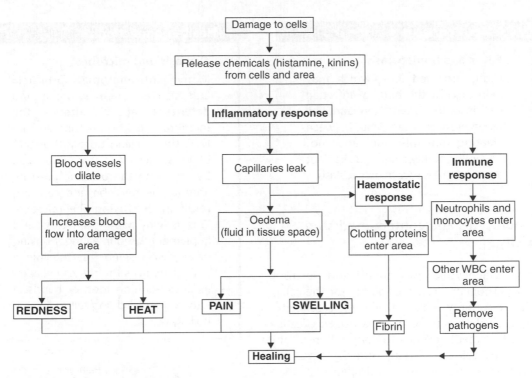

FIGURE 11.4 **Inflammatory response**

become more 'leaky' allowing cells and plasma to pass from the blood across the vessel walls to the area of tissue damage. Thus WBC and immune defence chemicals from the blood can enter the tissue space. Pain is caused due to the inflammatory chemicals and to tissues swelling (dilation) which puts pressure on nearby nerves. The inflammatory chemicals also attract other WBC such as neutrophils and monocytes to the area of inflammation. These start to remove microorganisms by phagocytosis or by de-granulation (discussed below). Macrophages clear the debris through phagocytosis. Further swelling caused by **pus**, a mixture of dead WBC, cell debris and dead micro-organisms also occurs.

Fever

As with inflammation, fever has a useful role in the battle against infection. It is characterised by an abnormally high temperature, which may result in sweating and fluid loss. The hypothalamus is the control area of the brain for temperature regulation. It can be reset by **pyrogens**, chemicals secreted by WBC. High temperatures inhibit the release of iron and zinc from the liver and spleen. These metals are essential for bacterial growth. Without their availability, bacterial growth is inhibited. Fever also increases the speed of tissue repair.

Health Connection

Aspirin
Aspirin is thought to inhibit prostaglandin actions. This results in the reduction of swelling and of pain.

Chapter Reference
Fluid regulation is discussed in Chapter 9, 'Eating and Drinking' (see p. 241). Temperature regulation is discussed in Chapter 5, 'Controlling and Repairing' (see p. 142).

Granulocytes and contact-mediated toxicity

While phagocytosis can engulf and destroy many pathogens some are too big for the cells of the immune system. Granulocytic cells (cells with granules) can destroy pathogenic cells by contact-mediated cytotoxicity where they kill (or are toxic or lethal towards) a pathogen. In this case, when a pathogen is recognised by a granulocyte of the immune system the granulocyte adheres to the pathogen and releases an array of chemicals (granules) from its lysosomes. These chemicals include oxidative chemicals such as hydrogen peroxide mentioned above. The chemicals pierce the cell membrane of the pathogen. This results in the lysis (the swelling up of a cell and its eruption) of the pathogen. It happens because once the membrane is destroyed other substances such as ions and water can enter freely. The pathogen thus swells up and explodes! Other WBC such as macrophages will then ingest the debris and clear the area (Figure 11.5).

Natural killer (NK) cells

These cells are activated by a chemical called interferon. They recognise our own MHC molecules. When they don't see our MHC they bind to the 'foreign' cell and release chemicals such as **perforin** that perforates the membrane of the pathogen and causes lysis. Natural killer cells also have a role in tumour surveillance. When

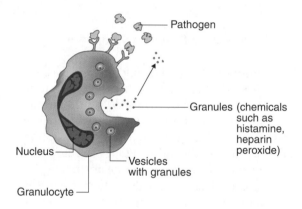

FIGURE 11.5 **Granulocytes and de-granulation**

tumours grow they may have altered proteins on their cell surface, including the alteration of the MHC molecule. They will thus be recognised as 'foreign' and destroyed by NK cells.

Complement

This is a series of chemicals that are released in response to B cell activation (discussed below). Like contact-mediated cytotoxicity, it results in the piercing of the membrane of the pathogen and thus the lysis of the cells as well as inflammation and **chemotaxis** (the chemical attraction of cells such as WBC to the area of infection).

The innate immune system (also known as the second line of defence) has, as stated, this huge arsenal of tools – both cellular and chemical – to destroy pathogens and prevent the spread of infection. It responds to any incoming invader. It cannot aid immunity, where one does not suffer twice from the same infection, nor can it fight virus infected cells. Those are the roles of the adaptive system discussed next.

Complement consists of a group of at least 20 proteins that are in the plasma of the blood (plasma proteins). They are in a 'silent' inactive state. They are activated when they encounter anything foreign and attach to cells (complement fixation). They then damage foreign cell surfaces which can result in the foreign cell lysing.

Other properties of some of the complement proteins include

- **vasodilators** – making blood vessels larger in diameter;
- **chemotaxis** – chemical attraction to a target area;
- **opsonization** – marking a target cell for destruction.

Box 11.3 Summary – Innate system

Our bodies have an innate system to rid us of pathogens.

The innate system has a number of mechanisms to do this. These include

- inflammatory response,
- fever,
- phagocytic cells,
- cytotoxic cells,
- NK cells,
- chemicals:
  - complement,
  - interferon.

Interferon

This is a protein that is secreted from virus-infected cells. It can bind to healthy cell surfaces to inhibit viruses from binding.

The adaptive immune system and response

The **adaptive** (or **specific**) immune system (also called the third line of defence) consists of two types of **lymphocytes** (cells of the lymph) and their effect on pathogens are

1. **B lymphocyte** or B cells, which consist of two types:
   (i) plasma cells, which synthesise antibody and
   (ii) memory B cells.
2. **T lymphocytes** or T cells, which consist of four types:
   (i)   cytotoxic T cells, which destroy pathogens;
   (ii) helper T cells, which activate the immune system;
   (iii) suppressor T cells, which suppress the immune system at the end of a response when the pathogen is no longer a threat and
   (iv) memory T cells.

Both B and T lymphocytes originate, as do all WBC or leucocytes, in the bone marrow. The B lymphocytes then mature in the blood and spleen. The T lymphocytes mature in the **thymus gland**. They both then enter the lymph nodes and other lymph tissues.

The type of immune response that each cell has is classified as

B lymphocytes

Humoral (antibody-mediated) immunity

- carried out by the B lymphocytes,
- antibody-mediated immunity,
- cells produce chemicals for defence.

T lymphocytes

Cellular immunity

- carried out by the T lymphoctyes,
- cell-mediated immunity,
- cells target virus infected cells.

Both types of lymphocytes are *adaptive* – they learn and are specific. While the innate immune system recognises non-self, each cell of the adaptive immune system recognises a specific foreign **antigen** (Ag) on the surface of pathogens. This recognition is called antigen recognition. We are capable of recognising 10^8 different antigens, that is 100,000,000 (one hundred million) different antigens. There are, thus, 10^8 different B lymphocytes or T lymphocytes each with its particular recognition *target*.

Once a single B or T lymphocyte has recognised its particular target antigen it will divide many times (**clonal expansion**) to form many B or T lymphocytes each with the same specificity for a *single* antigen type. These will then go on to react with the antigen in a number of ways. The B or T lymphocyte will also leave behind **memory** B or T cells. Any subsequent exposure to that particular antigen will result in a much more rapid and effective attack. So

effective, in fact, that you may not be aware of encountering the antigen again.

When a particular B lymphocyte recognises the antigen for which it has a specificity, it binds to it. The part of the B lymphocyte that has the specific binding region for an antigen is called an **antibody** (Ab). Once bound the B lymphocyte undergoes clonal expansion. A large number of B lymphocytes are produced, each a clone of the original one and each possessing the same antibody specific to that particular antigen. For instance, if antigen X comes along, then the B lymphocyte with the antibody X (anti X antigen) binds, but a B lymphocyte with antibody Z or Y or W will not bind. The large numbers of specific B lymphocytes produced are in three main types:

- B lymphoblasts,
- plasma cells and
- memory B cells.

The plasma cells secrete antibodies (also called **immunoglobulins** – globular shaped proteins of the immune system). The antibodies they secrete are of the same shape and specificity as the surface antibodies on the original B lymphocyte from which they are derived.

Antibodies inactivate antigens in a number of ways (Figure 11.6):

- neutralise toxins released by microbes;
- label pathogens for destruction;
- agglutination: this clumps pathogens together and makes them easy to attack;
- precipitation: by binding and clumping together;
- complement fixation: activate the complement cascade of proteins thereby enhancing inflammation and phagocytosis.

The plasma cells are thus part of the immune response to antigen.

The memory cells have the same surface antibody as the original B lymphocyte. They can circulate in the blood for years and retain the ability to respond in future to the same antigen. If the same pathogen with the same antigen that has been previously encountered and eliminated reenters our bodies instead of just

---

Box 11.4 Summary – B lymphocytes

- B lymphocytes with specific receptors bind to a specific antigen.
- The binding event activates the lymphocyte to undergo clonal selection.
- A large number of clones are produced (primary humoral response).
- Most B cells become **plasma cells**:
  - produce antibodies to destroy antigens,
  - activity lasts for four or five days.
- Some B cells become long-lived memory cells (secondary humoral response).

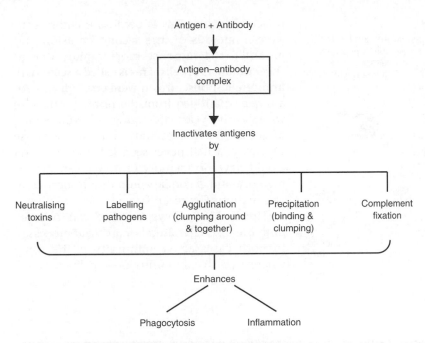

FIGURE 11.6 **Action of antibodies on antigens**

one B lymphocyte with a particular antibody on its surface being present, there are *many* memory B cells with that particular antibody on its surface to the particular antigen that first elicited a response. The pathogen is thus recognised and eliminated faster the second time.

It would seem logical to have lots of each type of B lymphocyte to speed up recognition and binding of antigen. However, given that we can recognise 10^8 different antigens we could not have many of each type of B lymphocyte circulating in our blood. Blood cells are mainly red blood cells for carrying oxygen. We need oxygen every minute. Hopefully we do not encounter pathogens every minute and certainly not 10^8 pathogens in our lifetime. It is not necessary for our blood to have many of each type of B lymphocyte. If we did our blood would become too viscous to flow and it could not carry all the other proteins and chemicals in the plasma as well as the red blood cells. Memory B lymphocytes are therefore expanded only in response to need. We have a large range of B lymphocytes, but not large numbers of each B lymphocyte and only expand the

numbers of a particular B lymphocyte in response to a particular infection.

Having encountered the pathogen the first time and having had the infection we have had the *primary* immune response. If we encounter the pathogen again we mount a rapid and effective *secondary* (exposure) immune response.

Having many memory B lymphocytes in our circulation we have become potentially immune to attack from the same pathogen. This is called **acquired immunity**. We are now **immune** to a particular pathogen. In this case it is acquired naturally, by reacting to the infection. We can exploit this in vaccination.

In the primary response very few B cells exist with the antibody that binds to the invading antigen. When it does bind it causes many identical cells to be made, a clone, all with the same antibody – clonal expansion (Figure 11.7). These attack the antigen. When the infection is over, some of the clonal cells remain as a memory. If the same antigen is encountered a faster secondary response will be mounted due to the presence of more B cells with the appropriate antibody. The response will be the same, but much faster.

If, in an experimental situation, you were injected with an antigen A on day 0 you would take about two weeks (14 days) to mount a strong immune response and to eliminate the antigen. This is a primary immune response. If you were challenged with the same antigen A again (injected again) five weeks or five years later, you would mount such a rapid immune response in two to four days rather than weeks that you may not even notice having had that

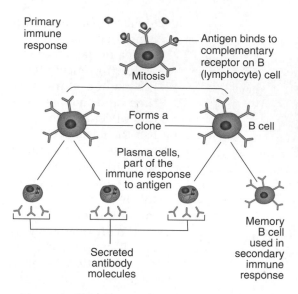

Primary immune response

Antigen binds to complementary receptor on B (lymphocyte) cell

Mitosis

Forms a clone

B cell

Plasma cells, part of the immune response to antigen

Secreted antibody molecules

Memory B cell used in secondary immune response

FIGURE 11.7 **Clonal expansion**

infection again. This is because memory cells were numerous on the second occasion and mounted the response more rapidly due to sheer numbers of cells. This is called a secondary immune response. If you were challenged with a different antigen from the primary one, five weeks or five years later, antigen B, you would, of course, have a primary immune response to it as you had never seen it before and you would have no memory of it. We can exploit memory and secondary immune responses in vaccination (Figure 11.8).

Figure 11.9 shows that we can become immune through natural or artificial processes. In both cases active immunity is life long, whereas passive immunity is short-lived.

Health Connection

Vaccination

This is the clinical **exploitation** of **acquired immunity**. There are various types of vaccination:

Naturally acquired

Active – where we get the infection and respond to it by making memory cells that will be present should we ever get the same infection again, as above.

Passive – through mother to foetus where some types of immunoglobulin can pass though the placenta to give some protection to the foetus or through the mother's milk, again passing some immunoglobulins from mother to baby. In both cases this is where we receive the antibodies without getting the disease. This is a short-lived protection as the source of the antibodies, B cells, are not actively making antibody. The antibody protein gradually wears out and new protein cannot be made due to the lack of activated B lymphocytes.

Artificially acquired

Active – acquired through immunisation or vaccination. This is where a version of the infection is given, but the pathogen has been attenuated (altered) so as not to cause disease. The B lymphocyte with the specific antibody recognises it and is activated, mounts an attack and leaves behind memory B cells. We are now 'primed' as we have had the primary immune response. If we encounter the live and active pathogen we are now able to mount a secondary immune response, rapidly and effectively.

Passive – where we receive the antibodies by injection without getting the disease. This is a short-lived protection as the source of the antibodies, B cells, are not actively making antibody. The antibody protein gradually wears out and new protein cannot be made due to the lack of activated B lymphocytes.

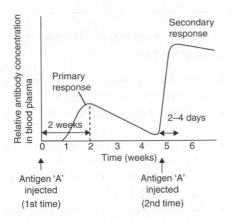

FIGURE 11.8 **Primary and secondary immune response**

We have one big pathogenic problem: viruses. When a virus is in the general circulation it can be attacked by a number of different leucocytes.

However, viruses are primed to bind onto host cells and inject their genetic material into the host cell, getting the host to make new viruses, as described above, like a sperm cell binding to an egg cell and injecting its genetic material.

Chapter Reference

Reproduction is discussed in Chapter 3, 'Growing and Developing' (see p. 64).

Box 11.5 Summary – T lymphocytes

- Antigens must be presented by macrophages to an immunocompetent T cell (antigen presentation).
- T cells must recognise non-self and self (double recognition).
- After antigen binding, clones form as with B cells, but different classes of cells are produced.
- **Cytotoxic T cells**
  - specialise in killing infected cells,
  - insert a toxic chemical (perforin).
- **Helper T cells**
  - recruit other cells to fight the invaders,
  - interact directly with B cells.
- **Suppressor T cells**
  - release chemicals to suppress the activity of T and B cells,
  - stop the immune response to prevent uncontrolled activity.
- A few members of each clone are memory cells.

Once the virus has 'infected' a host cell it is inside that cell. Our immune system can recognise foreign cells, but should not recognise our own cells. The virus is now inside a cell with our own MHC on it and should be immune to attack (Figure 11.10).

A virus cannot replicate itself and must use the replicative machinery of the host to reproduce itself. To do that it must 'infect' the host. It first adsorbs (sticks) to the host then injects its genetic material into the host. The host then replicates the viral genetic material and makes the viral proteins that form the outer coat of the virus and then release the fully assembled virus which can then go on to infect more nearby host cells.

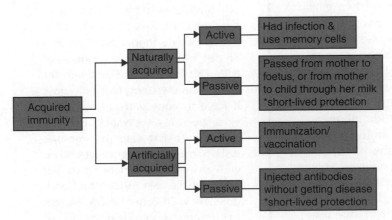

FIGURE 11.9 **Acquired immunity**

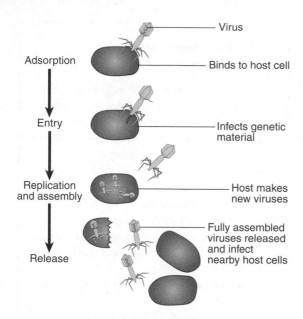

Virus

Adsorption

Binds to host cell

Entry

Infects genetic
material

Replication
and assembly

Host makes
new viruses

Release

Fully assembled
viruses released
and infect
nearby host cells

FIGURE 11.10 **Viral infection (this is not to scale –
viruses are smaller than eukaryotic human cells)**

Box 11.6 Summary – B and T lymphocytes

- The innate system can recognise a pathogen and inactivate it.
- It is not specific and does not have memory.
- T and B lymphocytes are part of the adaptive immune system.
- They are highly specific for their particular pathogen.
- They remember if they have seen that pathogen before as the first encounter leads to a clonal expansion of that particular T or B lymphocyte.

T lymphocytes come in a variety of forms. They all have a molecule on their surface that recognises our own MHC molecule. If they see our MHC they do not attack. Cytotoxic T lymphocyte (Tc) will attack our own cells if they see our own MHC in conjunction with viral proteins. Each Tc cell has an antigen recognition molecule specific for a particular antigen, similar to B lymphocytes. Once a Tc lymphocyte recognises and binds to a viral infected cell it undergoes clonal expansion in the same way as B lymphocytes. It then goes on to attack and destroy body cells with the virus in it and leave behind memory T lymphocytes to prevent a secondary infection (Figure 11.11).

The other types of T lymphocytes Helper (Th) and Suppressor (Ts) aid the function of the entire immune system both specific and innate. The Th lymphocytes send out chemical signals such as cytokines to stimulate the activity of NK cells, B lymphocytes and innate cells. They are involved in helping innate cells to present antigen to other leucocytes to increase the immune response. Ts cells slow down the T and B lymphocyte activity once the pathogen has been removed.

Health Connection

HIV

Viruses attack cells for which they have an entry point. Each virus has a specific protein 'key' that binds to a receptor on a host cell akin to having a key for a lock. Once attached, they inject their genetic material and take over the host cell. HIV happens to have a key to a human cell, a Th cell. It attaches to this cell and takes over the machinery of the Th cell so that is can no longer function as a Th cell, but merely as a producer of HIV. This is an added problem for the immune system. Not only does it have to cope with an incoming virus, but the virus knocks out one of the cells that help the immune system to function. Hence we end up with an immunodeficiency disorder, Acquired (i.e. not Innate) Immuno-deficiency Disorder, AIDS, where the immune system is depressed or not fully functional.

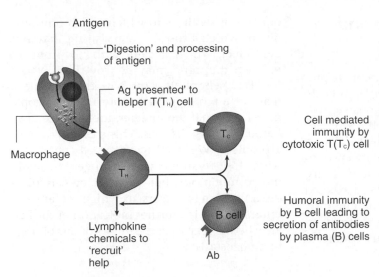

Antigen

'Digestion' and processing of antigen

Ag 'presented' to helper T(T$_H$) cell

Macrophage

Cell mediated immunity by cytotoxic T(T$_c$) cell

T$_c$

T$_H$

Humoral immunity by B cell leading to secretion of antibodies by plasma (B) cells

B cell

Lymphokine chemicals to 'recruit' help

Ab

FIGURE 11.11 **Antigen presentation and Th interactions**

Allergies and hypersensitivity

Not all foreign molecules are antigenic. All do not elicit an immune response. Many small molecules (called **haptens** or incomplete antigens) are not antigenic. If they combine with our own proteins the immune system may recognise and respond to this protein–hapten combination and mount a response. This can cause an inappropriate response to substances that are not pathogenic.

Our immune system can sometimes malfunction, as can any organ in our body. Autoimmune diseases discussed above are one such malfunction. Allergies where there is an inappropriate immune response to a hapten or allergen that is not dangerous, is another such malfunction. There are various types of **allergies** all resulting in immune responses. Two such allergic reactions are

- **Immediate hypersensitivity**
- triggered by release of histamine from a particular antibody, IgE binding to mast cells (similar to basophils);
- reactions begin within seconds of contact with allergen;
- anaphylactic shock – dangerous, systemic response.
- **Delayed hypersensitivity**
  - triggered by the release of lymphokine chemicals from activated helper T cells;
  - symptoms usually appear one to three days after contact with an antigen.

Changes during lifespan and lifestyle

During foetal development the foetus is protected from infection via the placenta. At birth, while the immune system is responsive, it is naïve, having never encountered the environment in which the newborn finds itself. Each encounter of antigen is thus a primary encounter and the newborn is susceptible to each disease afresh. As we develop we have been exposed to many antigens and have acquired immunity. In old age our immune system decreases in its responsiveness and we become susceptible to disease.

At birth the lymphoid organs are poorly developed and only the thymus and spleen are functioning fully. A newborn has no functioning lymphocytes at birth; only passive immunity from the mother. This immunity has been through the placenta and continues very briefly in the first milk that the mother produces. Gradually the newborn manufactures its own lymphocytes and antibodies.

The song 'Everywhere you go, you always take the weather with you' could be substituted for 'Everywhere you go, you always take your germs with you!' When we travel abroad we are often vaccinated against the diseases prevalent in the country we are visiting to protect ourselves against infection. What we forget is that we are taking the diseases to which we have acquired an immunity with us. It is estimated that more 'native Americans' died from the diseases brought into America by the various groups that went to live there such as the Dutch, Norwegian, Swedes, Poles, Spanish and British than by warfare. It must be remembered that more of us have died due to microbial infection than by war (see Chapter 13, 'Dying', for the numbers). When we travel we take our 'germs' with us to which we are immune but to which those we are visiting may not be. Travel, which is said, with no proof, to broaden the mind, may destroy those whom we visit. Xenophobia, the hatred of outsiders, may have a biological history in that people have learnt that the stranger, though nice, may harbour deadly diseases. This presents us with a problem. We need to outbreed (not breed with close relatives) with strangers to avoid inbred mutations, but we must be careful of diseases from strangers to which we are not immune. This is a further indication of the balance between costs and benefits of our biology in homeostasis.

Conclusion: Cleansing and dressing

Being able to be clean is not just a pleasure, but it also helps to prevent infection. Not being able to cleanse oneself or one's environment (clothing and home) can lead to feeling uncared for and isolated. We need to live in the external environment which provides all our nutrients, but it also contains other organisms that can infect us and be pathogenic. We have an immune system that cleanses our bodies of these infections. However, the microbes to which we are trying to become immune can mutate and become resistant. Due to their short lifecycles they change faster than we can produce antibodies (or antibiotics) and are therefore highly adaptable organisms. For this reason they are at the top of the food chain and can out-compete us. Basic hygiene, in the form of clean hands, clothing and dressing help to reduce the transmission of infections and reduce the chances of our cells becoming lunch on another species' dining table!

Chapter Summary

▶ We are not the only species on this planet.

▶ The species with the largest number of members are micro-organisms.

▶ Many micro-organisms (microbes) have no direct impact on our internal environment.

▶ Some are commensal and some pathogenic.

▶ We have lines of defences to keep invading pathogens out.

▶ If barriers are breached the immune system patrols and recruits cells to help in eliminating any pathogenic organism.

▶ The immune system can recognise self from non-self and some parts of the immune system has a memory.

▶ We are thus able to maintain the integrity of our bodies separating self from non-self.

▶ We can also remember previous infections and mount a more rapid response (secondary).

▶ A memory can be exploited in the manufacture of vaccines.

▶ The innate system is a rapid response system.

▶ The adaptive system is more specific and has a memory of its encounters.

▶ Viruses present particular problems to our immune system.

▶ T lymphocytes are especially adapted to recognise virally infected cells.

Healing is a matter of time, but it is sometimes also a matter of opportunity.

Hippocrates (450–380 BCE), father of modern medicine and the Hippocratic Oath all doctors swear at graduation

Chapter Outline

Introduction: Sleeping and healing as activities of daily living

Most of us have suffered sleepless nights, suffering from some form of *insomnia*, the inability to sleep. It upsets and disturbs our normal routines. We may be kept awake by worry, illness or excitement. All of us have different abilities to sleep. Some of us can sleep in noisy environments; some of us need complete quiet. We also need slightly different amounts of sleep from one another and during our lifespan, but we all crave a 'good night's sleep' if we haven't had one and feel that it has restorative values. We even talk about 'getting our beauty sleep' which implies that if we don't sleep enough we get baggy eyed and unattractive.

We humans sleep one-third of our lives; that is, in each 24-hour day we sleep, on average, one-third of the day, 8 hours. Why? What is the purpose of sleep? We know that *sleep deprivation*, lack of sleep, can have detrimental effects on **cognitive functioning**, our brain's ability to decipher complex ideas. We know that some animals sleep more or less than we do. But we know very little of the *purpose* of sleep. But being deprived of this ADL can make us feel very tetchy and irritable. Even during sleep many of our living processes are continuing.

This chapter looks at what sleep is and why we may need it. It then looks at pain, one of the most important symptoms in health.

The environment

The external environment

Time is a strange concept which many of us find difficult to understand. We feel that there is some external, objective time, which we can measure. These times include the spin of the Earth around its axis, which we call a day, and the orbit of the Earth around the Sun, which we call a year. All other times that we use, months, weeks, hours, minutes and seconds are our inventions.

We are also aware of seasonal changes from the summer to winter. Those of us in equatorial regions on the Earth will not notice much change in daylight, but those of us in Northern or Southern hemispheres will notice the long days of what we call summer and the short days of what we call winter. These external changes affect our internal environment.

We may also be aware of time in relation to motion – the physics of time set by the universe.

For most of us we experience time as part of our lifespan and our daily activities: what we have done in the space between waking and sleeping and how we have slept.

The internal environment

Time has a great influence on our lives. Our metabolism and rates of growth change during the day and during our lifespan. There may be central mechanisms measuring the day and the year for us. Just as hormone levels are known to change throughout the year in certain animals to bring them into the breeding season at the correct time for the supply of food and mates to be available, so our days are measured out for us. We too have hormone changes during the day and during our lives bringing on, for instance, puberty or increasing times of growth. Hormonal release is controlled by central mechanisms in the nervous system.

There appears to be a rhythm to life from the daily rhythm to that of one's lifespan. How do cells know time? How do we measure our lives? How do we know when to grow, rest, repair, age and die? Can we prevent some of these processes or reduce their effect on us? Does sleep anaesthetise us from carrying out all the living processes all the time? Is sleep there to remove us from pain and allow our bodies to rest, recuperate and regenerate?

Our bodies, our tissues and our cells keep the cycle of time dictated by that of our planet and its orbit around a star. If we are removed from any sense of day and night and are allowed to 'free-run' in an experimental situation, we find that our bodies run on a 25-hour cycle. Very soon we become 'out of sync' with those not in this situation. We have external cues called **zeitgebers** that re-set our internal clock so that our bodies are entrained to a 24-hour cycle rather than the 25-hour cycle we would run in without these cues.

The *rhythms* that cells go through vary due to demand for growth and new cells to replace old cells, the nutrients available for repair and growth and the metabolic rate of the cell which varies depending on the tissue and activity of the tissue during the day or lifespan. Sleep may reflect the needs of the individual cells' variations in activities. Hibernating animals slow their metabolic rates.

Health Connection

Routines

The activities of the medical ward may be 'out of sync' with that of the patient's daily activities and routines. The ward runs on the routine and convenience of the hospital rather than each individual patient. This can also be seen in residential homes. Cues such as hunger of the patient or client may be different from that of the ward or home.

Sleeping and dreaming

What is sleep?

We are all aware of what it is to sleep, to feel drowsy, to drop off to sleep. Sleep seems to be a time when our consciousness is lessened, when we are not as aware of our surroundings as when awake. During sleep, however, many of the biological processes that occur whilst awake continue such as respiration, cardiac cycle, transport of nutrients to cells, removal of waste from cells and cell metabolism. In fact cell metabolism, the chemical activities of the cells, must continue; if it stops the cell dies. During sleep, however, the *rate* (speed or frequency) of metabolism and therefore of supply and removal of products to and from cells may be reduced.

Sleep, therefore, seems to involve reduction in

- conscious arousal,
- metabolic rate,
- alertness.

Chapter Reference

Hormones and nervous system are discussed in Chapter 4, 'Communicating' (see p. 102). Growth and puberty are discussed in Chapter 3, 'Growing and Developing' (see p. 64).

The activity of sleep is brought about by changes in brain activity.

A group of cells in an area of the brain stem called the **reticular formation** are responsible for levels of arousal. These areas in the brain stem help to arouse us or depress our arousal.

These areas are, in turn, under the control of higher centres in the brain. In the **hypothalamus** is an area called the **suprachiasmatic nuclei**, a group of cells that appear to be responsible for our *daily cycle of wakefulness* and *sleep*. The rhythm is called the **circadian rhythm**. This rhythm sets up a cycle that *approximates* day length. As mentioned above, in experiments where the subject is not aware of changes in daylight and is kept in a constant light with no outside references to time, eating, drinking and eliminating freely, the body cycle is 25 hours rather than 24 hours.

Health Connection

Brain stem activity

Activity or arousal of the brain stem is measured in coma and death. Interestingly in much poetry and philosophy sleep is compared to death, a preparation for it or a 'mini death'.

What happens during sleep?

Generally sleep is thought of as a time of *muscle relaxation* and lessened *awareness* of external activity.

There are two main stages to sleep:

- **non-REM** and
- **REM.**

REM refers to 'rapid eye movement'.

Non-REM sleep

During non-REM sleep the heart rate and blood pressure fall. Four stages of non-REM sleep can be described and numbered in Roman numerals from I to IV.

We move rapidly from stage I through II, III and into IV, which is deep sleep and then back through to stage I in 90–100 minute cycles through the night.

We need less stage IV sleep as we grow older, the stage where talking, sleepwalking and nightmares may occur.

REM sleep

REM sleep occurs at intervals throughout the night interspersing with non-REM sleep cycles. During REM sleep we have, as defined, rapid eye movement. This is also the time when dreaming occurs. It is thought that, because of this dreaming cycle, muscle relaxation is at its most pronounced preventing us from re-enacting our dreams. There is an increase in blood pressure, pulse and breathing. The length of each cycle of REM sleep increases during the night.

Transition between REM and non-REM sleep is often accompanied by changes in body position and movement and electrical activity of the brain. Recordings of electrical activity in the brain can be taken by **EEG** (electroencephalogram) and matched to REM or non-REM.

The effect of lack of sleep

Sleep deprivation, lack of sleep, can lead to loss of concentration, irritability, drowsiness and sluggishness. Long-term sleep deprivation was thought to have serious health consequences; however, in experiments, it appears that subjects recover very quickly. Just as humans cannot go more than a few days without water, most people cannot manage to remain awake for more than a couple of days.

Sleep and car traffic accidents

The amount of traffic on the road tends to be lowest from 22.00 at night through to 08.00. Sleep-related car traffic accidents comprise up to a quarter of road traffic accidents and tend to be highest from 01.00 to 08.00. This obviously has an effect on staffing levels in the accident and emergency departments of hospitals.

Shift work

Many people do not work regular '9 to 5' jobs; they work in shifts, some long days, some short days or night shifts. When taking a history of a patient this is one health ADL that is asked. Shift working affects many other ADL such as sleeping, eating and eliminating. Wakefulness is one of the primary problems with shift working. Altering patterns of sleeping around shifts can have debilitating effects.

The function of sleep

Without sleep we can suffer, but we do not really know what the function is of sleep or of dreams. Many theories have been put forward.

The evolutionary explanation is that we humans do not have very good night senses, relying heavily on *vision* which is impaired in the dark. We are not, therefore, good night hunters, unlike some animals, but we are good night prey and are vulnerable to animals suited to night time activity. Sleep may encourage removal from vulnerable areas of the environment. Some mammals *hibernate* for long periods during unfavourable conditions.

Another reason proposed for sleep is to give the body a period of time for rest and *repair*. During activity we impose damage on our tissues and may suffer from low levels of pain. Sleep allows us to rest the affected areas and to be less aware of pain and for healing processes to occur.

Finally, sleep may not only have a restorative function, but also allow the brain to re-programme, assimilating *memories* and experiences. It may, therefore, be good for our mental health.

Sleep amount

How much sleep we need is also contentious. Evidence suggests that 7–8 hours per 24 hours is

Sleep deprivation

In certain circumstances we are prevented from sleeping and suffer sleep deprivation, being deprived of sufficient sleep. Within a few days we have severe physical and mental health problems. If sleep deprivation can have such severe effects in such a short time it points to the importance of sleep. We can 'make up' for lost sleep in quite a short time.

the average need. Studies suggest that those who sleep less than 4 hours or more than 9 hours per 24 hours have an increased chance of mortality from cancer, stroke or coronary artery diseases, but these studies may not be conclusive.

Changes during lifespan

The amount of sleep needed alters during our lifespan as does our style of sleeping. The sleep pattern of the foetus and newborn is about 18 hours in 24, while 6-year-olds sleep about 10 hours per night. Youths tend to sleep in a clear pattern between sleep and waking, while the elderly may break up this pattern and have many daytime naps and frequent night-time awakenings.

The amount of REM sleep also alters with newborns having the highest amount, about 50% of sleep time, which decreases during development. This suggests that REM sleep may have some function for the development of central nervous system (brain and spinal cord).

Children need more sleep per day in order to develop and function properly: up to 18 hours for newborn babies, with a declining rate as a child ages. A newborn baby spends almost 9 hours a day in REM sleep. By the age of 5 or so, only slightly over 2 hours is spent in REM (Table 12.1).

Dreams

During the REM phase of sleep if a person is woken they often report of having dreams. Some people also recall dreams from non-REM sleep. Dreams are usually visual so one would expect eye movement. People born blind tend to have auditory dreams rather than visual ones and do not show REM.

What are the functions of dreams? They may just be our usual conscious activity, but more jumbled due to the brain's altered electrical activity during sleep. They may be a way of cataloguing the day's events and laying some

> ### Health Connection
>
> #### Insomnia
> Insomnia is the subjective feeling of not being able to have a satisfying night's sleep. It can result in poor ability to concentrate, irritability, fatigue and moodiness. Causes of insomnia range from pain, changes in circadian rhythm due to altering life or work patterns (shifts), psychiatric disturbances, alcohol abuse and the side effect of some medications. However, we are told we need eight hours sleep per night and this may not be true. We can become stressed about not sleeping this eight hours and this may keep us awake. One treatment may be to accept sleeping less or only the amount needed by the individual.

down into our memories, or they may be a way of clearing them out from our memories. They may be important or totally random. It is hard to investigate them as one would have to have a group that dreams and a group that does not dream and compare physiological states of each group. The fact that we do not always remember dreaming does not mean that we have not dreamt, so the experiment would be hard to conduct. There are people that have survived appalling circumstances who suppress dreaming, presumably from fear of reminiscing on the events. They have completely normal lives otherwise, so dreaming may not be needed. However, many of us like to dream and to daydream! Or as the poet and playwright Shakespeare puts it, longing 'to sleep perchance to dream'.

Table 12.1 Amount of sleep needed during changes in lifespan

Age and condition	Average amount of sleep per day
Newborn	up to 18 hours
1–12 months	14–18 hours
1–3 years	12–15 hours
3–5 years	11–13 hours
5–12 years	9–11 hours
Adolescents	9–10 hours
Adults, including elderly	7–8(+) hours
Pregnant women	8(+) hours

Pain

One function of sleep may be for us to repair ourselves from tissue damage. Tissue damage tends to cause us pain. Pain is both a *sensation* and an *emotion*.

It is a sensation because there is a sensory aspect to it: physiological processes occur and our brain detects the event.

It is an emotion as we each have a different response to the same stimulus; an individual perception of how we feel.

Chapter Reference

The nervous system is discussed in Chapter 4, 'Communicating' (see p. 102).

The value of pain

Pain *warns* us that we have done *damage* to our tissues. Without the sensation we could continue damaging our tissue and may cause destruction of vital functions. There are people who do not have pain sensations and are constantly breaking bones and burning themselves without noticing. Pain notifies us of the damage and encourages us to *rest* the affected area, if possible, until it is healed.

Components of pain

Pain has many components.

The **descriptive** components of pain are

- sensory,
- affective,
- autonomic,
- motor.

The sensory is the sensation that you are feeling.

The affective is how it makes you feel.

The autonomic is how your internal mechanisms, your body, reacts to it.

The motor component is how you move to avoid the pain.

The **time components** of pain are

- acute,
- chronic.

Acute pain is sudden and may not last long. It is associated with trauma and is often described as sharp.

Chronic pain tends to be a pain that has continued for more than six months and is often described as dull.

Both can be very painful.

The **location component** is where the pain is felt. Pain can be felt as

- superficial,
- deep,
- visceral,
- referred.

Superficial pain is pain on the surface of the body and does not mean pain that is slight. Superficial pain can be extreme caused, for example, by burns on the skin or tears in the skin. The skin has many touch and temperature receptors and is very sensitive to both of these sensations.

Deep pain tends to be pain felt in the muscles, tendons and bones such as in strain, breaks and in bone cancers.

Visceral pain is pain felt in internal organs.

Referred pain is usually due to how tissues move during development. A pain felt in the left armpit, for example, is associated with a heart problem. This is because the heart developed near the left armpit in the foetus and during foetal development it moves towards the centre of the chest bringing its nerve supply with it. This means that when the heart is hurting the pain may be felt all along the nerve pathways into the left armpit. There are other anatomical links such as these formed during foetal development.

Health Connection

Observing pain

It is very hard to decide who has a pain, how much pain they have and how serious may be the cause of their pain. This makes assessing patients very hard. It is easy to blame medical staff, but it is difficult to know another's pain. For example if two patients arrive both with stomach aches, only a history and some investigations can distinguish acute appendicitis from constipation and both of them could be in the same amount of pain while one cause is life threatening and needs urgent treatment.

Puzzles of pain

Sometimes pain is felt when there should not be any, such as a pain in an amputated limb that is no longer there. This may also be due to referred pain as the nerve pathway in the remains of the limb may be present, but it cannot always be explained in this manner.

Sometimes pain should be felt and it isn't, such as when a soldier is shot in the leg and manages to suppress the pain to get off the battle field. The ability to suppress pain suggests that it is not only a *sensation*, but also an *emotion* so that higher brain functions can override it.

Measurement of pain

Can an emotion be measured? If you say you are happy how can we measure it? Sensations can be measured in the amount given, but if there is an emotive element to pain, how much is *perceived* will vary from person to person for the same amount given.

As mentioned above there are *subjective*, internal descriptive components of pain. We would like an *external*, *objective* measure. Physiologically, looking at the biological workings of pain detection, we all operate at the same levels for stimuli for the *thresholds* at which we detect a stimulus. However, we have different *tolerances*.

Some of the differences may be due to learning, how we are taught about pain and how people respond to us when we are in pain. If we are rewarded for pain each time we fall over as a child, with cuddles or sweets, we may learn pain differently from a child that is ignored. There are also different cultural conventions for pain: how much we can scream and shout. Different personalities may also influence the amount of pain perceived.

Health Connection

Measuring pain

One way pain is measured is by using something as simple as a ruler and asking the patient to point on the scale where they think their pain is. After treatment when asked again they should point to a lower scale if the pain has been lessened.

Treatment of pain

There are various ways in which pain can be treated. If they are to be used in evidence-based medicine they must perform better than a **placebo**. A placebo is an intervention that looks the same as that being tested but has no active ingredient or surgical use. A placebo is tested in a clinical trial called a double-blind clinical trial.

Box 12.2 Clinical interventions – The double-blind clinical trial

The clinical trial is a piece of **applied science**. It seeks to understand whether something works. It does not seek to understand how something works.

This clinical trial takes the form of a double-blind test. In this the patients are selected such that all have the same clinical problem. They are then divided into two groups and one is given the trial intervention, for example a new medicine, and the other group is given a 'placebo', an intervention that looks like the trial intervention, but, in fact, has no active ingredient. This is a blind trial as the patients do not know which group they are in so that their expectations of a drug do not interfere with how they think the drug has affected them. The trial is made double-blind by not letting the clinical staff administering and measuring the outcomes of the trial know whether their group is on the trial or the placebo. This is to avoid any influence by the staff on the patients. The trial drug or intervention must work better than the placebo. It is known that some people get better on the placebo, perhaps through belief. We cannot control the experiment against this, and perhaps a certain number of people self-heal. Some of those on the trial may also have got better, therefore, without any medical intervention, through their own homeostatic mechanisms. However, for an intervention to come to market it must work better than the placebo. All medicines and surgical interventions are thus tested in clinical, double-blind trials. They are not fully scientific as you cannot control all the possible variables in patients, but they are the best evidence-based medicine we can gather. They are used in all regulated medicines. Many 'alternative' and 'homeopathic' medicines have not been tested in this way or have not been shown to have a better effect than a placebo.

Treatments of pain include

- drugs,
- surgery,
- psychological help,
- TENS,
- acupuncture,
- hypnosis.

Drugs work by blocking the receptors that allow transmission of nerve signals from the damaged site to the brain.

Surgery can sever the neural pathways linking the site of pain to the brain detectors.

Psychological help can alter the perception of pain. If a person is in chronic pain the pain can become the centre of their lives and make them depressed. Altering their focus may help alleviate the pain. With acute pain, some of the pain may be down to fear of what is happening rather than the stimulus itself.

TENS is 'transcutaneous electrical nerve stimulation'. This works in the way that the old adage 'mummy rub it better' does and in the same way that acupuncture probably works. Pain travels along its own neural pathway, discussed below, separate from touch. Touch, however, travels along faster pathways. If one stimulates touch pathways by electrical stimulation in TENS or manually in massage or **acupuncture**, the touch pathways travel before the pain. It is thought that the touch pathways may be able to flood out the pain pathways by closing a 'gate'. This is discussed below.

Hypnosis works on about 30% of the population. They may be the same percentage that is susceptible to placebos. It may also be a learning experience where one is taught not to perceive the pain or to concentrate on something else.

Pharmacology

Pharmacology is the science of the therapeutic use of drugs, their synthesis and use. All drugs are made from chemicals and some chemicals are found in plants. Their therapeutic use has sometimes been known for centuries. Pharmacology studies their actions and properties to be able to make safe and effective drugs.

In general, drugs are medicines or chemicals that can

- cure a disease,
- arrest a disease,

- relieve symptoms,
- ease pain.

Types of drugs that can aid include

- analgesic pain relief, such as aspirin, opiates,
- anti-inflammatory,
- anti-emetic,
- supplements, such as hormone replacement, vitamins and minerals,
- contraception,
- antibiotics against bacteria,
- antifungal agents,
- anti-cancerous tumours,
- anti-coagulants, such as heparin and warfarin.

Drugs can be *administered*, given, into various *sites* or *routes*. Entry sites include

- respiratory,
- gastrointestinal,
- epidermally,
- intramuscular,
- intravenous.

The site where drugs are administered will affect their speed of action. If a drug is administered into blood or muscle there will be fast dispersion of the drug through the body and its transport systems. If the drug is administered in the GI tract it must survive passage through the GI to reach its target and there will be a slower dispersal of a drug going via the GI tract.

Most drugs must pass through the liver before they reach their target. This pass through is called the **first pass effect**. The liver alters (metabolises) the drug. This will alter the drug either into

- an active form (rate of action) or
- metabolise it into an inactive form for excretion (half life).

If a drug is given via the oral route it may be extensively metabolised by the liver before reaching the systemic circulation (high first-pass effect). The same drug given intravenously (IV) bypasses the liver, preventing the first-pass effect from taking place, and more drug reaches the circulation.

If it is into an inactive metabolite it will be excreted.

Mode of action of drugs

Drugs work by two general principles:

- **non-specific** and
- **specific**.

In non-specific actions a drug acts by altering general physical or chemical properties in our internal environment. For example,

- a laxative draws water from the GI tract to increase fluid volume, soften faeces, and aids peristalsis and defecation;
- antacids neutralise HCl in the stomach.

Neither of these examples are specific; they merely act to alter pH or osmotic pressure.

In specific actions a drug binds to its target receptor. This requires the drug to be the correct shape and therefore the particular subunits it is made from must be in a specific arrangement to fit into the target. The drug then binds to its target such as a large molecule and influences a chemical pathway or functioning in a cell.

Targets include

- enzymes,
- carrier molecules,
- ion channels,
- receptors – signalling pathways,
- micro-organisms,
- cancer cells.

For a drug to act it must bind to a target, often a receptor on a cell, and affect that cell. It can be blocked from binding by an antagonist, a chemical similar in shape that binds to the receptor of the cell but prevents the effect occurring. There are also agonists that act in a similar manner to the drug by binding to the receptor and having an effect on the cell (Figure 12.1).

Half life

The half life of a drug is a measure of how long a drug is active in our body before it is excreted. The time it takes for half of the amount of administered drug to be inactivated or excreted is its half life (T ½).

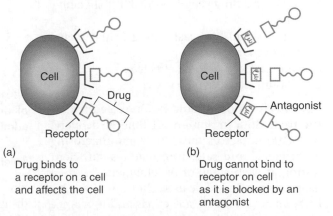

(a) Drug binds to a receptor on a cell and affects the cell

(b) Drug cannot bind to receptor on cell as it is blocked by an antagonist

FIGURE 12.1 **Action of drugs and antagonists**

Dosage and pharmacodynamics

The amount of drug administered is its **dose**. Doses vary during our lifetimes from childhood to old age. Many drugs are toxic at high dosages. In fact, nearly all chemicals that are therapeutic or nutritious for us are also toxic at high dosages, including substances such as vitamins. We need to administer the therapeutic dose, the dose that will have the required effect, without giving the toxic dose. What dose to administer also relies on **pharmacodynamics**, how long a drug takes to become active and effective.

Dosages are assessed taking into account

- route of administration;
- onset or reaction time – the time it takes for the drug to elicit a therapeutic response;
- peak – the time it takes for a drug to reach its maximum therapeutic response;
- duration – the time a drug concentration is sufficient to elicit a therapeutic response;
- how fast a drug is metabolised into an active form;
- half life and how fast a drug is inactivated and excreted;
- amount needed to be effective;
- amount needed to be toxic.

The effective dose should never exceed half of the toxic dose in amount of time of delivery. All of these factors mean that manufacturing an effective and safe drug requires sufficient testing at each stage of development before a drug is permitted to be used clinically. Even so, there may be *adverse side effects* and a balance may need to be struck between treatment and these effects. There are also **contra-indications** where having a pre-condition, such as pregnancy, may preclude a patient from a particular drug.

Drug interactions are the alteration of action of a drug in the presence of other drugs or foods. These other drugs or foods can be

- other prescribed drugs,
- over-the-counter medications,
- herbal therapies.

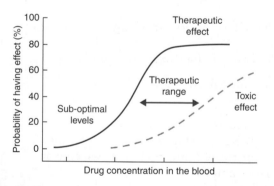

FIGURE 12.2 **Effective dosages and toxic dosages of drug must be calculated before the correct administrative dosages can be estimated**

Tolerance and dependence

Not only can we mount allergic reactions to drugs but we can also become tolerant to them. This is where there is a decreasing response to repetitive drug doses so that higher doses are needed to elicit the same response that was seen previously at lower doses.

Chapter Reference

Allergic reactions are discussed in Chapter 11, 'Cleansing and Dressing' (see p. 299).

We may also become dependent on a drug. This can be a physiological or psychological need for a drug, such as seen with some painkillers.

Health Connection

Monitoring

A patient given any medication may need to be monitored to avoid adverse drug events. These can be due to

- medication errors that result in patient harm;
- any reaction that is unexpected, undesirable, and occurs at doses normally used.

The biology of pain

Pain is usually generated in response to *tissue damage*, extreme mechanical or heat stimuli on the body. Pain, like touch, is a *contact sense*. The stimuli do not act directly on the brain. There has to be a *transduction* from the **stimulus**, the touch or pain on the body, which is converted (transduced) into an **electrical stimulation**, an action potential which is then conveyed to and **detected** by the brain.

Chapter Reference

The nervous system forms the basis of the biology of pain and is discussed in Chapter 4, 'Communicating' (see p. 102).

If pain is a sense in the way that sight, sound, smell, taste and touch are senses, then it must have its own **receptors**, **pathways** and **brain locations**.

Chapter Reference

The senses are discussed in Chapter 4, 'Communicating' (see p. 102).

Pain receptors

If pain is not only an emotion but also a sense it will have its own receptors. Receptors tell us information that the body needs to know about a signal:

1. the quality of the signal – what it is;
2. the intensity of the signal – how much or little;
3. the duration of the signal – how long it lasts;
4. the location of the signal – where it is.

The quality of the pain stimulus

We know what the signal is by having a range of receptors that each detect particular stimuli. For example, we have receptors that only detect electromagnetic waves at a small range of frequencies. These are called eyes and they can only see things within a particular 'human visual spectrum'. We have receptors that can detect airwaves at a certain range of frequencies. These are called ears. With touch we have receptors for light touch and thermoreceptors for warm and for cool on our skin. We know this because we can stimulate different receptors on the skin and follow their response.

We also have receptors on our skin for intense touch or heat called **nociceptors**. They detect noxious stimuli. They are tuned to their particular signal, just like any other receptor, and detect stimuli of *intense* frequencies but do not respond to light touch or warm/cool stimuli.

There are **mechano-nociceptors** for extreme mechanical stimulation and **polymodal nociceptors** for extreme temperature or mechanical stimulation.

The intensity of the pain stimulus

How can we know how big or small a stimulus is? When a stimulus such as touch, stimulates a receptor, if it reaches a threshold of detection an action potential is sent along the receptor's nerve fibre.

The action potential is an *all or nothing* response; either the current flows or it doesn't. So the size of the action potential cannot tell us about how large a stimulus is; it merely tells us that there is a stimulus.

Detecting the intensity relies on two events:

1. The threshold of the receptor. Nociceptors have higher thresholds than touch receptors. It takes more intensity of stimulus to pass their threshold for firing an action potential.
2. The frequency of action potentials increases with increasing intensity. The action potential size remains the same (the change in electrical potential) but there are more or less of them.

The duration of the pain stimulus

How long a stimulus is detected depends on receptor **adaptation**. If a stimulus remains on for a long time the receptor can cease to send action potentials. Some receptors are fast adapting such as the ones for light touch from, for example, your clothing. Your clothes are touching touch receptors, but they are not detecting your clothes. This is a useful adaptation. There is potentially so much information in the universe and you do not need to monitor all of it all the time. If your clothes were suddenly grabbed and moved, you would notice, but when they are just there, they are not a stimulus needing a response. Some receptors are slow in adapting. They tell you of the stimulus for a long time. Pain nociceptors may be one such **slow adapting receptor** to warn you of tissue damage.

The location of the pain stimulus

All information from the surface of the body is taken from the peripheral system to the spinal cord. This information is kept within **dermatomes**, areas of the body whose sensory information is then transmitted to one segment of spinal cord and up through a discrete pathway to one **topographical area** of somatosensory brain. In this way *where* the stimulus is from is *preserved* on its way to the brain.

Health Connection

Pain as a symptom

When feeling ill one of the most common signs is having a pain. One of the first symptoms that a health professional will ask us is 'Do you have a pain?' If we have a pain the health professional will want to know its

- **location** – here the pain is;
- **duration** – how long we have had the pain (acute or chronic);
- **intensity** – how much pain we have;
- **quality** – what type of pain, sharp, dull, burning or itching for example.

All of these help to diagnose what is causing the pain and therefore help in treatment.

Pain pathways

Nociceptors have their own nerve fibres. Touch receptors send their signal to large alpha myelinated fibres that convey messages fast, at up to 100 m/s. Nociceptors send their signals to small, unmyelinated C fibres that convey information at lower rates than touch. The C fibres enter a deeper part of the spinal cord than touch fibres and carry their information up the spinothalamic tracts to the brain, different to the touch tracts.

This means that touch and pain travel at *different speeds*, in *different tracts*. However, they appear to end up in the same part of the brain.

Pain thus has many components of a sense. It has its own

- sensory receptors (nociceptors),
- nerve fibres (C fibres),
- tracts to the brain (spinothalamic).

However, it does not appear to have a separate part of the brain from the touch areas – somatosensory cortex.

The Gate Theory

As mentioned above, the old adage 'mummy rubs the pain better' may work due to the different speeds of the touch and pain transmission. If a pain is detected and you rub the area affected you are sending up touch responses at the same time. These may arrive quickly and flood out the area of the brain detecting stimuli from that location. This is how TENS and acupuncture, mentioned above, may work. There is a detailed theory of how these events may occur called the **Gate Theory** developed by Melzack and Wall.

In this theory all the biology is used to explain how pain can be reduced in various ways including the actions of TENS, acupuncture and rubbing a wound better. It relies on the different speeds at which pain and touch travel in their pathways and the fact that the touch pathway can 'flood out' the pain pathway so that we no longer feel pain merely touch.

The stages of the Gate Theory and the transmission and interruption of pain pathways are

- Intense pain or tissue damage stimulates *nociceptors*. The nociceptors take the 'pain' signal up towards the spinal cord in small diameter slow 'pain' fibres.
- At the spinal cord the 'pain' fibres synapse with neurons in the spinal cord called **T** neurons (transmission neurons).
- The T neurons take the 'pain' message up to the brain and pain is detected.
- However, at the synapse in the spinal cord there is another neuron, an interneuron **I**.
- The I neuron is stimulated by large diameter fast 'touch' fibres.
- If the I neuron is stimulated it can close a gate between the 'pain' fibre and T and the signal can no longer ascend to the brain. No pain is felt.
- When I is stimulated it releases a substance, enkephalin.
- Enkephalin binds to T and prevents the transmission of 'pain' signals.
- If the gate is closed no pain is detected by the brain.
- The gate can also be closed by descending messages from the brain stimulating the I interneuron to release enkephalins (mind over matter!) (see Figure 12.3).

Enkephalins are the body's own **opiate**. Opiates are substances such as cocaine and heroin known to reduce pain. We produce chemicals with very similar structures to opiates. They bind to chemical receptors in our nervous system and reduce pain sensation.

Box 12.3 Summary – Gate Theory

In Gate Theory sensations caused by pain can be interrupted while ascending up to the brain by competition from

- ascending touch signals,
- enkephalins,
- descending signals from the brain closing the gate area.

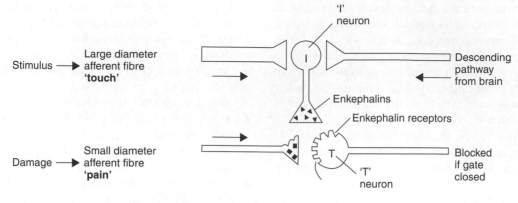

FIGURE 12.3 **The Gate Theory of pain transmission**

TENS

It is possible to purchase TENS in many outlets these days. The TENS comprise small pouches that deliver low level stimulation and are recommended for use for about 15 minutes. Anecdotal reports suggest that they give high levels of relief from chronic pain. They would not be advised for use in acute pain.

Inflammation

Not only does tissue damage cause pain, but the workings of the immune system – discussed in Chapter 11, 'Cleansing and Dressing' – also can cause pain. When the system is working inflammation can occur leading to a rising temperature and painful swelling around the damaged area. This is due to infiltration of the area by cells of the immune system. They enter from the blood vessels due to the local release of chemicals that make the blood vessels dilate and become 'leaky'. The chemicals and their effects can cause pain.

Box 12.4 Summary – Pain

- Pain may have a protective function to warn us of tissue damage so that we remove ourselves from the danger and rest the damaged part.
- There are pain receptors, fibres and pathways, making this a sense.
- The Gate Theory explains some mysteries of pain and some pain relief.
- Pain is a subjective sense and it is hard to objectively measure other people's physical pain. This makes assessing pain by the health professional very difficult and using pain as a symptom hard to describe and measure.

Conclusion: Sleeping and healing

A good night's sleep is what most of us need to remain healthy. Sleep acts as an escape from the worries of the day. It also enables us to escape from pain and rest our bodies, allowing healing by tissue repair and regeneration. Disruption to sleep can have very profound effects on our mental health, but both pain and sleep are areas of biology that have proved very difficult to understand. Pain is subjective and hard to assess.

Sleep is an activity we all need, but its function is unknown. However, nearly all of us know what they are and know that we want sleep and want to avoid pain!

Chapter Summary

- Humans tend to sleep at night when their vision is reduced.
- Sleep may have a protective factor, so that we rest when we are not so able to carry out activities such as hunting.
- Sleep may have a repairing factor, allowing cells and tissues to be replaced while resting from many other activities.
- It may also allow metabolic activities to be reduced.
- We have a normal sleep/wake pattern controlled by a clock in our brains.
- We can override the pattern, but we cannot survive for long without sleep.
- Damage to our bodies tends to cause pain.
- Pain tells us to rest the afflicted area and allow healing to occur.
- Without pain we do not know that we have done damage to an area of our body and may continue using it, exacerbating the damage rather than resting the afflicted area.
- There are many treatments, including pharmacological ones that do not cure tissue damage but can reduce pain from the damage.
- Part of homeostasis is our ability to heal ourselves.

13 Dying

Chapter Outline

Introduction: Dying as an activity of daily living

Unlike the opening sequence of the *Star Trek* television programme it is not space, but death that is the final frontier we must face in the narrative of our lives. There is a saying by Anatole France that 'The average man, who does not know what to do with his life, wants another one which will last forever.'

It may be a mixture of thinking there is no going back and not knowing what happens next that fills us with fear of death. Many of us would like to have greater **longevity**, to live a long time, but we do not want the signs and symptoms of **ageing.** Some of us will die through a gradual ageing process with all parts of our bodies gradually wearing out at the same rate. Some of us will die from pathologic conditions where certain organs may fail prematurely. Some of us will die young, before the time expected. However we measure our life expectancies, one thing seems certain, every living thing is *mortal* and we all die. This is one ADL that we cannot escape.

Without death we cannot live as we obtain our nutrients from other living things, plants or animals, killing them in the process. Death, therefore, seems to be a necessary part of life.

The aim of clinical intervention is to save lives, prolong life and delay or even prevent death, but ultimately the work fails and inevitability death occurs. Given that death will happen, **palliative care** is concerned with giving an individual a 'good death'. We must all face our own deaths and how we have a 'good death' varies as to what we want from this stage in our life and what is available at the time as we cannot choose when we are born or when we die.

In this chapter, we will look at what death is, how it occurs at the cellular level and how it manifests itself, what we die from, our **morbidity** rates, and when we die, our **mortality** rates, healthy ageing and the process of dying. There is no definition of what life is. Understanding what death is may help us to understand what life is.

The environment

The external environment

While we may find the necessary nutrients, gases and environments for us to survive and even thrive, as we said in Chapter 11, 'Cleansing and Dressing', the planet on which we live is merely permissive to our being here and is indifferent to our survival. We live in a fairly hostile environment full of physical and chemical properties that challenge our internal environment. To maintain our integrity, our bodily functions, requires the expenditure of large amounts of energy that we must find and make. When we are successful we are independent and healthy. However, eventually the external environment wins and we perish.

The internal environment

How many of us are on the planet depends on our ability to survive and reproduce and our offspring's abilities to do the same. In Darwinian evolutionary terms those that survive and thrive are called 'fit', but this does not mean that they are fit in our terms of the word. It means that they are well *adapted* to their environment. Also, the more of us that survive and thrive and reproduce the greater effect we have on the environment to which we originally adapted; we change our environments. As the environment changes, we humans don't. We are very slow to evolve; it takes nine months for our eggs to develop to birth and 12 years to reach sexual maturity in which we can repeat this development of the next generation. This compares to a species such as bacteria which is born and can replicate itself every 20 minutes. Any changes to our genes, therefore, take a long time to affect our offspring or to spread through the population, if it is a gene that confers viability.

Box 13.1 Darwin and evolution

Darwin's Theory of Evolution by **Natural Selection** is one of the most misunderstood theories. When we **breed flowers** we are artificially **selecting characteristics** that we want such as **colour** or **scent**. **Nature** also **selects**. When nature selects it is called natural selection and is the selecting of **individuals** that are well **adapted** to their external **environment**. Those that are well adapted will live (survive) and reproduce passing on those inherited characteristics. The characteristics that can be **inherited** are contained in our **genetic material**. This material **(DNA)** can **mutate** and **alter** some of the characteristics. The alterations can be good or bad for the individual carrying the mutation. If it is bad the individual does not thrive and reproduce. If the mutation is good the individual survives and reproduces, passing on this new mutant gene. If the gene confers many advantages to individuals possessing it in a particular environment those individuals survive and reproduce, so the gene **spreads** through the **population** and those with the gene are fitter than those without it. However, the environment can change and that gene no longer confers 'fitness'. So there is **no** 'absolute fitness' only 'relative fitness' compared to other individuals in the group. If the mutation spreads and alters the characteristics of those that have it then a new **species** may emerge: **natural selection** by **random mutation** leading to **evolution**. We who are here today are the result of useful mutations.

As stated previously, we are a slowly *evolving* species. We have also been a slowly *growing* or *reproducing* species. For most of our existence our numbers have been quite low, given the time we have been on the planet. Gradually we are doubling our population at far faster rates than in the past. This is due to a number of factors including lower infant mortality, more reliable food and water supplies. Since the Industrial Revolution we may have become somewhat divorced from nature, perhaps thinking we are above the environment. This is a false view. We are subject to nature, the external environment, and we are here due to it. We are not a separate thing from nature and we are limited by its resources. As stated before the environment in which we live is indifferent to our existence and merely permissive. We must adapt to it, not the other way around (it to us!). In the words of Mark Twain 'Don't go around saying the world owes you a living. The world owes you nothing. It was here first.'

Population numbers

The number of people on the planet has increased dramatically in the past 50 years. Our presence on the planet affects the planet, our external environments, and may make it less able to support us. This may put a strain on resources such as food and clean water which in turn will affect how long we live and how well we live and may be the single largest issue for the conservation and health of the planet. Wanting to live longer and breeding more may present conflicting interests where a balance between individual desires and society's needs may be mutually exclusive (Table 13.1).

Death and dying: Biological aspects

If you are involved in the health care profession it may be hard to maintain a perspective about the numbers of healthy versus ill people, but most of the time most of us are healthy. In the UK, for example, if five million people use the health services in a year 70 million don't! We evolved before the health care professions and before health care organisations. If we were not healthy we would not be here. We are healthy because of homeostasis; we build ourselves from

a single cell and maintain ourselves, our bodies, independently of others. When we are healthy we make our own energy, replace worn-out cells and tissues throughout our lives and have some capacity to repair our own bodies. However, we are mortal and eventually we die.

We die from one of four main causes:

1. Traumas such as car accidents and burns remove more tissue than we can replace.
2. Microbial infections destroy our cells and produce vast toxic waste in our bodies.
3. Hyperplasia produces more cells than needed and replace functional cells with undifferentiated growing cells (cancers).

Table 13.1 Estimated world population

Date	Numbers of people (millions)
BC	
40,000	2
10,000	4
7000 (settlements – farming)	4
3000	14
1500 (Moses –Torah)	25
500 (Buddha, Hippocrates)	100
AD	
1 (Christ – Gospels)	200
200	190
500 (Mohammed – Koran)	190
600 (Roman Empire ends)	200
1000	265
1100 (Crusades)	320
1500	415
1750 (Industrialisation starts)	720
1800	900
1850	1200
1900	1625
1950	2500
1970	3698
1990	5200
2000	6250

Source: Adapted from Goodwin (1997) *Human Biology and Health, Book 1 Conception to Birth*. Open University Worldwide (Fig 4.2)

4. Degeneration reduces the numbers of functioning cells through either malnutrition, or disease or ageing.

Whatever ethnic, religious, political, social, economic, geographic, gender or sexual group to which you belong, you will die mainly of one of these causes. The health and safety industries try to delay this and even prevent some premature deaths such as those from infections and accidents.

Many of the living processes we carry out have harmful side effects; they not only keep us alive, but are also reasons for our death. For example:

1. The production of energy has carbon dioxide (CO_2) as a side product which must be expelled from the body before it causes changes in pH. Changes to pH affect our enzymes which are very sensitive to these changes and cannot function at the incorrect pH.
2. Producing muscular activity has the side effect of producing lactic acid, a waste product that needs to be expelled, and heat which can warm the body, but can also overheat the body.
3. Producing energy in the mitochondria of the cells also produces free radicals, very reactive atomic species with a spare electron which can start a chain reaction damaging the contents of the cell.

Life itself is risky; it kills us.

The nature and causation of disease

The main causes of death rely on a number of factors. These factors are used in the area **epidemiology**:

- **epi** – from the Greek meaning **upon**,
- **demos** – (as in 'democracy', which is an ancient Greek invention over 2000 years old) meaning **people** or **population**,
- **logos** – (as in logic) from the Greek meaning **science**.

Epidemiology

Epidemiology is the science of what is visited upon people, and what is visited upon the people is disease. Disease is a disorder or abnormal functioning of body cell, tissues, organs or systems. The factors that effect the diseases to which we succumb include

- gender,
- age,
- genetics (ethnic/racial),
- lifestyle,
- environment,
- pre-existing conditions,
- predisposing factors.

These factors can be grouped into two types, **nature** and **nurture**:

- who you are (your **genes**) i.e. nature;
- what you do, where you live and how you live (your lifestyle) i.e. nurture.

These two factors, nature and nurture, will have an impact on the diseases to which you succumb. There is a lot of debate in biology of the role of each in homeostasis and the role of each in health.

Epidemiology is the science of diseases in populations, how *often* they occur, to *whom* they occur and what are the *causes*. It proposes, from its findings, risk factors that *increase the chance* of getting the disease and therefore helps in public health and health promotion. However, it can only tell you about the risk to a population, not to an individual. It measures the rates of occurrence of a disease in a population. A rate is how often something occurs, its frequency.

Rates are ratios of one thing to another, how often one thing occurs within a group or compared to another group or the whole group and can be expressed, therefore, as one number (the numerator) divided by another number (the denominator). For example,

A **crude rate** is presented for an entire population; for example, Birth Rate is the number of live births per population:

Birth Rate = Number of live births/population

A **specific rate** is a rate in a specific population; for example, Fertility Rate can be measured as number of live births per number of women of reproductive age (15–44):

Fertility Rate = Number of live births/number of women aged 15–44

A **standardised rate** is used to compare two or more populations with a confounding variable (see below) removed; for example, Infant Mortality Rate is the number of infants that die before age one against the number of live births, rather than against all births or all ages:

$$\text{Infant Mortality Rate} = \frac{\text{Number of infant deaths}}{\text{Number of live births}}$$

Dependent and confounding variables

What we see in the universe are effects. We may wish to work out what causes them. For example, if you say eating fats causes heart disease, the **dependent variable** (the effect) is heart disease, the outcome. There is also an **independent variable** on which the dependent variable depends. In this case the fats are the independent variable that can be varied and the effect it has on the dependent variable (heart disease) is observed. This is an attempt to find the cause of an effect. There are also **confounding variables** that may influence the dependent variable such as the genetic makeup of the individual or the amount of exercise they do. Many experiments are hard to carry out as confounding variables are hard to control. They literally confound or confuse the results and may gain the credit for the cause of an effect when they merely occur alongside it or contribute to it. This is where correlation masks the effect of causation.

The epidemiological causes of ill health and death are therefore very hard to prove as there are so many variables in our lives.

Box 13.2 Correlation, coincidence and causation

Unfortunately many health studies rely on correlation or coincidence rather than causes so confounding variables, variables which occur systematically in the observation, are easily allocated the role of causal agents. Correlation or coincidence is when two things occur together, but do not necessarily cause one another to happen. For example,

- In summer more people drown in Britain than in winter.
- In summer more people eat ice-cream in Britain than in winter.
- Correlation: eating ice cream makes you drown?

Now this is obviously nonsense. The two things happen together (coincidence or correlation) for other reasons such as it is hotter in summer in Britain than in winter and one way to cool down is swimming and another is eating ice-cream. The more people swim the more there is a likelihood of some people getting drowned. So the increase in numbers of drowning may be in proportion to the increase in numbers of people swimming; i.e. if 3% of swimmers drown in summer perhaps 3% drown in winter. There could be other causes, however.

'Coincidence does not prove causation'. Most statistical tests employed in research are to try to prove that two things occurred together at a higher rate than would be expected by chance; i.e. that there is some causal relation between the two. This is why so much research is later disproved when the real cause is elucidated.

Nature, nurture and epidemiology

We would like to know what the cause of a disease is so we can prevent it or treat it. For instance, we have seen increasing obesity in the developed world. Is this due to the genes we have (nature) or to the lifestyle we lead (nurture)?

In epidemiology we try to see what causes a disease. For instance, in Japan one of the common cancers in the 1980s was esopharyngeal (of the oesophagus), while stomach cancer was rare. In America in the 1980s one of the common cancers was stomach cancer while esopharyngeal cancer was rare. Are these conditions nature or nurture?

To answer this we can look at populations. Japanese populations are more homogeneous (similar) than are American populations, making a comparison difficult. However, if we look at Japanese people emigrating to America or vice versa, we get a clue. When this occurs the people take their genes (nature) with them! They change lifestyle. When Japanese people moved to America their rates of esopharyngeal cancer decreased and their rates of stomach cancer increased. This demonstrates that there is not something inherent, a gene, causing these cancers. They are lifestyle related, something perhaps in our diet. We can then look at foods and pollution to find the causes.

Morbidity

Morbidity rates are the patterns of disease within a population. In many developed countries many diseases and degeneration of the body are compressed into the last few years of life. 'The compression of morbidity' is when the body fails or wears out. This would be the hope for many to live a healthy life with everything wearing out at the end, all together. However, this is an unusual scenario at present.

For infectious diseases there are a number of epidemiological parameters to describe the spread of the disease:

- **endemic** – is where the disease is confined to local region;
- **epidemic** – is where the disease spreads to many individuals at the same time;
- **pandemic** – is where the epidemic spreads to large geographical areas;
- **syndrome** – a collection of different signs and symptoms.

All of these measures are to help in a **diagnosis**, which is the identification of disease or disorder or condition and the **aetiology**, which assigns a cause to a given outcome. For us as individuals we present to our doctors with **symptoms**, subjective abnormalities. The doctor then takes measurements to find **signs**, objective abnormalities, such as raised temperature or high blood pressure. A diagnosis can then be made so that a **treatment**, an intervention to alter the course of the disease or condition, can be prescribed. We will be monitored to see the **pathogenesis**, the pattern of disease development and to see if the treatment halts the pathogenic outcomes. During treatment a **prognosis**, an estimation of the likely course or outcome of the disease, may be made.

Life expectancy

Life expectancy is a statistical measure of the average length of survival, usually from birth, of a given population, including infant mortality rates. Currently the world average life expectancy at birth is 67. We often talk about life expectancies increasing, but this is based on previous life expectancies. Life expectancy can only truly be calculated in the generation that has already died. While it may see trends such as that previous life expectancies have increased, it is not truly predictive of the life expectancies of future generations as we cannot see the future, what diseases may affect us and how the environment may change.

Mortality rates

Mortality rates are a measure of the number of deaths in a population over a particular time period.

The mortality rates are calculated as Standardised Rates to account for the structure of a population, multiplied by 100 to get a percentage point:

$$\text{Standardised Mortality Rate (SMR)} = \text{No of deaths occurring (No)/number of deaths expected (Ne)} \times 100,$$
$$\text{i.e. SMT} = \text{No/Ne} \times 100$$

The standard population has an SMR of 100%. In other words the number of observed and expected deaths are the same. More than 100 is an unfavourable mortality, while less than 100 is a favourable mortality rate.

Main causes of death

Different causes of death can be calculated against the total (100%) death rate. For the year 2003 there were 57,029,000 recorded deaths worldwide. The main causes of death for that year are presented in Table 13.2.

The deaths fall into the four main causes mentioned above degenerative diseases, infectious disease: traumas (accidental or intentional) or hyperplasia (the overgrowth of cells, cancers) (Table 13.3).

This demonstrates that in the developing world you are more likely to die of an infectious disease than a degenerative or hyperplasic or hyper nutrient disease. In the developed world clean water supplies and sewerage treatments have reduced many microbial infections. Immunisations have also contributed to their decreasing effect on mortality. The developed world may have longer life expectancies, but the population are now more likely to die of degenerative diseases or hyperplasia.

Table 13.2 Main causes of death worldwide (2004)

World	Deaths in millions	Percentage of deaths
Ischaemic heart disease	7.25	12.8
Stroke and other cerebrovascular disease	6.15	10.8
Lower respiratory infections	3.46	6.1
Chronic obstructive pulmonary disease	3.28	5.8
Diarrhoeal diseases	2.46	4.3
HIV/AIDS	1.78	3.1
Trachea, bronchus, lung cancers	1.39	2.4
Tuberculosis	1.34	2.4
Diabetes mellitus	1.26	2.2
Road traffic accidents	1.21	2.1

Source: WHO (2011) Factsheet no 310. The 10 leading causes of death by broad income group (2008) (updated June 2011) http://www.who.int/mediacentre/factsheets/fs310/en/index.html. Reproduced with permission.

Table 13.3 Top causes of death in low-, middle- and high-income countries

	Deaths in millions	Percentage of deaths
Low-income countries		
Lower respiratory infections	1.05	11.3
Diarrhoeal diseases	0.76	8.2
HIV/AIDS	0.72	7.8
Ischaemic heart disease	0.57	6.1
Malaria	0.48	5.2
Stroke and other cerebrovascular disease	0.45	4.9
Tuberculosis	0.40	4.3
Prematurity and low birth weight	0.30	3.2
Birth asphyxia and birth trauma	0.27	2.9
Neonatal infections	0.24	2.6
Middle-income countries		
Ischaemic heart disease	5.27	13.7
Stroke and other cerebrovascular disease	4.91	12.8
Chronic obstructive pulmonary disease	2.79	7.2
Lower respiratory infections	2.07	5.4
Diarrhoeal diseases	1.68	4.4
HIV/AIDS	1.03	2.7
Road traffic accidents	0.94	2.4
Tuberculosis	0.93	2.4
Diabetes mellitus	0.87	2.3
Hypertensive heart disease	0.83	2.2
High-income countries		
Ischaemic heart disease	1.42	15.6
Stroke and other cerebrovascular disease	0.79	8.7
Trachea, bronchus, lung cancers	0.54	5.9
Alzheimer and other dementias	0.37	4.1
Lower respiratory infections	0.35	3.8
Chronic obstructive pulmonary disease	0.32	3.5
Colon and rectum cancers	0.30	3.3
Diabetes mellitus	0.24	2.6
Hypertensive heart disease	0.21	2.3
Breast cancer	0.17	1.9

Source: WHO (2011) Factsheet no 310. The 10 leading causes of death by broad income group (2008) (updated June 2011) http://www.who.int/mediacentre/factsheets/fs310/en/index.html. Reproduced with permission.

Lifespan

Maximum lifespan

Maximum lifespan may be a fixed sum for a species. For humans it appears to be 122, the highest recorded age of a person. If this is so then it would appear that there is a 'programmed' lifespan. This could be a genetic programme that tells cells when to die or a cellular programme that kills cells after a certain number of divisions. The latter is hard to explain as we are composed of functional end cells that do not divide. Somehow they must die out of their own accord. Environmental damage may be harder to repair in older cells or the problem may lie with stem cells which replace worn-out older cells. Stem cells may be less efficient in older humans.

Chapter Reference

Cell repair is discussed in Chapter 1, 'Maintaining a Safe Environment' (see p. 1) and in Chapter 3, 'Growing and Developing' (see p. 64).

All of these mechanisms contribute to ageing, which is discussed below.

Increasing lifespan: life extension

Many of us would like to live longer, increase our lifespan. Increasing lifespan has many biological, health and ethical issues. We need to balance **quantity**, how long you live, with **quality**, the health of the individual. Currently we **prolong morbidity.** We extend life by clinical intervention. We have more years, but not necessarily good health.

As mentioned above, if our lifespan is fixed we would like to have a healthy life to the end to **compress morbidity.** Medical research and resources would also have to eliminate premature death and debilitating diseases.

There are those who wish to concentrate resources on extending life, not merely delaying death, by delaying the ageing process. Scientists are looking at the causes of ageing and trying to alter their effects, either by altering genes, cells or by the use of drugs. Others think that we have moved away from acceptance of nature and that we need to limit our longevity for the sake of the next generation.

Ageing

Biological explanations of ageing

How we age may be due to many factors including the genes we inherited, damage through biological processes such as to our genetic material or the effects of free radicals or our lifestyle, particularly diet. There is also an evolutionary theory of ageing.

Genetic ageing

Evidence for a genetic involvement in ageing is twofold. Genes can be altered in animal studies that result in the animal having a prolonged life. This suggests that we have genes that age us. Another piece of evidence for genetic involvement is the disease of **progeria**, where the body ages very rapidly. This disease suggests that there are a number of genes that effect the onset and development of the disease. The question then is, can we alter these genes (gene therapy) to reduce the effects of ageing while increasing longevity?

Every time our cells form new cells through cell division the genetic material DNA must be replicated. During this process mistakes can be made, mutations, that affect the functioning of the genes and therefore the proteins produced. As we age our cells have divided many times and more mistakes may have been made to our DNA. This may affect lifespan. Mutations to our **somatic** cells (cells of the **soma** – body) can cause the cessation of function of a cell and therefore its death or it may alter its behaviour so that it does not respond to homeostatic controls on cell numbers and grows unregulated, becoming a cancer. This is part of the disposable soma theory – the soma being the body. Our bodies may die, but our germ cells, our egg or sperm cells, are more protected against damage so that our offspring will live.

Chapter Reference

Cell division and growth is discussed in Chapter 3, 'Growing and Developing' (see p. 64).

Cell cycle ageing

The end of our genetic material, DNA, is protected from damage by a mixture of nucleic acids and proteins called **telomeres**. These in turn are maintained by an enzyme called **telomerase**. The telomeres shorten during each cell division. Telomerase is active in germ cells and early embryonic cells and in cancerous cells – it is now a target for anti-cancer drugs, but its activity reduces in somatic cells.

Environmental damage and ageing

Free radicals are the by-products of normal cellular mechanisms such as oxidation to make ATP. They are highly reactive atoms that are normally short-lived, reacting with other atoms. They are normally deactivated by enzymes such as catalase and super-oxide dismutase, but if they are not deactivated they can have damaging effects on other molecules by oxidising them. Evidence has shown that free radicals may oxidise other proteins and cause damage and the effects of ageing.

Chapter Reference

The formation of ATP is discussed in Chapter 2, 'Working and Playing' (see p. 35).

Diet may also have an effect on ageing. Evidence has shown that reduced calorific intake may prolong life. Certain constituents in our diets, such as saturated fats, have been shown to have damaging effects on our vascular system which would result in reduced health. Perhaps anything that reduces our health is ageing.

Exercise may have beneficial effects for health and well-being. Excessive exercise, however, damages tissues and produces more free radicals during oxidation to produce the energy for exercise.

Health Connection

Wound healing

Cross-linked collagen has less elasticity which may affect wound healing. This may help to explain the observation that ageing has an effect on wound healing, discussed in Chapter 5, 'Controlling and Repairing' (see p. 142).

Cellular changes occur during ageing, but it is hard to decide whether they cause ageing or are a consequence of ageing. Cellular metabolism may slow down during ageing and the recycling of cellular constituents may also slow down. **Lipofuscin** is a yellow pigment which is a by-product of inefficient recycling. It is found in old cells and interferes with metabolism. **Lysosomes** in cells contain digestive enzymes which are used to break down products in the cell such as old organelles or microbes. The number of lysosomes in a cell increases with age. While they have a use in the cell they are also potentially destructive. The protein collagen has an altered structure in ageing becoming more cross-linked, meaning the molecules of collagen become enmeshed together. This is due to **glycation** where sugar molecules on collagen react with the collagen.

Evolutionary ageing

One way to counteract mortality is to reproduce, passing on your genetic characteristics to another generation. Our bodies, soma, may die, but our genes live on. Evolution by natural selection favours those that are well adapted to their environment – they are fit. As discussed above, fitness is a measure of survival and reproduction. How then can we explain the evolution of ageing? One theory is the 'disposable soma' where our somatic cells, our bodies, are sacrificed in favour of reproduction. In other words, once we have reproduced we have performed our biological function and can die. However, women usually survive past the age of reproduction, going through a menopause. In this case, survival and reproduction are separated. So perhaps fitness, the ability to survive *and* reproduce, may not be the driving force. It is hard to explain how ageing evolves as it reduces individual fitness.

Chapter Reference

Development and reproduction are discussed in Chapter 3, 'Growing and Developing' (see p. 64).

Normal ageing

From birth to 20 we are *developing*, from 20 to 50 we are *maturing* with some organs already having reduced capacity, but, generally in health, we can compensate for this. After 50 this *compensation* decreases and damage and deterioration increase. In ageing viability decreases and there is a failure to maintain homeostasis after physiological stress. In other words, our ability to maintain homeostasis decreases. We normally restore our bodies to the ranges in Table 13.4.

The normal ageing body organs

Skin

Collagen elasticity decreases as we age, probably due to the cross-linking with sugars (glycation) mentioned above. The proportion of collagen increases in skin while the proportion of water and the fat layer below the surface of the skin decreases. Our skins thus become dry and loose with increased wrinkles.

Chapter Reference

Skin is discussed in Chapter 5, 'Controlling and Repairing' (see p. 142).

Muscles and bones

Up to 30% of our muscle fibres appear to be lost as we age from 30–80. Strength is also, therefore, decreased. Exercise may help to alleviate some muscle loss by improving muscle performance.

Bone mass reduces with age due to mineral loss, such as calcium, and loss of the organic matrix of bone. With the loss of calcium bone

Table 13.4 Normal ranges of some important constituents and physical characteristics of the body

	Normal value	Normal range	Approximate non-lethal limits
Oxygen (pp mmHg)	40	35–40	10–1000
Carbon dioxide (pp mmHg)	40	35–40	5–80
Sodium ion mmoles/L	142	138–146	115–175
Potassium ion (mmoles/L)	4.2	3.8–5.0	1.5–9.0
Calcium ion (mmoles/L)	1.2	1.0–1.4	0.5–2.0
Chloride ion (mmoles/L)	108	103–112	70–130
Bicarbonate ion (mmole/L)	28	24–32	8–45
Glucose (mmole/L)	85	75–95	20–1500
Body temperature (°C)	37.0	37.0	18.3–43.3
pH	7.4	7.3–7.5	6.9–8.0

density decreases. The loss of calcium in older people may be due to poor absorbency from the GI tract and from vitamin D deficiency. Vitamin D may also be poorly absorbed from the older GI tract. Vitamin D facilitates the transport of calcium and controls the deposition of calcium in the bones. Lack of vitamin D therefore will slow down bone growth.

Chapter Reference

Muscles and bones are discussed in Chapter 6, 'Moving' (see p. 163).

◤ **Health Connection**

Osteoporosis

When the bone mass falls below a critical level there is an increased risk of fractures. There is some evidence that calcium counteracts this effect. Other evidence suggests the use of hormones in post-menopausal women increases bone density.

Lungs

Lungs have a reserve capacity on top or the tidal volume of air that enters and leaves during inhalation and exhalation which could be used to maintain their efficiency. The lungs fill and empty due to the movement of intercostal muscles. The muscles are attached to the ribs via cartilage and cartilage can be less flexible in ageing. Lungs are made of elastic (elastin) fibres, mainly collagen, which can be less elastic in ageing. All of these factors could reduce the efficiency of breathing during ageing and therefore limit activity.

Cardiac

The cardiac output (CO) of the heart varies during different activities normally. When needed it can increase by about 400%. If there was a 30% reduction of cardiac output in age there would still be sufficient output, although the heart muscle may have to work harder to maintain this output as 30% of 400% = 120%, and 400–120% = 280% reserve in a healthy 70 year old.

In a healthy 70-year-old person their cardiac efficiency is about 70% of a younger person and they have 50% of respiratory efficiency. We can survive with one lung and one kidney so presumably these efficiencies, while compromised, are sufficient for normal living.

If one looks at 60 year olds, 75% of males and 25% of females will have a narrowing of the coronary arteries supplying the heart. Fifty per cent of the older adult population do not have normal heart functions

Blood vessels

Tissues age as the protein elastin, which forms part of the connective tissue layer in many organs, becomes less elastic and results in the vessel wall becoming less compliant (able to expand and contract). This means that greater pressure will be needed by the heart to pump blood; the muscle tissue of the heart will have to work harder to compensate through cardiac output. The heart will require more oxygen and nutrients to supply energy to the heart muscle for its contraction. If the coronary arteries supplying blood to the heart narrow as other vessels do, there could be a problem with cardiac output which could not be compensated by changes in blood pressure in the peripheral vessel as they are less compliant.

Brain

The cardiovascular system supplies blood to the brain. A poor supply can lead to cells of the brain not receiving enough nutrients to maintain themselves resulting in loss of neurons.

Chapter Reference

Blood supplies are discussed in Chapter 7, 'Breathing' (see p. 184).

Senses

The lens of the eye grows throughout life adding crystalline protein fibres. These gradually reduce the ability of the eye to change focus. The pigments found in the rods and cones are formed of retinol, a lipid similar to vitamin A, coupled to opsin proteins. Lipofuscin accumulates decreasing the amount of pigments in the eye reducing vision.

The sensory cells in our ears may degenerate causing reduction in hearing. Loud noises can cause breaks in the sensory hairs in the inner ear, reducing our capacity to hear across many frequencies of sound.

Chapter Reference

The senses are discussed in Chapter 4, 'Communicating' (see p. 102).

Temperature regulation

Sensory receptors rely on oxygen supplies to maintain their ATP levels for electrical potentials. Oxygen levels rely on blood supply. This can decrease in the ageing skin and lead to reduction in sensitivity to temperature. Vasoconstriction and dilation may also be compromised. In cold weather this can lead to hypothermia.

Chapter Reference

Body temperature is discussed in Chapter 5, 'Controlling and Repairing' (see p. 142).

Kidneys

The kidneys regulate pH which, as shown in Table 13.4, needs to be kept within a very strict limit. pH is a measure of hydrogen ion concentration. Hydrogen ions are formed during metabolism. They are neutralised by binding to bicarbonate ions in the extracellular fluids and blood and are then excreted by the kidneys. Bicarbonate ions formed from carbon dioxide and water via carbonic acid:

$$CO_2 + H_2O = H_2CO_3 = HCO_3^- + H^+$$

The circulatory system transports buffered ions to the kidneys can. Any failure in the circulatory system or the kidneys can, therefore, have very serious effects on pH and acidosis of the body fluids.

Health Connection

Ageing and disease – Links to practice

Not all older people will get the diseases discussed below, but these are quite common in ageing. The disease of Alzheimer's and dementias are probably an over-diagnosed group of diseases and may reflect how older people are treated rather than clinical diagnosis. Living in old people's homes or being in hospital wards reduces independence. Care is not always high and many people are probably suffering from dehydration (the effects are similar to dementias) and malnutrition rather than some of the clinical diseases below.

Diseases of ageing

The diseases of ageing are

- degenerative diseases where the homeostasic mechanism of balancing cell numbers to need is no longer maintained and more cells are lost than are replaced;
- traumas, such as stroke and myocardial infarction;
- excess, hyperplasia, for instance fat cells and fat storage;
- infections.

The causes of these diseases can be a

- genetic predisposition, where there is a gene that makes us more susceptible to a disease, but may not act in youth or may need other factors such as lifestyle choices;
- lifestyle and environmental factors.

Atherosclerosis

This is caused by a build-up of lipids in artery walls. The lipids combine with calcium and cell debris to form plaques on the artery walls, narrowing the arteries regardless of blood pressure. This can lead to hypertension, which increases blood pressure. Diabetes and obesity are major contributors to atherosclerosis.

Type II diabetes mellitus (adult onset diabetes)

This can make one insensitive to insulin and leads to increase in blood glucose and decrease in cellular glucose. It can lead to the dehydration of tissues due to altering osmotic pressure and the loss of glucose in urine due to changes in osmotic pressure in the kidney renal tubules and the decrease in tubular re-absorption of glucose back into the blood. It can lead to reduction in blood volume and inadequate blood flow to tissues. The heart then pumps more to try to compensate. If there is atherosclerosis as well in the vascular system the heart will need to compensate further.

Obesity

This can be associated with type II diabetes. There is a reduction in the effect of insulin and, therefore, in the regulation of glucose levels in the body cells. A high fat diet is associated with atherosclerosis. As blood supply to heart decreases the risk of ischaemic heart disease increases leading to myocardial infarction or heart attack. While some of the world is suffering from a lack of nutrients (malnutrition) it must be remembered that one can have too many nutrients – hyper-nutrition.

Stroke

This is caused by a rupture of the blood vessel wall. A clot forms in the vessel (haemostasis – discussed in the blood section of Chapter 7, 'Breathing'). The effect is a lack of oxygen reaching cells in the brain. The cells die. It can be associated with intracerebral bleeding, which can lead to death. It again can lead to coronary or vascular problems.

Cardiovascular shock

This can lead to an insufficient blood flow to tissues. It is caused by heart attacks or haemorrhage.

Haemorrhage

This is a sudden loss of blood volume. It will lead to a drop in blood pressure and a decrease in blood supply to all tissues; a reduced supply of oxygen and nutrients and a build up of waste. This form of trauma has a severe effect on other homeostasic mechanisms.

Respiratory acidosis

Ventilation is controlled by the respiratory centre in the medulla. It increases ventilation when extracellular carbon dioxide levels rise. Respiratory insufficiency (inability to get rid of waste carbon dioxide) in many pathologies is not caused by lack of inspired oxygen, but by some abnormality in the exchange of gases across the pulmonary membrane or by failure in oxygen transport from the lungs to the tissues. Increasing inspiration does not alleviate situation. Air hunger – **dyspnoea** (gasping for breath) – can also lead to mental anguish.

The pulmonary system removes carbon dioxide from the blood and transports oxygen from the lungs to the heart for the systemic and cardiac circulation. Pulmonary ventilation is needed therefore to control carbon dioxide levels. If pulmonary ventilation decreases, the concentration of carbon dioxide increases in extracellular fluid and the equation shown in the kidney section above moves to the right:

$$CO_2 + H_2O = H_2CO_3 = HCO_3^- + H^+$$

This results in decrease in pH with an increase in hydrogen ion concentration and the acidity of the body fluids increases. This is **respiratory acidosis**.

You can induce respiratory acidosis by holding your breath. This will reduce pulmonary ventilation and the exchange of gases in the alveoli of the lungs will be slowed down. Carbon dioxide will be produced at same rate from cellular respiration:

$$O_2 + glucose = ATP + CO_2 + H_2O$$

But as the carbon dioxide is not being removed in the lungs it will remain in the plasma and then it will rise in the extracellular fluid. The pH drops to a dangerous level. Your respiratory centre in the medulla of your brain will encourage you to start breathing!

During ill health respiratory acidosis is caused by blockages of airways and the reduction in efficiency of gas exchange. This can be seen in bronchitis and pneumonia. It can also result from kidney failure as hydrogen ions are not excreted (discussed above).

Other causes include diarrhoea where faeces are excreted from the large bowel too fast for water and ions (electrolytes) to be re-absorbed back into the blood. This leads to excessive loss of bicarbonate ions and the equation again moves to the right with hydrogen ions being released into the body fluids:

$$CO_2 + H_2O = H_2CO_3 = HCO_3^- + H^+$$

Box 13.3 Summary – Ageing

- Normal ageing may result in the slowing down of many body processes. As this occurs one becomes aware of the interactions between all the body's various control systems and the narrowness of the normal range for constituents of intracellular fluids, extracellular fluids for cells to survive.
- Values outside these ranges lead to death.
- Ageing may lead to loss of function, less reserve capacity and the body can easily be pushed beyond the line between competence and failure.

Another cause of respiratory acidosis is diabetes. Here glucose uptake is insufficient so fats are broken down instead. This leads to the release of fatty acids and the acidity of extracellular fluid rises.

There is thus an interdependence of many different bodily functions to maintain pH.

Dying

Immediate cause of death

From the table of main causes of death and the fact that many countries issue death certificates, death is categorised by cause and old age does not appear to be sufficient. Many death certificates state the cause of death as cardiovascular complications due to the interactions of many body systems. It may be over-diagnosed, therefore, as a cause of death (as may dementias, discussed above). In fact, as stated above a 70-year-old person has a decreased cardiac output compared to a 30-year-old person, but it may be sufficient for normal functions. The causes of deaths and their percentages are listed in Table 13.2.

Clinical death

For a few minutes after the heart has stopped beating and breathing has ceased it is possible to revive the patient. Even with sudden death from haemorrhage or cardiac arrest, most cells are still viable and first aid may succeed. This makes it hard to say when death occurs.

The **agonal** (struggle) phase of death is where the muscles spasm. These spasms of muscular activity can include the tightening of laryngeal muscles in the larynx as air in lungs is expired, but the dying person is probably unaware of it. This is because the brain fails first if circulation ceases. The brain can only use glucose to combine with oxygen to make ATP energy and it has no stores of glucose, needing a constant supply from the blood brought by the cardiovascular system. Without a sufficient supply of glucose the person therefore will be unconscious.

At death the face changes colour. A **corpse** (dead body) looks different from an unconscious person. The choice to attempt resuscitation relies on medical experience. Often looking in the eyes helps to make that decision as they go glassy dulled with dilated pupils, then the eyeballs flatten out. There is a lack of a pulse as the cardiovascular system ceases. The skin becomes dull as oxygen gives the skin its bloom and it is no longer being inhaled. The cells stop functioning although some tissues, e.g. kidney, can survive half an hour and heart cells can survive 15 minutes, which means that nowadays they can be transplanted. Anaerobic processes (metabolic processes not requiring oxygen) continue; for example the liver continues to break down alcohol. Within hours of death the body shrinks due to a loss of air which is expired.

Newly dead muscle is flaccid; it becomes rigid within hours (**rigor mortis**) due to the cross-linking of actin molecules in muscles. Aerobic metabolism has ceased and the bonds are not broken, as ATP is needed to break bonds and the formation of ATP requires oxygen. Eventually, a few days later, stiffness leaves the muscles of the corpse as lysosomal enzymes from resident commensal bacteria break down actin cross-links.

Defining death

Defining life is hard; defining the moment of death is equally hard as many biological processes occur in each. They are continuous processes rather than sudden.

There are various legal and clinical definitions of death. For many years the definition from Judaism, the cessation of breathing for half an hour, was used. For the past 30 years brain stem death has been used. In the UK brain stem death is the major criterion for defining death. It is characterised by absent brain stem activity and absent tendon reflexes. Brain death and death of the central nervous system in general define death for many. This is characterised by

persistent apnoeic (no breathing) and an electrically silent brain with no electrophysiological activity in the superficial or deeper parts of the brain. The irreversible loss of brain stem functions results in

- inability to be conscious,
- inability to breathe.

Coma is also part of the characteristic. Coma can show many of the same signs as death:

- absence of cerebral responsiveness,
- absence of induced or spontaneous movement,
- absence of spontaneous respiration,
- absence of brain stem and deep tendon reflexes.

Hypothermia and drug intoxication might resemble brain death. Comatose patients are tested over 24 hours to ensure persistence of their condition. However, there can be a recovery completely or partially from coma such as seen in **persistent vegetative states** (PVS). In this state the individual can breathe and appear conscious, but they do not react to any stimuli. The vegetative state needs a medical diagnosis. In the vegetative state

- the cerebral cortex has died;
- there may be some brain stem function;
- they may breathe unaided;
- the heartbeat is spontaneous;
- the individual can live for years.

'They may cyclically awaken and sleep, but express no behavioural or cerebral metabolic evidence of possession of cognitive function or being able to respond in a learned manner to external events and stimuli' (Walton, 1995).

A higher brain functioning ability may be needed to define this state versus death.

This contrasts with the **locked in syndrome** where the individual:

- may appear conscious and alert,
- may be unable to move any body part,
- may be unable to speak or swallow.

- may only be able to communicate through blinking or voluntary eye movement.

Their recovery may be unlikely, but these people are conscious and aware.

Death rather than coma blurs a clear defining line. With increasing medical intervention we can maintain a non-homeostatic life.

Health Connection

Euthanasia

Euthanasia, the voluntary aiding of death, is a very problematic area for clinical practice, going, as it does, against the main aim of clinical practice, to save and prolong life. The decreasing quality of life is used as an argument for the ending of a life that is in terminal illness and no longer deemed to have much quality. Of course this is very problematic for two reasons:

1. All of us are going to die and a terminal illness should not be an automatic reason for ending a life.
2. Who decides what lives are worth living? Health care professionals need to be aware of some of the dangers of this route, which could have enormous impact on those with any form of disability or terminal illness of ageing.

The arguments in favour of euthanasia include

- The human right of the person to decide when to die;
- Not wanting to prolong pain in a person in terminal decline.

Health Connection

Palliative care and care of the elderly

With an increasing ageing population more of us may suffer from long-term decline and morbidity. Palliative care is the care of the dying, rather than the ageing. With an increasing population in general there will be increasing demands for better palliative care for all.

Health Connection

Suicide

Suicide, the deliberate taking of one's own life, is a very hard decision to make and a very hard outcome for others to live with. The survivors, family and friends, are left with guilt and even resentment. The person committing suicide must be in the most desperate situation to think that death is the only way of resolving their problems. Not long ago it was illegal everywhere and only recently have some countries changed their laws. There are charities to help those feeling suicidal such as the Samaritans.

Clinical investigations

Normal homeostatic mechanisms usually correct fluctuations in the internal environment, but if the internal environment alters too much or for too long these mechanisms fail and clinical intervention is needed. Clinical intervention aims to save or prolong lives. To do so requires diagnosing what is not working. This is done by carrying out various tests such as

- Temperature measurements to see if an infection has occurred that would lead to inflammation and a temperature rise while the immune system tries to kill off the invading micro-organism.
- Blood gas measurements to monitor breathing and blood flow.
- Blood pressure measurements to monitor the systemic blood system and assess if there is haemorrhage.
- Heart beat measurements to assess the fitness of the heart.
- Urine constituents to measure the functioning of the kidney and liver.
- Neurological measurements to assess the functioning of the brain and consciousness.

The results are then analysed and a decision made as to what is malfunctioning. Appropriate intervention is then administered such as antibiotics to kill off bacteria, blood or saline to alter blood pressure or electric stimulation to start the heart beating. The point is that it is very difficult to make a rapid and accurate analysis as to what is the cause of the problem. Death is the likely and normal outcome of extreme variations in the internal environment. Clinical intervention goes against this natural course of events.

Conclusion: Dying

It seems that part of being alive is being mortal. Our bodies grow and maintain themselves and finally cease to do that, cease to maintain homeostasis. When this occurs we become ill and dependent. If we cannot survive we die.

There are many causes of death; each organ and tissue can fail. Clinical interventions attempt to put off death and **care** of the ill, the disabled, the elderly and the dying is one of the measures of a civilised society. As an ADL we all want a 'good death'. For many of us that means pain free, comfortable and having had time to sort out our lives and come to some conclusion.

Chapter Summary

- All living organisms are mortal and have a limited lifespan.
- Within an organism such as a human, different cells have different lifespans.
- Cells and tissues are constantly being replaced as they degenerate.
- Degeneration may be part of a normal 'ageing' process.
- Eventually it seems that more cells need replacing than there are cells, such as stem cells, to replace dying cells.
- When too many cells die, life is compromised.
- Biological causes of death relate to organ failures.
- There are various stages of clinical death.
- Deciding when somebody is dead relies on both measurements of clinical organ function and definitions of lack of function.
- Coma and persistent vegetative states blur the line between healthy homeostatic people and dependent and incurable patients.
- Euthanasia presents many problems for clinical practice.
- Palliative care in an ageing population is increasingly needed.

Finale

The biological living processes and their activities of daily living, which are a measure of health, include dying. How you live, the aims and purpose you give to your life, can also make an impact on your health. It is not just what we do, but how we do it. We can survive or we can thrive and there is science and art in that. Many political and economic movements as well as health are interested in 'thriving'.

Unfortunately, many of us only come to appreciate our life and health when we have gone through a life-threatening situation or diminished health. I hope you all appreciate your lives without needing to be in that situation and get great joy from it. Enjoying work and study forms the basis of thriving for many people. As Confucius says

> Choose a job you love and you will never have to work a day in your life.

If you intend to become a professional in the health field and are interested in helping people to live, and particularly helping people to live well, to thrive, I hope you have good fortune in your aim and I send you much heartfelt thanks.

Index

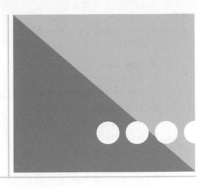

NOTE: Page references in *italics* refer to figures and tables.

S/NVQ Level **3**

Technical Certificate

18·89
✗

Business & Administration

Carol Carysforth

Maureen Rawlinson

Alison Chadwick

www.heinemann.co.uk
✓ Free online support
✓ Useful weblinks
✓ 24 hour online ordering

01865 888058

Heinemann

Inspiring generations

Heinemann Educational Publishers
Halley Court, Jordan Hill, Oxford OX2 8EJ
Part of Harcourt Education

Heinemann is the registered trademark of Harcourt Education Limited

First published 2006

10 09 08 07 06
10 9 8 7 6 5 4 3 2 1

British Library Cataloguing in Publication Data is available
from the British Library on request.

10-digit ISBN: 0 435 463 34 9
13-digit ISBN: 978 0 435463 34 2

Typeset and illustrated by 🖊 Tek Art
Original illustrations © Harcourt Education Limited, 2006
Cover design by Wooden Ark
Printed in the UK by Scotprint
Picture research by Chrissie Martin and Natalie Gray

Contents

Optional units on the CD

Unit 314 Word processing software

Unit 315 Spreadsheet software

Group A option units

(Units repeated from Level 2)
110 Ensure your own actions reduce risks to health and safety
204 Manage diary systems
205 Organise business travel and accommodation
213 Use IT to exchange information
216 Use database software
217 Use presentation software

Answers Section
Notes on punctuation and use of English
Index

Acknowledgements

The authors would like to record their personal thanks to all those friends and associates whose advice and expertise proved so invaluable to the writing of this book.

We are particularly indebted to the following people for their assistance with our case studies: Linda Barton, FIQPS and Chairman of the Institute of Qualified Professional Secretaries; Rachel Bretherton; Alison Henderson, BA (Hons), GIPD; and Carolyn Lee. Thanks, too, are due to Christine Blackham for her help and advice on the IT units.

We are also extremely grateful for the guidance provided by Margaret Reid, a Consultant in Administration, Technical Certificates and Key Skills to a leading awarding body. She is also a Lead EV in a number of business-related awards for the same awarding body. Her input helped to ensure that all the evidence guidance provided in this book is accurate, up-to-date and meets all the latest scheme requirements and her positive and efficient contributions throughout the project were very much appreciated.

As ever, we would like to thank all those at Heinemann who have worked so hard to make this book into a reality. Especial thanks are due to Mary James, publishing manager, for her constant support and encouragement; to Jilly Atwood, our publisher on this project, for her enthusiasm, energy and efficiency; to Roger Parker for his expert editing; and to Melissa Greaves, Alistair Nunn and Liz Evans, editors, for their forbearance and attention to detail.

Carol Carysforth, Maureen Rawlinson and Alison Chadwick
April 2006

Dedication

This book is dedicated to Holly, the newest member of the Carysforth clan. May you be blessed with an open and encouraging mind, a warm heart and the confidence to believe that you can achieve your dreams.

The author and publisher would like to thank the following individuals and organisations for permission to reproduce material:

Oxfam – page 58
ACAS – page 58
Employer's Forum on Disability – page 163
Copyright Licensing Agency – page 174
IQPS – page 349

Photo acknowledgements
Getty – pages 1, 7, 14
Corbis – pages 33, 171, 203, 216, 330, 381
Alamy – pages 37, 41, 71
Corbis/Paul Handy – page 94
Courtesy Mackies – page 111
Natalie Gray – pages 114, 281
TopFoto.co.uk – page 125
Jon Feingersh/zefa/Corbis – pages 135, 190
Getty Images/Photodisc – pages 140, 197, 270, 273, 285, 319
Digital Vision – page 161
Ingo Boddenberg/zefa/Corbis – page 199
Kevin Wilton; Eye Ubiquitous/Corbis – page 211
allOver photography/Alamy – page 223
M. Thomsen/zefa/Corbis – page 228
Stone/Getty – page 229
Image Source/Alamy – page 236
Image Source/Rex Features – page 239
ImageState/Alamy – page 254
Jack Sullivan/Alamy – page 259
Nicholas Bailey/Rex Features – page 266
ITV Granada – page 289
Janine Wiedel/Photolibrary/Alamy – page 294
The Photolibrary Wales/Alamy – page 300
Bill Varie/Corbis – page 309
Startraks/Rex Features – page 330
A. Inden/zefa/Corbis – page 333
BBC Panaroma/Corbis Sygma – page 342
Phanie/Rex Features – page 345
AFP/Getty – page 355
Aflo Foto Agency/Alamy – page 359
Richard Cooke/Alamy – page 365
Duomo/Corbis – page 371

Getty Images – Unit 314 page 1, Unit 315 page 1
Steven May/Alamy – Unit 314 page 4

Introduction

Welcome to NVQ Business and Administration level 3. If you are new to NVQ awards then you need to take time to understand the scheme and what you have to do. This is because there is quite a difference between the way you achieve an NVQ and other awards, such as GCSEs.

If you have already taken an NVQ award, such as NVQ level 2 Business and Administration, then you can safely skip most of this section, unless you took your award some time ago and need to refresh your memory. However, you may still find some other sections useful, particularly those that relate to the structure of this book and the accompanying CD-ROM and how these have been designed to help you (see page xii).

Understanding NVQ awards

- NVQs are qualifications designed for people in the workplace. At level 3, all your evidence to prove you are competent at carrying out specific tasks must be generated through undertaking real workplace activities.
- NVQ awards are offered at different levels. The level you take usually depends upon how much responsibility you have. Level 1 is the first level for junior staff; level 5 is the top level and taken by senior managers.
- Business and Administration NVQs cover tasks carried out by administrators working in different businesses and the skills that they need.
- All NVQs consist of a number of units, each covering a specific area of work. To obtain your level 3 award you have to complete six units. *Two* units are compulsory because they cover skills required by all administrators. You then choose a further *four* units. These should be the ones that most closely link to your job role so that the evidence you provide occurs naturally as you do your job.
- There are two groups of option units in the Business and Administration scheme, A and B. At least *three* of your option units must be from group B.
- You are assessed on tasks you can do competently. This means that you can demonstrate or provide evidence to show that you can consistently carry out those tasks to a high standard.
- You must prove that you understand what you are doing and how it relates to your job. You will also be asked how you would adapt your skills if you changed job or worked in a different type of office.
- Most NVQ candidates provide evidence in a portfolio. This is normally an A4 file that contains documentary evidence relating to your work. Electronic portfolio packages are now becoming more popular so, if you are expected to store and record your evidence electronically, you will be shown how to do this. You can find out more about types of evidence on page x of this introduction.

 For advanced apprentices only

If you are on an Advanced Apprenticeship scheme then you will also be taking Key Skills qualifications in Communications level 2 and Application of Number level 2 as well as a Technical Certificate at level 3. The Technical Certificate will also test your knowledge of many areas of business and administration (see page xiii). The Council for Administration (CfA) also recommend that you complete at least one IT unit from the optional units available.

Working to achieve your NVQ

You will be guided through the scheme by your tutor, trainer or workplace supervisor, depending on where you work and where you are studying for your award. This person will be responsible for helping you to learn new skills and understand the administrative tasks you will be carrying out, as well as finding out more about your organisation and other important aspects of work, such as your employment rights and responsibilities.

You will prove your competence at certain tasks to your assessor who will check your evidence to make sure it meets the requirements of the scheme. For example, your assessor will visit you at work to watch you perform some tasks and carry out professional discussions. This simply means your assessor will want to discuss certain aspects of your job role with you. It is called a *professional discussion* to differentiate it from a casual chat, because it is much more important. You can prepare for this by following the advice given throughout this book and, of course, by carrying out any preparation your assessor has requested on your assessment/action plan for a particular discussion. At the end of the professional discussion, your assessor may decide that more information is needed about your knowledge and understanding, and either verbal or written questions will follow the discussion. If your assessor is then satisfied, you will be judged competent.

At certain intervals an internal verifier will also sample and check your evidence. This is normally done as you progress and when you complete the award. Then a final quality check is made by the external verifier who is sent by your awarding body. This is the organisation that will issue your final NVQ certificate, such as EDI, City & Guilds, OCR, Edexcel, IMI or SQA.

You will not know which units may be checked by a verifier, but if your assessor has judged you to be competent in those units, this normally means that there are no problems.

You may like to note that in certain circumstances one person may act as both your tutor/trainer and assessor. That person will be extremely careful to ensure that your training is kept completely separate from any assessment that takes place and this will be monitored by an internal verifier.

Providing evidence

You will need to provide evidence to your assessor that you are competent at each area of performance specified in a unit as well as understanding the knowledge items that are listed. There are two main ways in which you can do this.

- **Performance evidence** is direct proof of how you work. There are two types of performance evidence.
  - **Work products**, such as documents you have created. This could be a diary page or telephone message, email or typed document – depending on the unit you are doing. It is even better if it has your own notes on it or if you have your draft notes together with a final version. Alternatively you can keep a work diary or work log of tasks you do and then use this as a basis for a professional discussion with your assessor (see below).
  - **Observation by your assessor** when you are at work, such as when you are dealing with a customer or sending a fax or email. In this case it is better if your assessor visits you at a time when you are busy doing various jobs – and you just act naturally and get on with your work.
- **Supplementary evidence** is used in situations when there is no direct performance evidence, such as when you are trying to prove that you behave in a certain way or understand something. Again there are different types of supplementary evidence.
  - **A professional discussion** between you and your assessor will give you the opportunity to demonstrate how you behave, or demonstrate your competence, in your present job role. In addition, this method of assessment will be used when you have not had the opportunity in your current job role to prove competence and you will need to show how you would behave in certain situations or circumstances. Your assessor will identify which situations or circumstances you need to be prepared to discuss.
  - **Witness testimony** is a signed and dated statement from your line manager, supervisor or colleagues to confirm something you have done. It is often easier to write a full description yourself and then ask your boss or supervisor to sign and date this statement to confirm it is true.

A dedicated task might be set by your assessor to enable you to demonstrate your knowledge of a situation that you may not meet during the actual assessment period.

Key facts about evidence

For your award you do not collect evidence separately for the core units. Instead you use the evidence you collect for your option units to count twice, wherever possible. This means, for example, that you prove that you can communicate information (core unit 301) through the tasks that involve communications in your option units. You then cross-reference this evidence to both the option unit and to the appropriate sections of core unit 301.

Two features in this book will help you to do this more easily, as you will see on page xii of this introduction.

Many administrators think that they must always provide a piece of paper to prove what they have done. This isn't true! As you will see with the suggestions for evidence in this book, there are several other ways. For example, you can note the location of documents that are used by everyone – such as the procedures to follow if you receive a customer complaint or if you carry out a risk assessment. You do not need to make a copy for your portfolio. Similarly, if you produce documents on a computer there is no need to print out dozens! Simply include one or two examples in your portfolio and include a reference to say where other examples are saved on your system. You can then show these to your assessor if requested.

 IMPORTANT!

Make sure that you read all the information and guidance notes issued by your awarding body so that you understand:

- the performance indicators for the units you are doing
- the knowledge that is required
- the recommended evidence suggested by your awarding body
- the way in which you must record your evidence.

Don't hesitate to ask your tutor or trainer to explain anything that you are unsure about. This is particularly important if you choose optional units that have been imported from other schemes which may include additional elements. For example, if you select a unit imported from the Management Standards you will have to demonstrate specific behaviours as well as your understanding of certain types of contextual knowledge. You may also find that some of the assessment requirements for the IT units, imported from e-skills UK, are slightly different depending on your awarding body.

The structure of this book and features to help you achieve your award

This book has been written to help you to achieve your award as smoothly as possible. It covers all the information for the two core units and the most popular option units. If you are on an Advanced Apprenticeship scheme and are studying for a Technical Certificate at the same time, you can cover key topics as you go, to save you covering the same areas over and over again. You can find out more about the links to the Technical Certificate on page xiii.

Features in this book to help you

In addition to the knowledge and information you need to be able to carry out various tasks, the following features have been included to help you achieve your award more easily.

- **How to...** features summarise the steps to do a task properly. These features link to many of the performance indicators (PIs). These are the tasks you have to prove you can do competently.
- **Evidence planning** sections in the core units help you to prepare for the way you will link the core units evidence with the evidence you will collect in your option units.
- **Evidence collection** sections in the option units suggest appropriate evidence that you can collect that is not always paper-based!
- **Core unit link** features show you how the evidence you may be able to collect in the option units will link to the core units so that you can cross-reference the evidence to both units.
- **What if...?** features tell you what to do if you are unable to provide any particular type of evidence during the time you are being assessed.
- **Snapshots** and **case studies** in the option units enable you to see how specific tasks are carried out in different types of organisations.
- **Changing places** features give you examples of other ways in which certain tasks may be undertaken. This is important because your assessor will ask you questions to check that you would be able to transfer your skills if you changed your job in the future.
- **Over to you** sections enable you to check your own knowledge of the information given so far and investigate some aspects further on your own.

... and on the CD-ROM

As well as additional Group A optional units and the IT units 314 and 315, the CD-ROM also gives you suggested answers to the 'Over to you' features and case studies as well as an invaluable Use of English section to help you to check and improve your communication skills.

Links to Technical Certificate

Don't forget!

If you have already achieved one of the Group A optional units at level 2, you can count this again towards your level 3 award.

If you are also studying for a Technical Certificate at level 3 then you should note that many certificate topics are covered in this book. Those on which you need to focus will vary, depending on the scheme issued by your particular awarding body. You can look up any topics you want to find in the index at the end of this book, but you might also like to note the main sections where you can find specific types of information. These are shown in the table below.

Topic	Units and pages
Business purpose and values	Unit 302, pages 95 – 119
Change management	Unit 302, pages 83 – 5
Communicating verbally and in writing	Unit 301, pages 2 – 31
Communicating by email	Unit 213, pages 2 – 24 (CD)
Confidentiality	Unit 302, pages 170 – 178
Continuous improvement and personal development	Unit 301, pages 54 – 70
Contract of employment	Unit 302, pages 141 – 4
Data Protection and copyright legislation	Unit 302, pages 129 – 131, 174
Dealing with other people	Unit 301, pages 71 – 92; + Units 303, 305, 320 and 321
Diversity	Unit 302, pages 161 – 8
Employment rights and responsibilities (including employment legislation)	Unit 302, pages 131 – 156
Health and safety legislation and risk assessments	Unit 301, pages 126 – 9, Unit 302, pages 179 – 89 and Unit 110 (CD)
House style	Unit 301, page 13; Unit 217, page 13 (CD)
Internet software	Unit 213, pages 24 – 32 (CD)
Leading a team	Unit 321
Planning, targets and meeting deadlines	Unit 301, pages 32 – 50
Productive working relations with colleagues	Unit 301, pages 71 – 92 and Unit 320
Researching and reporting information	Unit 310
Security of property and information	Unit 302, pages 170 – 78
Self-development/improvement	Unit 301, pages 54 – 70
Sources of information	Unit 310
Supervising an office facility	Unit 303
Systems and procedures	Unit 302, pages 113 – 155
Time management and working effectively	Unit 301, pages 40 – 43; Unit 204 (CD)
Working with other people	Unit 301, pages 71 – 92; Units 303, 305, 320 and 321
Workflow management	Unit 301, pages 32 – 50

Links to Key Skills

At the end of each unit you will find a reminder to check whether any evidence you have collected for that unit can be cross-referenced to a Key Skills award. It is sensible to check the matrix issued by your awarding body which shows where possible Key Skills opportunities occur in the Business and Administration core units and your chosen option units. However, you should check carefully with your assessor before assuming that the evidence you are offering will definitely meet the requirements of both.

Carol Carysforth, Maureen Rawlinson and Alison Chadwick
April 2006

Carry out your responsibilities at work

Unit summary and overview

This core unit is divided into four sections:

- communicate information
- plan and be accountable for your work
- improve your own performance
- behave in a way that supports effective working.

Your ability to communicate effectively and to get the right information to the right people at the right time is all-important in a smooth-running office. You also need the skills to get people to listen to you and act on what you're saying, and to be able to persuade them to read and understand what you have written. You must be able to be selective about the information you read and extract what to pass on to others. In addition, you will be expected to contribute to discussions and have the ability to develop useful points and ideas.

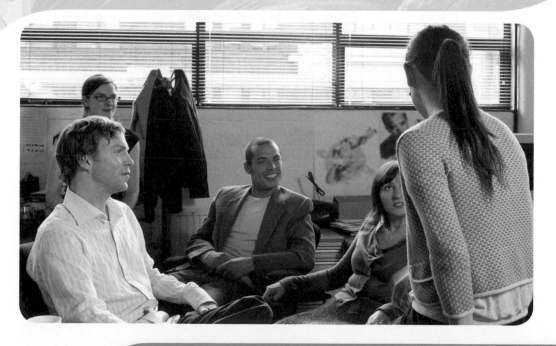

Link to option units

Your evidence for this unit will be generated and assessed through the option units that you select. This is because your option units should reflect the main areas of your job role so your evidence will occur naturally as you carry out your day-to-day work. For each option unit in this book, therefore, you will find guidance notes to show how evidence can be cross-referenced to this unit.

Within this unit you will also find suggestions to help you plan your evidence. These will help you to make the most of opportunities for obtaining evidence as you progress through the scheme.

Your planning skills will also be vital to your efficiency and to success in your job. You have to be able to set and achieve targets, prioritise these and help others to do the same. You have to be a problem-solver, to know when to get help if you need it and to take responsibility for your own work, but you must also realise when it is essential to obtain advice or check specific guidelines or procedures to follow.

No matter how well you can do your job, complacency is never a virtue! Encouraging feedback from other people, evaluating your own work and identifying how you can make improvements will all help you to set, and work towards, long-term career goals.

Even if you have high standards, regularly show that you can cope with pressure and are willing to accept a challenge, you need also to be aware of the way in which your behaviour can affect other people. The ideal is when you work efficiently and effectively yourself but still make time to help and support other people and always treat all your colleagues considerately.

Developing all these skills isn't easy but is all part of the challenge to you as you learn to carry out your own responsibilities at work.

Communicate information

You might have been on a training course where, as an ice-breaker, your group was asked to put together a puzzle without speaking to each other or using any non-verbal communication. If so, you probably found it a bit difficult. That's hardly surprising given that not many of us go through a day without talking or writing to someone else.

Why effective communication is important

It's easy enough to communicate. Whatever form you use the person listening to you is getting some information. What he or she may not be doing, however, is getting the right message, the message you want to communicate.

If you constantly snap at people rather than speaking to them pleasantly they might not want to hang around long enough to make sure they know what you want. If you send someone a badly written email full of spelling mistakes he or she might get the impression that you're not all that bright and that what you've written isn't worth reading.

How to... Make sure people listen to you

- **Use language that fits the occasion.** When the late Mo Mowlam addressed people as 'babe' during meetings in Northern Ireland, she did it for a purpose – she wanted to avoid too much formality. In most other top-level meetings you would probably use a more formal mode of address.

- **Use the right level.** You would talk to primary school children in a different way from speaking to a group of university students.

- **Allow people to respond to you.** If you never allow anyone else to speak you are missing out a vital part of the communication process. If you send an email but take no notice of any responses you are only involving yourself in one part of the communication process.

- **Get attention.** Interest your listeners in what you are trying to tell them and engage their attention.

Focussing actively on what others are communicating

Have you ever tried to talk to someone about something that really interested you and been disappointed at the lack of response? Have you ever suspected that in some cases they aren't *really* listening to you? Have you ever been guilty of doing exactly the same thing if someone is trying to communicate with you? Nowadays a lot of emphasis is put on 'active' listening – as distinct from staring at someone with a glazed expression hoping he or she will shut up soon so that you can get a coffee. *Listening with a purpose* can actually be quite hard work.

Blocks to listening

At one of your meetings your line manager arranges for a member of the health and safety team to come to update you about recent developments. Some of you find it useful. Others don't – partially because they are blocking out the information.
- Charlie judges the speaker too quickly – 'She seems a bit too sure of herself', 'I don't like people who say "you know" after every second

Did you know?

You may have heard the old saying 'We are given two ears but only one mouth, because God knew that listening was twice as hard as talking.'

Did you know?

Researchers have found that it takes 50 per cent more effort to listen than to speak. Apparently you can speak without really understanding what is going on, but not listen!

word', 'Come on, come on – get to the point!'. The speaker may not have been very good at expressing herself but that doesn't mean that she doesn't have something valuable to say.

- Raies keeps second guessing her – 'Here we go again', 'She's singing the usual tune', 'Well I won't learn anything from her'. By thinking in advance that you know what someone is going to say you might be cutting yourself off from useful information.

- Sandy keeps trying to reinterpret the information to make it something she wants to hear. She doesn't want to have to worry about having an accident at work so she concentrates on the figures that say the possibility of that happening is very low.

- Henry has definite likes and dislikes. He takes a dislike to the speaker because he thinks she is too much of a know-it-all. He allows his listening skills to be affected by his emotions. If you don't like someone you're less likely to take on board what he or she is saying, however sensible.

Being an effective listener

You have to try to avoid blocks to listening.

- **Be willing to listen.** Practise paying attention no matter how boring the topic might be. Try to shut out any distractions, either physical or mental. If you have any control over the situation try to minimise these distractions. If the room is too hot, put on the air conditioning or open a window. If it is too noisy, switch off the equipment, put a hold on telephone calls, shut the door etc. If you feel your attention wandering, make a conscious effort to tune back into the conversation.

- **Encourage the speaker.** Good listeners give both verbal and non-verbal signs that they are listening. Staring out of the window with

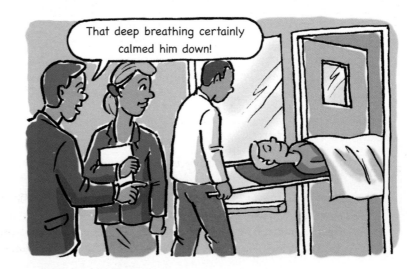

That deep breathing certainly calmed him down!

your feet propped up on the edge of a chair won't help the speaker to feel at ease or to give of his or her best. The occasional smile or nod helps. So too does good eye contact. Not only are you being polite to the speaker, you are also picking up his or her non-verbal signals, which helps the whole communication process.

- **Avoid over-reacting.** The speaker may say something that triggers a strong emotion in you. If, for instance, you happen to be strongly in favour of building a new motorway and the speaker makes a disparaging remark about it, don't let your emotions get in the way of what otherwise might be some very relevant information.

 How to... Actively focus on information other people are communicating and question parts you are unsure about

- **Pay particular attention** to certain key phrases such as 'What I must get across…', 'What really concerns me…', 'I'd like you to…', 'The key date is…'. These tend to signal 'must know' information.

- **Be prepared to respond** when required. It not only lets the speaker know that his or her message is being received, it also allows you to clarify your own thoughts. The act of speaking out loud what you have heard helps you to understand and remember the information. Obviously it can be mildly irritating to the speaker if you parrot every sentence he or she utters, or if you constantly interrupt; but, if used wisely, asking works.

- **Give direct feedback** on what you think. 'Fine, I'll get on to it' shows that you have fully understood the message. 'I think I understand what you want but can I get back to you if I have any further questions?' This tells the speaker that you have taken on board most of what has been said but there are one or two points you might not have fully understood.

 Did you know?

A quarter of all workers questioned for a recent Investors in People survey complained that their managers took little or no notice of their views and failed to consult them when making decisions. Most of them said they longed for the chance to be listened to!

Focussing actively on written communication

It's easy to miss the point or drift into a daydream if you are looking at written communication. Later on in this unit is some guidance on how to prepare written documents that help the reader to understand. Not all writers, however, are willing to take the time and effort in making sure that what they have written is reader-friendly. In such cases you, as the reader, have to avoid the temptation to skim read or – worse – give up half way through and throw it in the waste paper bin or delete it. You never know what you might miss.

Structuring and presenting information clearly and accurately

Tempting though it is to sit down and write something off the top of your head it does help if, before you start, you think about what you want to achieve by sending it and what you think is the best method. Sometimes it's a good idea to follow the checklist below to make sure you're getting it right first time.

Communication checklist

Do I know?
- Who is going to read this and why – customer, colleague, boss etc.
- What I want him/her to do – read it, understand it, take action on it etc.
- How I'm going to persuade him/her to do it
- The format I am going to use – email, letter, report, telephone call etc.
- What language I am going to use – relaxed, informal, formal etc.
- How much the reader knows already
- Anything that might stop him/her from reading and/or acting on it

Have I?
- Given the reader enough time to read and act on it
- Avoided sending it the day before his/her holiday, an important meeting etc.
- Avoided thinking too far ahead and expecting him/her to do the same

---

Did you know?

The use of language is constantly evolving and it is quite possible that the apostrophe will disappear at some time in the future, because people are unsure where to put it and it is said that it does not make any difference anyway. For the time being, however, it should be used correctly! If you are unsure, check the Use of English notes on the CD-ROM.

Other than telephone messages or very brief notes between colleagues, most office documents are word processed. In addition they are normally expected to be:
- laid out in a particular way
- normally in sentence (not note) form – although nowadays the use of email is changing this a bit

- grammatically correct, properly spelled and punctuated and free from jargon
- written in the correct style – formal or informal as the case may be.

Each business document requires a different format and structure.

Letters

Letters are now a less used form of communication. In an informal world they are still quite formal and there is still a recognised way of producing them. The Plain English Guide to writing letters recommends the following:

- A letter needs a beginning, a middle and an end.
- The beginning depends on whether you are sending or answering a letter. If you are answering one, then you should start with 'Thank you for your letter of…', not 'I acknowledge receipt of your letter of…'. If you decide to use a heading, don't use all capitals or put 'Re' at the beginning. Use lower case and bold for a simpler result.
- If you are on first-name terms with the reader use 'Dear Ray'; otherwise use 'Dear Mr Smith', 'Dear Mrs/Miss Smith'. If you are writing to a woman and don't know whether or not she is married use 'Dear Ms Smith'.
- In very formal letters or letters where you don't know the name of the reader you can use 'Dear Sir', 'Dear Madam' or 'Dear Sir or Madam'.
- In the middle part of the letter you should put your points, answers and questions in a logical order. If it is a long letter, use sub-headings. You should also paragraph throughout – generally about three to four sentences to each paragraph.
- The end doesn't need to be a summary of what you have already written. All you need is a final sentence – 'I hope you find this of use', 'If you want any further information please let me know', 'Thank you for your help' etc.
- If you begin your letter with a person's name you should end it with 'Yours sincerely'. Otherwise use 'Yours faithfully'.

Find out

Some organisations use a computer program to store standard letters, such as requests for payment or account information, paragraph by paragraph. If you want to send a particular letter all you do is key in the numbers of the paragraphs for a final result. Check to see whether you have this facility in your own organisation.

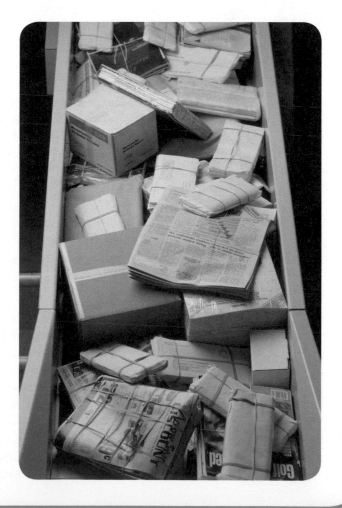

You probably use a style of your own or house style when you are sending out your own work letters. However, the table below gives you some examples of good opening and closing lines.

Types of opening and closing lines in a letter

OPENING LINES

Do say:

- Thank you for your letter of 8 June
- In reply to your letter
- I should like to enquire about
- After having seen your advertisement in …, I should like
- I recently wrote to you about
- I should be grateful if you would give me the following information
- Is it possible for you to let me know
- I wish to complain about
- I should like to thank you for

Don't say:

- I am writing to say
- Re your recent letter

CLOSING LINES

Do say:

- If you require any further information, please let me know
- I look forward to your reply
- I look forward to hearing from you
- I look forward to meeting you
- I look forward to hearing from you shortly
- I should be grateful if you would look into this matter as soon as possible

Don't say:

- Looking forward to hearing from you
- Hope to hear from you
- Awaiting your reply

Emails

Traditionally the email has been regarded as a very informal type of communication. This is changing, however, particularly since people have begun to realise that they can be held just as responsible for any defamatory or stupid remarks they transmit by email as they can for those made in a letter or report. In addition certain rules for structuring emails have begun to be widely accepted:

- Where possible restrict the information to a small number of short paragraphs or a list of numbered points. If you want to transmit a lot of information, consider using the attachment facility – although current thinking is to avoid doing this as many receivers are becoming more reluctant to open attachments because of the increased prevalence of viruses that can come through them.

- Use the subject line to clearly describe the topic of your email. This is helpful for both the recipient and you if you want to find a message you've sent.
- Include only one subject per email message. It makes email filing and retrieval simpler.
- For a lengthy or complicated email, create the message in your word processing program and then copy to your email. Then if there is a problem in the sending process, you can easily retrieve the information.
- When replying to an email, attach enough of the old message for the recipient to remember the content of the original email but delete unnecessary information.
- It used to be thought that no email should be signed. However if you want to hit a particularly informal note there's no harm in adding your name or an email signature. Be careful, however, with the more formal emails. They are still regarded as 'letters on screen'.

If you feel you are receiving too many emails, there are various options to consider:

- Get off as many lists as possible (e.g. unwanted 'cc' lists).
- Try to get a separate email address that you use only for the important communications you wish to receive – in the same way that you might get an 'unlisted' telephone number to be shared only with those to whom you want to give access.
- Stop checking so often! Discipline yourself to check your email once or twice a day only unless you have been alerted that an important email is on its way.

Did you know?

The average business person is getting around 80 emails a day and many feel that about 80 per cent of the messages are of no value.

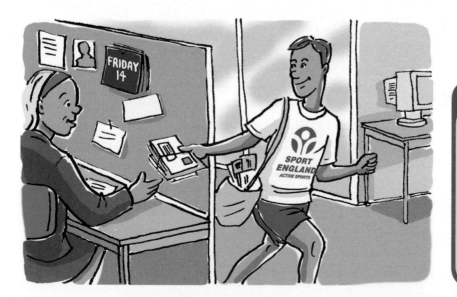

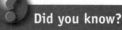

Did you know?

Emails can make you fat, according to Sport England, because they encourage people to be lazy and stay at their desks rather than speaking to their colleagues. Sport England want 'email free Fridays' to improve communications, fitness and health at the same time!

- Don't let emails pile up. As you open each email decide whether it requires a quick response and, if so, respond to it. If it requires a longer response but it is not a priority, try to delegate it to someone else if possible. If this cannot be done and it is going to take some time to respond to, then either flag it and move it to a pending folder (if you are using a program like Microsoft Outlook) or make a note in your planner to respond to it when you have made the time to do so.

Snapshot – Beware of emails!

Email has many advantages. It allows rapid internal and external communication and encourages people to communicate with each other. It's very simple and informal to use. But because it is so easy to use it has caused a huge increase in 'written' communications in the workplace, some of which have been unwise to say the least.

One recent case hit the news when there was an email row between a solicitor and a secretary in the same firm. He sent the secretary an email asking for £4 to cover his dry-cleaning costs because he alleged she had spilt some tomato ketchup on his trousers. The secretary apologised by email for the delay in replying, saying that this was because her mother had just died. However, she also copied in other members of the firm, which caused widespread amusement.

What was less amusing was the firm's reaction to this. Both employees were regarded as being guilty of using the firm's email system for personal rather than work matters. However, other staff were regarded as being equally to blame in forwarding the emails to others – particularly to those outside the firm. The firm could rightly claim that it damaged its public image.

Most larger organisations nowadays have a written email policy warning staff exactly what will happen if they misuse the email system.

- They set out their policy in the staff handbook, contract of employment or other stand-alone document so that employees are made well aware of it.

- They let employees know the legal implications of email and the fact that improper statements in emails may give rise to personal or company liability.

- They remind employees of their duty of confidentiality.

- They state expressly whether employees are allowed some restricted personal use of email or whether it is completely forbidden.

Find out

Check to see whether your organisation has an email policy. If it has, obtain a copy to see what it says.

- They state how they intend to monitor email use. Employers have a number of legal duties under the Data Protection Act 1998, the Human Rights Act 1998 and the Regulation of Investigatory Powers Act 2000.

The next time you have a bit of exciting news to tell, don't email it!

Memos

Nowadays memos can get a bit sandwiched between letters and emails. However, thousands of them are sent each day. Some of them are merely written versions of emails. Some of them can be much more formal particularly if, for instance, they are memos to or from senior managers.

Find out

Check the way in which you lay out your memos with the information opposite and/or with any memos you get from other areas of your organisation.

- A typical memo contains the following information in the heading – To:, From: and Date:. In this case the names of the sender and receiver do not require courtesy titles (Mr, Mrs, Ms etc.).
- That is followed by the subject heading or line. It should be as specific as possible so the reader is clear about the purpose of the memo. Long subject lines are easier to read if they are in single line spacing and centred.
- The body of the memo is again usually single line spacing and paragraphed. As with letters there should normally be three to four sentences per paragraph.
- Whereas letters are always signed, memos need not be. Many memo writers simply put their initials at the end.

Reports

A lot of very bright people find reports scary! They don't need to. Reports are really quite easy and, unlike a lot of other documents you might have to prepare, there's normally a set format to follow.

Suppose, for instance, you are helping your boss to prepare a report about the reasons for the recent high staff turnover of the reception staff. She asks you to undertake some research and then to draft a report. All you need to do is to take your time and either follow a series of straightforward steps laid down by your organisation or use those suggested in the 'How to...' section on page 12.

What you might also have to do, however, is to check that your language and style are suitable. Generally speaking, you will have to be more formal both in the words you use and in the layout of the document itself. For instance, you will almost certainly be expected to use a standard numbering system The most popular are a combination of figures and letters or the use of the decimal system of numbering. Some examples are shown below.

Some standard numbering systems		
1...	A ...	1.0 ...
a ...	1 ...	1.1 ...
i ...	a ...	2.0 ...
		2.1 ...
		2.2 ...
		2.2.1 ...

You might also have to use different language from what you use, for instance, in a memo:

- **Avoid using abbreviations** such as don't, can't, isn't etc.
- **Avoid slang or jargon.** You might have to translate 'The staff are going up the wall at having to deal with all the nosy parkers from the HSE' to 'The staff expressed concern at the frequent visits from members of the HSE as they felt it interrupted their work flow.' If you have a boss who insists on using slang there is little you can do about it other than putting quotation marks round the words to minimise the impact – e.g. The staff are 'sick as parrots' at having to change their hours.
- **Avoid first names.** In reports, 'Robbie' becomes Robert Eddison, the Sales Manager.

How to... Write a business report

- **Write down what you've been asked to do.** You might want to use a heading ('Possible causes of the recent high staff turnover in the reception area') or give a bit more detail ('As requested I've now looked into the possible causes of recent high staff turnover amongst the reception staff').

- **State what you have done.** You might have gone to the reception area to talk to the staff and have a look around. You might have seen certain incidents occurring in the area over the past few months. You might have been in touch with other organisations to check on their rate of success in keeping reception staff, or contacted a job centre for views.

- **Summarise what you've found out.** The reception area might be very cold. The staff might regard it as a bit unsafe because members of the general public wander in and out at will. The pay may not be very good. The staff might feel that no one even notices them and they like the idea of having a uniform. Other firms may pay higher rates and have security guards situated in the area.

- **If asked, make certain recommendations.** Examples are 'There should be a meeting with the staff to discuss their problems'; 'The area should be renovated and the heating improved' and 'Higher rates of pay could be considered'.

- **Sign and date it** – or in this case leave that for your boss to do.

- **Attach a circulation list if appropriate.** Much depends on the level of confidentiality. If it is very confidential then circulation will be restricted.

House style

Most organisations have a house style they apply to all their documents, particularly those that will be going to clients or customers. Some of them give 'corporate identity guidelines' to staff on:

- the preparation of stationery and templates – so that the paperwork of each department or area is identical
- how to set out not only letters, reports and memos but also the positioning of logos and the style to be used for compliments slips and business cards
- the typefaces and fonts to be used.

Did you know?

The University of Kent has a house style even for photography. It wants photographs to reflect university life and, as a rule, be close-ups of people doing something rather than standing in stiff poses looking like a 'firing squad'!

Oral presentations

Nasreen works in the Equal Opportunities Unit of an organisation and has been asked to give a talk to the new members of staff about her work and the work in her area. She says 'yes' to her boss, comes out of his office and then has a panic attack! She wonders about either resigning or trying to palm the job on to her junior. She's overreacted a bit. Giving a talk for the first time can be daunting, but once you've done it you normally feel absolutely wonderful. You might not have been the second Davina McCall but at least you've managed to say something!

Find out

Check to see whether your organisation has its own 'corporate identity guidelines' and, if so, what documents they apply to in your own work area.

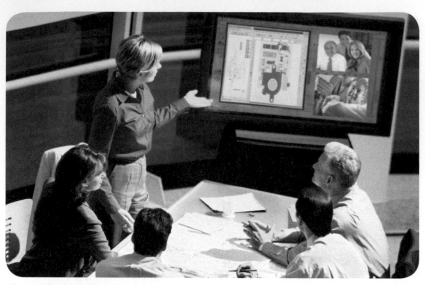

Thorough planning is the key to a good presentation

Even if you're not likely to be asked to actually give a talk there might be a number of occasions when you have to talk to people on a semi-formal basis. You might have to:

● talk about something you're doing at a team meeting
● help your boss to entertain customers or clients at a sales conference
● explain what your work area does to a group of interview candidates.

As with nearly everything else the secret lies in the planning.

How to... Speak to a group of people

● **Think about what you've been asked to do.** Who are you going to be talking to? How much do they know already? Do they know you? What effect are you aiming for?

● **Check up on the practicalities.** How long have you got? Do you have to follow a certain format? Where are you going to be?

● **Decide on what you are going to say.** A lot depends on what you have been asked to do, but a general rule is not to say too much. Concentrate on one or two main points.

● **Decide whether you are going to show anything.** Will you use charts or graphs, handouts, slides or video clips, objects (e.g. a first aid kit) for them to look at?

- **Think of a good ending.** Don't just break off suddenly. Summarise what you have said, ask for questions – if you feel you'll be in a strong enough state to answer them. Get a friend to come in with you and ask the first question if that would help.

- **Ask for feedback.** This could be from someone you can trust and whose opinion you value – particularly if it's your first time.

After the planning comes the practice. Very few people are good at talking unrehearsed – especially those who think they are! If it is your first time you might think about these things:

- **Decide what you want to use as notes**. Do you want to write down every word? That might make your talk a bit stilted. Do you want to use cards on which you write key words, phrases or facts? Do you want to write out everything you want to say but then highlight key points to glance at as you are going along?

- **Practise giving the talk on your own**. Only you will be able to hear your mistakes, and you can burst into tears, kick the furniture, tear up your notes without anyone knowing.

- **Decide whether there will be handouts**. If you are using handouts or any other visual aids, pick appropriate times to introduce them – and mark this in your notes.

Did you know?

Professional sports people, barristers and actors frequently use breathing exercises to calm themselves before they start to perform. They breathe in slowly and deeply, then breathe out getting rid of as much air as possible. They repeat this five times. Try it!

 Over to you

1 One of your jobs is to keep your team up to date about what is happening in the organisation. You:

- have occasional meetings with them

- send them frequent memos and emails

- make sure that you circulate all the information you get from your own line manager and other senior managers.

However you are a bit disappointed when you overhear one of them saying that she never knows what is going on and that she just hasn't the time to read everything that lands on her desk.

Decide what changes you think you should make in the way you let them have information. Discuss your ideas with your tutor or trainer and/or check them with the answers on the CD-ROM.

2 When you do hold meetings you know that on some occasions you are not getting through to individual people:

Over to you Continued

- Lauren doesn't like the HR manager so if you ever try to discuss a personnel issue she is critical of it no matter what.

- Winston has a very short concentration span. If you take longer than a few minutes on any topic he switches off.

- Damian just doesn't like meetings. He says very little and keeps looking pointedly at his watch if they run on.

- Tara tries to be helpful by commenting on every topic, but she holds things up particularly at the end of the meeting when everyone else is preparing to pack up and leave.

Discuss with your tutor or trainer how you would deal with each of these problems and/or check your ideas with the answers on the CD-ROM.

3   Nasreen comes to you to show you a draft of her talk to the new staff about work in the Equal Opportunities Unit. She asks for your comments.

> *Hello. I do a lot of things in this department. I do the post, answer the telephone, word process, take notes at meetings and do what David wants me to. Martia helps me. The unit is responsible for a lot of things. Here's a leaflet showing you what we do. It makes sure that the firm looks after the employees and doesn't break the law. It looks at all the documents everyone produces to see they are not discriminatory. It has someone on all the interview panels. It's very interesting and if you want to contact us at any time we'll be pleased to hear from you.*

List the suggestions you might make to improve this introduction. Remember it's Nasreen's first time at preparing a talk, so be tactful! Check your ideas with the answers on the CD-ROM.

Evidence planning

You will obtain your evidence for this unit through the option units you select. However, you should find this easier if you start to plan opportunities for evidence collection now, whilst this section is fresh in your mind. That is because it will be easier to obtain evidence relating to your verbal communications (such as your listening and questioning skills) in option units where you regularly deal with other people face to face, rather than those where you don't.

If you haven't yet chosen your option units, it is time you discussed your ideas with your tutor or trainer. Remember that you need to choose four, at least three of which must be Option B units. One can be an Option A unit that you may have already achieved if you have previously taken the NVQ2 Business and Administration award. There may only be a few units that fit your job role, but it is likely that you will have a wider choice. In that case you may find it better to look at option units that cover the different types of skill you need to demonstrate in the core units. Remember that the earlier you choose your option units, the sooner you can start to plan how to obtain your evidence, as you will see on page 22.

Adapting the way you communicate to different audiences

Read the following extract from a conversation between the new receptionist, Kylie, and the managing director:

Kylie:	Hi there.
MD:	Good morning, could I speak to Miss Stalker, please.
Kylie:	Who?
MD:	Miss Stalker, she's your line manager isn't she?
Kylie:	Oh her, we call her the 'Squawker'.
MD:	Indeed?
Kylie:	Yes, we give a nickname to everyone round here. Some of them are hilarious. We call Derek Delboy, and Ellie's Nellie the elephant – behind her back of course.
MD:	(*Coldly*) Really. Well if you would just let Miss Stalker know I'm here.
Kylie:	OK, no problem.

Even Kylie has a vague idea that the conversation didn't go as well as it might have done. However, she's distracted by the next visitor who's asking about possible job vacancies.

Kylie:	What do you want?
Visitor:	(*Hesitantly*) To see someone about a job. Sorry, my English is not very good.
Kylie:	Oh, you'll need the Human Resources Department. (*Very rapidly*) Go out of this door, walk 50 yards along the mezzanine corridor, take the stairs up to the fourth floor and check the noticeboard for directions to Room 403. If you've got a resume of your qualifications and CV you can hand them in to one of the personnel in that room.
Visitor:	(*Silence*)
Kylie:	Over there. (*Points to the door*)
Visitor:	(*Silence – he then wanders slowly out*)

Kylie doesn't think that went as well as it could have done either. It didn't. She turns her attention to the correspondence on her desk. There's a note from Miss Stalker asking her to draft out a letter to a customer who doesn't like the new system of having to check in and out of reception by signing a visitors' book and a notice to all staff reminding them that Christmas is nearly here and would they let her know what sort of staff party they would like. Kylie has a go. Unfortunately her written communication is about as good as her verbal communication, as the following extracts show.

> *I'm sorry you don't like the new system. It can't be helped as if we don't do it, people could sneak in and out without anyone knowing.*

> *Miss Stalker would be very grateful if you would kindly let her know your views on the most appropriate method of celebrating Christmas this year.*

Kylie has fallen into the common trap of failing to adapt the way she communicates with different people.

How to... Communicate with different people

- **Think about your audience:**

  - Is it a senior manager, an important client, a colleague, a group of people from different backgrounds?

  - Is it someone who is nervous, shy, angry, aggressive, critical?

- **Think about the type of communication to use** (if you have a choice):

    - Is it best if you talk to someone face to face?

    - Should you use the telephone?

    - Are you better at putting it in writing? If so, should you write a letter, send an email or prepare a report?

- **Think about the approach** you should use:

    - Are you tactful, polite and controlled in all situations?

    - Are you careful to use simple language, take time to explain, be formal with one person and less formal with the next and so on?

How non-verbal communication affects the impact you have on other people

Did you know?

According to the public affairs manager of the Chartered Management Institute, 90 per cent of the messages we convey are through body language.

You might remember the now famous photocall with Prince Charles and his sons at the skiing resort Klosters. His body language said it all! His smile was fixed, his eye contact was limited and his whole posture told everyone he really wanted to be somewhere else. Prince William, on the other hand, smiled readily, looked to be in a good humour and conveyed an entirely different impression. You can communicate either well or badly with another person even if you don't open your mouth.

Negative body language

Farouk doesn't want to be in a particular meeting. Every time anyone speaks he:

- gives them a blank stare
- keeps his head down
- avoids eye contact
- fidgets and drums his fingers on the desk
- shrugs his shoulders every time he is asked something
- leans back in his chair
- constantly looks at his watch.

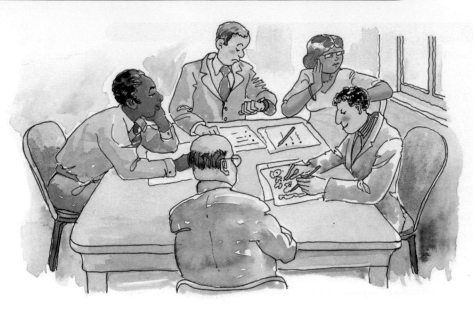

Is your body language more positive than this?

He isn't the most popular member at the meeting. Nor is he getting anything out of it.

Positive body language

Jeni likes being at meetings. She:

- smiles
- nods encouragement when relevant
- makes eye contact with the speaker
- keeps her head up
- sits still.

She's regarded as a good listener and, in turn, everyone listens to her.

You can use body language to work for or against you in different situations. What you must do is be aware of it and how you want to use it to help you.

Snapshot – When you believe your own message, your body language will reflect this

Nowadays a lot of top executives regard courses in non-verbal communication as essential. One specialist firm in communication and body language trains managers first of all to believe in what they are saying. Otherwise their body language is almost certain to let them down and their listeners will react badly to what they consider to be a false message.

Once that's established, the managers are then taught how to use both their voice and their body to communicate what they want to say. The training covers:

- the way in which they should use their voice – not too low so that no one can hear; not too high so that everyone is backing away

- the pace of speaking – again not so slowly that everyone has lost interest or so fast that no one can understand a word

- the way in which they should walk, sit down, show different facial expressions and use eye contact to control a particular situation.

 ## Over to you

1   Kylie is no better at body language than she is at dealing with people verbally. One day you walk into the reception area to find it full of people. Kylie is obviously fed up and is leaning back on her chair balancing it on two legs. She is trying to find someone on the phone and is pulling a face because she can't do so. She doesn't look at the visitor even when she eventually directs him to the office. When he goes and she turns to someone else she still doesn't smile. In fact she sighs noticeably and sags wearily in her chair. The visitor is a bit taken aback and rushes through what she has to say. Kylie tells her that the person she wants is out. When she asks when he will be back she shrugs her shoulders and says nothing. You realise that Kylie is going to lose you a lot of customers if you're not careful.

You decide to have a quiet word with her. Discuss with your tutor or trainer how you will go about this as tactfully as possible and say how you will make the best use of your body language to try to get the message across. Alternatively check your ideas with the answers on the CD-ROM.

2   Set aside a day in which you make a note of every occasion when you see someone using body language, such as raising eyebrows or pointedly looking at a watch. Note also what reaction you had to it. Did it please you, annoy you, upset you, make you work harder etc? Discuss your findings with your trainer or tutor – or talk them over with a colleague.

Evidence planning

Think about the times at work when you do each of the following activities:

● receive verbal information and instructions, and have to ask questions if you are not sure of something

● have to provide clear information, confidently, to other people both in writing and verbally

● have to adapt the way you communicate to meet the needs of other people.

For each of these, think about the type of information that is involved, the type of written documents you prepare, the occasions on which you provide information verbally and the option unit to which they relate.

Now start a communications log sheet on which you can record these occasions. Each time put the date, what you did, the subject matter and the option unit you have chosen to which each one relates. Attach to your log sheet any relevant written communications you have received or written.

You can then use this information in various ways:

● You can use it as a basis for a professional discussion with your assessor about the way you communicate at work.

● You can use it as a basis for asking for witness testimony from your supervisor or colleagues to prove what you did.

● You can use it to help identify future occasions on which your assessor can observe you or during which you could produce a tape or video to prove what you did.

How to contribute positively to discussions

You have a weekly staff meeting that is quite informal and meant to be an occasion where everyone can talk, exchange ideas, raise issues etc. Your manager normally starts the ball rolling but he then looks round for a response. Some of your colleagues aren't good at this.

● Gareth is painfully shy and says nothing. If the manager asks him directly for a contribution he goes bright red and mumbles the first thing that comes into his head.

- Monica does contribute. In fact, she contributes too much too often. She's very difficult to shut up.
- Parveen doesn't listen properly. She hears the first few words and then jumps in with suggestions or comments that aren't really relevant.
- Dan always has his own agenda. Whatever the topic under discussion he tries to hijack it. Last week, for instance, when everyone else was talking about the installation of the new computer system, he started complaining about new systems in general and then introduced what he really wanted to say – that he didn't like the new car parking procedures.
- Leslie is a bit of a yes-man. No matter what the manager says he agrees with it. He never offers an independent suggestion.
- Dawn is just the opposite. As a matter of principle she never agrees with what the manager has to suggest and tries to start an argument about it.

No wonder the manager feels like lying down after each meeting!

If you want to make a positive contribution to a discussion you need first of all to look at yourself.

Find out

At the next meeting you attend, try to identify any of these characters among the other members.

How to... Improve your contributions to a meeting

- Are you comfortable in a meeting or are you a bit nervous at speaking up in front of everyone? Don't worry if you are. It's quite common. Try, for instance, to have a look at the agenda to see what is going to be discussed and plan what you might say or what questions you want to ask. Write this down if it makes you feel more comfortable. Try to think of what the possible response may be and plan your reply to that.

- Are you naturally talkative? If you are, it's very difficult to keep quiet for a long time even if you notice people around you getting restive. Try to control what you say by, for instance, limiting yourself to one contribution per topic or even asking a friend to signal to you when he or she thinks you've said enough!

- Are you a bit of a day-dreamer? You listen to the first few remarks and then your attention wanders. If so, you could practise concentration techniques such as deliberately making notes. The act of writing might stop you contributing at first but at least it forces you to concentrate on the topic.

How to... Continued

- Are you a bit impatient? If someone makes a remark that irritates you do you let it show? Count to ten if someone is making what you think is a particularly stupid remark and, unless you are convinced that he or she is leading the discussion totally the wrong way, try to stop yourself arguing. The same applies if you have a particular hobby horse. Say your piece and then keep quiet.

You then need to consider how you would deal with others in group. Even if the senior person is trying to encourage some people to speak and others not to, he or she needs some help. You can do this by:

- refusing to become involved in arguments
- listening politely to someone else's point of view and genuinely trying to consider whether it is useful
- training yourself not to get exasperated because someone is being particularly silly, argumentative or uncommunicative
- changing the subject if the present discussion is going nowhere
- bringing back everyone's attention to the matter in hand
- offering imaginative or creative solutions to a problem – even if it's just a way to get everyone talking
- not taking offence if your best suggestion is not acted on!

Did you know?

A recent survey of office staff found that 70 per cent of them never opened their mouths at meetings because no one took any notice of what they said. Forty-five per cent said that there was no point because the manager got irritated with them if they interrupted!

Giving other people the chance to contribute ideas and opinions – and showing you have taken account of these

It could be very tempting for your line manager to give up on these meetings and simply to make every decision alone. If that happened, he or she would be missing out. For instance, the manager might never find out these things:

- Gareth eats, sleeps and breathes computers. There's not much he doesn't know about both the existing system and the ways in which it could be improved.
- Monica is hyperactive but very thorough. If she contributes to a topic she'll know what she's talking about as she'll have done her homework the night before.
- Parveen is particularly good with figures. Give her a budget and she'll tell you exactly what the bottom line means.
- Dan's great interest is marketing. He's absolutely full of ideas.

- Leslie is an admin man. Tell him you want the filing system improved and he's away.
- Dawn understands how people tick. She'll know how any new scheme or procedure will go down with the rest of the staff.

However annoying people can be, nearly everyone has something to offer to a discussion and the end result is nearly always better. Even if it is exactly the same result as your manager would have reached alone, because he or she has consulted the staff it is less likely that there will be a need to defend the decision or to have it ignored.

However, having listened to staff opinions and adopted some of them, your manager shouldn't leave it there. Although it may be tempting to listen to someone else's idea and then represent it as your own, he or she isn't a good manager if that happens. Obviously the manager isn't going to heap someone with praise every time he or she suggests that there should be a new towel dispenser in the washroom, but generally speaking, credit should be given where it's due. Otherwise the suggestions will start to dry up.

Providing written information in a way that meets the needs of different audiences

Did you know?

The Government's curriculum 'watchdog' has recommended that children should learn how to send text messages and surf the Internet rather than read books or write essays, to reflect the impact technology has had on the way written information is provided nowadays. Do you agree?

If your boss asks you to find some information on credit card fraud and how to deal with it, he or she won't want a long description of which banks offer which credit card facilities. If what is needed is a brief eye-catching few sentences for a notice about the new menus to be offered in the staff dining room, you've obviously got to avoid coming up with a two-page document on the benefits of a good diet. Before you actually start to compose any document you should consider these points:

- Find out exactly what your boss wants.
- Check on the type of document required – and check also that you know the required format, whether house style or otherwise.
- If it's not immediately obvious, find out to whom the document is going to be sent – to a client, the chief executive, staff, a newspaper, an individual, a group of people.

Selecting the right material

The next stage is to actually get your hands on what you need to know. Even with the vast amount of information now available on the Internet, your Intranet or the library, information may not be readily

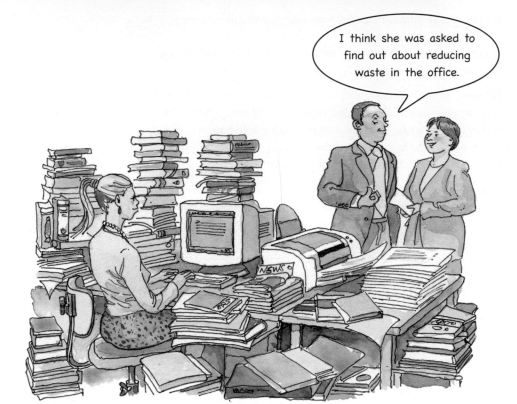

available. You might need to rummage through your files, talk to a number of colleagues, persuade senior members of staff to give you some information or make numerous telephone calls before you finally get what you want.

Be sure to give yourself enough time to do this and, if you think it's going to be a long job, alert your boss to this fact so that he or she isn't expecting a quick turnround. Further information on how to research information is available in unit 310 page 255.

The final stage is equally tricky. You may have pages and pages of information to check through, read and understand and from them you then have to select the information your boss actually wants.

At this stage good reading skills are a must.

How to... Read for a purpose

- Write down exactly what you want to know.
- Come up with a number of possible sources.
- Check that the information is up to date.

- Check also who has prepared the information. If it looks lightweight, forget it.

- Look at the list of contents if there is one and make a note of any relevant chapter, section or page numbers.

- Check the index for key words.

- Scan or skim read the contents. If you have marked down a particular section use the fingertip method (or cursor) and flick through it to see if anything jumps out to you. If it does, make a note of the page number or numbers.

You're then in a position to assess the selected information:

- Check whether it answers your questions and helps you to prepare your document.

- If you are using a photocopy, mark the relevant sections with highlighter so that you can refer back to them.

- Alternatively start making relevant notes – not just a complete rewrite.

- At certain points stop and mentally review what you have written or selected to check that you are still on track and haven't wandered off the point.

Identifying and extracting the information you need

When you are sure your information is as complete as you can get it you then have the final task of reproducing it. Very few bosses want a verbatim (word by word) account of anything unless it is going to be used as a direct quote. In most cases a summarised version is required. That's normally up to you! Again it's a case of sticking to a few rules.

How to... Identify and extract the main points from written material

- Skim read all the information you have collected, document by document.

- In each case, list your findings in note form.

- Check your lists against the original documents to see that you haven't left out anything important.

Remember

Don't use over-complicated language. One of the annual Golden Bull awards for 'spouting nonsense' was given to the Department of Trade and Industry for defining a pram as 'a wheeled vehicle designed for the transport in a seated or recumbent position of one or two babies or infants, any carry-cot or transporter thereof'.

How to... Continued

- Start drawing together all the information on the same topic. For instance you might find that several of the documents you have read and made notes on contain information about one particular aspect of your research. Now is the time to re-list the information under one common heading.

- Start to draft your summary from your notes – not from the original documents.

- Check what you have written:

  - **Accuracy.** Is there anything that stands out as being wrong, needing further checking, or not completely understandable?

  - **Relevance.** Yet again, check that you are giving your boss what he or she wants.

  - **Completeness.** Have you covered all aspects of what you have been asked to do?

  - **Grammatical correctness.** Is it spelled properly? Is the punctuation correct? Is the language used appropriate? Is the tense the same throughout? Is it in sentence form?

  - **Logical order.** Is the information set out logically and therefore easy to follow? Are all the points on the same topic contained in the same paragraph or paragraphs – or are they dotted about all over the place?

  - **Length.** Is it too long or too short? Does anything need adding or taking away?

The final check

You have gathered together the information you need and prepared a first draft. However you're not completely satisfied with it:

- It's not the right length. In this case don't try to cut corners by taking out odd words or phrases or adding a few 'howevers', etc. If it's too short read the whole summary again and decide where you think you could put in additional material. Go back to your original information and pick out some relevant material to use. If it's too long take a paragraph at a time and see whether you can rewrite it to make it shorter. Check also to see whether you can leave out any examples or illustrations.

- It seems to be 'bitty'. Read it through again and number each different point 1, 2 etc. Check to see whether you need to combine or rearrange any material by putting, say, 3 and 5 together or by leaving 6 out. Sometimes reading aloud can give you the 'feel' of how it will sound to others. If there's a bit you're not satisfied with, leave it out or rewrite it.

Summarising can be a time-consuming business!

How to... Provide written information accurately and clearly

The Plain English Campaign has some advice on the most effective way to communicate.

- **Keep your sentences short**, with an average sentence length of 15–20 words. Don't keep all sentences the same length but vary them. Follow the basic principle of sticking to one main idea in a sentence plus perhaps one other related point.

- **Use short rather than long words** and everyday English wherever possible.

- **Use active rather than passive verbs.** Say, for instance, 'About 10 000 people watched the programme' rather than 'The programme was watched by about 10 000 people.' Remember, however, that you can use a passive if you want to soften a message (e.g. 'A mistake was made in the bill' rather than 'Mr Malcolm made a mistake in the bill').

- **Use 'you' or 'we'** wherever possible.

- **Use words the reader will understand.**

- **Use positive language.** Rather than saying 'Either pay up in two weeks or you will lose your membership', say instead 'If you pay within two weeks we can then renew your membership.'

- **Use lists where appropriate,** preferably with bullet points rather than numbers or letters which can be distracting.

Did you know?

Not everyone welcomes positive language. There's recently been a fuss about the way weather forecasters 'talk up' the weather to put the best possible slant on it. One writer has suggested that rainy spells should now be called 'deferred sunshine'.

Over to you

1 Katie, your boss, wants to liven up a staff training day which is aimed at encouraging women to apply for high-level executive posts. She has seen an article in the paper on 'body discrimination' which she wants to use. However, she wants it reduced to about half

its length so that the women can read it quickly. She asks you to do this.

A recent university study has found out that more than 90 per cent of UK bosses rate the right attitude and appearance including looks and dress sense above skills and experience. The researchers conclude that this means that some men and women could become unemployable if they are not sufficiently good looking. Women might be passed over as being too fat, old or ugly. Men might be passed over as being too hairy or stooping too much. Apparently the technical term for this is 'body fascism' and is likely to be found in industries such as the retail industry where the attractive personal appearance of employees is considered vitally important to the company's image. However it is also spreading to industries such as banking which traditionally have been more interested in an employee's brains rather than his or her looks. In the USA, for instance, a 44-year-old female Wall Street executive was awarded £15.5m damages from her banker employer who called her 'old and ugly'. The Equal Opportunities Commission also gives an example of an employer telling a pregnant woman that she couldn't go to breakfast meetings because she looked so awful.

The university study was based on a survey of 150 bosses and 128 male and female workers working in service industries. Some female celebrities were also asked for their views. These differed in that one woman thought that looks have always mattered but it mattered more nowadays because people were so much more interested in looks. Another said that others thought she was quite odd looking but that hadn't seemed to harm her career. A third said that looks might have been one of the things but not the only thing that helped her get promotion.

Check your final version with the example on the CD-ROM.

2   One of the new members of staff sends you the following email:

Katie has asked me to summarise the article in the staff magazine about marketing to women. I've done my best but it doesn't seem very good. Can you be a sweetie and tell me what you think. I honestly don't mind criticism!

Advertisements don't relate to women. Breweries and car manufacturers particularly. They are too geared to men.

Particularly the car manufacturer's. They talked about car features such as engine size and performance. The women would like to know about things such as storage space safety & comfort. Ignoring the fact that women made up a large proportion of car buyers. Also ignoring the fact that women influence car buying decisions by persuading husbands or partners what to buy. Breweries are also guilty of ignoring the needs of women when designing pubs. They don't offer family friendly services.

Rewrite the summary to make it read better. Discuss the result with your tutor or trainer and/or check it with the answer on the CD-ROM.

Evidence planning

Identify occasions when you carry out the following activities at work:

- make useful contributions to discussions and develop points and ideas

- encourage others to contribute their ideas and opinions and take these into account

- select and read written material that contains information you need

- identify and extract the main points – either for yourself or for other people

- prepare and provide accurate, clear written information to other people.

Now look at the type of information you prepared in each case and decide to which option units these documents relate. This is likely to depend on the topic of the material and/or the reason you were asked to provide it.

Include copies of these documents in the evidence you collect for each option unit and make sure that you do this for any future written material you prepare and provide. These are valuable work products that are invaluable as evidence of your written communications.

Plan and be accountable for your work

Your line manager calls you into her office and asks you to take over the planning of the next staff development away-day. You will probably be quite happy doing this if:

- you have carried out the same plan before
- it is quite simple
- you are given enough time
- you and only you are involved in the planning (other than those people you choose to consult and ask for advice)
- you feel confident about your role.

You might be less happy if:

- you are tackling something new
- the task is quite complex
- there is a tight deadline
- you need to involve other people in the plan
- you just don't want to do it
- you get off to a bad start.

Everything is made a bit easier if you establish exactly what you are supposed to be doing, to what standard and to what time limit.

Planning your work and being accountable to others

In the case of the planning for the staff development day you might decide first of all to **work out your plan and devise your objectives**:

- Talk to a trusted senior colleague and get an overview about what you should be doing.
- Talk in more detail with your boss to find out exactly what she wants. Make sure that you clear it with her that you can carry out periodic checks as the plan begins to take shape. If relevant get hold of a copy of the programme for the last staff development day and try to find out whether it has been a success. If it has, follow the same formula. If not, think of something different.

Then you need to **prepare your schedule linked to a deadline**:

- Make a preliminary list of what you think you need to do. At this stage it can be as detailed as you wish and you don't need to put it in any particular order. Nor do you need to hesitate about whether or not to put anything in. Put it in and delete it at a later stage if necessary.

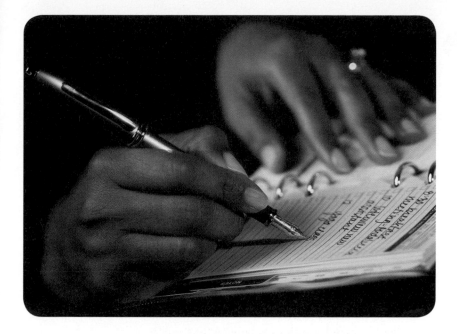

- Include names of people who are going to be at the staff development day plus their email addresses and contact telephone numbers.
- Start thinking about venues and contacting speakers, internal and external trainers.
- Establish time limits. In this case it's quite easy. Everything has to be done by the date set for the staff development day. However, try to set a few 'in between' dates as targets for certain parts of the plan so that you don't wake up in a panic two days before the event only to find that there is just too much to do in the time.

Next you must **follow the schedule taking action to achieve objectives**:
- Find out what resources are needed – staffing, a budget etc.
- Have an early check with your boss just to see whether you are on the right lines. Make any relevant adjustments.
- Check regularly to see if you are on target.
- Review the plan if necessary. Use your office planner to remind you to make periodic checks of the plan. If certain things are going wrong (e.g. you cannot get the trainer you originally wanted), start again and try to find someone else.

Make certain that you know to whom you are accountable. In this case you already know. It's your immediate line manager and you would be silly not to keep her informed throughout the process, not only because she is ultimately responsible for the success or otherwise of the day but also because you might need support and reassurance that you are doing what you should be doing.

Did you know?

One of the first things a well known and highly successful businessman says to a new member of staff is 'Surprise me at the rehearsal.' He wants to be prepared, not to be taken by surprise.

The importance of negotiating realistic targets for your work

Good targets are ones that meet the SMART test. They are:

- **S**pecific – they say exactly what you intend to do
- **M**easurable – you can prove you've reached them
- **A**chievable – they are not beyond your reach
- **R**ealistic – you haven't been over optimistic
- **T**ime-related – you have a deadline for completion.

Ideally too they should be:

- easily understood – so that not only you but everybody else understands them
- have the support of your line manager and colleagues.

Knowing where to start is crucial. It's easier, of course, if your line manager has set targets for you or if they have been decided as a result of a team meeting. Read the checklist below to see what people should ideally consider during the target setting process.

Example of a target-setting checklist

Questions to consider
- Is the target a completely new one?
- Can it be based on what already exists?
- What has a similar target achieved elsewhere (in other parts of the organisation, in other sectors or industries, nationally)?
- Can we do the same thing?
- If we use an existing target, have we got the same resources and help?
- Have staff providing services been consulted?
- Does the target take account of what they say?
- How will we get staff on board?
- Does the target represent value for money?
- Is it worthwhile?
- Will achieving it be satisfying?

There may be occasions when you have to try to follow the SMART rules on your own. If, on a personal level, you decide to set some targets for yourself in relation to what you want to achieve in your career, you can make vague statements to yourself such as 'I'll have to be more efficient because I'd like to be promoted' but that doesn't get you much further. You've stated your long-term goal but not made any realistic plans about how to achieve it. What you need to do is to break down your long-term goal into a number of specific targets. You may, for instance, decide that within the next six months, you will:

- improve your IT skills
- go on a customer services training course
- complete your NVQ 3 Business and Administration qualification
- meet all your deadlines.

Then break each target down a bit further. One might be 'I will learn how to use spreadsheets by the end of December.' That's a good target because it's *specific* – you want to know how to use a spreadsheet; it's *measurable* – you and everyone else will soon know whether or not you can be trusted to prepare a spreadsheet; it's *achievable* – you haven't said that you will become the office expert on all things computer related; it's *realistic* – you haven't over-estimated your capabilities or set too rigid a timescale for yourself; and it's *time-constrained* – if you don't have a definite end date in mind, it's surprising how easily you can let things slide and mentally allow yourself another week, month etc.

Although you might want to think about your targets on your own first, it's a good idea not to keep them entirely to yourself. In some cases you'll have agreed them with your line manager. In other cases you might have prepared them for your own personal use. Whatever the case, talk them over with a trusted friend – one who will neither scream with laughter nor agree slavishly. An honest opinion is very helpful.

Negotiating targets and why this is important

It's best right from the start to establish certain targets in relation to the job in hand. Ideally if you are given a job to do you should do all of the following.

- Discuss with your boss as precisely as possible what you have to do – either verbally or in writing if it's a bit more complicated. If you don't fully understand what you have to do, ask. It's sometimes a bit difficult to do this if you are very new, wanting to impress or if your boss is very senior to you or can be a bit off-hand.
- Pick your time. Don't choose the beginning of an important meeting or at the end of a very fraught day. Be positive. Say that you really want to do a good job but you need to be clear that you are going about it the right way.
- Try to establish a series of progress checks if the target looks quite complicated. Your boss will probably expect that to happen and be quite willing to agree to this.
- Steel yourself to go back to the boss if things are beginning to go wrong and, if necessary, try to renegotiate a target. Most bosses

Did you know?

When setting yourself targets be sure to say that you 'will' do something rather than you 'might' do it. It encourages you to focus on the outcome. Think also about other helpful words you are going to use – such as 'learn', 'improve' and 'update'. Always say what you are 'going' to do not what you are 'hoping' to do.

are much happier to renegotiate a target rather than be faced with one that has not been achieved and there is no time to do anything about it. It's wise not to do this too often of course!

Prioritising targets and setting timescales

Prioritising sounds just a matter of common sense. Obviously something that is urgent must be done before something that is not. Life isn't always so easy, however:

- You could be trying to achieve a number of targets all of which are urgent.
- You could be working for a number of people, each one expecting you to achieve a different target.
- As you are trying to achieve one urgent target, another even more urgent one might land on your desk.
- You might be constantly interrupted.
- Targets that weren't initially very urgent might have been allowed to pile up so that eventually they've become urgent too.

You need a plan – if only to preserve your sanity!

How to... Prioritise targets and agree achievable timescales

- Have a master list on which you write every target you need to achieve – which often tends to be the completion of a certain number of jobs during a specific period.

- Don't be tempted to put everything into a 'pending' or 'jobs to do' file.

- Classify your targets into those that are:

  - both urgent and important (class 1)

  - urgent (class 2)

  - important (class 3)

  - neither (class 4).

- Highlight any specific deadline dates.

- Set certain 'milestones' along the route. The more you manage to break down the work involved in achieving a target into manageable periods of time, the more in control you will feel.

- At the outset, identify any targets that may be difficult to achieve and will take extra time and effort.

- At the start of each day plan to tackle your targets in 'class' order.

- Make an early check on resource issues or people you need to speak to so that you can then have a clear pathway.

- Try not to panic if you have to re-order targets because an even more urgent one suddenly crops up. Just slot it into the most appropriate place on the list and then keep going.

- At the end of the day always reschedule your targets for the next day.

- Make sure that you move forward targets with specific deadline dates and try, if possible, to complete at least some of them one day in advance of the deadline.

Snapshot – Targeting crime

Nowadays even the police have to achieve targets. For instance, Crime Concern has produced a document for police on how to set and monitor targets for tackling crime and disorder.

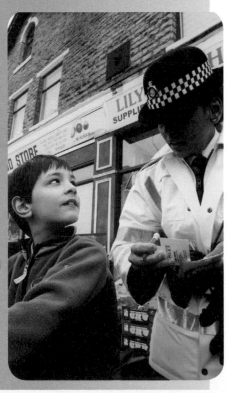

- Decide on the target. Is it to reduce the number of people committing crimes?

- Gather together the facts. How many people were convicted of a crime last year?

- Decide how the target should be expressed. Is it going to be:

  - an actual reduction in the number of crimes (e.g. 500 fewer crimes committed)

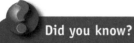

Did you know?

If you work with husky dogs in the Arctic you've either to decide how long they should work each day or how much they should get through in a certain time. Too long and they are tired and bad-tempered. Too short and they haven't done enough.

Problems that may occur during your work – and how to solve them

You've had a bad day. Your bus was late. At the staff meeting you sat next to Gordon who commented under his breath about everything everyone said, ignoring the boss's irritation. When you get back to your desk you find that someone has 'borrowed' a file. You accuse Roseanne who sits in the next workstation only to find that she is completely innocent and it's the boss who has taken the file. You start work on a report but are constantly having to get up to find files because you haven't all the information to hand. You try to cram in one or two jobs before lunchtime but know that you are not doing them thoroughly.

In the afternoon your boss asks you whether you've time to take a group of interview candidates round the building. You don't like to say no. You race them round. It's about 3 p.m. and you haven't even glanced at your 'things to do' list. You waste a bit of time reading all the junk items that have appeared on your email. You then panic and launch into another fairly major job about 15 minutes before the end of the working day. You miss the bus home. You're exhausted and frustrated – and you're not looking forward to tomorrow.

That's hardly surprising. In every organisation you will encounter different types of problem throughout the course of a working day including those involving:
- conflict between you and another person
- a crisis or emergency
- a self inflicted problem.

If you looked back on the day you would probably realise that you were involved in all three types of problem. Again bearing in mind what you already know about setting and achieving targets, it's not a good idea to lie awake that night making promises to yourself not to be late, to get through more work and not to get so easily upset. What you should try to do is to analyse the situation.

Problem-solving

In theory you should follow a four-step approach in which you:

- decide what the problem is
- choose a solution
- implement the solution
- check it has worked.

Like many things, it's easier said than done. What follows is one suggested approach.

Stage one: Find the key factors

Start by writing down every key factor associated with the problem. In the case of the problem between you and your colleagues it might be:

- you and the way you were feeling when the problem occurred
- the overall relationship between you and your colleagues
- any past history between you
- your relationship with your boss.

Stage two: Look for related areas

The next stage is to find 'sub areas' that fit in with the factors you've listed. With the present problem you might identify:

- the fact that you were late and flustered and not in the best of moods
- your irritation and embarrassment at the way Gordon behaved in the meeting
- the importance of the file you thought was lost

Find out

If you are having a bad day, try to find a friend to sit down and relax with you – even for a ten-minute coffee break. Your problems might not seem so bad after that.

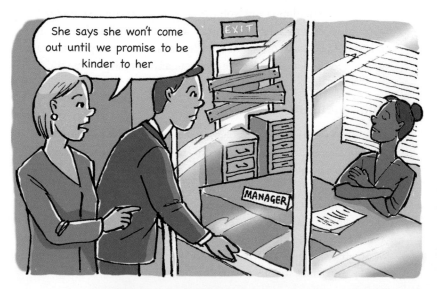

Did you know?

A US survey of office staff found that the reason most of them gave for not liking work was fear of their immediate boss. The same survey found, however, that a number of managers gave as their reason for not liking work the fact that they were frightened of their staff and the way they could make life awkward if they were criticised in any way!

- the fact that you were not very organised and couldn't afford to spend time looking for the file
- previous occasions when Roseanne has actually borrowed a file without asking
- you are in fact frightened of your boss.

Stage three: Analyse your notes

Study what you have written, being as honest as possible with yourself but remembering that the cause of the problem may not be completely your fault but partially the fault of others.

Stage four: Find any common factors

You might find that you can spot a recurring theme. You might, for instance, just not get on with Gordon in any area, not just in meetings.

Stage five: Ask someone else

You might want to talk the problem over with a friend.

Stage six: Communicate

Sometimes this works, sometimes it doesn't. You might want to think about approaching Gordon directly and saying that you are uncomfortable about the way he speaks to you in meetings; or Roseanne, asking her to let you know before she borrows anything. You might also find it helpful to say sorry to her – most people melt a bit if they are given an apology.

Stage seven: Find some common ground

You'll be very lucky if you find a perfect solution. If you can't, try to reach a situation which is the least you can live with. You might never like Gordon but you could make sure you never sit next to him in meetings. If you don't think you can trust Roseanne not to borrow files, you can arrange to keep all important files under lock and key. You might not be able to overcome your fear of the boss but you can train yourself to think twice before agreeing to anything she wants, and so on.

Time management

You may have solved the problems you have had when dealing with your boss or colleagues, but that still leaves you with the problem of how to organise your work more effectively. You obviously have a problem managing your time. You can't guarantee that you'll arrive at work on time or that you will be able to get through your workload by the end of the day. You can't even guarantee that you'll leave work on time! That's quite important because you haven't been able to protect your 'quality time' – which is the time you need to spend with your family or friends, to pursue a leisure interest or merely to relax.

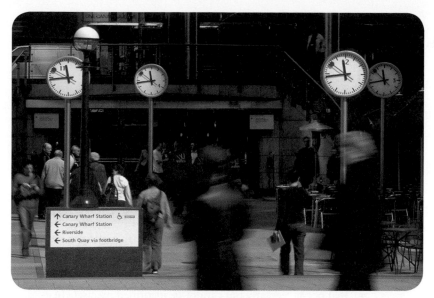

Time management skills are well worth developing

How to... Make the best use of your time

- **Don't** make unnecessary trips.

- **Don't** frequently lose information and spend ages trying to find it.

- **Don't** waste time playing about with trivial, unimportant jobs because you cannot motivate yourself to tackle anything larger.

- **Don't** over-use your email and access it every half hour to see whether you've received anything new.

- **Don't** chat to anyone who happens to be around – or telephone a colleague and waste half an hour gossiping.

- **Don't** be frequently visited by the office time waster and be unable to get away.

- **Don't** get so overwhelmed with what you have to do that you simply sit there doing nothing.

- **Don't** put off jobs you don't like doing.

- **Don't** dither – and be unable to decide what to do first.

- **Don't** try to deal with a dozen things all at once.

- **Don't** take on too much.

- **Don't** schedule badly so that if anything unexpected occurs the whole plan collapses.

Remember

Make sure you take into account the tips you were given on how to cut down on any over-reliance on email, on pages 8–11.

Once you have decided what stops you from managing your time well, the next step is to do something about it.

Task management

If you find that your main problem is that you are not organised, try to analyse your working practices. Find a free space in your diary and try to shut yourself away from other distractions. Then do this:

- List all the tasks you have to do. At this stage it doesn't matter how large or how small they are. If you do have junior staff, make a similar list for them.
- Separate these tasks into those:
    - that don't happen often and which can be planned well in advance (e.g. an annual general meeting – AGM)
    - that occur more frequently but which are also expected (e.g. monthly updating of staff absences)
    - that occur regularly but cannot be identified precisely (e.g. dealing with visitors, producing word processed documents, being called to the boss for a meeting).
- *Then* introduce a time element. What can you plan on a monthly or yearly basis?
- Think then about planning on a weekly or daily basis. This usually requires a bit more skill and you might want to think about:
    - allowing for the unexpected – the last-minute request by your boss to take a party of visitors around wouldn't have been quite so traumatic if you'd scheduled your other work to allow yourself a bit of a breathing space
    - establishing some priorities which ideally you would like to stick to but which are not so rigid that they don't allow you to reorganise in case of an emergency.
- You might also find it useful to make a list each week of:
    - work you *must* do
    - work you *should* do
    - work you *could* do – if, miraculously, you have a free moment
    - work you could delegate to someone else.
- Then examine each job in turn. It's often a good idea at this stage to prepare a 'jobs to do' list against which you can put a tick every time you complete a job.
- Plan major tasks in advance so that, for instance, you are not constantly walking backwards and forwards to the photocopier every time you start a new job.
- Identify when you are most productive. You might be a lark or an owl. You might flag just after lunch. Recognise this and plan your most difficult or important jobs when you are feeling most productive.
- Pick up a piece of paper and deal with it there and then.

- If you find you have a few moments between planned jobs, fit another small job in. It's not only a productive use of time, it's very satisfying to tick another job off your list.

People management

However well organised you are, people can get in the way! If your boss interrupts you there isn't much that you can do about it (although, even then, if the job is really urgent you can mention that fact). If other people interrupt you there are a few more options. Check first of all whether or not you are dealing with 'time-wasters' or 'askers'.

- **Time wasters**. They always appear just when you're in the middle of an urgent job and expect you to sit back and listen to what they have to say. You really have to be a bit ruthless. Try one of these approaches:
  - Encourage them to phone rather than just turn up. You can then always use the excuse of a call on another line or the appearance of a visitor.
  - Explain politely that you are snowed under but will contact them later in the day/week etc.
  - Look a bit distracted when they arrive and keep your eyes firmly on your word processor, document etc. – to give them the hint to disappear.
  - If desperate, arrange with another colleague to interrupt with an 'urgent message' if the unwanted visitor stops for more than five minutes.
- **Askers**. You might find that you are constantly being plagued by people asking you to do them a favour. Obviously you don't want to get a reputation for being unhelpful. Equally, you don't want to spend all your time doing other people's work for them at the expense of your own. Learn to know the person who is doing the asking. If it's a one-off, try to help. If it happens over and over again perfect the art of saying 'no' nicely.

Delegation

An important lesson to learn is that you're probably not the only person in the office who can carry out a particular job. There might be any number of people who can either help you or even take over from you. Wherever you can, try to delegate those jobs that don't require your own particular skill. However, don't just grab your office junior as you are on your way out of the office and tell him or her to take over the preparations for the next health and safety meeting. The junior might not have a clue where to start and might make such a mess of it that you end up with more work than you had at the start.

Did you know?

When a top PA was asked what her biggest time-waster was, she replied – hopefully as a joke – her boss!

Remember

The saying 'If you don't ask, you don't get' should not be taken to extremes!

How to... Delegate

- **Explain clearly what you want** and what standard is required. You might just want the office junior to type up a pre-prepared agenda. You might want more and expect him or her to prepare the agenda from notes you have left or by looking at the minutes of the previous meeting.

- **Check that the junior has understood** by encouraging questions.

- **Be realistic about what you want done.** It's unfair to expect the newest office junior to have a detailed knowledge of the office and all the systems and to give him or her a job that needs that sort of information.

- **Be equally realistic about a timescale.** Just because you've left a job to the last minute it's not going to help by giving your office junior an impossibly tight deadline.

- **Be there for help and guidance.**

- **Don't check up every five minutes** that things are going to plan.

- **Give constructive feedback.** If the junior hasn't done a good job it's no use ignoring it. However, it's equally useless demolishing the person's confidence by being too critical. Compliment whenever you possibly can.

Stress management

Did you know?

The number of working days lost through stress has increased by nearly 20 per cent over the last ten years.

You've sorted out all your office problems but one – you. Very often problems can be caused not because you can't cope with the work but because you can't cope with your reaction towards it. When you shouted at Roseanne were you genuinely annoyed at her for apparently borrowing a file without permission, or were you just reacting to your bad start to the day? When you were sitting at home exhausted, was that physical or mental exhaustion?

Problems can cause stress, and so can overwork and conflict. You will learn more about how to recognise the symptoms and how to cope with pressure at work on pages 75–81.

Over to you

1 Your boss has asked you to talk to your office juniors about the importance of achieving targets. No matter how you try to explain what a good target is, one of the juniors cannot seem to grasp it.

Eventually you write down a few targets that have not been properly thought out and which you intend to show your junior. They are:

- I'll try to finish off all my work as soon as I can.

- I'm going to be the best administrator ever.

- I'm going to work very hard.

- I'm going to do better than anyone else.

Make a few notes about how you will explain to her why each of these targets needs altering and how each could be improved.

2   The same office junior isn't very good at managing her time. You talk to her in general terms about time management but during the course of the conversation she says:

- 'I'm a slow starter. It takes at least two cups of coffee to get me going in the morning.'

- 'I think a tidy desk is the sign of a sick mind.'

- 'I like going into my email – it keeps me up to date with what's going on in the organisation.'

- 'I'm not actually chatting with people all day – I'm picking their brains.'

Discuss with your tutor or trainer what you will say to her to convince her that she's wrong, and/or check your ideas with the answer on the CD-ROM.

3   You've arrived at work at the beginning of the week and look through your diary entries plus your 'jobs to do' list:

- You're booked for a staff meeting that day.

- You're in the middle of making arrangements for your boss's trip to London next week and you've to see her about some urgent staffing issues.

- The chair of the monthly finance subcommittee is pestering you for the minutes of the meeting held last week.

- The Health and Safety Office is also pressing you to carry out a routine health and safety check.

- The staff database is out of date.

- You've told the junior staff that their staff appraisal interviews are coming up but you haven't yet told them when.

Over to you Continued

- The reprographics technician is warning you that photocopying supplies are getting dangerously low.

- You also realise that there is going to be a fairly large number of visitors to the office during the course of the day.

- You haven't done any filing for a week although you think there might be one or two important documents in the basket that you will have to refer to pretty soon.

- There's a pile of routine correspondence.

Discuss with your tutor or trainer how you will prioritise these jobs. You might want to re-classify them into jobs that you (a) must do, (b) should do, and (c) could do. Say too what you think you could delegate to a fairly experienced junior.

Discuss with your tutor or trainer what action you would take if, despite your best efforts, you couldn't get through all you planned that day. Alternatively check your ideas with the answers on the CD-ROM.

 Evidence planning

You can now practise your planning skills by thinking about the evidence you will need to prove that you plan and are accountable for your work. You are likely to find that you produce this evidence more easily if you think about more complex tasks you have to do as part of your job that involve each of the following:

- negotiating and agreeing realistic targets, either for partial completion or for the whole task to be completed

- prioritising your targets and agreeing timescales you can achieve

- planning how to make the best use of your time and resources on a day-to-day basis

- identifying and solving problems when they arise.

Ideally, select four or five complex tasks and keep a record of the way in which you plan and prioritise the work. In addition, keep your 'to do' lists, diary, notebook and other relevant documents safely. Instead of throwing away notes or emails you receive that make you change your plans, keep them. Note alongside the targets that apply and how you negotiate these, in addition to any problems you encounter. Remember to include how you solved each problem and who you asked for support, when this was necessary.

Ideally you should present this information as part of your evidence for at least one of your option units, but you can also use it as the basis of a professional discussion with your assessor about the way you plan and are accountable for your work.

The importance of keeping other people informed about progress

Very few people work entirely on their own. Even fewer are responsible to no one but themselves for the work they do. Most of us have to make sure that other people know what we are doing and, in many cases, approve it. If you don't keep them informed you're going to make both your life and theirs that bit harder.

It's quite easy to let people know about the end result of your actions. You send a memo to each member of staff telling him or her of the time of the staff appraisal interview. You hand the boss a file containing all the relevant travel documents. You tick the completed box on your list of 'jobs to do' and that's that. What is equally important is keeping people informed on an ongoing basis as a particular job progresses, particularly if it is long and complicated. Here are some reasons for this:

- You might not be completely clear about what you are supposed to do and don't want to go any further because you might be taking the wrong route.
- Something unexpected turns up that might alter what you have to do, such as not being able to book your boss on the flight she wants.
- You might urgently require some advice. For example, a particular project on which you are working looks as if it might be heading for an overspend so you need to update your boss with what has gone on so far.
- The person for whom you are doing the job needs a regular progress report for his or her own boss.
- The job is so big that a number of people have to be kept informed on a regular basis of what everyone else is doing so that they feel confident that they can continue carrying out their part of the plan.

Did you know?

In the recent Iraq war one of the most important parts of the army was the intelligence section. Staff there had to try to keep track of the movements of the US and coalition forces in various parts of the country. They then had to make sure that everyone else knew where they were – and where they were going to next.

If the regular progress checks are built into the job itself all you need to do is to use a reliable planner system – or your diary – to remind you when they are required. In some cases sending an update email to those involved should be fine. In more complex cases you might have to prepare a progress report for discussion at a meeting of all those involved. An example of one type of progress report is shown below.

Progress report on the Sales Conference to be held on 20 February

A meeting was held on 14 November to discuss the arrangements for the above event.

Present: Stephanie Burns, John Kelly, Dominic McGlynn, Corrine Masters, Neelam Rani

Arrangements already agreed:
- The event would be held on 20 February
- An outline programme had been decided
- Conference rooms had been booked
- The technical and administrative staff had been informed and their duties agreed

Arrangements to be made before the next meeting	Action by
All staff to be informed of the event	JK
Catering arrangements to be agreed with the hotel	SB
Outline presentation to be available	CM
Design of presentation packs to be available	NR
Conference programme to be finalised	DMc

The next meeting would be held at 2 p.m. on Friday 9 December in Room T45

Giving people sufficient notice if you need to revise your plans

You are preparing for an important sales presentation to be given to existing customers, potential customers, the board of directors and senior management. The press have been invited.

- The computer graphics staff have prepared a sophisticated presentation.
- External printers are preparing the presentation pack to be given to each invited guest.

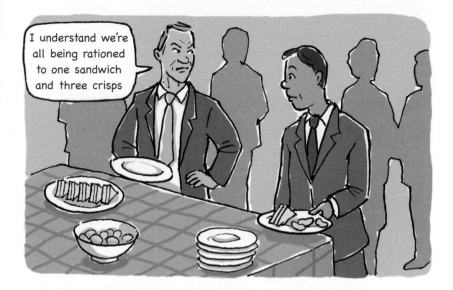

- External caterers have been asked to put on a cordon bleu buffet.
- A conference suite has been booked at a hotel through the conference events manager.
- The sales team have been rehearsing for weeks.
- Your own team are going to be there to give administrative and reception support.

As always with events of this size, not everything goes to plan. A couple of weeks before the event:

- one of the sales team goes off on long-term sickness
- the number of invited guests has risen from the expected 60 to 100
- the conference events manager asks you if you would mind changing the event from the Blue Room to the Gold Room.

You think you are taking this in your stride. You arrange with the sales team to replace the sick member of staff. You let the hotel know about the change in the number of guests. You agree to using the Gold Room.

What you haven't done is give everyone else sufficient notice to change their plans to take your changes into account.

- The presentation pack gives the name of the original not the substitute member of staff.
- The press have been given the wrong information about where the presentation is going to be given.
- The caterers have planned for 60 not 100 people.

Again it's a question of task management. What you need to do at the start of each job involving a number of people is to make sure that you prepare a circulation list and/or group email containing all their names

Did you know?

A wedding magazine says that the most frequent complaint it gets from its wedding dress manufacturers is that brides don't keep them informed of their dress size. Brides tend to lose weight as the wedding day draws nearer but they don't think to warn their dressmaker until dangerously near to the day itself.

so that each time you or someone else within the group makes a change to the agreed procedures or plans, you can then automatically inform everyone else. It will save you endless time and upset.

The importance of acknowledging and learning from your mistakes

Remember

Can you remember the occasion when the football manager, Sir Alex Ferguson, was alleged to have thrown a boot at David Beckham during a dressing room row? No matter how reporters pressed him, Sir Alex absolutely refused to say sorry. David Beckham is now elsewhere!

Very few people like saying sorry. Nor do they like even admitting to themselves that they have made a mistake. How often have you heard someone saying 'It's not my fault because...

- I wasn't given the right information
- the photocopier is on its last legs
- I was off sick when the instructions came through
- the computer staff don't know what they're doing
- that clown at reception would let an armed gang through the door without looking up from her magazine.'

It might boost your morale in the short term to blame everyone but yourself when a mistake is made. In the longer term, never admitting a mistake can cause problems.

Acknowledging your mistakes can help both you and the person you're talking to. He or she will:

- recognise that you have admitted your mistake without trying to lay the blame on anyone else
- be immediately in a position to try to correct the mistake because you have not tried to be obstructive about it
- try to ensure that the same mistake won't occur again by giving you extra training, assistance or support
- appreciate your honesty.

Did you know?

Some years ago there was a TV programme called 'Sorry'. The main character was a middle-aged man still living at home with his mother. Every time he opened his mouth he said 'sorry' whether he meant it or not – just to keep his mother quiet.

You, on the other hand, can hope for:

- a sympathetic hearing – unless you have a very unreasonable boss – because most people know that anyone can make a mistake
- improved work performance, because if you recognise you have made a mistake you are not as likely to make the same mistake in future
- recognition that you are not the sort of person to lay the blame on others.

Obviously you would be a bit unwise to relax completely and think that if you've done anything wrong, all you have to do is to admit it, apologise and all will be forgiven and forgotten. You have to really intend to try to improve!

Guidelines, procedures and codes of practice relevant to your work

The types of guideline and procedure you will be expected to follow depend on where you work. In a large firm you will probably find that there are procedures and guidelines for a large variety of tasks. If you work in a smaller organisation you may have to make up your own. In a larger organisation, procedures often follow policies.

- An organisational **policy** is a statement of the standards expected in certain areas. It tells you about the firm's values, as you will see in unit 202 (page 112).
- **Procedures** state how policies will be put into practice. For instance, an organisation may have a policy that outlines its strong support of equal opportunities in the workplace. To support that policy it then needs sets of procedures for those in charge of recruitment, training and promotion to ensure that the principles laid down by the policy are being carried out in practice.
- In addition to procedures you might find that you are expected to follow **guidelines** in areas such as dress, the way in which to talk to any visitors from overseas, what to do if you feel you have been subjected to sexual harassment in the office, and so on.

Codes of practice

Codes of practice can be both internal and external. They are often specific to an industry, and many organisations are members of associations that have codes of practice intended to safeguard and promote the interests of consumers.

The idea behind a code of practice is that it states what people can expect from an organisation. A person who is not satisfied with the way he or she has been treated by that organisation can approach the relevant association and ask for further assistance. Much depends on the individual association, but normally an unhappy customer can ask it to:

- provide conciliation procedures – i.e. to see whether, after discussion, an agreement can be reached
- arbitrate in the dispute – i.e. come up with an agreement that both sides must agree to.

A lot of organisations use the fact that they have a specific code of practice to show their commitment to providing a first-class service and their willingness to try to resolve any difficulties. Below you can see a list of some of them.

Associations with industry-wide codes of practice	
ABTA	Association of British Travel Agents
AMDEA	Association of Manufacturers of Domestic Electrical Appliances
BDMNA	British Direct Marketing Association
CCA	Consumer Credit Association UK
CCTA	Consumer Credit Trade Association
DSA	Direct Selling Association
FDF	Footwear Distributors Federation
FLA	Finance and Leasing Association
GGF	Glass and Glazing Federation
LAPADA	Association of Art and Antique Dealers
MOPA	Mail Order Publishers' Authority
NAMSR	National Association of Multiple Shoe Repairers
NCCF	National Consumer Credit Federation
RETRA	Radio, Electrical and Television Retailers' Association
RMIT	Retail Motor Industry Federation
SMMT	Society of Motor Manufacturers and Traders
TSA	Textile Services Association
VBRA	Vehicle Builders and Repairers Association

Find out

In your workplace check to see what policies, procedures and guidelines are in place. Make a note of their location so that you can show these to your assessor if necessary. Check also to see whether your organisation has a code of practice and, if so, obtain a copy of it.

In addition, many public organisations and government agencies have their own codes of practice. Some are legally obliged to do so. Section 62 of the Care Standards Act 2000, for example, requires social care employers to produce codes of practice to ensure that everyone who works in social care conforms to a particular set of standards. The Disability Rights Commission has produced a number of codes of practice explaining the legal requirements under the Disability Discrimination Act 1995. There is an approved code of practice in respect of the Workplace, Health, Safety and Welfare Regulations 1992; and so on.

Over to you

1   It has been a very busy few months and the last week in particular has been frantic. Your boss is a bit concerned at the way some of the staff have been reacting to the pressure:

- Tara absolutely refuses to take responsibility for anything, believing that then she will not be blamed for anything.

- Jaz is too quick to make excuses for anything he's done wrong.

- Elena makes sure that everyone knows if someone else has made a mistake.

- Tony is not very good in a crisis. If one arises he says he has migraine and goes home early.

- Muspha keeps everything to himself. He doesn't see why he should have to tell anyone what he's doing so long as he's doing it properly.

- Kim's junior is quietly going mad. Every time he gives her something to do, he spends the whole time hanging over her shoulder to see what she's doing.

Your boss asks you to try to improve the situation as you work with them every day. You decide, therefore, to talk to each one of them individually. Make a few notes about what you would say to each one and discuss them with your tutor or trainer and/or check them with the answers on the CD-ROM.

2 Try to be honest with yourself. Look at the way in which the rest of the staff have been behaving and decide if you are guilty of doing any of those things. If you are, discuss with your tutor or trainer – or a colleague – what action you intend to take or have taken to try to improve matters.

Evidence planning

On page 46 you started planning by identifying four or five tasks where you have needed to plan, agree timescales and solve problems. Now check that for each of these tasks you have the following information:

- The type of targets that relate to that task, such as the deadline(s), quality or quantity of work to be completed and the resources that you can use.

- Any guidelines, procedures or codes of practice that you must consider when you do each task.

- The working methods you will use (or used) to achieve the agreed result – such as how you will do the work, use equipment, obtain information or communicate with other people. Remember that you will need to prove that these were effective. You could do this by deciding whether or not they could be improved – and if so, how.

- The problems that could occur. You might have identified these in advance in a contingency plan. If problems actually occur when you

Evidence planning Continued

are doing your work, make a note of these together with the action that you took at the time.

● Records of any progress meetings you attend, even if these are just informal discussions with your boss or colleagues.

● A note of any mistakes you made and the action you took to put matters right.

● Any documentary evidence that relates to this task and witness testimony to support your claim that you worked effectively and achieved your targets.

Remember that you will be expected to link this evidence to the option units you have chosen. Do this by identifying the option unit to which each task best relates.

What if...?

What should you do if either:

● no problems arise during your assessment period

● your organisation has no codes of practice?

In either case, talk to your assessor who can arrange to observe you at work doing a dedicated task to cover the knowledge and understanding required or seek confirmation of your competence during a professional discussion when you can explain how you would perform in such a situation and the type of evidence you might obtain.

Did you know?

The Campaign for Learning says that learning can improve:

● customer satisfaction

● dealings with overseas customers if staff can speak the language

● absenteeism rates and employee turnover – happy staff don't take time off or leave

● accident prevention

● productivity – a motivated workforce is a good workforce.

Improve your own performance

Knowing that you are getting better at something feels good. Sometimes this happens just because you get more and more experienced at doing it. At other times it needs someone to show you how you can improve on what you're doing. Your first step is to decide where you are now and where you want to get to.

The importance of continuously improving your work

It's your first week in your new job. You're bursting with enthusiasm and keen to make a good impression. After a few days your enthusiasm starts to disappear. Although most of your colleagues are hard working and well motivated, some of them are not. When you dash back from your coffee break early they raise their eyebrows. When you take a lot of time preparing a document they pretend to be surprised at the trouble you're taking. When you say you're looking forward to the induction training, they laugh.

It's easy to be put off by that sort of attitude. However, if they refuse to accept that they can learn anything new or improve existing skills they might be sorry. Bosses notice the people in the office who are working hard, are receptive to new ideas and are willing to learn. Those are the ones who tend to get the promotions.

A lot of organisations try to encourage their staff to 'continuously improve' themselves, often referring to it as 'lifelong learning' because they feel that it can help them to improve the organisation's overall performance.

It's just as important that you try to continuously improve for your own satisfaction. If you think about a day at work when you felt you achieved nothing and compare it with a day when everything went well and you went home in a glow of satisfaction, you'll recognise the difference.

Did you know?

You go into a shop and ask for a particular type of shampoo. The shop assistant shakes her head and says that she doesn't stock it as there's no demand. That's the fourth time today she's been asked the same question. If she won't learn, she won't learn!

Did you know?

Seventy-seven per cent of the respondents in a business survey said they preferred to work for an employer who offered them time and support for training rather than one who gave big salary increases but offered no training.

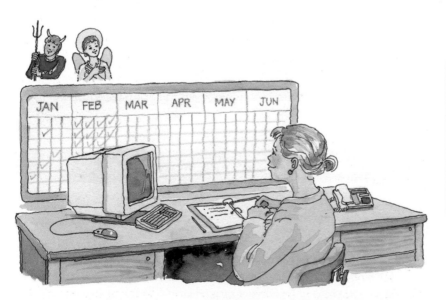

Personal Improvement

The importance of encouraging and accepting feedback from others

You're getting constant feedback when you're at work even if you don't realise it at the time. You give your boss a report that's taken you hours to prepare. He is pleased and thanks you. You're dealing with an awkward customer on the telephone. When you've finished your colleague at the next desk says 'Well done – you handled her beautifully.' You pluck up your courage to say something at a meeting and when you've done so one of the other members gives you the thumbs up sign. You take some photocopies to a senior member of staff who says she can't read them very well.

You don't need anyone to point out where you have succeeded and where you haven't. If you're smart you'll learn from it.

You may find that you will sometimes be given more formal feedback, normally during your appraisal sessions with your line manager. In most cases these sessions will follow a standard format:

- You will be told in advance that the session will take place. That gives you the chance to think about what you are going to say.
- Unless you are completely new, your manager will probably review what you agreed to do at the last session, the targets that were set and how far you think you have achieved them.

You should then be given the opportunity to raise any issues about things that worry or puzzle you.

You can then agree on what your new targets are. If you genuinely feel you can't meet them, say so. Your manager is then given the opportunity to offer you extra help, training, resources etc. if required.

Your manager will normally then end the session with an overall summary of your strengths and 'possible areas for improvement'. At this stage you can either float out on a cloud or trudge out muttering to yourself.

Remember

If you haven't achieved a particular target it's better to be honest about it rather than try to dodge out of it. Look back to page 50 for information on how to acknowledge your mistakes.

Did you know?

In many financial organisations, specially trained compliance officers spend all their time evaluating everyone else's work to see that they are following (or 'complying with') the rules and carrying out the correct procedures. They are meant to prevent problems from occurring.

How to... Deal with negative feedback

- First of all decide what sort of person you are. If you think your reaction will make matters worse, try to prepare a strategy for yourself.

- Try to understand that most people don't really like criticising – they much prefer to give praise. If your boss is one of these people try to accept that the criticism might be justified.

- Respond actively but calmly to what is being said. Don't just sit there silently, fly into a rage or get tearful. If your boss says that one of your colleagues has difficulty in working with you don't start raving on about that fat useless lump who's too busy eating crisps all day to bother getting on with anyone.

- If you can't understand why you are being criticised, ask for an explanation. It gives you time to consider what is being said and perhaps the chance to correct some wrong assumptions there and then.

- If you feel the criticism is totally unjustified, say so but give reasons.

- However irritating it might be, try to avoid blaming other people. Even if you have a point it doesn't usually put you in a good light. Of course, there's nothing to stop you tackling that other person later on and asking him or her to set the record straight.

- Grit your teeth and accept the criticism if you know it's true. If you know that you have difficulty in this area, ask for help. At this stage your boss might be very happy to give it to you.

- When the feedback is over, boost your morale by concentrating on the positive points made about you (assuming there were some!). Then actively consider how you can improve on the rest.

Evaluating your work

You are evaluating your work all the time. If you finish word processing a report and read through it before handing it over to your boss, you're making a mental evaluation of how good you think it is. If, after a meeting, you sit down to think over how well you've contributed, again you're trying to assess the quality of your input. Self-evaluation is very important. If you don't know whether or not you are doing a good job, you've little chance of improving your performance.

Sometimes, however, a more formal approach is needed. Suppose, for instance, it's the first time you've made some travel arrangements for your boss. Some things have gone perfectly, others have not. It's easy to heave a sigh of relief and to move on to your next job. Here are some tips:

- Make a note of everything that went well so that you can repeat the process next time.
- Make yourself write down what problems occurred. Did you forget to check on foreign currency? Did you find out only at the last minute that your boss's passport was out of date? Were

Find out

If you regularly have formal evaluations, obtain copies of any paperwork you or your line manager use in the process.

Remember

If you work as part of a team you might be evaluated twice, once as an individual and once as a team member. Teamwork is discussed in more detail in unit 321 page 355.

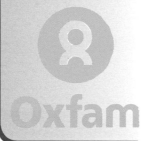

you thrown into a bit of a panic when your boss gave you some different instructions a week before the trip was scheduled to start?

- Ask yourself why. Was it simply your inexperience? Were you unwilling to keep approaching your boss to ask her still more questions? Didn't you think to ask someone more experienced than you in making travel arrangements for some help? Were you not given enough time?

- Analyse each of the problems and ask yourself whether any of them could have been foreseen or prevented.

- Recognise that some problems were beyond your control and that you could do little to prevent them re-occurring other than to expect the unexpected. If your boss's plane was held up for 12 hours because of weather conditions, there's nothing you can do about that!

Evaluation by others

You're not likely to be the only person who is going to be evaluating your work. Your boss will obviously be interested in the quality of the work you produce, so too will your colleagues, particularly if they are affected by what you have done. Again you can have informal evaluation – a comment from your boss that your minute-taking skills are really improving – or formal evaluation in the shape of a performance appraisal interview (look back to page 56 for further details).

Evaluation can start right at the top. A lot of organisations evaluate their performance in publicity material, reports to annual general meetings, auditor's reports etc. Most of them evaluate their work by checking progress against objectives or targets – have they achieved what they set out to do or have they fallen short?

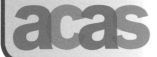

Testing out possible improvements to your work

You know you really should try to improve your computer skills because you're beginning to irritate the colleague sitting at the next desk by constantly asking for help. You make this one of your targets. You book onto an advanced level IT course and you now find your colleague is coming to you for help and advice!

It's a bit different when your improvements affect other people. Suppose, for instance, you work in reception a few times a week. One Friday you decide to make a few changes:

- You get the caretaker to help you to move some of the furniture around.
- You buy some large plants out of petty cash.
- You get one of the computer staff to change the computerised appointments system.

You go home rather satisfied with yourself. The next time you go into reception you find some rather bad-tempered colleagues:

- One of them was on duty first thing Monday morning and couldn't understand the computerised appointments system.
- The cleaner pops in to complain that no one told her about the changes to the furniture layout and she needs a new vacuum cleaner to get into the corner. She also asks who is going to look after the plants. She hasn't the time and isn't being paid for it anyway.

You are a bit disappointed because you thought you had improved things. You have. All you've forgotten to do is to keep other people informed and to consult those most likely to be affected by your changes. In most cases they'll be more than pleased to cooperate. At the very worse they can't complain that you haven't let them know.

Did you know?

Don't carry out a major improvement all at once. You'll lose track of what you are trying to achieve. One management writer recommends that you make one small improvement each time. That encourages you to take the next step.

How to... Test the effectiveness of any improvements you have put into practice

- ***Don't*** make improvements and then forget about them and move on to something else. Think about them as plants – however nice they look now, they'll wither and die if you don't look after them.

- ***Do*** build into your planning system a periodic review of the improvement, at least for the first few months.

- ***Do*** ask your boss, your colleague, a friend or someone who is affected by the improvement to give you some feedback. If, for instance, you've reorganised the reception area, ask the staff and the customers for their views to see whether or not they like the changes.

- ***Do***, if possible, test out the improvement yourself by becoming your own service user. If you have reorganised the office filing system, try finding an awkward document quickly. If you've tried to improve your spreadsheet skills, give yourself the target of producing one within a specified period of time. You'll soon know whether the improvement has been effective!

Find out

The competition for customers in the magazine world is now so fierce that editors are looking for all sorts of ways to attract new readers. Many editors have found that advice columns of any kind – on health, love life, careers – are very popular, and more and more of them are using them as regular features. Check your own favourites to see if that's the case.

How learning and development can help you to improve your work and further your career

Read the following extract from a letter to the careers advice column in one of the so-called 'girlie' magazines.

'I left school at 16 with a few GCSEs and went straight to work in a small office. I had used a computer at school and could word process a bit. I could have gone on a word processing course but didn't want to take the exam. A woman who's worked there for years showed me what to do but it's only recently that I found out that she's completely out of date. She's also a bit lazy and does the minimum. The manager did ask me if I would take notes at some of the meetings but I panicked and started making excuses not to attend. Someone else took over. At the time I was quite happy doing all the routine stuff – and I knew I was going to see my friends every night. One of them tried to persuade me to come on a holiday Spanish course but I couldn't be bothered.

'Two years on and I'm bored rigid. I've started to apply for other jobs but I've got a hopeless CV. I can't even get an interview.'

Obviously the writer has some decisions to make. She can resign herself to the fact that as things stand she isn't going to get a better job and she has to remain where she is for the next 40 years – a prospect she obviously isn't looking forward to. Alternatively she can start to think of improving her skills and her knowledge. There are various possibilities:

- **She could update her skills.** If she can't face taking an exam she can try to find a course that is either entirely or mainly based on coursework.
- **She could look for some internal support.** If the senior member of staff is really not much good, she can perhaps try talking to other colleagues. She might want to talk to her line manager to explain that she now feels ready to take on further work, undergo further training etc. – and hope he doesn't bear her a grudge for dodging out of the meetings!
- **She could do some reading.** If she skims through a newspaper she'll probably find that there are one or two articles in the magazine section in particular that will interest her – information about successful women managers, rights at work, time management, and so on.
- **She could find a leisure interest** – one that she can enjoy and at the same time benefit from. She may not need to use a language skill in her present job, but who knows when and where else it might be very useful.

Did you know?

Learndirect (www. learndirect.co.uk) is meant to help people learn new skills online. In many instances they don't have to sit an actual exam. They can also get free online advice on funding, childcare, courses and careers and even match skills and interests with possible suitable jobs.

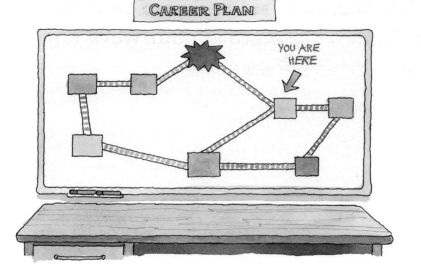

Did you know?

Many famous people have made use of their 'transferable skills' to move easily from one successful career to another. Gary Lineker has used not only his football knowledge to make himself a career in television journalism, but also the skills he learned on the pitch – quick thinking, always checking on the next move, avoiding getting into arguments, and not scoring an own goal!

Main career progression routes available to you

There are two basic choices to make when deciding what career route to take:

- You can move *vertically* – i.e. go up your chosen career ladder step by step.
- You can move *laterally* – i.e. check to see what other careers are open to you given your existing qualifications and experience.

You don't have to pick one in favour of the other. You'll have plenty of time during your working career to do a bit of 'mixing and matching'.

Administrative experience and qualifications are great to have. No matter what the type of industrial sector or public authority, there will almost certainly be a need for staff to give administrative support to it. Unless the organisation is very small there is generally a structure to it and you can see quite clearly what your next step could be. You can also take a look at other organisations in the same sector to investigate opportunities there.

Most administrators also have 'transferable skills':

- You may be experienced in preparing all the documentation and making arrangements for interviews and preparing training programmes for junior staff. If so, you could think of personnel work as a possible future step.
- You may be very skilled at preparing audio-visual presentations. If so, you might be a very effective member of a sales team.

Find out

Check in the business journals that relate to areas of work which you are interested in to see if they have a 'situations vacant' section. If so, keep a regular check on the types of jobs being advertised and the skills they need.

- You may be very good with figures. Accountancy could be the next career step.
- You may have experience in dealing with equal opportunities issues. Increasingly nowadays both private and public organisations are setting up equal opportunities units and need people to staff them.

The same could not be said if you had chosen a career in deep-sea diving or glass blowing!

It is sometimes difficult to decide the way ahead. Here are some tips:

- You need to pinpoint where you are on the career ladder. If you are not sure, take a look at your organisation's management structure and try to work out how many people are senior to you and what their responsibilities are. Then try to decide if any of their jobs would suit you.
- Talk to your line manager either at a convenient time or at your next appraisal to find out whether there are any suitable career opportunities for you in the organisation.
- Consider talking to someone from the Careers Advisory Service if you think you would like a change or if you don't feel there are any career opportunities for you in your existing organisation.
- Check the newspapers and business journals to see whether there are any interesting jobs you think you might like or be suitable for – again if you want to look outside your organisation.

Learning and development opportunities that are available to you

You have found the job of your dreams only to discover that you haven't yet got all the skills or qualifications it asks for. That's OK. What you now have to do is to obtain those skills. Nowadays many employers encourage their employees to consider learning and development from the beginning to the end of their careers.

You might therefore want to:

- discuss with your line manager what opportunities are available within the organisation and what assistance, if any, you might be given if you decide to undertake further study or training
- look outside the organisation to see what other options are available.

At the end of the process you might discover these courses:

- **Workplace training courses**. If your organisation has its own training unit you will probably find that you can take part in a wide range of training activities. These could include information

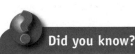

Did you know?

Ever since David Brent got the sack in the comedy series *The Office*, the BBC has been swamped with requests from companies wanting to show the video as part of their 'how not to' training.

updates on changes taking place in the organisation or the introduction of new policies or procedures, or they could be more general and cover issues such as interviewing or meeting skills.

- **College based courses**. They offer nationally accredited qualifications such as NVQs, GCSEs and A levels, skill qualifications in IT, professional and management qualifications in areas such as human resources, accounting and supervisory management. You need to check whether these are offered on a part-time or distance-learning basis.

- **Private training courses**. These offer short specialist courses either on the organisation's premises or in hotels or conference centres. They cover a huge range including updates on how to handle redundancies, health and safety issues, interviewing and recruitment, assertiveness, stress management, time management etc. These courses can be quite expensive, so it might be as well to look round for other options before asking your boss to pay out a few hundred pounds for a two-day course!

- **On-the-job training**. This covers a specific skill. If, for instance, you want to learn how to access a database or use a computer graphics package you could learn this from an experienced colleague. More sophisticated on-the-job training includes secondment to another department to find out what goes on there, or work shadowing where you spend time with a senior colleague observing what he or she does.

Choosing the right course

Sometimes you just don't have a choice. You might be expected to go on a one-day training session on telephone techniques. Your line

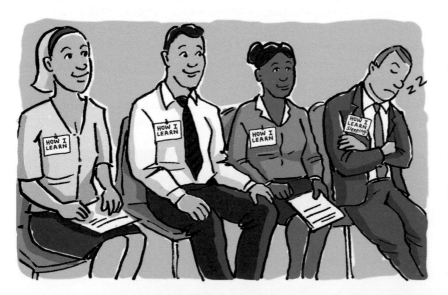

Did you know?

A group of primary school children in Cheshire now wear badges to show what style of learning they like best – hearing, doing, seeing. The teachers then adjust their teaching to meet all those needs at some time during the lesson.

manager really wants you to attend a part-time day-release course to improve your IT skills. You've just got to get your head around the new telephone answering system. Even so, it sometimes helps to know what sort of learner you are.

How to... Decide how you learn

Management writers Peter Honey and Alan Mumford set out the following classification of learners.

- If you prefer taking action to talking about it and like new challenges and experiences you are an **activist**. You might feel better taking a course involving a lot of hands-on work rather than one that requires you to do a lot of research and reading.

- If you are task-based rather than people-based and always want to have a solution you are a **pragmatist**. You might want to undertake a course that leads to a definite result – such as a job-related qualification – rather than one that is intellectually challenging but of no immediate benefit – such as a degree in fine arts.

- If you like to think carefully about things and see situations from different perspectives you may be a **reflector**. You'll enjoy the challenge of a full-time course or one with both an academic and problem-solving bias.

- If you are a born academic you are a **theorist**. You like to know the why as well as the how, and the deeper you have to dig the better. Again you'll probably enjoy a long-term rather than a short- term course of training.

Remember that you are thinking of a lifetime career plan. What is available to you – and how you feel – can differ whether you're 18, 28 or even near retirement age. At some time throughout the course of your career you're likely to be able to undertake the type of learning that best suits your style and which you really enjoy.

Snapshot – There's more than one way of reaching the top!

A job for life isn't nearly as common as it used to be. Nowadays most employees are expected to re-skill at least two or three times during their careers. In most cases this helps their climb up the ladder.

ILEX, the Institute for Legal Executives, has recently pointed out that many top lawyers have not followed the traditional route of school and university followed by a training contract in a firm of solicitors. Instead they have worked in an administrative capacity in an organisation, followed by a spell in a legal firm during which they picked up their 'paralegal' ILEX qualification and have eventually progressed to solicitor status.

It's a route that a number of people really enjoy. ILEX gives the example of Carina who is 19 and is training to become a legal executive. She likes the balance between working and studying even though it's hard work. She especially likes the fact that she is being paid while she is training! At present she is working in the immigration department and has been involved with a lot of high-profile cases on suspected terrorists who were unlawfully detained. Her firm represented some of them and, when the case went to the House of Lords, was successful in getting them released. Later on when she is fully qualified she hopes to specialise in media and entertainment law.

Other institutes such as AAT (Association for Accounting Technicians) and IPD (Institute for Personnel and Development) can give similar examples. They also say that many employers nowadays are only too willing to employ someone with different work experiences because of the added dimension they often bring to their new role. They can work in a team, they know how to deal with people, they're used to pressure – and so on.

You'll never know until you try.

Developing a learning plan

You know what sort of person you are, don't you? But have you ever taken the time to really analyse your personal strengths – and also those areas that perhaps need a bit more attention. If you haven't, you might find it useful to read the chart below and decide how you rate in each of the categories. If you have been totally truthful with yourself you will probably find that, although you have a number of low scores, you might also have one or two high scores.

The next step? You could just have a laugh or congratulate yourself on how good you are. Alternatively – and particularly if you are thinking about your career – you might decide to concentrate on improving your high-score areas by setting yourself some appropriate targets. Remember the SMART formula and try to apply it to each of the targets you set yourself. Look back to page 34 if you need to refresh your memory.

You should then be ready to build all your targets into a **learning plan**.

Key areas for analysis	
Score yourself from 1 to 5 in each of the following areas, where 1 is excellent and 5 is poor.	
Skills, knowledge and abilities	**Areas to think about**
Organisational skills	Ability to plan, find items stored easily, meet deadlines, prioritise, juggle several jobs effectively, coordinate a job and keep people informed, keep in control of tasks
IT skills	Ability to use PC software including word processing, spreadsheets, databases and presentation packages effectively Ability to use Internet, email and on-line services appropriately; undertake Web page design/website maintenance; use hardware such as scanners and ZIP drives
Information-handling and decision-making	Find and research information, check information, storage and retrieval systems (manual and electronic), extract and summarise, obtain and analyse appropriate facts to solve problems and make decisions
Communication skills	Good written English and oral skills, telephone manner, face-to-face communications Good listener, appropriate use of body language, negotiating skills
Self-management	Self-disciplined, takes responsibility for own actions and learns from mistakes Committed to giving best in a situation, knows self and reaction to stress/negativity from others, schedules time for personal interests, values own appearance and fitness
Money management	Able to plan and stick to a budget Financially self-aware Good financial knowledge/judgement
Numeracy skills	Can carry out basic numerical operations with or without a calculator Can understand basic statistics and trends in a financial document
Interpersonal skills	Sociable and approachable Good conversational skills plus ability to start a conversation with strangers Genuine liking for people and ability to identify different needs Cooperative and helpful
Organisational awareness	Understands aims and needs of employer Knows products and services Knows organisational structure and management responsibilities Sensitive to culture and 'office politics'
Personal skills	Positive attitude; uses initiative; self-confident with belief in own ability, flexible, open-minded
Miscellaneous skills	Good memory for facts and names; technical expertise in areas such as audio-visual presentations; knowledge of a foreign language; good with graphics; good at training junior staff

How to... Draw up a learning plan

- For a simple plan all you need to do is list a number of action points and the completion time for each one. An example is shown below:

Extract from a learning plan based on achieving a target	
Target: To meet deadlines	1 August
Action points	**To be done by when**
Check that I have a suitable diary	Now
Check all my existing jobs and the deadlines for them to be completed	Now
Enter those dates in the diary	Now
Make a note each time a job is completed	
Each time a new job is given to me, enter the deadline in the diary	
Set weekly reminder dates in the diary so that I can check that I am not falling behind with any jobs	
Review progress at the end of each month	31 August

- If you want to achieve something a bit more time-consuming, such as getting higher level IT qualifications, add extra information such as what help or additional resources you are going to require.

Extract from a learning plan – where meeting the target requires additional resources			
Target	**Help required**	**Additional Resources required**	**Time of completion**
To achieve Advanced word processing	• Time off to study *(state how much)* • Gather information • Attend college *(state when)* discuss with tutor	• College fees *(state how much)* • Access to photocopier, folders, textbook, stationery	• Milestone check with tutor every month *(specify dates if you have them)* • Date for final completion – 31 December

How to... Continued

- Break it down even further and list the individual units together with the help, resources and the time you are going to spend on each one. Normally the smaller the target the more easy it is to manage.

- Decide how often you are going to check progress. Make sure your planning system is up to this, whether it be a diary, a computerised reminder system or a wall planner.

Over to you

1   You are responsible for a small team of administrative staff but are becoming quite concerned about its newest member, Becky, as her work isn't up to standard. You arrange to have a quiet word with her. However, the meeting doesn't go as planned.

> *You*:   We have a bit of a problem here.
>
> *Becky*:   Well you might have. I don't think I have.
>
> *You*:   Well, let me tell you why I do have a problem. Your work is below standard, you never meet any targets, you refuse to go on any training courses, you won't even try to learn new skills. Everyone's sick of you, including me.
>
> *Becky*:   Everything else OK then?

You could have handled that better. Your first instinct is to go to the boss and demand that she sack Becky. However, when you're going out that night you hear Becky crying in the cloakroom. She might not be as tough as she appears. You decide that a different approach is needed. You sit down with her over a cup of coffee, start to talk things through and find out various things about Becky.

- Becky didn't do as well in her GCSE results as everyone thought she would. She was too disappointed to resit them and lost her nerve about applying for a business studies course at the college.

- The staff at the Job Centre insisted that she applied for this job. She got it but doesn't know why because all the other applicants looked much more capable than she was.

- She was really good at maths at school and what she likes best about her current job is working with figures and spreadsheets.

- She's also rather artistic and, if given the chance, would spend hours working on the presentation of a document. This causes problems because she spends so much time doing that that she gets behind with all her other work.

- She has no idea how to work the photocopier or fax machine.

- She's a bit shy – despite her manner – and doesn't know what to say in a meeting or whenever a group of people get together to discuss something.

- She doesn't like answering the telephone because she doesn't feel she knows enough about the organisation to deal with any enquiries.

You decide to sort out a plan of action to try to overcome some of these problems. You feel that first of all Becky needs some targets to try to reach over the next 12 months. You also agree that she might need to develop those targets into a learning plan. Before the next meeting with her you decide to:

- list the sort of courses or subject areas you think Becky might be interested in, based on what she has already told you

- check with the local colleges and training centres to see what they can offer that might suit Becky (remember that most of them are online nowadays)

- if there is anything relevant, obtain full course details

- check www.learndirect.co.uk/ to find out the courses that may be suitable for someone wishing to progress an administrative career

- check with www.google.co.uk if you want to find out about a specific course

- list any shorter courses Becky might benefit from in case they are available in-house or through a private trainer

- list any workplace training she might find useful

- draft out a list of possible targets, including any relevant courses

- draw up a first version of a learning plan, including realistic timescales.

Over to you Continued

Discuss your results with your tutor or trainer and/or check your ideas with the answers on the CD-ROM.

2   If you haven't already done so, carry out the same exercise for yourself – i.e. produce a learning plan to cover the next 12 months. Discuss your results with your tutor or trainer, your line manager or a friend, or check the suggestions on the CD-ROM based on the learning plan formats on pages 67–68.

 ## Evidence planning

For this section you can use evidence from any performance reviews or appraisals you attend. You will need to provide evidence that you:

● receive feedback from other people

● evaluate your own work

● have identified how to improve your work, put your ideas into practice and tested their effectiveness

● have noted how further learning and development could improve your performance.

● develop and follow through a learning plan that meets your own needs, then review your progress and update this plan.

The easiest way is to keep all your evidence related to your personal development and future ambitions in a special folder that you can refer to in professional discussions with your assessor.

Behave in a way that supports effective working

You may think that a section on behaviour is more suited to new or junior employees than it is to you. Interestingly, it is quite easy to argue exactly the opposite. This is because the greater your responsibilities at work, the more your behaviour can influence or affect other people. You know this yourself. If the youngest or most junior employee is in a strop, everyone will ignore this behaviour or just tell the person to stop. If the boss is in a dreadful mood then that is much more serious. It is likely that everyone is tip-toeing around, trying not to make matters worse. In an organisation where staff are made to feel miserable or hounded because of someone's behaviour, it is doubtful that any of them are working very effectively.

Hopefully you will be fortunate at least once, during your career, to work for someone who is not just a good boss but also an inspirational one – someone who trusts you, believes in your abilities and constantly encourages you to do your best. This will (or should) spur you on to try to achieve things you never thought possible before. In other words, your boss's positive behaviour then not only helps you to work effectively but also motivates you to set your sights higher than before.

This is why the higher you climb the more important it is that you behave in a way that supports people at work. You owe it to your boss to be loyal and focused; you owe it to your colleagues to be reliable and honest; you owe it to people who are your juniors to help and inspire them to do their best. On a lovely day, when everything is going well, this may seem simple. When it's teeming with rain, you are running late, your computer is playing up and you suddenly hit another setback, it isn't easy at all. Some of the hints and tips in this section will help you to rise to the challenge!

Did you know?

A **role model** is someone we want to copy because we admire them. Role models can be celebrities such as Joss Stone or Keira Knightley, or sporting personalities such as Kelly Holmes or Freddie Flintoff. Or they can be people we know and respect because of their attitude and achievements. Do you have a role model? If you can't think of anyone, what attributes should your role model have? What personal characteristics do you need to develop to become more like them?

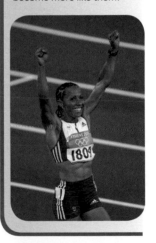

Did you know?

Soft skills relate to people's behaviour at work. They are different from 'hard skills' that you acquire when you learn to do something, such as use a computer or drive a car. We start to learn soft skills as children and continue to develop them all our lives. You can test some of yours in the activity opposite!

Over to you – Soft skills quiz

If you can remember your parents telling you not to fight, to share your toys, not to fidget or interrupt and to say 'please' and 'thank you', then you are remembering the first stages in your soft skills training. If – or when – you have children yourself, you will no doubt say the same things to them!

Such skills are important because they help us to become responsible adults who can interact positively with other people. Adults who lack soft

Over to you Continued

skills need to rethink their attitudes if they want to do well in life. So check out yours now by doing the quiz.

1   You are asked to do a job with two other people. Are you:

   a   nervy, until you know they are people you like

   b   annoyed – you work best on your own

   c   pleased – you enjoy working with others.

2   You are interrupted by the phone ten times in an hour. Are you:

   a   pleased to have an excuse to chat

   b   irritable – and it shows

   c   already working out how to reshuffle your priority list.

3   You've hit a problem trying to book accommodation for a trip your boss will soon be making. Do you:

   a   immediately ask a colleague for help

   b   tell your boss he will have to change his dates

   c   enjoy the challenge of finding a solution.

4   A colleague has let you down three times now, despite promising to email you a document with information you need. Do you:

   a   shrug and manage without it

   b   ring up or email and give the colleague a piece of your mind

   c   go and see your colleague to get what you need.

5   It's dreadful at work at the moment. There's too much to do, three people off with 'flu and a crisis virtually every day. Do you:

   a   work hard for a day or two but then make it clear you need extra help

   b   ring in sick yourself – last night's headache could well be the start of 'flu

   c   use the opportunity to prove you deserve both a pay rise and promotion.

6   Your boss has asked you to change the staff rota – but this needs the cooperation of two other members of your team. Do you:

   a   plead with them to go along with the plan

   b   tell your boss that his idea won't work

   c   persuade them by identifying the benefits they will gain.

7   Your boss chooses you to represent the firm at a formal event involving some important customers. Do you:

   a agree nervously and ask for help on what to wear and do

   b refuse – you've better things to do in your spare time

   c agree happily and research the customer files to find out more about them.

8 A student on work experience from a local school has started to arrive later and later each morning. Do you:

   a talk to her for at least half an hour about the importance of punctuality in today's workplace

   b tell her she's a waste of space and report her to her tutor

   c ask for her mobile number so that you can ring with an alarm call every day.

9 Your boss thinks that the office would be more productive if you changed things around a bit. Do you:

   a listen with growing alarm – you can't cope with the amount of extra work involved and hope she'll lose interest

   b listen with amusement – she's suggested this twice before and both times you've ignored her

   c listen with interest and contribute to the discussion with a few ideas of your own.

10 You have been on holiday and a temp has been covering for you. On your return you can't find an important file. Do you:

   a send an email to tell everyone the temp has lost the file

   b ignore it because it's not your problem – you weren't here

   c check all the likely places, then email to ask if anyone has borrowed it.

Did you know?

A 2005 survey on careers in business found that the most important ingredient to be successful and do well was to really enjoy the work you are doing. Do you?

Answers

- Mainly (a): Your main problems relate to lack of commitment and lack of confidence. Although you may be popular with your colleagues, you will be less valued by your boss, who may find it frustrating that you don't work as well as you could.

- Mainly (b): You are not a people person and your lack of soft skills is scary! Your colleagues are likely to try to avoid you and have probably long since given up expecting you to help or support them.

- Mainly (c): You enjoy your job and like working with other people. You show commitment and have good ideas. Remember that if you are ambitious and want to get on, then consideration for others is twice as important!

Setting high standards for your work

There are several important reasons for setting high standards for your work.

Find out

At what times do you arrive in the morning and leave at night? Are you last on most days, arriving in a mad rush? Or do you arrive in good time so that you are mentally calm and ready for a new day? And are you ready to go 'on the dot' no matter what? Now think about how your time-keeping contributes to your standards at work!

- Your boss and your colleagues can rely on you to give a professional impression of yourself and your organisation.
- Your boss and your colleagues know that they can trust you with complex and/or responsible tasks and to cooperate with them to achieve shared goals.
- If you lead a team, you must lead by example. You can hardly expect the members of your team to work harder or better than you do!
- You will work quicker because you will be far less likely to have to redo work because you have made a mess of it.
- You will be under less stress because you will do tasks more quickly and never have to take the blame for a serious error.

Setting your own standards

Did you know?

The standard you set should be realistic but it should also stretch you. It should be achievable if you work hard and focus on doing your best.

Setting high standards for yourself doesn't mean setting unrealistic targets that you can never achieve. If you do this, you will rapidly become demotivated and give up. Equally, you shouldn't set vague, meaningless standards that neither you, nor anyone else, can tell whether you've achieved.

You may set standards in one of two ways:

- You may set yourself personal challenges that you want to achieve.
- You may set standards for specific types of work during performance reviews or appraisals with your supervisor or line manager (see page 56).

Whichever method you use, the way to set them is shown below.

Remember

Try to see a mistake or failure as an opportunity to grow and learn rather than a problem. Focus on analysing what went wrong so that you never make the same mistake twice.

How to... Set high standards and show drive and commitment in achieving these

- **Identify specific standards** that are appropriate to the work you do. For example, accuracy and speed would both apply to document production; accurate communications or complete discretion would apply to your dealings with other people.

- **Decide the target** you want to achieve (see page 34). Examples are zero errors in a one-page word processed document produced in ten minutes; all emails replied to or acknowledged within 24 hours; greater cooperation between team members.

- **Decide how you will measure your achievement**. Examples are no documents returned for re-typing; achievement of team goals; ability to resolve difficult customer issues more smoothly and professionally.

- **Identify the time frame** over which you intend to achieve the standards you have set for yourself. Remember, if you are already achieving them then this isn't stretching you!

- **Identify your priorities**. You may not be able to achieve every standard you set yourself at once. Start by focusing on the most important for your job and your own personal development.

- **Identify any additional training or assistance** you may need to achieve your standards and discuss this with your supervisor or line manager.

- **Seek out opportunities** for practising your skills.

- **Revise your standards** at regular intervals so that they continually stretch you.

Did you know?

Business activity is rarely a steady flow. In virtually all jobs there are quiet times and very busy times. This will depend on the type of business and its seasonal variations. So you can expect to be under pressure in any job from time to time.

How to cope with pressure

Remember

Challenging work should motivate you. You should enjoy both the process (what you are doing) as well as the outcome. If you don't, something is wrong.

It's a frantically busy week at work. The phone is ringing, your in-tray is piled high, emails are arriving by the dozen. Every day you and your colleagues have worked flat out to cope. How do you feel about this? Are you exhilarated – the variety and pace has been much more enjoyable and challenging than quiet, routine days? Or are you exhausted and fed up – you work to live, you don't live to work and you've had enough, thank you. Or are you a nervous wreck, completely stressed out and seriously considering finding a different job because you just can't cope with that sort of pressure?

We all need a certain amount of pressure in our lives, otherwise we would become bored, frustrated and apathetic. Couch potatoes aren't under any pressure, but they don't achieve anything either and if you worked in a job where there was hardly anything to do you would be unusual if you wanted to stay longer than a few days. However, there is a balance. We all need some pressure to keep us stimulated, but too much can be harmful. The problem is that people vary in the amount of pressure they can tolerate, so what might be stimulating for you may be very stressful to someone else.

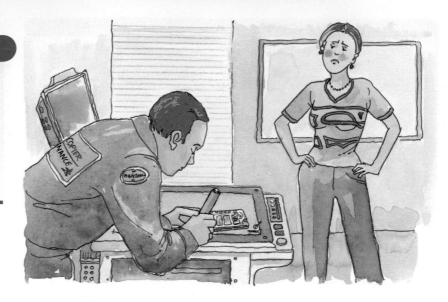

Coping with pressure at work

You will usually deal with pressure at work more easily if the following circumstances apply:

- You know your job well and are good at the tasks you have to do.
- You have the support of your boss who is realistic about what can be achieved.
- You and your colleagues can rely on each other for help and support.
- You have good organisational skills so that you work efficiently.
- You have some control over the work you do and how you prioritise it.
- You are not under pressure in your private life, as well.
- You can rationalise the situation and know that the current situation is short-term. If it isn't, then you also know your boss will arrange for you to get more help.

This means, of course, that if these circumstances don't apply, you are far less likely to cope. In this case then you can start to feel stressed. In this situation you need to know how to recognise and cope with the problem. This involves three stages:

- understanding the relationship between pressure and stress
- recognising the symptoms that show you are struggling to cope
- taking appropriate action, when necessary, to reduce the pressure.

The relationship between pressure and stress

We encounter pressure whenever we are faced with a new or challenging situation – trying to meet a deadline, having an argument, changing our job, meeting new people, travelling to new places, trying to do a lot in a short space of time. All these events make our lives more interesting. They also create pressure and can cause stress. These events do not relate just to work but also to our private lives, as you can see from the table below.

Factors that increase pressure and cause stress	
Work related	**Home/personal**
Lack of support from management	Relationship problems
Harassment or bullying	Family demands, commitments and responsibilities
Conflict with colleagues	
Negative atmosphere	Home/work conflicts (e.g. over hours, domestic arrangements or work commitments)
Excessive workload	
Too many urgent deadlines	
Long or unsociable hours	Stressful life events outside work, e.g. bereavement, relationship problems or divorce, health problems (self or family)
Insufficient training for the tasks/ responsibilities you are given	
Poor working conditions	
Lack of control over your job content	Financial worries
Job insecurity	
Lack of clear guidelines/proper instructions	
Change – both good (getting married, having a baby, moving house) and bad (death of a member of the family, personal illness or injury)	

Find out

Two American psychologists, Holmes and Rahe, devised a scale of 43 life events that are stressful and assigned values to each of these. A score of over 200 in any one year is likely to cause most people to feel stressed. Some examples are:

Death of partner or spouse	100
Divorce	75
Personal injury or illness	53
Marriage	50
Dismissal from work	47
Pregnancy	40
Change in work responsibilities	29
Trouble with boss	23
Holidays	13
Christmas	12

Find out more and score yourself online at www.covenanthealth.com/aboutus/pbh/pbh-lifechange.cfm.

However, different events affect people in different ways. Whereas you may feel faint at the thought of speaking to 200 people at a conference, it doesn't faze Tony Blair one bit! If you felt totally overwhelmed – even trapped – by the situation then you might display physical symptoms of stress. There is also a relationship between what is going on in your personal life and your response to work pressure. So whereas you might cope well with a new challenge at work or deal effectively with a problem involving a colleague, your response may be very different if you are under serious pressure at home too.

Recognising your reaction

People's responses to excessive pressure can vary. You might get a migraine and your friend may struggle to sleep at night. You will also have emotional as well as physical reactions and your behaviour is likely to change. All of the symptoms and behavioural changes shown below can be caused by too much pressure.

Remember

You should watch for signs of stress in your colleagues, too, and take account of personal difficulties that may have lowered their ability to cope with pressure at work.

Remember

Coping with pressure is like keeping balls in the air. Developing your coping skills enables you to juggle more balls at the same time. Asking for help enables you to throw some to someone else for a bit!

Emotional reaction

Lack of concentration, mood swings, weepy or tearful, anxious or angry, lack of confidence, irritable, feel overwhelmed and want to run (or hide) away

Physical symptoms

Headaches, dizziness, skin rashes, sleep problems, tiredness, nausea, digestive problems, chest pains or palpitations

Effect on your behaviour

Forgetful, accident-prone, make more mistakes, drink and/or smoke more, cannot relax, jump to conclusions, lose ability to make decisions, start to have negative thoughts and become depressed.

In this situation many people try to cope by relying on 'props' to help them, such as drinking endless cups of coffee or cans of Coke, drinking more alcohol or smoking. These actually make the situation worse – because getting more sleep and eating properly are two essential components in coping with increased pressure.

Taking action

There are two actions to take. First, you need to do something about the amount of pressure you are under. Second, you need to do something about your emotional and physical reactions.

Remember

If you are struggling to decide between priorities, and feel overwhelmed with work, list all the jobs you have to do and ask your manager to decide the order in which you should tackle them. It will then be immediately obvious if you have too much to do in the time allowed.

Reducing the pressure:

- Start by identifying the aspects of your job that are causing you pressure.
- Assess – with help if necessary – whether you can work more efficiently. Should you have a daily 'to do' list, use time management techniques (see pages 40–44), prioritise your workload and learn to negotiate deadlines more realistically?
- Remember that it is best to focus on one task at a time, complete it properly and get rid of it than only partially complete a series of jobs.
- Assess whether any problems are caused through lack of skills. Then ask for your manager's support to reassess your training needs.
- If your workload is too great, talk to your manager and ask for someone to help you or find out if some of the jobs can be reassigned to other people.
- If your deadlines are too tight, discuss with your boss how these can be renegotiated. If the deadlines are immovable, then you will need help to achieve them.

Changing your reactions

Only you know whether you have a low or high tolerance to pressure. If it is very low – or if you are going through a bad patch – then there are a few techniques you can use to try to reduce negative reactions and increase your resilience. This is dealt with in the next section.

The importance of being resilient when you experience setbacks

Resilience is the ability to bounce back when something goes wrong. It goes hand in hand with learning how to cope with pressure because both are attributes found in people who have found ways of managing when things get tough in their life.

Resilience is important because, unless you are very unusual or incredibly lucky, you will have to cope with life's knocks just like everyone else. Some of these might just be minor setbacks, others may be more serious. Unless you are going to give up at the first hurdle, you need to develop a strategy for coping.

Research has shown that life's best survivors display certain attributes or qualities. These are shown in the table below.

The attributes of life's survivors			
	What they do . . .		**What they don't do . . .**
✓	Realise everyone encounters difficulties from time to time	✗ ✗	take setbacks personally agonise for days if something goes wrong
✓	Know that setbacks are temporary, not permanent	✗	insist on perfection when it isn't necessary
✓	Adapt quickly	✗	think they can please everyone all the time
✓	Are positive and optimistic	✗	wallow in self-pity
✓	Have good supportive network of family and friends they can talk to	✗	agonise over things they can't change
✓	Learn from experience	✗	play the martyr
✓	Are professional and self-confident and prepared to try new things	✗ ✗	ignore the feelings and views of other people think that asking for help is a weakness
✓	Have a sense of humour		

Remember

If life is hectic you need to look after yourself. Drink lots of water, take exercise, have plenty of leisure breaks, eat well and get enough sleep so that you have the energy to cope. If *you* don't look after yourself, who will?

Did you know?

Life's survivors have the knack of turning disasters into triumphs. Think of the administrator who, after being unfairly dismissed from a routine job, studied for higher level qualifications and then applied for a top-level PA job. She said that getting the sack had been her wake-up call to do something more with her life!

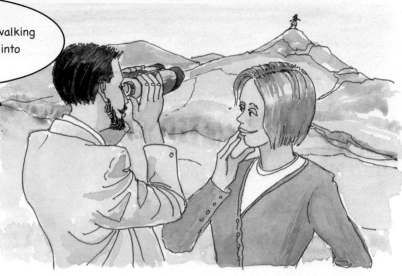

She said she was going to keep on walking until she got things into perspective

Remember

Never take action of any kind when you are furious, distraught or upset. Get away for a while on your own. If necessary, go for a walk and breathe slowly and deeply. Look out to the horizon – or up at the stars – to put things into perspective.

How to... Cope with pressure and overcome setbacks

- Identify the types and amounts of pressure you enjoy.

- Recognise when pressure levels start to become too much for you or out of your control.

- Identify when your emotional and physical reactions are telling you that you are under too much pressure.

- Don't indulge in negative thoughts or behaviour. Think positively and look after yourself.

- Reassess the way you are working to see if you can improve your efficiency.

- Talk to your manager if your workload is excessive and ask for support.

- Ask for training if a task is beyond your skills or abilities.

- Talk to a close friend or colleague if you are very worried, depressed or feel as if you cannot cope.

- Analyse each difficulty or setback to see whether you could have done anything better and what you can learn from it for the future.

- Keep difficulties and setbacks in perspective and learn to take them in your stride. They happen to everyone.

- Hold on to your sense of humour!

Snapshot – The power of GTD (or the art of stress-free productivity)

GTD stands for Getting Things Done and is being hailed as the new answer for coping with the age-old problem of having too much to do and not enough time to do it in. This is a combined time/stress management technique, established by management guru David Allen. It claims to enable you to reduce your stress levels by working far more effectively.

Allen argues against working out what to do by assigning a priority order. Instead the lists should be made to reflect different contexts – at home, on the computer, out shopping – so, in every context, you can move a project forward even if you only have a minute or two. That way, even large projects become manageable.

You can find out more online at www.davidco.com/what_is_gtd.php or by Googling 'Getting Things Done David Allen' and reading more at any of the thousands of hits you'll get!

Situations when it is important to be assertive

Remember

The right to refuse to do something doesn't extend to the work you are paid to do as part of your contract of employment!

If you are assertive, this means that you can state your point of view calmly and without upsetting other people. You are not someone who can be pushed around and will agree to anything for a quiet life; nor someone who regularly rants and raves to get your way.

The idea behind assertiveness is that everyone has certain rights. You have the right to:

- consider your own needs
- refuse to do something without feeling guilty or selfish
- make mistakes
- express yourself – provided that you don't upset anyone else when you do so.

Other people have these rights too. This means they have the right to ask you something, just like you have the right to refuse. So you should be assertive when any of your own rights are being denied:

- Your own needs are being ignored. This would be the case, for example, if you are struggling to cope under pressure or if you had asked for help and nothing has been done to assist you.
- You are being asked to do someone a favour without the time, resources or skills to do it; or are being asked to do something unethical or which would compromise your principles.
- You are being victimised or bullied for any reason.
- You are being harangued or made to feel embarrassed in front of your colleagues for making a mistake.
- You are being unfairly accused of something or treated unfairly in any way.

In any of these situations, it is no good being passive and simply hoping the problem will go away. Neither is it effective or appropriate at work to lose your temper and get in a rage. Being assertive enables you to raise the issue in such a way that you keep control of the discussion and of the situation. How to do this is shown below.

Remember

If you lose your temper with someone who is making your life difficult, you will lose any advantage you might have had. The person may use your outburst as evidence that it is you who is hard to work with.

Find out

Test your assertiveness skills in the presence of someone whose feedback you trust. Don't expect to get the words and the balance right at the start – it takes practice to do it well.

How to... Assert your own needs and rights when necessary

- Think about what you are going to say before you start to speak.
- Speak calmly and unemotionally. Don't shout or mutter.
- Look at the person you are speaking to.
- Be prepared to give a reason for what you are saying. This is different from long defensive explanations or feeling that you have to justify yourself.
- Start with the word 'I' (to own the statement), not the word 'You' (which is inflammatory and accusatory).
- Get to the point quickly.
- Refer to your own views and feelings, not someone else's.
- Make it clear that you consider that your own views are as important as everyone else's.
- Ask questions, if necessary, to obtain clarification.
- If you are refusing to do something, explain the reason clearly and don't feel guilty afterwards.
- Act in an adult manner and don't resort to childish tactics or personal criticism to get your way.

How to... Continued

- If you feel you are starting to lose control because the other person won't accept what you are saying, repeat your main points and end the discussion.

Did you know?

The type of organisation you work for will influence the rate of change you experience. Organisations that operate in a relatively static environment include solicitors and funeral directors. Those that operate in a dynamic environment include IT and telecommunication companies.

Taking on new challenges and adapting to change

On page 77 you learned that change can be a major cause of stress. It may seem logical to think that it should therefore be avoided at all costs. In the business world this is neither practical nor realistic. In any case, if you consider for one moment a world without change, the idea is quite horrific. We would presumably still be trying to scratch letters on tablets of stone, let alone have paper or use computers!

There are two types of change that are likely to affect you most at work:
- major organisational change, over which you have no control
- change relating to your own job role, over which you should be consulted.

Both may give you the opportunity to take on new challenges, depending on the reason for the change and how it is being implemented.

Did you know?

The term **restructuring** means that the organisation has changed the way it is structured or organised; so the number and names of the departments, branches and/or managers will probably be different.

Major organisational change

All organisations have to change constantly to survive. They may have to change to remain competitive and to continue to attract customers. Or they may change because they have identified more effective ways of working or adopted new types of technology. Alternatively, they may change because they are struggling to survive. In this case the changes could involve staff cuts and the reallocation of jobs amongst the remaining staff.

Changes are seen as a threat by many people because they fear the unknown. They may worry they will be worse off, or that they will have to do a different job, work with new people or even lose their existing job status. They may be scared they will lose their job altogether and struggle to find another, or that they will not be able to cope with more work or new responsibilities.

Good planning and good management can help to reduce these fears. If change takes place over a reasonable timescale, so that people are

Did you know?

Employers who want to make changes to any existing contracts of employment must discuss and agree the proposals with the unions, staff association or employees. They must then inform employees who are affected in writing within a month of any changes being made.

Find out

Some people like change because they have a low boredom threshold. If this is very pronounced they may 'job hop' quite a lot, especially when they are young with no ties. Other people prefer a known routine. If this is very pronounced they may easily get stuck in a rut. Do you prefer change or do you like things to stay the same?

consulted and know what is happening, it has a greater chance of success. Change that is enforced or done in a hurry is always more traumatic, and time has to be allowed for people to adjust.

Changes to job roles

Your job role may change in one of three ways.

- Your current job role may change because of an organisational restructure, because of new technology, because of new activities being undertaken by the business, or simply because your boss (or you!) wants to try something new.
- You may change your job but continue to work for the same employer – either because you move department or are promoted, in which case you will be expected to take on more responsibility to go with the higher pay cheque.
- You apply for another job in a different organisation and are successful. In this case you will need to be prepared to meet a host of new challenges and opportunities in your new role.

Remember

If you ever hear yourself saying 'But I've always done it like this' then you are rejecting new ideas – even if these might be better.

Responding to change

Employers always value staff who take a positive view to changes at work and do their best to adjust. They are usually even more delighted to find a member of their team who actually welcomes new challenges and different ways of working. Someone who not only suggests new ideas but will help to try to implement them is usually worth his or her weight in gold.

This isn't very easy, though, if you are basically a creature of habit and prefer the known to the unknown. In this case you may start to dig in your heels the minute someone suggests that you should do something differently. In this case, try the strategies in the 'How to...' box below to work out why you are doing this.

How to... Respond positively to change and new challenges

- Remember that you need time to adjust to changes. The more dramatic the change, the longer you need, so be patient with yourself.
- Find out as much information as you can. This removes fear of the unknown.

- Analyse new ideas and suggestions objectively. What are the strengths and weaknesses about the idea? If you ran the organisation, would you be in favour of it?

- Analyse your feelings. If you are feeling negative or resisting new ideas then why is this? Is it because you like a known routine or are scared you may fail if you do something new?

- List all the advantages and benefits you may gain from the change.

- List any worries or concerns you have and discuss these with someone who can advise you.

- Rather than turn down a new challenge, offer to do it for a trial period instead. This gives you adjustment time! At the end of the trial you may find you've enjoyed it more than you thought.

- If you are naturally resistant to change, work at becoming more flexible and developing your self-confidence. Remember, the more new things you accomplish successfully, the more your self-confidence will grow. You might even find you start to enjoy trying new things.

Snapshot – Do you work for a learning organisation?

Even if you relish new challenges and change, many of your colleagues might not. In this situation you may need to help and support people who are nervous or struggling. Some organisations manage change better than others – management writers have called these **learning organisations**. They view change positively and encourage continuous personal and organisational development. The benefits are staff who are less likely to feel stressed and a more productive and happier workforce.

You can see the extent to which your organisation would qualify by checking out the attributes of learning organisations which are listed below.

- Group and team working is encouraged with many teams setting their own goals and targets and monitoring their own performance.

- There are good communications at all levels and networking across the organisation.

Snapshot Continued

- Employee welfare is considered important, but high standards of performance are also expected.

- There is a strong emphasis on product quality and/or customer service.

- There is continual staff training and development.

- The company expects staff to collaborate and support each other over problem-solving and doesn't encourage competition and rivalry.

- New ideas and experimentation are welcome and mistakes are accepted. These are treated as 'positive learning experiences'.

- All employees are encouraged to share in decision-making processes in the organisation.

- Change is viewed as an opportunity, not a threat.

- Everyone is proud of the organisation and its achievements.

Did you know?

Andrew Carnegie was a Scottish entrepreneur who knew the value of good staff. He said that if he lost everything – his house, money and factories – but kept his staff, he would be able to get everything back again within 12 months.

The importance of treating others with honesty, respect and consideration

One of the good things about meeting people in your social life is that, if you don't like them, you can just walk away. Life isn't as simple when you work with them! In every organisation in the land, employees are expected to work productively alongside a variety of other people, many of whom will have completely different backgrounds, ideas and attitudes.

In the worst workplaces, this mixture becomes a witch's brew of intrigue, arguments, power games and back-biting. In others, staff just about tolerate each other by saying very little, doing their jobs and avoiding people they don't like. In the best workplaces, staff are mutually supportive. They have a shared purpose and common goal. Individual differences are welcomed and accepted because they enrich the team as a whole. In this situation everyone benefits. The business wins because staff are more productive; the staff win because it is a pleasure to work in a positive and supportive atmosphere.

All these benefits, though, don't just occur naturally. They are possible only if all the staff in the organisation – from the top downwards

– treat each other properly. And this means being honest, showing respect and having consideration for the views and feelings of other people.

Honesty

Being honest doesn't just mean being able to be trusted with other people's property or money. It also means being honest in dozens of other ways. While you might be indignant if anyone implied that you couldn't be left to guard her handbag or be anywhere near an open petty cash box, do you have the same type of principles about more minor types of theft? What about arriving late, taking too long for a break or emailing your friends at work? All of these could be seen as stealing *time* from your employer. What about doing private photocopying, sending personal letters in the firm's mail and 'borrowing' a few pens from the stationery cupboard?

And how honest are you if you make a mistake? Would you blame someone else or keep quiet, rather than own up? Or do you prize honesty so much that you would bluntly give someone your views whether these were hurtful or not?

Honesty with other people's property is straightforward. You are either honest or dishonest. Honesty about feelings is a greyer area. We all accept that we shouldn't tell lies, but that doesn't mean being tactless or trampling over other people's feelings. The skill of diplomacy means converting 'honest' remarks so that they are more acceptable for the recipient. That does not mean lying! So if your boss says 'Tell him I'm out' when she is next pestered by Andrew in accounts for some figures he needs, you don't actually need to lie to Andrew. Just saying 'I'm sorry, Sue can't take your call at the moment' is the diplomatic (and honest) answer.

Respect

You probably first learned about respect from your parents and at school. You may have been told to respect people older than yourself, or respect other student's views in your class. You might have accepted this without question or, at times, you may have challenged the idea. What about people who you don't agree with? Do you need to respect everyone – no matter what they think or how they behave? And what if they don't show much respect for you?

Although it may sound tough, respect is not supposed to be conditional. If you show respect for someone it means you acknowledge their right as a human being to have views different from yours. This is because you don't know the reason why they think or act

Did you know?

The Retail Fraud Survey 2005 claimed that research showed 25 per cent of employees are totally honest, 25 per cent are totally dishonest, and the remaining 50 per cent are swayed by opportunity. The GMB union, which represents many of the 28 million retail staff in Britain, was furious. Paul Kenny, Acting General Secretary, argued that 'any claim that seven million workers are totally dishonest and another 14 million would rob you blind if they got the chance is both insulting and utter nonsense'. What is your opinion?

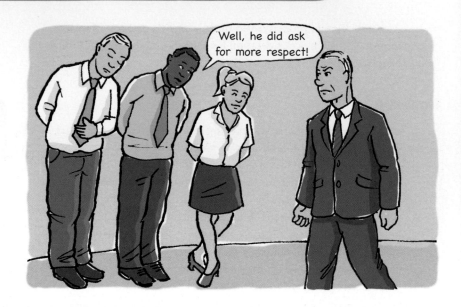

as they do, but (as long as what they are doing is not against the law) you can accept that they have the right to express themselves as they wish.

Consideration

If you respect someone then you are far more likely to show consideration than if you don't. If you respect your neighbours and accept they have a right to a peaceful life – even if you are a night owl – then you are far less likely to play loud music at midnight. You are therefore also being considerate.

Consideration simply means being thoughtful and, on occasion, putting other people's needs before your own – even if this is inconvenient. There is therefore an element of self-sacrifice in being considerate. It may mean depriving yourself of something you want or having to adjust your plans to fit in with other people, rather than insisting on having your own way.

Types of behaviour that show you are honest, respectful and considerate and those that show you are not

The key point about all these values is that they affect our behaviour. If you are honest, respectful and considerate then you will behave in a different way from someone who isn't. You will not, for example, exaggerate something to impress the boss. Neither will you pretend to be busy when you are not, make a colleague look foolish in front of other people, or 'rubbish' someone's idea – simply because you didn't think of it. In fact, there are quite a lot of things you would not do – and several you would, as you can see in the table below.

Types of behaviour			
If you are honest, you		**If you are honest, you don't**	
✓	Can be trusted with money and other people's property	✗	Think that a box of CDs or two notebooks won't be missed
✓	Arrive punctually and do the work you are paid to do.	✗	'Stretch' your breaks and lunch hours or spend half the day gossiping/doing personal work
✓	Admit your mistakes and apologise	✗	Shift the blame or fudge the issue
✓	Admit your feelings and motives	✗	Say one thing and do the opposite
✓	Keep secrets you promised not to tell not to tell	✗	Drop hints so that people 'guess' what you know
If you respect someone you		**If you respect someone you don't**	
✓	Pay attention when he/she is talking	✗	Ignore, interrupt or talk over him/her, dismiss his/her ideas
✓	Defer to him/her, temporarily, by putting your own feelings to one side	✗	Discount his/her feelings as unimportant in relation to your own
✓	Value his/her views as worthwhile, whether you agree or not	✗	Devalue his/her ideas by only taking heed if it helps you to achieve your own ends
✓	Behave appropriately, e.g. exchange ideas, obey an instruction, cooperate, protect or help him/her	✗	Behave inappropriately, eg manipulate, lie, hurt, poke fun at him/her
If you are considerate, you		**If you are considerate, you don't**	
✓	Show respect for others	✗	Think about other people negatively or disrespectfully
✓	Ask people for their opinions	✗	Tell people what you think and ignore their views
✓	Take other people's views into account when you are making plans or coming to a decision	✗	Think you are always right and your own needs are paramount
✓	Are prepared to make sacrifices or inconvenience yourself to fit in with other people.	✗	Insist people always do things your way

Helping and supporting others

At first sight the terms 'help' and 'support' indicate that you should have a key aim of looking around for anyone in trouble so that you can lend a hand. So you should, but help and support in a working environment goes a little deeper than that. It also implies other values, such as group loyalty and kindness. It is important because it means everyone can work more effectively and productively because they can rely on each other, all the time. It is also important because it helps to engender team spirit – and the fact that everyone is 'in it together' and working to achieve the same thing.

Find out

Check whether any of your organisation's policies relate to staff behaviour at work and assess how these should influence the way you treat your colleagues.

There are three ways in which you can provide help and support:

- begrudgingly – accompanied with huffs, puffs and sighs
- acceptingly – you just do it when asked
- pro-actively – you are sensitive to the needs and feelings of other people and instinctively know when they need your help or support.

When you offer support proactively you don't wait to be asked. Needless to say, this is the one you should be aiming for!

How to... Help and support other people

- If you ever have time to spare, look around to see whether you can help someone else.

- If someone is struggling or has a lot to do, offer to lend a hand whenever you can.

- Do favours for people when you can – such as collecting a cup of coffee or picking up their dry cleaning or a sandwich because you are passing the shop.

- If someone is alone, offer to have coffee or lunch together.

- If someone is new on the team, offer to help him or her learn the ropes.

- If you know someone has a problem, allow the person space but offer the opportunity to talk it over.

- If someone offers to help you, accept the offer generously and say thank you for favours received.

- If someone apologises to you, accept it graciously and tell them to forget about it. And you do the same.

- Be sensitive to body language, so that you can be aware that someone is stressed or struggling to cope.

- Give moral support. Commiserate when someone is 'down' or has a problem. Give compliments when he or she has done well.

Over to you

1 Check out your own stress levels and how well you are contributing to effective working by doing the self-assessment below. Discuss the result with your tutor or trainer and decide the best way of

improving your score. This is particularly important if you score less than 60.

Stress self-assessment

Score yourself from 1 to 5 on the degree to which each statement is true. 1 = never true; 2 = rarely; 3 = sometimes; 4 = mostly; 5 = always true.

1 I feel secure in my job.
2 I far prefer going to work than staying at home.
3 I really enjoy the work that I do.
4 I am involved in discussions and future plans about the organisation/my department.
5 I feel optimistic and positive about life.
6 I am good at coping with everyday setbacks.
7 I rarely worry or lose sleep over work.
8 I have lots of energy.
9 I can cope with my workload.
10 I get along well with my colleagues.
11 I know I am valued by my colleagues.
12 I can 'switch off' from work easily when I go home.
13 I have some control over the way I do my job.
14 There are people I can turn to when I have a problem at work.
15 I rarely get angry.
16 I am not devious or underhand.
17 The atmosphere at work is great – friendly and supportive.
18 I don't like getting into a rut.
19 I enjoy listening to the views of other people.
20 I work hard, but play hard too.

---

2 State the action(s) you would take in each of the following situations, (i) immediately, and (ii) to show you can learn from the experience! Compare your ideas with other people's and check them against the suggestions on the CD-ROM.

   a You are on your way to a job interview when you get stuck in a traffic jam. It looks as though you will be at least 20 minutes late.

   b Your colleague makes a huge fuss at the end of each month when she has to check expense claims and argues she cannot do her normal work and process all the claims in time, too.

Over to you Continued

c   In a team meeting, a colleague puts forward as her own brainwave a good idea you told her about yesterday.

d   Your boss loses her temper when she spots three mistakes in a document typed by one of your colleagues that she needs to take to her boss. Your colleague is nowhere to be found so she takes it out on you.

e   You have set yourself the goal of learning PowerPoint and are trying to prepare a presentation for your boss but are stuck trying to understand some of the instructions in the book you have.

f   A junior colleague asks you to check the contents of a letter you thought had been posted two days ago.

g   Your boss asks you how you feel about coordinating your department's contributions to your organisation's Intranet. You hardly know what she is talking about, let alone know whether you want to do it.

h   You do work for three managers, one of whom is very disorganised and often has urgent work that needs doing at the last minute. You stayed late once or twice to help him out but you now suspect he's taking advantage of your good nature as tonight he has arrived with another 'emergency' job at 5.15 p.m., fifteen minutes after your official leaving time.

Evidence planning

Identify the times when you have been involved in any of the following:

- You specifically set yourself high standards and had to show drive and commitment to achieve these.

- You experienced difficulties and setbacks and had to overcome these.

- You had to cope under pressure and/or handle stressful situations.

- You asserted your own needs and rights.

- You were asked to take on new responsibilities or challenges.

- You adapted to change. This could be a change of location, colleagues or a change involving the work you do.

● You gave other people help and support.

Now check the evidence you have. Do you have memos, emails or personal development plans to support your claims? Will your supervisor or colleagues give you witness testimony?

Finally, identify the option unit(s) under which you can appropriately place this evidence.

Key skills reminder

If you are taking Key Skills awards, remember to discuss with your tutor or trainer how your evidence for this unit could also count towards those awards.

Work within your business environment

Unit summary and overview

This core unit is divided into five sections:

- work to achieve your organisation's purpose and values
- apply your employment responsibilities and rights
- support diversity
- maintain security and confidentiality
- assess and manage risk.

As an administrator you may work for a variety of business organisations during your career. They could produce goods or provide a service, deal only with other businesses, with private individuals or with both. They may be large or small, owned by the state or by private individuals. They may operate in a high-tech, leading-edge environment or offer a traditional service that has changed little over the years. Appreciating how these differences will affect your job is crucial if you are to help your organisation to achieve its own particular purpose and values.

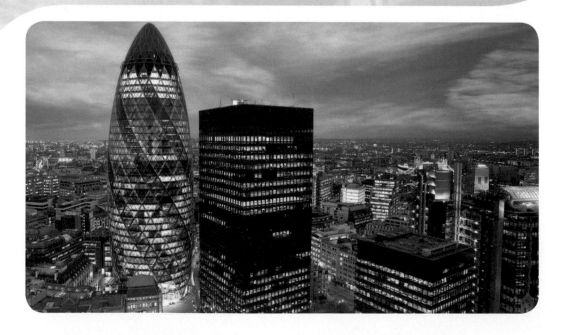

All organisations have certain factors in common. They must be law abiding – and so must you! Both you and your employer have certain responsibilities and rights. One of your employer's rights is to expect you to work towards the objectives of the company. This includes working productively and harmoniously alongside all your colleagues. Legislation prevents discrimination against anyone because they are different in some way. Beyond that, you will be expected to appreciate the benefits that a diverse workforce can bring to an organisation.

Working towards the objectives of a business also includes maintaining security and confidentiality. The greater your responsibilities at work, the more your employer can reasonably expect you to handle sensitive information with discretion. Finally, you will be expected to work safely and have the ability to identify and manage the risks that relate to your job.

Throughout this unit you will be involved in learning more about your current organisation, as well as the terms and conditions of your employment. You will find out about the laws that apply wherever you work in relation to issues like discrimination, security, confidentiality and safety. Your wider knowledge of your working environment will help you to understand your current organisation better and help you to identify ways in which you can work more effectively within your business environment.

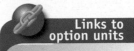

Links to option units

Your evidence for this unit will be generated and assessed through the option units that you select. This is because your option units should reflect the main areas of your job role so your evidence will occur naturally as you carry out your day-to-day work. For each option unit in this book, therefore, you will find guidance notes to show how evidence can be cross-referenced to this unit.

Within this unit you will also find suggestions to help you plan your evidence. These will help you to make the most of opportunities for obtaining evidence as you progress through the scheme.

Work to achieve your organisation's purpose and values

All organisations exist for a purpose. In this section you will learn how this can vary between individual businesses, depending on the industries they are in, the type of activities they carry out and their ownership.

You will also find out about mission statements, which set out the aims and purpose of an organisation and, often, its values or beliefs. These can affect company policies that control the type of activities that take place and how these activities are carried out. All employees must keep to the policies and follow any systems or procedures that state exactly how certain tasks must be done.

By the time you have completed this section you should understand how your job fits into the organisation, how you can help to achieve your organisation's purpose and apply its values, and what to do if you are unsure about any of these aspects.

The sector in which your organisation operates

Did you know?

Business organisations are grouped into **sectors**, based on their activities. To find out more about your business, you need to know the sector in which it operates.

All organisations are different, but some are more alike than others because they carry out the same, or very similar, activities. This is commonly used as a way of grouping different types of organisations by their industrial sector.

There are two main benefits of grouping business organisations into sectors, based on their activities. First, any information that is obtained will be more specific and relevant – builders aren't usually interested in whether or not farmers are thriving, or vice versa. Second, different types of organisations can be compared more easily, for example in relation to the numbers of staff they employ or their safety records.

Find out

The Health and Safety Executive uses SIC categories to present many of its statistics on accidents, injuries and other health matters in the workplace. Find out more at www.hse.gov. uk/statistics and check out the statistics for your type of organisation.

The main method of grouping industries in the UK is the **Standard Industrial Classification of Economic Activities** – SIC for short. SIC is regularly revised because, over time, new products and industries emerge and others may wane. The most recent version was issued in 2003 but a further update is due in 2007. If you are doing your NVQ award after 2007, check whether any changes relate to your organisation.

SIC categories are used by the Office for National Statistics (ONS), the government department that produces statistics relating to many aspects of life in Britain. These range from how many people own a dishwasher, to birth, marriage and death rates in different regions – and even the marital prospects for women in the twenty-first century! Many business-related statistics are grouped into SIC categories, for ease of reference and comparison – such as average earnings and weekly hours of work.

Did you know?

The word 'statistics' scares many people. It just means sets of figures, such as the number of boy and girl babies born each year or the number of people who work in different industries.

SIC categories

These divide businesses into three main sectors, with 17 sub-sectors. The main sectors follow the natural sequence of production for many goods.

- The **primary sector** covers all the industries that extract or produce raw materials from the land, such as the Forestry Commission which plants, grows and cuts down trees.

- The **secondary sector** contains all the industries that process and produce items, such as saw mills and furniture manufacturers which would turn the wood into tables and chairs.
- The **service sector** includes wholesalers and retailers, such as those who stock and sell wooden furniture to customers. It also includes business services like banking, insurance and distribution, and personal services like hairdressing and healthcare.

You can look up the full classification system online at the ONS or in any library and find out exactly which sub-sector includes the activities undertaken by your employer. To help you, a summary is shown on page 98 and more details on service industries are given below.

Did you know?

In 2005, the working population of Britain was over 30 million people. Eighty per cent worked in the service sector, 18 per cent in the secondary sector and 2 per cent in the primary sector. Therefore the odds are that you work in the service sector.

Service industries and business sub-sectors

Wholesale and retail trade – e.g. all wholesalers and retailers, including market stalls and dispensing chemists, plus repair/maintenance businesses such as garages and watch repairers

Hotels and restaurants – e.g. camping sites, youth hostels, holiday centres, take-away food shops, pubs and bars

Transport, storage and communication – e.g. taxis, furniture removals, freight transport by road, rail, sea, canals and air, passenger transport, pipelines, cargo handling and storage, travel agencies and tour operators, post and courier services, telecommunications

Financial intermediation – e.g. banks, building societies, finance houses, insurance companies and pension funds

Real estate, renting and business activities – e.g. estate agents, car hire firms, all rental firms, computer consultants, software developers, office equipment repairers, solicitors, accountants, market research companies, quantity surveyors, architects, advertising agencies, recruitment companies, security firms, industrial cleaners, photographers, secretarial agencies, call centres, debt collectors, exhibition organisers

Public Administration and defence – e.g. government agencies which oversee healthcare, education and other services, defence activities, the justice system, the police and fire service

Education – e.g. all schools, colleges and universities, driving schools, private training firms

Health and social work – e.g. hospitals and nursing homes, doctors, dentists, vets, social workers

Other community, social and personal service activities – e.g. sewage and refuse disposal, professional organisations and trade unions, religious and political organisations, film and video production and distribution, radio and television, theatres, fair and amusement parks, news agencies, libraries, museums, sports centres, dry cleaners, funeral directors, hairdressers, beauty therapists, gyms and fitness centres, nature reserves

Did you know?

If you work for a public limited company its name will end in 'plc'. You can then quickly check which sector you work in by looking for its share price in a national newspaper. The shares are grouped by sector, so when you find your company's share price you find out the sector at the same time! If you don't know what company shares are, ask your tutor or trainer.

PRIMARY SECTOR		SECONDARY SECTOR			SERVICE SECTOR
Agriculture, hunting, forestry and fishing	Mining and quarrying	Construction	Electricity, gas and water supply	Manufacturing	Services
✓ Farming (all types), Landscape gardeners, Horticultural firms, Animal breeders, Catteries and kennels, Gamekeepers, Tree growers, Forestry businesses, Logging companies, Fishing fleets, Fish farms	✓ Water extraction companies, Bottled water companies, Mining companies, Quarries (stone, slate etc.), Gravel and sand pits	✓ Earth-moving and demolition firms, Building and civil engineering companies, Highway/road builders, Electrical fitters, Plumbers, Plasterers, Joiners, Painting, Window firms (glaziers)	✓ Electricity generation companies, Electricity supply companies, Oil and gas manufacturers, Water treatment companies	✓ Food products, beverages and tobacco (e.g. bread, pet food, sweets); Textiles and textile products (e.g. carpets); Leather and leather goods (e.g. footwear); Wood and wood products (e.g. boxes) but not furniture; Pulp, paper products, publishing and printing (e.g. wallpaper and books); Coke, refined petroleum products and nuclear fuel processing; Chemicals, chemical products and man-made fibres (e.g. soap, glue, blank CDs); Rubber and plastic products (e.g. tyres); Mineral products (e.g. glass and ceramic goods – sinks, baths etc.); Basic and fabricated metal products (e.g. cutlery, central heating radiators, screws); Other machinery and equipment (e.g. domestic appliances); Electrical and optical equipment (e.g. computers, cameras, office equipment); Transport equipment (e.g. cars, boats); Other manufacturing not covered above (e.g. games and toys, sports goods, furniture)	✓ Wholesale and retail trade; Hotels and restaurants; Transport, storage and communication; Financial intermediation; Real estate, renting and business activities; Public administration and defence, social security; Education; Health and social work; Other community social and personal service activities; Private households employing domestic staff; Extra-territorial organisations and bodies (e.g. armed forces)
✗ Vets, Production of pet food, Fishmongers	✗ Builders' merchants, Stonemasons	✗ Estate agents, Architects, Interior designers	✗ Water-cooler maintenance firms, Garden centres	✗ Film and television production companies	✗ Growing of herbs and spices; Salt extraction; Newspaper, book and magazine publishing/printing; Production of blank videos, CDs and DVDs

Over to you

1 a Study the tables on pages 97 and 98 to locate your own industry and identify the main sector (primary, secondary or services) in which your organisation operates.

b Each of the industries marked with a cross in the bottom row of the first table has been placed in the wrong sector. Identify the sector in which it should be placed and give a reason for your decision. You can check your ideas with the answers on the CD-ROM.

c Sam has had four jobs as an administrator. First she worked for Barratts, the house builders, then she moved to UK Coal. Next she worked for a local paper-making company and now she works for her local college. In order, identify the sectors in which she has worked.

d If you work in the service sector, state the specific industry in which your organisation operates.

2 Explore the National Statistics site yourself at www.statistics.gov.uk to see the type of information that is available. To find out more about employment in your industry, click on Employment under Key Statistics. Explore some of the alternatives available on the summary screen. Try to find out at least three new facts about your own industry and discuss your findings with your tutor or trainer.

3 Find out more about your own sector at www.dti.gov.uk, the website for another government department – the Department for Trade and Industry. On the home page you can search for a particular industry. Click on the arrow and select your own industry to find out what it says. Note that the headings for each sector and industry are slightly different from the SIC categories but still cover broadly the same areas. If your own industry does not seem to be listed, talk to your tutor or trainer.

Your organisation's mission and purpose

An organisation's mission is a short, preferably memorable, statement about its main purpose or goal. Sometimes, rather than call it a 'mission statement' you may just see 'our aims are' or 'our goal is'. This means the same thing.

The mission or aim of a business may be linked to the type of activity it carries out and its sector. However, it is far more likely to be linked to the type of ownership of the organisation. And this brings us to another way in which businesses can be grouped by sector.

Sectors, ownership and aims

Remember

All businesses in the private sector aim to make a profit, otherwise they will not survive. Profit is the money remaining from sales income after buying stock and paying all the costs and expenses involved in running the business.

- **The private sector**. If you owned your own business, and had to decide on an aim or goal, you would be very unusual if the thought of making money did not come into your head. You would also be very silly. Unless you were very rich you would need to earn enough to live. So your main purpose, if you had invested your savings in an enterprise, would be to make a healthy profit. If you work for a privately owned organisation, then it will be very surprising if this goal is not uppermost on your employer's mind, too!

- **The voluntary (or charity) sector**. If you work for Oxfam, Barnados or any other major charity, the last thing you would expect is to find that the trustees aim to get rich. In fact, that would be illegal. The trustees of a charity have to identify its main aim and can have charitable status in law only if this purpose matches one of the legal definitions for charitable enterprises. This includes providing specific benefits for identified groups of people.

Did you know?

In the voluntary sector, the funds remaining after costs have been paid are called *surplus* (not profit) and must be spent on supporting the main aims of the organisation.

- **The public sector**. Although your GP, health centre or hospital also provide benefits for people, none of them is a charity. They are all funded by public money, collected through taxation, to provide essential services to the community. So their main goal is to provide an efficient and effective service so that taxpayers obtain value for money. This is the same aim you would find if you worked in education, for the police or for your local town hall.

Ownership and mission statements

The ownership of an organisation affects its main purpose and aims, and therefore the content of its mission statement.

Remember

You are more likely to find mission statements used by public sector and voluntary organisations than the private sector – particularly small businesses. But they all still have aims and goals!

Many large organisations have a mission statement, especially in the public and voluntary sectors. Some organisations call this their **vision statement**. Others have both a mission statement and a vision statement, and some have separate statements about their principles, goals or values and the activities being done to achieve the aims. There may even be more than one mission statement – Ben and Jerry's ice-cream Statement of Mission is in three parts – its product mission (related to what it supplies), its economic mission (which includes finances and profit) and its social mission (the way it links to society). The key point is there is no rule about mission statements, so there are many differences between organisations.

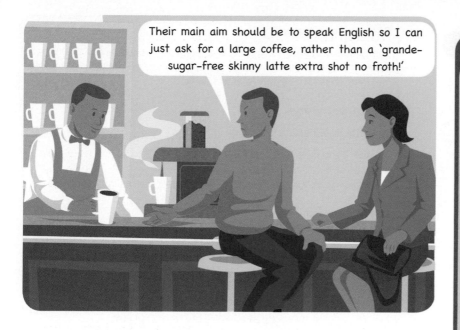

Did you know?

A good mission statement should be brief and easy to understand. But this does not mean that people will always agree with it. In 2005, British Airways had problems when many staff at Gate Gourmet, its meals supplier, were sacked by their employer. Some BA staff went on strike in sympathy, many flights had to be cancelled and, even after BA staff returned to work, customers had to take their own food on flights for several months. This didn't match the BA mission statement: 'To be the undisputed leader in world travel'!

- **Private sector organisations** normally mention customer relations, providing high-quality goods or services, giving value for money or employee relations in their mission statement. Starbucks Coffee Company is a private organisation and its mission statement reads: 'To establish Starbucks as the premier purveyor of the finest coffee whilst maintaining our uncompromising principles while we grow'.

- **Public sector organisations** usually stress that they are keen to provide a quality service, be efficient and give good customer service. The BBC is a public sector organisation because it is funded through the television licence fee. Its mission statement is: 'To inform, educate and entertain'.

- **Voluntary sector organisations** describe the service they provide and talk about the specific aims of the organisation and the types of people they aim to help. Oxfam is a voluntary organisation and its purpose is: 'Oxfam works with others to overcome poverty and suffering.'

Find out

Although many people (volunteers) work for charities for nothing, 2 per cent of the UK workforce – about 570 000 people – are employed in the sector as salaried professionals, many of them administrators. If you would like to work in an area like animal welfare, social care or international development, check out www.charitypeople.com to find out more.

Business values

Another word for business values is 'ethics'. Both relate to what the business believes in and the way it operates. An ethical business would never deliberately mislead or deceive its customers or suppliers, as you will see on page 112.

The mission statement, vision and values of Samaritans in 2005, as shown on their website, were as shown on page 102.

Find out

Do you know how your organisation is owned? Find out and then decide how this affects its main purpose.

Samaritans' mission

Samaritans is available 24 hours a day to provide confidential emotional support for people who are experiencing feelings of distress or despair, including those which may lead to suicide

Samaritans' vision

Samaritans' vision is for a society in which:

- fewer people die by suicide
- people are able to explore their feelings
- people are able to acknowledge and respect the feelings of others

Samaritans' values

Samaritans' values are based on these beliefs:

- The importance of having the opportunity to explore difficult feelings
- That being listened to, in confidence and accepted without prejudice, can alleviate despair and suicidal feelings
- That everyone has the right to make fundamental decisions about their own life, including the decision to die by suicide

Over to you

1 a Find out more about Samaritans at www.samaritans.org and then identify the sector in which it is placed in terms of its ownership.

b Samaritans now offer their clients an email service. Do you think this fits with their mission statement? Give a reason for your views.

c As an administrator who regularly uses email and the telephone you may consider helping the Samaritans in your spare time as a volunteer to deal with clients. What other skills do you think you would need to do this work that would also be useful for an administrator? If possible, compare your ideas with other people at work or in your group.

2 Sport England states as its vision: 'Making England an active and successful sporting nation'.

a Access the website at www.sportengland.org and click on 'about us' and 'Who we are and what we do' to read its mission statement, role and business objectives.

b From the way its role and objectives are worded, decide whether it is in the private, public or voluntary sector in terms of its ownership. Give a reason for your answer. Check your ideas with your tutor or trainer or with the answers on the CD-ROM.

3   Read the following private sector mission statements online
    and say whether you think they are clearly written and easy to
    understand. Give reasons to support your opinion. List any words
    that are new to you and find out what they mean.

    a   The Ben and Jerry's mission statement and values can be seen
        in full at www.benjerry.co.uk/missionstatement.

    b   Sainsbury's goals are at www.sainsburys.co.uk, on the About
        our Company FAQs page.

    c   The Starbucks mission statement and guiding principles can be
        seen at www.starbucks.co.uk/en-GB.

4   Virtually all educational establishments have a mission statement,
    so it is likely that your college or training organisation has one.
    Obtain a copy and identify three ways in which the administrators
    who work there may help to contribute towards achieving its main
    purpose. Compare your ideas with other members of your group
    and with the suggestions on the CD-ROM.

Evidence planning

You will obtain and present your evidence for this unit to your assessor
through the option units you have chosen. However, you should find
this easier if you start to plan opportunities for evidence collection
now, whilst this section is fresh in your mind. You need to prove to
your assessor that you understand this section and how you can work
towards achieving your organisation's objectives.

Start by preparing a description of the organisation you work for and
your job role within that organisation. This will also help you to decide
how best to relate your evidence to your option units and can also form
the basis of a professional discussion with your assessor.

Choose your own title and layout. Bear in mind that if your document
is clear and easy to understand it may also contribute towards your
evidence for unit 301.

1   Start with the name of your employer, the main activity of the
    organisation (i.e. what it does) and the sector it is in. This should be
    the main sector related to its activities, but you should also state
    whether it is in the private, public or voluntary sector as this will
    affect its main purpose.

2   Find out whether your organisation has a mission statement. If it
    does, obtain a copy and read it carefully. Is it short, memorable
    and easy to understand? To what extent do you think it accurately
    reflects the main purpose of the organisation?

    If there is no mission statement, talk to your supervisor or line
    manager about the purpose and aims of your organisation. Then
    draft out your own statement to explain these to your assessor.

Save your work – you will add to this document as you progress through
the section.

How your organisation compares with others in the sector

When organisations want to gauge how successful they are, they do this
by comparing themselves with other organisations in the same sector.

Private sector organisations

These organisations are in direct competition with others in the same
sector and industry:

- Ben and Jerry will want you to buy their ice-cream rather than
  Häagen Daz or Walls.
- Sainsbury will compare its performance and results to that of Tesco,
  Asda and Morrisons.
- Starbucks is in competition to outlets such as Costa Coffee, Coffee
  Republic and Caffe Nero.

These organisations compete to increase their **market share** in their
own particular market – for ice-cream, supermarkets or coffee. The
'market' is the total consumer market for a product or service. Market
share is usually shown as a percentage of the total market and can
be calculated by finding out the value of the sales made by different
suppliers. Large organisations will buy reports from market research
companies such as Euromonitor International (www.euromonitor.com)
and Keynote (www.the-list.co.uk). These companies provide in-depth
reports and up-to-date statistics on all the major firms in a sector or
industry and compare their performances. In many cases, sectors are
divided into different groups, known as segments. For example, two
major segments of the ice-cream market are impulse ice-cream (which
includes wrapped products such as Magnums) and take-home ice-
cream (the type sold in tubs in your local supermarket).

In 2004, the UK take-home ice-cream market, by global brand owner, based on retail sales, was as shown below. You will find out more about one of these brands, Mackie's, on page 110–11.

UK take-home ice-cream market in 2004	
Manufacturer	**UK market share**
Unilever	29.6%
General Mills Inc.	7.1%
Mars Inc.	3.1%
Mackie's	2.8%
Nestlé SA	1.5%
Cadbury Schweppes plc	0.9%
Hill Station Ltd	0.2%
Yeo Valley Organic Co Ltd	0.1%
Richmond Foods plc	0.1%
Private label	33.9%
Others	20.7%

Table reproduced with permission of Euromonitor International

Small organisations, such as hairdressers, solicitors and estate agents, are interested in increasing sales and profits too. They are not interested in national market share because they mainly compete on a local or regional basis. They will not be able to find out details of the financial affairs or sales of their competitors but their accountants will be able to tell them whether they are making better than average profits for their own sector or industry.

Voluntary sector organisations

Oxfam and the Samaritans do not compete in terms of supplying their services, but they do compete with other charities to obtain donations. They would not want to be left behind because they were not successfully competing with the fund-raising efforts of other charities. For this reason large charities operate on a highly professional basis and are often structured and organised very similarly to large private sector companies – as you will see on page 108–9.

All charities are aware that a series of major catastrophes can result in 'compassion fatigue', where the level of donations falls rapidly. In ten months between December 2004 and October 2005, a series of crises from the Asian tsunami to the earthquake in Pakistan resulted in

Remember

Small producers may get taken over by larger organisations, so names are not all they seem! Ben and Jerry's is now owned by Unilever, which also owns Bird's Eye Walls. The Häagen Daz brand is owned by US giant General Mills Inc. If you are doing option unit 310, which involves researching information, remember that you can check out this type of information in the *Who Owns Whom* reference directory.

Did you know?

The Internet has enabled many small, local (or remote) firms to sell their goods internationally and challenge some larger established suppliers.

Did you know?

Many charities have more staff and handle more money each year than many large companies. For example, the children's charity Barnardo's has 6500 staff, 11 000 volunteers and an annual turnover of over £100 million.

hundreds of millions of pounds being donated by Britons. The danger is that there is little left for the smaller charities unless they have some very original fund-raising ideas.

Public sector organisations

Many types of public sector organisation have their performance highlighted annually in published league tables. Facts and figures on their performance are normally obtained from relevant statistics or by visits from inspectors – or both:

- Your GP must provide a summary of the treatments discussed and given after each consultation with a patient. These form the basis for both payments to the practice and the practice's performance ranking, which you can check out online.
- Your local police force has to provide statistics to show how successful it is at fighting and solving crime, and is then ranked against other police forces in the country.
- School and college league tables are based on statistics from SAT tests and examination results. Inspectors also visit educational establishments, such as those from Ofsted and ALI. Your college or training organisation will check its performance and results against similar organisations in your area.

Supporting your organisation's mission and objectives

All employees have a legal responsibility to work towards achieving their employer's main aims (see pages 131–3). You already know that these are often identified in a mission statement. Even if they are not, you are still expected to know that your employer is in business for a purpose and to cooperate in helping to achieve the long-term goals.

Many public sector organisations review their long-term goals (and even their mission statements) at regular intervals and involve all their staff in the process. They may then publish a strategic plan and an operational plan.

If you work for an organisation that produces operational plans, then this will state the **objectives** of your department over the next 12 months. Objectives are different from aims because they are short-term targets. They are less overwhelming and are significant because their achievement means that progress is being made towards the long-term goal. It is exactly the same for personal goals you set for yourself. For example:

- If you want to save money, it's better to aim for £10 a week than £500 a year.

Did you know?

Not everyone agrees that inspections accurately reflect performance. When fire authorities were first ranked in a league table in 2005, Merseyside came out on top, followed by Kent and Medway. The Isle of Wight and Lincolnshire came last, rated poor. The Fire Brigades Union attacked the figures because they didn't include emergency response times or lives saved but were based on corporate management, modernisation, fire prevention and value for money.

Did you know?

Long-term goals are rather like New Year resolutions. Ambitious, easy to make but very hard to keep over any length of time! That's why businesses set short-term objectives that identify 'milestones' to achieve along the way.

Did you know?

A **strategic plan** sets out organisational aims over the next three to five years. An **operational plan** states how these will be achieved and what each section or department will do to help.

- If you want to complete this award, it's easier to plan to obtain evidence for one unit every two months than to think about the whole qualification at once.

These objectives then become your targets. At work you may have specific targets to meet and know what these are. If you work in a small organisation, your boss may know exactly what targets there are – but may not have told you. Just because you do not know what aims, objectives and targets there are, that doesn't mean that there aren't any!

Your main responsibilities at work

Most people are issued with a job description when they start work. In many cases this may be sent out to job applicants so that they can see the work they will be doing if they succeed in their application. This deters anyone applying for a job if they wouldn't want to do the work or be qualified to apply. An example of an administrator's job description is shown below.

Find out

Find out whether your organisation has strategic and operational plans. If it does, check how they affect your department and job role.

If not, talk to your supervisor about his or her aims, objectives and targets over the next 12 months. Then discuss how you can help to achieve these.

CAPITAL SERVICES LTD

Job description

Department:	Human Resources
Job title:	Administrator
Hours of work:	37.5 per week, normally 9 a.m. – 5.30 p.m. Monday to Friday
Salary scale	£14,000 – £17,000
Responsible to:	Human Resources Manager
Responsible for:	Assistant Administrator
Job purpose:	To provide administrative support for the human resources team and oversee key administration requirements of the human resources department

Duties and responsibilities

1. Assist with the preparation and placing of job advertisements in selected newspapers.
2. Log requests for application forms, send these to enquirers and log completed, returned forms.
3. Maintain all files and records relating to job applications, shortlists, references and interviews.
4. Arrange job interviews and contact candidates as requested by the human resources team.
5. Log all test and interview results.
6. Oversee the effective and prompt processing of general enquiries and ensure departmental files and records are kept up to date.
7. Oversee other routine administrative duties carried out by the Assistant Administrator.

Find out

Surveys have shown that most administrators do the following tasks at work:

- They communicate with other people.

- They produce, store and retrieve documents.

- They use IT systems and software.

- They answer the telephone.

- They operate standard office equipment.

Does this accurately reflect your job? What else do you do? What additional responsibilities would you expect to carry out if you obtained a more senior administrative job in the future?

Did you know?

In a well-organised business, the organisation should run like a well-oiled machine. The staff are the individual components who all have specific jobs to do, yet work in harmony with all the rest.

8 Record staff leave requests, maintain absence records and keep the staff database up to date.

9 Prepare general correspondence as required by the Human Resources Manager.

10 Attend any training course or team events as requested by the Human Resources Manager.

11 Maintain staff confidentiality at all times and be aware that breach of this could lead to instant dismissal.

12 Undertake any other relevant duties which may be identified.

This job description will be the subject of regular review and possible amendment in line with company priorities. The post holder may also be required to undertake related tasks that are not specifically mentioned above.

If you compare advertisements or job descriptions for a number of administrative jobs you will find certain similarities. These relate to the core skills and abilities required by almost all administrators. There may also be specific tasks related to a particular job, department or organisation. The main difference you will find is between levels of job – which will affect the rate of pay. In the job description above, the administrator is responsible for an assistant who has less responsibility and would therefore be paid less.

Your role and contribution in your organisation

Even the smallest organisations have some type of **structure**, even if this is not immediately obvious. If the business is operating effectively then, when you watch people at work, you should be able to identify several factors in operation:

- All staff have specific responsibilities linked to their skills and qualifications.
- All staff know what they are responsible for doing.
- They also know what their colleagues are responsible for doing.
- Jobs do not overlap, so people don't get in each other's way.
- Staff know the type of decisions they are allowed to make – and those they must refer to someone else for.
- Someone is responsible for doing every job that is needed for the organisation to achieve its goals.

In a small business this should be relatively easy to achieve. If you work as the only administrator in a small firm, then you will know exactly what you have to do. The directors or managers would be responsible for managing the business; you are responsible for administration; the sales or technical staff would be responsible for selling or maintaining the product or service.

As the business grows and more staff are employed, there is a danger that things may start to get in a muddle unless everyone is clear about what they are doing and how much responsibility they have. This is why, in all medium-sized and large organisations, there is a specific structure of some type.

- **By functional department**. Many large organisations are structured into departments based on the main functions carried out by staff, such as: Purchasing, Sales and Marketing, Finance (or Accounts), Production, Human Resources (or Personnel), IT and Distribution.
- **By specialist area of work**. In some types of organisation the work is more specialist and the departments will have different titles to reflect this.
  - Newspapers often sub-divide areas of work into news, features and advertising.
  - Book publishers may have an editorial department, a design department and a production department.
  - Charities may have a campaigns department and/or a membership services department as well as IT, admin, marketing and finance sections.
- **By product or service**. Many organisations have specialist terms for their departments, which relate to the type of work carried out there.
  - Pharmaceutical companies may have separate divisions for drugs, toiletries and hospital supplies.
  - Large legal firms divide their operations into different areas of law such as employment, property, probate etc.
  - Your local council will name its departments after the services it offers, such as Housing, Education and Social Services.
- **By market or customer**. Other organisations structure themselves by different markets or types of customers.
  - Banks, computer firms and telecommunications businesses often have separate divisions for private accounts and business customers.
  - Hospitals have departments such as radiography, physiotherapy and maternity to reflect specialist services for patients.
  - Very large organisations that operate all over the world, like Ford and IBM, have different geographical divisions (e.g. North American, European, SE Asian).

Your role and the structure of the business

The size of the business, its main activities, its structure and the type of department that you work in will all affect the tasks you will be expected to carry out.

If you are the only administrator in a small firm you will be expected to provide a wide range of support services to all, or most, of the staff. If

Did you know?

Organisations that deal with private individuals may have a Customer Service Department, or may use a call centre to deal with customer queries. Organisations that deal only with business clients may have a Technical Department that provides specialist help and advice.

Did you know?

When companies are struggling to make profits they often **restructure** to try to save money. This often involves reassessing jobs to see whether any reductions can be made. When IBM restructured its European operations in 2005, over 1000 people lost their jobs.

you work in a small team some tasks will probably be shared and other more specialist jobs will be the responsibility of certain individuals. In both cases some of the specific tasks you do will vary, depending on the main activities of the organisation.

In a large organisation your duties would vary depending on the specific department you work in. As you saw on pages 107–8, the job description for a human resources administrator specifically related to job applications and maintaining a staff database, because HR departments are responsible for all staff issues. By contrast, administrators in other departments will carry out different duties.

- In a **sales department**, administrators may liaise with representatives and other sales staff, prepare correspondence, keep the customer database up to date and arrange sales conferences and other events.
- In a **finance department**, administrators may keep financial records that might involve using special accounting software, preparing spreadsheets and/or processing expense claims and payments.
- In a **customer services department**, administrators will keep customer records (probably on a database), log complaints with reasons, prepare correspondence and deal with customers over the telephone unless specialist staff are employed to do this.
- In a **specialist department** in a public sector organisation – such as in social services at your local authority or in the administration section of your local police authority – you would undertake a range of support services. This would usually involve using Microsoft Office software, interacting confidently with specialist colleagues and the public, organising meetings and coordinating training events.

Did you know?

Wherever you work, a key part of your role will include liaising with your colleagues in other areas of the organisation. In a large firm they may be in another town or even in another country. In a small firm they may be sitting at the next desk. You will be more successful if you have established productive working relationships with them. You will find out more about this if you study option unit 320.

Snapshot – Licking the competition

Ice-cream producers are as keen as any other type of business to keep a watchful eye on their competitors, especially as total sales in the UK were worth a cool £1.65 billion pounds in 2005. Euromonitor International considers that this market will grow to be worth nearly £1780 by the year 2010.

Big companies can easily dominate these markets because they have huge production resources, can produce goods more cheaply and spend millions of pounds on advertising. So how can a small producer compete? One way is to join forces by merging. Hill Station, a small producer of exotic ice-creams, merged with two other small-scale firms and now makes own-label ice-cream for supermarkets.

Another strategy is to focus on a smaller specialist market – known as a niche market – such as that for luxury ice-cream. This is what

Mackie's of Scotland has done. Mackie's was originally a farming and milk retailing business which put its links with supermarkets to good use when it diversified into making luxury ice-cream, made with cream from Jersey cows. It now has 12 per cent of the luxury ice-cream market with ambitions to sell far more. Its vision statement is: 'To be a Scottish global brand from the greenest company in Britain created by people having fun'.

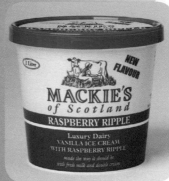

So if you worked as an administrator for Mackie's how would you have fun? Well, you could work for one of the five directors – of marketing, sales, production, development and personnel and administration, or for the chairman or MD. A crucial role of administrators at Mackie's is checking orders and ensuring that stock is distributed promptly, as required, from its depot to the stores. The target for this is 100 per cent – which means that no stores anywhere should ever be left with empty shelves in their freezer cabinets while they wait for a Mackie's delivery.

Find out more about Mackie's, the ice-cream it produces, how it is organised and – if this has whet your appetite – your nearest store at www.mackies.co.uk.

Policies, procedures, systems and values of your organisation that are relevant to your role

You already know that one of your main responsibilities is to help your organisation to meet its goals and that you do this by helping to achieve your department's (or your team's) objectives. You will also need to do this by following the policies, procedures, systems and values relevant to your organisation and your own job role.

Policies and values

All reputable organisations must take steps to ensure that their staff do not do anything illegal, such as deliberately lying about the features of a product they are selling, driving without a valid licence or fiddling

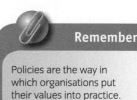

Remember

Policies are the way in which organisations put their values into practice.

Find out

Ethics is another word for values. The Institute of Business Ethics (IBE) argues that 'doing business ethically makes for better business'. In its 2005 survey *Ethics at Work* it found that, while women had stricter ethical standards than men, those aged under 35 were less ethical than older employees. Find out more at www.ibe.org.uk.

their expense claims. Wherever you work, you are likely to find there are rules that all employees must observe, otherwise they may be subject to disciplinary action which could result in dismissal.

The difference between rules and policies is quite simple.

- **Rules and regulations** focus on preventing bad or illegal behaviour.
- **Policies** focus on encouraging ethical behaviour, linked to the company's values.

Examples of illegal, unethical and ethical types of behaviour to customers, suppliers and employees are shown in the diagram below.

Types of behaviour			
	Illegal	**Unethical**	**Ethical**
To customers	Lying about product features/ selling unsafe product	Misleading a customer about performance or delivery date to make a sale	Being honest, even if this means losing a sale
To suppliers	Not paying suppliers' bills	Making small suppliers wait a long time for payment	Paying all bills promptly
To employees	Paying below minimum wage rate	Cutting hours of staff when minimum wage rate is increased	Paying fair and competitive wages

Many organisations go one step further. In addition to having stated values they support named charities or even operate their own charitable foundation. Or they may demonstrate a commitment to the

Find out

You can find a list of charitable foundations, such as those operated by Lloyds TSB and Nationwide, online at www.acf.org.uk/linkstrusts. htm. Click on any of the links to see the types of grant and award made by businesses.

You can read company case studies on the carbon neutral site at www.carbonneutral.com/pages/casestudies.asp.

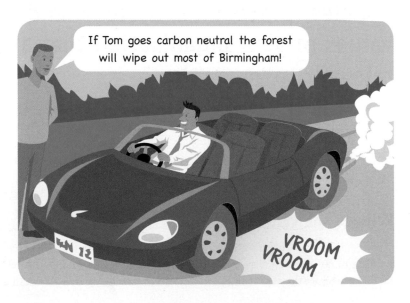

environment, such as those organisations involved in carbon neutral activities where trees are planted to offset the emissions related to their business activities.

Systems and procedures in business

Once a business has decided its objectives (and its values and policies) it then needs to have a practical way of making sure these are achieved. This is where systems and procedures are invaluable.

A **system** is a process by which a specific result is obtained. Your central heating system heats your water and radiators, your respiratory system keeps you alive, an audio system enables you to listen to CDs, and your computer system gives you the facilities to create documents, surf the Internet and send emails.

The main point about a system is that it can be changed or reorganised to get a different result. You could replace your audio speakers to get better sound quality, buy a faster processor for your computer or upgrade your central heating system. You could avoid smoky environments and do cardiovascular exercises to improve your respiratory system.

At work there will be a number of systems you will be expected to use. These will have been designed to get the best possible result, consistently, by all the users. As an example, a complaints system should ensure that all complaints are dealt with in the same way, no matter how they are received.

Procedures support a system because they tell users what to do, usually in a list of step-by-step instructions. You use procedures every day. You follow a specific procedure when you want cash from a cash machine, send a text message or log on to your computer.

Procedures vary in their importance.

- An **important (mandatory) procedure** that must be followed is written down because there are usually penalties for not following it. An example would be failing to buy a parking ticket. For that reason, clear signs are positioned that explain exactly what you have to do on every car park you visit.
- A **recommended procedure** is usually based on the best way to do something, established by other users. If you find a more effective way of doing something you may then be able to suggest improvements (see page 121).
- A **suggested procedure** enables you to do your own thing if you prefer – such as whether to read this book from cover to cover or just dip into it when you need information by using the index at the back.

Remember

A small firm may have no written policies but still operate ethically. There may be no need for formal policies if all the staff share the same high standards and values.

Remember

Systems are just another way of describing processes that have a result. So a bee is a system for making honey and a clock is a system for telling the time. Can you add to these examples with two 'systems' of your own?

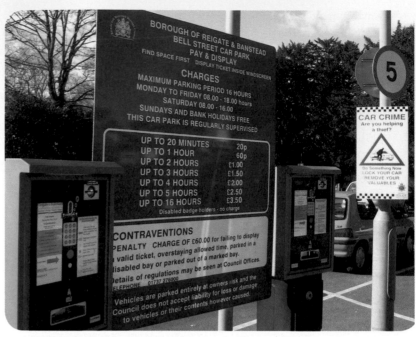

Pay & Display – unless you want a fine!

Further examples are given in the table below.

Types of procedures			
Type	**Meaning**	**General example**	**Business and admin example**
Mandatory or prescribed	'Must do' to comply with rules and regulations	If driving a car, stop at a red traffic light	Evacuation procedures in an emergency
Recommended	'Should do' to get best results	Recharge mobile phone every two days	Remove jammed paper from a printer
Suggested	'Could do'	Route to travel from town A to town B.	Organising your paperwork and desk drawers

How to... Follow the systems and procedures relevant to your role

- **Identify the systems that relate to your role.** Often these relate to aspects of work such as security, health and safety, maintenance, purchasing, staff recruitment, stock control, communications and information. Talk to your supervisor or line manager if you need help.

- **Identify the relevant procedures that relate to these systems** and your job role. Examples can include safety procedures, how to operate items of equipment, how to process financial documents, how to deal with visitors, how to check and record new stock, how to format certain documents, how to file documents and so on.

- **Check the office handbooks and manuals** you refer to and your firm's Intranet. These may include procedures that you follow every day without thinking – such as sending a fax, or taking multiple photocopies.

- **Identify examples of procedures** that are mandatory as well as those that are recommended or suggested.

- **If very few written procedures seem to apply to you**, think about why you do particular tasks the way that you do – such as filing documents, taking a telephone message or dealing with visitors. This is probably because you are following a procedure that someone has shown you, even though it isn't written down.

 Over to you

1 Find out the businesses with which your organisation compares itself by undertaking the following activities:

  a Decide whether your employer provides goods or services locally, nationally or internationally.

  b Identify other businesses in your sector that compete in exactly the same market.

  c Check any market research reports that are available or league tables, if you work in the public sector.

  d Check your ideas with your supervisor.

2 Your boss has the following objectives for your organisation over the coming year. Suggest three ways in which you could contribute to each one:

  a Reduce waste.

  b Improve response times for customer enquiries.

  c Improve the quality of written communications.

  d Encourage staff ideas for improvements.

Over to you Continued

3 Study the job description on pages 107–8 and answer the following questions as if it were your own job. You can check your ideas with the answers on the CD-ROM.

    a Identify four duties that directly relate to the function of the human resources department.

    b Identify three duties an administrator could be asked to do in any department.

    c Identify three responsibilities that are likely to be included in every job description at Capital Services.

    d Assuming Capital Services didn't have job descriptions, suggest two problems this could create for the administrator and his/her assistant.

    e Job holders at Capital Services are expected to carry out other relevant tasks. Suggest one additional task that would be relevant for an administrator and one that would not be.

    f The more you are paid, the greater your responsibilities in relation to the preservation of confidentiality. Why do you think that is?

4 Check how the content of administrator jobs varies depending on sectors and size of organisation. Do this by looking in your local paper, by checking jobs online at a newspaper website such as http://jobs.guardian.co.uk/browse/secretarial/index.jsp or by looking at a recruitment agency website, such as www.fish4jobs. co.uk or www.secsinthecity.co.uk.

5 How do you cope if you are faced with an ethical dilemma? Do the quiz below and say what you would do if each situation occurred. Ideally compare your ideas with other people at work or in your group before checking the suggestions on the CD-ROM.

Ethical dilemmas quiz

How would you cope? Decide what your reaction would be in each of the following situations.

a A friend has applied for a job in your firm and been given an interview. You think she's good fun but know she is very slapdash in her ways. At the interview she says she knows you. Your boss now asks you for a character reference.

b Yesterday, one of your team suggested a better way of dealing with customer enquiries. This afternoon, your boss asks if you can suggest any good ideas for encouraging new business.

c You think everyone should recycle printer cartridges and paper but no one else is very interested. If you go ahead it is likely that this will give you extra work each week.

d One of your team is a PowerPoint wizard and agrees to help you prepare an important presentation. The next day she is late for the fifth time this month and your boss says drastic action is required. You are worried that if you say anything she will refuse to help you with the presentation.

e One of your friends often sneaks out of the fire door at the back for a cigarette. As a member of the safety group you have just been asked to suggest improvements to safety and security.

f You have reluctantly agreed to attend the birthday party of a colleague you don't much like. Two days later you receive a much better invitation for the same night.

g Your organisation needs a new state-of-the-art photocopier and you are talking to suppliers. One rep arrives with a huge box of chocolates just – he says – for the honour of talking to you.

h Staff in your department receive a bonus if sales exceed £50 000 in any month. A large firm is sent an incorrect invoice for double the correct amount which it pays in full. If you say nothing you will all meet this month's target.

i One of your colleagues is very critical, difficult to work with and currently bragging that she was chosen to prepare the MD's presentation because she's the only one with any decent IT skills. When you glance over her shoulder you immediately spot two dreadful spelling errors on her 'final' version.

j You are mentoring a junior employee who is struggling to do the job. You have promised the junior that everything she tells you is in confidence. She then says that she lied about her qualifications in her desperation to get the job, which is why she is having a problem.

Evidence planning

Continue the notes you started on pages 103–4 by adding the following information.

1 Write a statement explaining how your organisation compares itself to others in the sector.

2 a If you have a job description, obtain a copy and highlight all your main responsibilities at work.

b If you don't have a job description, start a work diary to summarise the tasks you do each day. This should be a summary rather than a detailed account, so just spend five or ten minutes at the end of every day keeping your record up to date. Do this

Link to option units

The option units you choose should reflect your main responsibilities. You will probably have chosen these already. If not, talk to your supervisor, tutor or trainer about those you are thinking of selecting. You can check this by looking at the titles and content of each one you are considering and checking this against the contents of your job description and/or work diary.

Evidence planning Continued

for three or four weeks – or until it gives a good picture of the work you do. Include information, too, on when you worked with other people to achieve specific goals. Ask your supervisor to countersign and date your diary to confirm that it reflects your job role; then you can use it as witness testimony.

3 From the information in your work diary, and your job description if you have one, note down the main aspects of your job and your responsibilities.

4 Write a brief description (or draw a chart) to show how your organisation is structured and how your role fits into this.

5 **a** Identify the objectives or targets that apply to your department or team, or to your own job role, and explain how these support the overall purpose of the organisation. If there is no official document, find out what your supervisor considers are the current objectives for your own team or department.

b For each objective or target, identify the tasks you do to contribute towards its achievement. Then decide which option unit these tasks relate to. This will then help you to identify the option units where you can best obtain your evidence for this section.

Applying your organisation's values and policies

You should apply your organisation's values and policies automatically, as a fundamental part of your job, no matter what particular tasks you are doing. This may mean obeying simple instructions or rules, such as keeping fire doors closed, to more complex issues such as how to respond if you are faced with some of the ethical dilemmas you read about on pages 116–17.

How to... Put your organisation's values into practice

• Make sure you know what your organisation's values are by reading the written policies that relate to your job role.

- Check that you understand your organisation's values by discussing these with your supervisor or line manager and checking you know what action to take if you are faced with a dilemma or difficult situation.

- Aim to treat everyone you deal with – customers, colleagues and callers – with the same degree of respect and courtesy, regardless of status.

- Don't cheat your employer by misusing business supplies, equipment or time when you are paid to work.

- Treat other people as you wish to be treated yourself. This includes keeping secrets and never saying something about colleagues you wouldn't be happy for them to hear.

- Don't tell lies, even little white ones. There is a difference between misleading someone and being tactful! In a difficult situation, take it as a challenge that you can handle the problem without telling a deliberate lie.

- Remember the magic words of 'please' and 'thank you', no matter who you are dealing with and repay favours whenever you can.

- Always lead by example. This means you never expect junior staff or other members of your team to do something you wouldn't be prepared to do yourself.

Working with outside organisations and individuals to protect and improve the image of the organisation

You may put your organisation's values into practice all the time but you will always have additional responsibilities when you are dealing with outside individuals and organisations. This is because, in this situation, *you are your organisation*. To all intents and purposes, when people deal with you they are not talking to you as an individual but to a representative of your firm. The same applies when you are sending emails or even posting a brochure or a price list. If you are professional, courteous, polite and efficient than this is how your organisation is viewed. Conversely, if you are abrupt, forgetful, careless or immature then this also has an immediate effect. It is no use your organisation spending money on advertising and cultivating clients if you operate as a one-person demolition squad to good customer relations!

How to... Protect and improve the image of your organisation

- **Insist on high standards for yourself** and every member of your team, from basic office tidiness to error-free documents and impeccable behaviour in front of customers or clients.

- **If you make a promise, keep it** – or make sure the person concerned knows exactly why it was not possible.

- **Make sure all your business emails are formatted correctly** and worded professionally.

- **Always keep your emotions in check.** This means keeping your temper and not becoming over-emotional. Walk away from a confrontation if you are struggling. If you have a personal worry or problem that is affecting you then talk to your supervisor or line manager in private.

- **Take a pride in promoting your organisation**, your boss, your colleagues and your team positively to outsiders.

- **Act and look professional.** If you are visiting an outside organisation or regularly deal with visitors, you will both feel and perform better if you are confident about your appearance.

- **Never embarrass a colleague** in front of an outsider. Protect your colleague's reputation as you would want your own reputation to be protected. Take the person to one side if you wish to point out that he or she is wrong about something.

Who to consult about policies, objectives, systems and values

Any systems and procedures you use regularly should be familiar to you. Similarly, if you regularly have to refer to certain policies, it is assumed that you understand them. Occasionally, though, you may be involved in doing something new, be covering for a member of staff who is on leave or simply be involved in a situation that rarely occurs in your workplace. You should then check what you need to do.

If you work in a large organisation, there may be documents or manuals you can refer to in your office or you may be able to find the relevant information on your organisation's Intranet. You may wish to check these sources first, before you ask someone for advice. At this point, the person to contact will vary, depending on the specific type of guidance you need. So if you need guidance about dealing with a customer, contact Customer Service or Sales. If there is a problem relating to a colleague then Human Resources would be best. If the query relates to money, contact Finance or Accounts. The golden rule is not to take any action on your own initiative if an issue is outside your job role or area of responsibility.

In a small organisation it may be best to speak to the person responsible for a particular area. Otherwise you will probably be expected to check with your supervisor or line manager. Do remember that it isn't advisable just to rely on a quick word from your colleague at the next desk, who may be able to give you a glib response but, in reality, is no wiser than you!

Helping to improve policies, objectives, systems and values

Your personal involvement with organisational policies, objectives, systems and values will depend on your job role. For example, if you were doing the job of human resources administrator specified in the job description on pages 107–8, you are likely to be involved with:

- **organisational policies** related to aspects of work such as recruitment, salaries, data protection, discrimination, harassment and bullying
- **objectives** relating to improving staff retention, minimising staff absences and staff training opportunities
- **systems** relating to the way job applications are received and processed, how staff absences and staff leave are logged, and the updating of staff records
- **procedures** for doing things
- **values** in relation to how staff are treated, welfare policies, and whether staff counselling services are available for staff under stress or with personal problems.

If you work in sales, customer service or accounts, for example, then your involvement with all these aspects of your organisation's operations will be different.

If you work in a small organisation it may be more difficult to identify improvements that are specifically related to your own area of work.

Remember

Failing to check what you should do can, at best, create extra work and make you look foolish – such as having to ring a customer who made a verbal complaint because you did not realise there was a form to complete with all the details. At worst, it can cause serious problems for your employer – such as if you tell the customer that you think your organisation was in the wrong!

Remember

Before you can start to suggest improvements, you need to be able to recognise the policies, objectives, systems and values that relate to your own job role.

Remember

Unless a procedure is mandatory or prescribed, you should be able to suggest improvements if you find a better way of doing something.

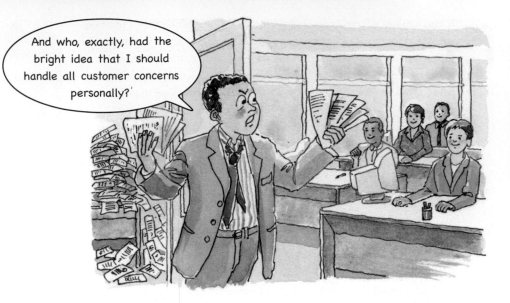

However, you will have more involvement with the work of the business as a whole. This may mean that you can make suggestions that relate to another area because you look at a problem from a different point of view. Just make sure you put forward any bright ideas tactfully, rather than trample over anyone else's feelings.

Remember

Some organisations have an annual review process and encourage staff suggestions for improvements. Others include this in the appraisal process. But this shouldn't stop you making positive suggestions on other occasions, too!

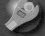

How to... Contribute to improving objectives, policies, systems, procedures and values

- Understand the difference between each of these aspects of your organisation's operations (see page 121).

- Identify the specific objectives, policies, systems, procedures and values that relate to your own job role.

- Refuse to let difficulties and problems go unchallenged! If you or your colleagues decide that something is not working properly, or are constantly receiving complaints, then don't just ignore it. Identify what is causing the problem.

- Think about how the problem could be solved and be positive. Do not just moan that things are not right.

- Don't keep good ideas, or better ways of doing things, to yourself.

- Talk to your supervisor, outline the problem and make your suggestions for improvements.

Over to you

1   Make a list that summarises the policies, procedures, systems and values of your organisation that relate to your own job role. Some of these may have been given to you at induction, others may be in a staff handbook or on the organisation's Intranet. If you are unsure about these, ask your supervisor or line manager to discuss the matter. Then check who else could help you with a query when that person is not available.

2   You have encountered several problems in your first few weeks in a new job. In this organisation you are the office administrator with two admin assistants who are junior to you. For each problem state:

   i   what you would do immediately

   ii what improvements you would recommend to the objectives, policies, systems, procedures and values that relate to your role.

   Discuss your suggestions with your tutor or trainer and/or check your ideas with the answers on the CD-ROM.

   a   When the phone rings in the office, everyone seems to ignore it except you!

   b   The two admin assistants regularly talk about other people in the organisation in derogatory terms.

   c   There is a cupboard full of old umbrellas, scarves and other paraphernalia that has been left in reception over the last few months.

   d   You have spotted both admin assistants franking personal mail on at least three occasions this week.

   e   Customers who access the company's website are offered the opportunity to make contact by email. To your knowledge, no one ever checks or answers these.

   f   Last week you ran out of envelopes, this week there are no file folders left.

Evidence planning

1   Start a work log on which you note occasions when you actively do each of the following:

   ●   follow policies, systems and procedures as part of your day-to-day tasks

Evidence planning Continued

- put your organisation's values into practice

- protect or improve the image of your organisation when you are dealing with outside organisations or individuals

- ask for guidance because you are unsure about your objectives, policies, systems, procedures and values.

2   When you think of a way to improve an objective, policy, system, procedure or value that relates to your job role, put your recommendation in writing to your supervisor. Or make a separate note of it on your log.

3   For each of the policies, systems and procedures that relate to your role, decide the option unit(s) to which each one relates. Bear in mind that some may relate to more than one unit. You can then plan to supply evidence that you follow the policies, systems and procedures that are relevant to your role in those units.

Ask your supervisor to countersign your log and date it to confirm its accuracy. You can refer to this log when you are gathering evidence for the option units you have chosen or use it as the basis of a professional discussion with your assessor.

What if...?

What should you do if:

- your organisation doesn't have a written mission statement

- your organisation has no stated values

- you think you may struggle to obtain some of the evidence bearing in mind your organisation and job role?

Your assessor will be aware that not all candidates work in businesses with written mission statements and stated values. You should ask your employer for guidance, as you saw on pages 104 and 118.

If there are any other parts of this section that don't seem to apply to your organisation or your job role, then talk to your tutor or trainer who may be able to help you to identify evidence opportunities linked to your option units.

Applying your employment responsibilities and rights

A hundred years ago there were few benefits available to anyone unfortunate to be old, ill, pregnant or unemployed, so having work was very important. The balance of power then was firmly in the favour of your employer, who could almost dictate your pay, hours of work and working conditions. If you were dismissed, that was that. If the business collapsed you were out of work with no way of getting any compensation. If you were a woman, disabled or black you might not even be offered work and there was little you could do about it.

Even then, though, you had *some* protection. In 1871 trade unions achieved guaranteed legal recognition and trade union officials worked to improve conditions. Enlightened employers also realised that a workforce that was treated properly would be more effective than one that wasn't. The other factor that began to change the situation was the beginning of government intervention in the field of employment and the passing of certain laws. These protected employees from exploitation and formalised many of the existing agreements between employer and employee in relation to rights and responsibilities at work.

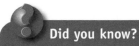

Did you know?

The law tries to keep you safe, to protect your privacy and to make sure you don't work for nothing!

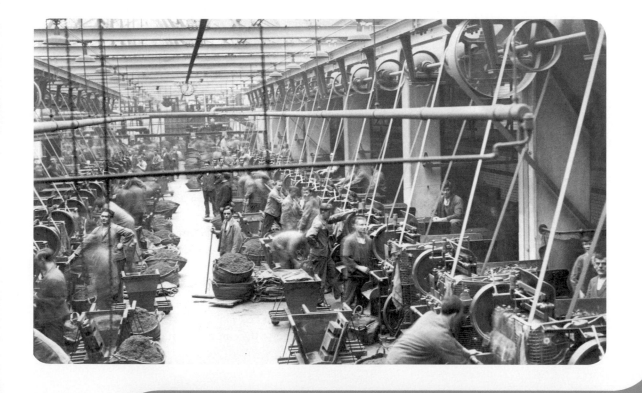

Aspects of employment that are covered by law

The aspects of employment covered by law can be divided into four different sections:

- health and safety at work (including fire safety and first aid)
- data protection
- employment rights and responsibilities
- pay and pensions.

Each of these areas will now be discussed in more detail.

Health and safety at work

Your employer must ensure, so far as is possible, your health, safety and welfare at work. In turn, you must cooperate with your employer and take reasonable care not only of your own health and safety at work but also that of anyone you work with.

Under the **Health and Safety at Work etc. Act 1974** your employer has certain duties:

- The employer must provide you with information about basic health and safety requirements, either in the form of a poster displayed in the workplace or as a leaflet distributed to all employees. This information must also contain details of those responsible for enforcing the health and safety requirements in the workplace.
- The employer must make sure the workplace is safe and without risk to health by:
  - keeping dust, fumes and noise under control
  - ensuring that plant and machinery are safe and regularly maintained
  - ensuring that articles and substances in the workplace are clearly identified and moved, stored and used safely
  - providing adequate welfare facilities
  - providing protective clothing where necessary
  - reporting certain diseases, injuries and dangerous occurrences to the relevant authority
  - providing adequate first aid equipment and facilities
  - taking precautions against fire, and providing adequate means of fighting fires and escape
  - assessing all dangerous substances and introducing substitutes, safety measures or protective clothing and equipment
  - drawing up a health and safety policy statement and bringing it to the attention of the employees (if there are more than five employees).

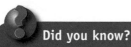

Did you know?

Good employers look after their employees as a matter of course. Poorer ones might find that if they don't, an officer from the Health and Safety Executive (HSE) or the local authority environmental health department (EHD) will be knocking at their door asking why they aren't complying with the law. The HSE covers work activities where there are serious hazards such as factories, mines, farms and building sites. The EHDs cover less hazardous work environments such as shops, offices and hotels.

- Employers have other obligations under the **Management of Health and Safety at Work Regulations 1999**. The table below gives its main provisions.

Main provisions of the Management of Health and Safety at Work Regulations 1999

Employers have to:

- Avoid risks to the health and safety of employees and anyone else affected by the employer's work activity.
- Where risks cannot be avoided, assess the risks so that protective and preventive measures can be arranged. An employer with five or more employees must make a written assessment.
- Arrange measures to deal with health and safety issues arising from the assessment.
- Provide appropriate health monitoring for employees.
- Appoint at least one person to help the employer enforce health and safety requirements.
- Set up emergency procedures and nominate people to help evacuate the premises in an emergency.
- Provide any temporary worker with health and safety information to meet any special needs he or she may have.
- Adapt the workplace to the individual employees, especially as to the design of the workplace, the choice of work equipment and the choice of working methods with a view particularly to alleviating monotonous work and work at a pre-determined rate.
- Replace the dangerous by the non-dangerous or less dangerous.
- Develop an overall prevention policy.
- Ensure that any necessary contacts with external services are arranged, particularly regarding first aid, emergency medical care and rescue work.

In addition, in most workplaces employers must ensure that these:

- are not overcrowded and generally well ventilated and lit
- have floors, stairs, ladders and passageways that are well constructed and maintained and kept clear of obstructions
- are clean
- are free from hazardous noise levels
- provide sufficient lavatories, washing facilities and drinking water
- provide suitable seating
- have rest facilities
- are of the correct temperature
- have enough space safely to accommodate the people working there
- have first aid facilities
- provide machinery and equipment which does not put the employee at risk.

Safety representatives

The **Safety Representatives and Safety Committee Regulations 1977** say that employers should consult safety representatives appointed by a trade union, and the **Health and Safety (Consultation with Employees) Regulations 1996** require them to consult any employees not in groups covered by trade union safety representatives. This means that all workers, not just those represented by a trade union, have the same protection.

Members of a safety committee are involved in several activities, including:

- keeping their employer informed of concerns about possible risks and dangerous events in the workplace and any general matters affecting the health and safety of employees
- finding out about changes that may affect employees' health and safety at work, for example in procedures, equipment or ways of working
- discovering what information employees must be given on the likely risks and dangers arising from their work, as well as measures to reduce or get rid of these risks and what employees should do if they have to deal with a risk or danger
- being consulted about the planning of health and safety training
- checking on the health and safety consequences of introducing new technology.

Related health and safety issues

The following are now considered to be health and safety issues:

- **Smoking at work** will be banned in all work places from mid-2007. In the meantime employers must ensure that rest rooms are arranged so that employees can use them without others having to breathe in smoke. Otherwise the employer may be in breach of the **Human Rights Act 1996**. In two cases, one employee was awarded £25 000 and another £15 000 because each felt their health had been damaged by other people's smoking at the workplace. One employee had complained about the heavy smoking of the solicitors with whom she had worked for years. She was situated next to the smoking room and the poor ventilation system meant that the smoke filtered through. Despite her protests nothing was done and she eventually resigned. Her claim for constructive dismissal (see page 146) was upheld.
- **Stress at work** is a major issue. An employer must look after his or her employees' mental as well as physical well-being. In one case a secondary school teacher who had a nervous breakdown because of pressure at work was awarded damages (i.e. financial compensation) even though the employer maintained that all the

Find out

Check to see whether your organisation has a safety committee. If it does, you may think about becoming a member, as this will help you to obtain evidence towards the final section of this unit (see pages 170 and 189). If it doesn't, try to find out who is responsible for looking after the health and safety of everyone at work. Find out also who that person liaises with – is it the HSE or EHD or both?

Find out

Find out more about the effects of passive smoking from the Action on Smoke (ASH) website at www.ash.org.uk, and investigate stress at the UK National Work Stress Network's website at www.workstress.net.

other staff worked under the same pressure. He was expected to recognise that someone was under undue pressure even if no one else felt the same way.

- **Violence at work** is growing in importance. An employer who has failed to foresee a potential danger and has not carried out a proper risk assessment is likely to be in breach of his or her duty of care.

Snapshot – It's as safe as houses where I work!

You might think that an office is a violence-free environment, but a British Crime Survey showed a different picture. Of working adults, 1.7% have been the victim of a verbal or physical assault. In one year alone there were an estimated 849 000 incidents of violence at work and approximately 376 000 workers reported experiencing at least one violent incident at work.

Workers most at risk included police officers and healthcare professionals including nurses and dentists. Most incidents were carried out by males between the ages of 16 and 40.

Even though levels of concern are still quite low, the number of workers who are worried about being assaulted by a member of the public is growing each year. Some workers say that worrying about workplace violence has a great deal of impact on their health.

Whether it will ever happen to you may depend on where you work. The Health and Safety Executive has recommended that employers should train staff to spot early signs of aggression and to know how to avoid or cope with it. In addition, the workplace should be made as secure as possible (see pages 170–9).

Did you know?

There are a large number of regulations that relate to health and safety. One relevant to most administrators is the **Health and Safety (Display Screen Equipment) Regulations** which state how computer workstations should be set up, how computers should be used, rest periods and free eye tests for regular users (see page 187). You can find out more about other regulations that may be relevant to your own job by referring to unit 110 on the CD-ROM.

Data protection requirements

Computer databases have made it easy for data about individuals to be stored and accessed by a wide variety of people. A lot of filing cabinets, too, are bursting with information. Normally this causes no problems but human beings can make mistakes. Someone can be listed as a bad credit risk and refused a bank account – perhaps just because of a keying-in error that has listed unpaid bills or a bad debt against his or her name. Under the **Data Protection Act 1998**, people can see their credit records and insist that any errors be corrected.

Similarly, anyone at work has the right to see the information that is held in a personnel file, for a small administrative charge. Again,

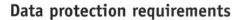

Did you know?

If you work in the public sector you may have heard of the **Freedom of Information Act 2000** which grants any person or organisation a general right of access to information held by public authorities, including government departments and local authorities. You can obtain further information from www. informationcommissioner. gov.uk.

Did you know?

The **Employment Practices Data Protection Code** gives guidance on keeping information about employees.

It covers information job applicants might be asked to provide unnecessarily. For example, applicants should not be asked whether they are members of a trade union or whether they have a driving licence when the job does not involve any driving.

It specifies that 'pre-employment vetting' used by some employers to enquire about job applicants should be used only when necessary, such as when it is a legal requirement under the Protection of Children Act 1999.

anything incorrect or damaging, which may unfairly jeopardise future promotion chances, must be deleted or amended. If the employer refuses to make any changes, then the employee can apply to the court to obtain an order requiring a data controller to correct inaccurate data and to seek compensation where damage and distress have been caused as a result.

The Data Protection Act also means that organisations have a legal responsibility to keep information secure, as you will see on page 174. The main provisions of the Act are given in the table below.

Main provisions of the Data Protection Act 1998

The Act requires all organisations and businesses that process personal data on individuals (data subjects) to give notification that they should be included in a register of data controllers.

The term 'data' relates to:

- information recorded or processed by computer
- information that is part of a relevant filing system or forms part of any accessible record (e.g. health records, social services records).

All data controllers must comply with the eight principles of the Act in relation to the handling of personal data:

- Data must be obtained and processed fairly and lawfully. Normally this means the individual has given his/her consent. Explicit consent is required for 'sensitive' data relating to religious or political beliefs; racial origin; trade union membership; physical or mental health or sexual life; criminal convictions.
- Data must be held only for one or more specified and lawful purposes and should not be processed for another reason.
- Data should be adequate, relevant and not excessive.
- Data must be accurate and kept up to date.
- Data must be kept no longer than is necessary.
- Data must be processed in accordance with the rights of data subjects – i.e. the individuals (see below).
- Data must be stored to prevent unauthorised or unlawful access, loss, destruction or damage.
- Data must not be transferred outside the EU unless the country to which it is being sent also protects the rights of data subjects.

The rights of data subjects include:

- the right to access data held about them
- the right to prevent processing which would cause damage or distress
- the right to prevent processing for direct marketing purposes
- rights in relation to automated decision taking (e.g. evaluating job performance or credit worthiness on the basis of personal information)

- the right to take action to correct, block, erase or destroy inaccurate data
- the right to compensation if damage is suffered through contravention of the Act.

Exemptions

Broadly these include data held for:

- purposes of national security
- crime detection and taxation purposes
- health, education and social work
- research, history and statistics
- domestic use only.

Employment rights and responsibilities

Imagine starting work in a new job and finding that your salary will be half as much as you expected, because nothing had been formally agreed. Similarly, your employer would get a shock if you didn't bother turning up one day but sent your best friend to do the work instead! Quite obviously, if such behaviour were acceptable, the workplace would be chaotic for everyone.

Being employed therefore carries with it both rights and responsibilities. You can expect certain things but in exchange you have to do certain things. Similarly your employer must expect both to give and to get.

It is both easier and also a legal requirement that you have a contract of employment (often referred to as 'legal terms and conditions of employment') that both you and your employer must agree and which sets out what you both expect. In that contract you might find a combination of express and implied terms.

Express terms

These are terms that are explicitly agreed between you and your employer. For example, if she says that she will pay you £13 000 a year there is little room for disagreement. On pages 141–3 you will read more details about the information that must be in your contract of employment.

Implied terms

Implied terms are those not specifically agreed between you and the employer. They are terms that a court would presume reflected the intention of both employer and employee even though they have never been expressly agreed or written down.

Did you know?

Both employers and employees must fulfil their legal responsibilities to each other. If one fails to do what has been agreed they are said to be in breach of the law.

They can be *general* terms that are implied in most contracts of employment:

- **A mutual duty of trust and confidence.** Neither you nor your employer must act in a way that is likely to destroy or seriously damage your relationship. If your boss shouted at you every time you asked for help or picked on you unfairly then you are hardly likely to trust, or have confidence in, her.

  Similarly, if you sneak in and out of the office when you want and hope she doesn't catch you, ring in sick when you want to go shopping for the day, are rude about her to your colleagues or to customers, and regularly do sloppy work then you are also in breach of your implied contractual duty.

- **A duty of care to each other.** If you work in an office that is cold and noisy and electrical equipment is never checked, your boss is obviously not bothered about your well-being and your safety. If you don't bother reporting a kettle with a dodgy plug and refuse to leave your desk in a fire drill you are obviously not worried about your own safety nor whether you are putting anyone else at risk. You are therefore in breach of the duty of care.

- **A duty to obey reasonable instructions.** Unfortunately there is no legal definition of what is meant by reasonable, but most courts would not find it reasonable if, for instance, you were asked to drive an uninsured or untaxed car.

- **A duty not to act arbitrarily, capriciously or inequitably without good reason.** An employer must be seen to be fair. If, for instance, everyone is given a pay rise except you, without any good reason, it is likely there will have been a breach.

- **A duty of good faith and fidelity**. Similarly you must not act in a way that is contrary to the interests of your employer. If you work for a travel agency, for instance, but in your spare time you arrange holidays for people at cut-rate prices, you are not acting in good faith.
- **A duty on the part of the employer to pay you agreed wages and to provide you with work**. In reality this is always covered by your written terms and conditions of employment. However, although an employer must always pay you, there is no law that says your employer must give you work. Even though that sounds great, it can prove to be a problem. If you have a very valuable IT skill, for instance, and need to use it constantly to make sure you are at the cutting edge, your employment prospects would be seriously damaged if your boss refused to let you use them – and you might be able to claim breach of this implied term of your contract.

Custom and practice

Some terms can be implied by custom and practice. For example, you may work for a firm that, for the past ten years, has always allowed its employees additional time off to go to weddings or funerals. You ask for leave of absence to attend your sister's wedding but are told you cannot go. You may be able to claim that by custom and practice this right has been established.

Negotiated agreements

Some of the terms of your employment may have been reached through a negotiated agreement between a union and your employer. The employer will then normally make sure the term is included expressively in each individual contract. If this has not been done, it would still be regarded as an implied term.

Pay and pensions

If you work you expect to get paid and in most cases the details of how much you are to be paid and at what intervals is contained in your contract of employment (see page 141). It does not matter what you are doing or where you work. However, there are certain groups who have additional protection, either because they have been discriminated against in the past or because they belong to a particularly vulnerable group. Examples are pregnant women, young people or very low-paid workers. In addition, nowadays many more people have access to sick pay and holiday pay. To make sure that you know exactly how much you are going to be paid, the **Employment Rights Act 1996** states that you must be given an itemised payslip showing your pay and deductions.

Equal pay

Before 1970 women could be paid a lower rate than men even if they were doing the same job. The **Equal Pay Act 1970** and **Equal Pay (Amendment) Regulations 1983** put a stop to that. Nowadays, if a woman believes that she is not being paid the same as a man she can make a claim in the following situations.

- She is doing **like work** (i.e. the same work as a man working in the same organisation) and there are no significant differences, such as the man working antisocial hours, having extra responsibility, doing additional duties or working in less pleasant conditions.
- Her work is **rated as equivalent**. In this case a job evaluation scheme rates the two jobs equally.
- She does **work of equal value**. In this case, even though the work is not the same the value of each job is the same. This helps women who work in segregated areas such as assembly work, cleaning and catering where it is sometimes difficult to find a man doing the same work.

National minimum wage

The **National Minimum Wage Act 1998** obliges employers to pay a minimum hourly wage to workers over the age of 18 regardless of where they work, the size of the firm or the worker's occupation. From 1 October 2004 the national minimum wage was extended to workers aged 16 and 17, but this does not extend to Apprentices aged 16–18. Apprentices aged 19 and above qualify for the minimum wage after the first 12 months of their Apprenticeship.

Sick pay

Unlike most employees in the past you can now expect to be paid when you are off sick. Statutory sick pay (SSP) is the minimum amount employers must pay to employees who are off work. It is paid for up to 28 weeks in any period of sickness (i.e. either a continuous spell of sickness of at least four calendar days or different spells of sickness of at least four calendar days that are not more than eight weeks apart). It is not paid for the first three days of sickness (known as 'waiting days'), but if an employee has a second spell of sickness within eight weeks then he or she will not have to repeat the three waiting days before getting SSP again.

Holiday pay

Under the **Working Time Regulations 1998** most workers have a statutory right to four weeks' paid holiday. They may also have a contractual right to more if that is what has been agreed with the employer.

Maternity pay

Statutory maternity rights are covered by the **Employment Rights Act 1996** and the **Maternity and Parental Leave Regulations 1999** (as amended). All pregnant employees are entitled to 26 weeks' leave (known as 'ordinary maternity leave'). Women who meet the qualifying conditions are entitled to statutory maternity pay or maternity allowance during their ordinary maternity leave. In addition most fathers can now take up to two weeks' paid paternity leave following the birth of the child.

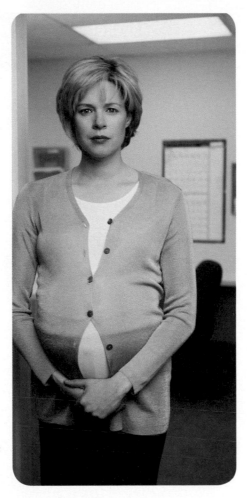

Did you know?

The **Work and Families Bill**, published in October 2005, included plans to extend maternity and paternity leave and provide leave for workers caring for sick or elderly relatives. New mothers will be entitled to nine months' paid maternity leave from April 2007 and a year from 2009. New fathers may be given the legal right to six months' unpaid paternity leave during the first year of their baby's life from April 2007. Some business leaders are against it, saying it will be disruptive and expensive, particularly for small firms.

Redundancy

Redundancy is a situation where a person is dismissed because there is no work for him or her to do. In law, redundancy must be fair. An employer cannot pick and choose which employees to make redundant and must consult fully over the criteria for selection with the trade union and follow an agreed process. If there is a staff association, it must be consulted when more than 20 jobs will be affected.

An employee who is made redundant and has worked for the employer for more than two years must receive redundancy pay at or above a minimum legal level based on age, length of service and weekly pay up to a specified amount. The employee must also be offered free counselling or retraining and given time off to attend interviews for a new job.

Did you know?

Many organisations try to avoid compulsory redundancies – first by **natural wastage**, when staff who leave are not replaced, then by offering a financial package to tempt some employees to opt for **voluntary redundancy**.

Snapshot – The changing face of employment law

Employment law is constantly changing and this can cause problems for small firms who do not employ legal specialists or advisers, as they need to be aware of laws that relate to employer rights and responsibilities as well as those aimed to ensure equality of opportunity and treatment (see pages 139–51).

Some important Acts relating to rights and responsibilities are summarised below. You can read about discrimination laws on pages 149–51

- **The Employment Protection (Consolidation) Act 1978** was one of the first Acts that brought together employees' rights at work under one heading. This made it easier for both employers and employees to check their rights and duties, rather than having to look through a number of individual Acts such as the Employment Protection Act 1975.

- **The Trade Union Reform and Employment Rights Act 1993** did much the same thing. It brought together all the trade union rights previously contained in other Acts. Now all major employment provision is contained in the Employment Rights Act 1996.

- **The Employment Rights Act 1996** gave all employees the right to a written contract within two months of starting work, covered maternity leave, the right to 'opt out' of Sunday working, the right to a minimum period of notice depending on length of employment, and the right to redundancy pay after two years' continuous employment. Many of these rights have since been extended through subsequent maternity and paternity leave regulations and amendments.

- **The Employment Relations Act 1999** improved maternity leave, introduced parental leave and gave workers the right to take time off in a family emergency. Further changes include a 'no surprises culture' so that employees are consulted about key decisions that affect them, such as redundancies.

- **The Employment Act 2002** introduced 'family-friendly policies' and the right to request flexible hours, outlawed discrimination against temporary workers, and covered the ways in which disputes should be resolved at work.

Over to you

1 You have become a member of your organisation's safety committee. Word about this has got round and your colleagues have begun to approach you with their concerns:

a Jeanette is complaining about the long hours she spends in front of her word processor. She says it is making her eyes hurt.

b Lance works in the laboratory and is often expected to handle corrosive chemicals. He frequently gets burns on his hands.

c Dival is tired out. Because of an absent colleague, he has been working on reception from 6 a.m. to 9 p.m. for the last four weeks and he doesn't think he can go on much longer.

d Khalid is a temporary worker. He wants to know whether he has any legal health and safety protection.

Before you raise their concerns at the next meeting you decide to find out more about their rights. Do this by checking the following laws and regulations, by referring to the information in this book, on the CD-ROM and on the HSE website at www.hse.gov.uk:

● Health and Safety at Work Act 1974

● Management of Health and Safety at Work Regulations 1999

● Health and Safety (Display Screen Equipment) Regulations 1992

● Personal Protective Equipment at Work Regulations 1992

● Working Time Regulations 1998

Make notes for each person on their main rights related to their concerns.

2 You work for the human resources manager of a large organisation. Various disputes have arisen that your boss has put in a file to discuss with the HR director. When you pick up the file the Post-it notes she has attached fall off. Match up the notes (shown below) with the cases and say why you have done so.

a Patrick wants to take some paternity leave. His manager tells him not to be so soft.

b Mariska is complaining that she is doing exactly the same job as Frank but is not being given the same rate of pay.

c The reception staff don't use the signing in and out book, so no one knows where they are and, although they were told all electrical equipment used on the premises must be checked, one receptionist keeps her hair straighteners in her desk to use before she goes out in an evening.

Over to you Continued

d Wallis has complained that the new manager has not allowed her to carry the remainder of her annual leave over until the next year. The previous manager always allowed her to do this.

e Haram's manager keeps asking him to move her car if she has parked in a restricted zone even though she knows he hasn't got a full driving licence.

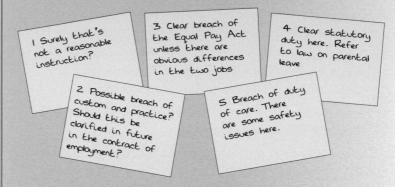

1 Surely that's not a reasonable instruction?

3 Clear breach of the Equal Pay Act unless there are obvious differences in the two jobs

4 Clear statutory duty here. Refer to law on parental leave

2 Possible breach of custom and practice? Should this be clarified in future in the contract of employment?

5 Breach of duty of care. There are some safety issues here.

3 Georgie is a very popular journalist working for a national newspaper. She has had a disagreement with her boss and is now talking about leaving. The editor has decided not to allow her to write anything further for the time being. Explain why Georgie's employers want to employ her, pay her and yet not let her do any work.

Evidence planning

For your evidence for this unit you will need to prove to your assessor that you act within your responsibilities and rights. You will do this through the option units you have chosen. You may find it useful to start to collect information that relates to your responsibilities and rights as you progress through this section. This can include information you were given when you started work and at induction as well as information you collect related to this unit. Note, too, the location of other information relevant to your job role on health and safety, data protection and the other employment rights that you have.

Store personal paper-based information in a file folder. Electronic information – such as downloaded, researched information – should be saved into a specific folder on your computer. Both should be easily available and accessible during a professional discussion with your assessor.

Industry-specific legislation and regulations relevant to your role

By the very nature of their work, some industries are regulated by additional legislation and a number of **industry-specific regulations** have been passed over the years. Here are some examples:

- The retail industry has to follow the rules laid down in legislation such as the Sunday Trading Act 1994.
- The transport industry has to take note of the Working Time Regulations 1998. So too has the aeronautical industry in respect of its cabin and flight crew and the agricultural industry in respect of agricultural workers.
- The transport industry has to be aware of the provisions of the Goods Vehicle (Licensing of Operators) Act 1995.
- Travel agents and tour operators must take note of the Package Travel, Package Holidays and Package Tours Regulations 1992.
- Anyone who works with children, old people or any other vulnerable section of society must abide by the rules laid out in the Protection of Children Act 1999.
- The publishing industry must be careful to avoid breaching the copyright rules laid down in the Copyright, Designs and Patents Act 1988 as amended by the Copyright and Related Rights Regulations 2003.
- Anyone handling other people's money has to abide by the legislation in the Proceeds of Crime Act 2002 and Money Laundering Regulations 2003.

Obviously, if you work in one of these areas you should be aware of what legislation applies to your organisation.

The importance of legislation in upholding and protecting the rights of both employer and employee

Legal procedures

Even though some people may criticise the legal system, it has many advantages. It gives some protection to the weaker members of society, offers a legal framework in which both employer and employee are made aware of their rights and obligations, and tries to solve the problems when those rights and obligations are ignored. Without it the most powerful would always win. Nowadays if the employment relationship goes wrong there are certain clear routes to follow to try to resolve the situation.

Find out

Check and make a note of any specific legislation that applies to your own particular organisation.

Did you know?

Over a hundred years ago London and other European capitals went in fear of bomb attacks. Then the terrorists were anarchists – of all nationalities – who believed that all forms of authority interfere with individual freedom and that the state should be replaced by communities in which no one has any control over anyone else. Some experimental communities were established but most did not last very long. With no rules or restrictions chaos reigned.

Suppose that you work part time. You work alongside a full-time employee and find out that she has better terms and conditions than you, even though, apart from working fewer hours, you do exactly the same job. You realise that under the Part-time Workers (Prevention of Less Favourable Treatment) Regulations 2000 and the Fixed Term Employees (Prevention of Less Favourable Treatment) Regulations 2002 you should be treated in the same way as your full-time colleague and have the same opportunities. Your problem is how to achieve that goal in practice.

The legislation allows you to take the following actions:

- **Talk to your employer informally.** If that does not work you can go into grievance and follow the standard grievance procedures. For further information about grievance procedures see page 145.
- **Turn to arbitration if your employer is still unwilling to help you.** Acas, the Advisory, Conciliation and Arbitration Service, will arrange for someone to talk to both you and your employer to try to resolve the situation quickly. If that fails, this person can act as an arbitrator by listening to both sides of the argument and making a decision. If both you and your employer agree, that is the end of the matter. If you cannot agree, then you have the right to take your claim to a tribunal.
- **Attend a tribunal.** If the claim proceeds, the tribunal panel will be convened which normally consists of a legally qualified chairperson and two lay members. It will try to keep the proceedings as simple and informal as possible – although if you ever attend a tribunal hearing you might disagree with that! Both sides can represent themselves, although mostly they have a lawyer or trade union representative to assist them.

Did you know?

Before a tribunal hearing there may be a pre-hearing review. If it is decided that the person bringing the case is unlikely to succeed, the tribunal may order that person to pay a deposit of up to £500 as a condition of being allowed to continue.

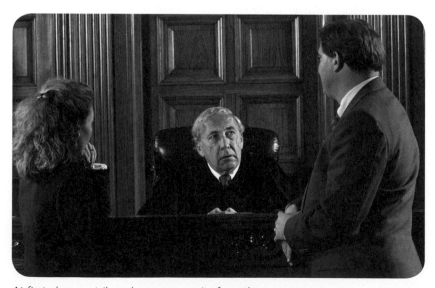

At first glance a tribunal can seem quite formal

A tribunal listens to both sides of the argument, taking into account witness statements and whether or not the correct grievance procedures have been followed. It then makes its decision which is binding unless the unsuccessful person decides to appeal to the Employment Appeal Tribunal. From then on there is a possibility that the case can be taken to the Court of Appeal or even, on rare occasions, to the European Court of Justice.

If the tribunal finds that your employer has not given you the same rights as your full-time colleagues and is therefore in breach of the regulations, it can insist that you are given these rights. If you have been dismissed because of this dispute and the tribunal holds the dismissal unfair, then you could be offered re-engagement or reinstatement and/or some compensation.

Main terms and conditions of your contract of employment

Written statement

The **Employment Rights Act 1996** says that you must be given a written statement of the terms and conditions of your employment within two months of starting work. The written statement must cover:
- the names of the employer and the employee
- the date when the employment began
- pay and the intervals at which it is to be paid
- hours of work
- holiday entitlement
- entitlement to sick leave, and any entitlement to sick pay
- pensions and pension schemes
- entitlement of employer and employee to notice of termination
- job title or a brief job description
- where it is not permanent, the period for which the employment is expected to continue or, if it is for a fixed term, the date when it is to end
- either the place of work or, if the employee is required or allowed to work in more than one location, an indication of this and of the employer's address
- details of the existence of any relevant collective agreements (i.e. normally union negotiated agreements) which directly affect the terms and conditions of employment
- reference to disciplinary and grievance procedures.

Because some of the information is quite detailed (see pages 145–6 for information on grievance and disciplinary procedures), employers are allowed to include a brief outline only in the statement itself provided they ensure that the employee is aware of where this information can be located, such as in the staff handbook.

Find out

Although most of the terms and conditions of your employment will be contained in one document, other documents may contain relevant information. These include a job advertisement, notes of questions and answers given during the interview, letters of offer and acceptance, a staff handbook, information given during induction training, and so on. Check that you have all relevant documents contained in one folder or have noted the location of each item.

Changing your terms and conditions of employment

Work constantly changes. If you start work at age 16 it is unlikely that you will be carrying out the same duties when you are 65. That's probably a good thing, otherwise you might suffer from dreadful boredom. However, during the course of your working life you might find that you welcome some changes and are less pleased about others.

If your employer says that your working week will be shorter and you can now leave early on a Friday, you're happy. If you are told that because of a reduction in demand someone has to leave and everyone else has to take on extra work, that's not such good news. One of the things you have to learn when starting work is to try to be flexible and to adapt to different circumstances. What you do not have to do, however, is accept *any* change to your contract your employer decides to make. If that change is major it might constitute a breach of your contract and, in particular, the implied duty on your employer's part to behave reasonably.

Terms in your contract that should not be altered without your consent normally include these:

- pay
- holiday entitlement
- sick leave and sick pay entitlement
- maternity rights
- redundancy rights
- major changes to job duties and responsibilities
- hours of work.

If a change makes you unhappy, first check your contract. It may contain what is known as a **variation term** – one that allows your employer to change a term without prior agreement from you. For example, if your contract says your 'normal working hours are 37 a week but these may be increased if circumstances call for it', then you may have little choice but to go along with the change. If the proposed change is not part of your contract you can either choose to accept it, check the situation with your trade union representative or register a grievance (see page 144).

One of the changes you may be asked to accept is to work under a zero-hours or key-time contract:

- **Zero-hours contracts** do not specify any number of hours that you will be required to work. The contract states that, instead of working a specific number of hours per week, you must be ready to work whenever asked.
- **Key-time contracts** guarantee you some work but not at guaranteed regular hours each week.

Both types of contract could involve you in waiting at home by the phone to see whether you are needed to come into work, or arriving at work each Monday and being told then your working hours for the week, or waiting on the works premises to see whether there is any work to do. One of the problems used to be that as you were paid only for the time you worked you might not be paid for the waiting time. However, the European Court of Justice has held that an employee on a zero-hours contract who has to be on site waiting for work to arise should be paid at the appropriate hourly rate or, at the very least, at the statutory minimum rate.

Find out

Find out whether anyone in your organisation works under a zero-hours or key-time contract and, if so, what his or her actual terms and conditions are. Bear in mind, however, that the terms and conditions might be confidential information.

Snapshot – Work till you drop!

You may have heard the old saying that 'hard work never killed anyone'. It's not strictly true. In extreme cases long hours, and the exhaustion it causes, has led to people committing suicide or collapsing under stress. Indeed, in Japan, 'karoshi' or 'working yourself to death' has become a legal issue and death by overwork lawsuits are common with victim's families demanding compensation payments. Some people think that Britain is going the same way. One survey has revealed the following facts:

- Many UK employees are working about 43.6 hours a week, compared with Europe where the average is 40.3 hours.

- In the last seven years the proportion of employees working over 48 hours a week has risen from 10 per cent to 26 per cent.

- Since 1992 there has been a rise of 52 per cent in the number of woman expected to work 48 hours a week.

- Even lunchtimes are changing. The traditional one-hour break is disappearing and the average time for a break is now 27 minutes.

What might be even more alarming is that some workers are so work-conscious that they don't take the time off they are owed. Another recent survey found that only 44 per cent of workers take their full entitlement to annual leave, either because they have too much work to get through or because they are frightened of upsetting the boss!

Have you got the right balance between work and play?

Over to you

1   A new employee starts work in your office. He has just been given his contract of employment and he is not too impressed with it. He asks you the following questions. Make notes of how you would reply to him.

   a Why do I need anything in writing? I've agreed to it and so has the boss.

   b Why is there a disciplinary procedure? I know when I've done something wrong – I don't need to read a lot of rules about it.

2   Study the terms and conditions of employment in your own contract carefully. Check each item against the list on page 141. Find out your sick pay and holiday entitlements. Check whether your contract contains a variation term or whether – for example – your employer could vary your hours of work to suit the needs of the business without your agreement. List your findings and discuss these with your tutor or trainer.

Evidence planning

As part of your evidence for this unit, you will need to prove to your assessor that you carry out your responsibilities to your employer in a way that is consistent with your contract of employment.

Prepare for this by looking at your option units to see whether you can identify examples of related responsibilities linked to your contract of employment.

Put a copy of your contract of employment into the file folder you started on page 138 and note where other relevant documents are stored.

Grievances at work, and guidance or support

Imagine that you work in the finance section of a large organisation. You like your job and your colleagues but your manager is giving you problems. You think she doesn't like you because she wasn't there when you were interviewed for the job and that she resents not having had a say in your appointment. She seems to tell you off for the slightest reason. If you are five minutes late coming back from a break she tells you off in front of others even though she doesn't say anything to anyone else. She is very critical if you make even a small mistake. You have also heard that she has said that she would like you to start looking for another job. Then she says that she is thinking about taking disciplinary action against you because of poor work performance.

What can you do about it? First of all, if you can bring yourself to do this, you should talk to the person who is causing the problem – in this case your manager – and explain how you feel.

- **State facts.** Rather than saying 'You're always picking on me' refer to a specific instance – e.g. 'In the last two weeks you've told me off three times in front of the other staff.' If you think it will help, either keep a diary for a time before you raise the matter with your manager so that you can refer back to the incidents as they occurred, or prepare a summary of them.
- **Avoid confrontation.** Give your manager the chance to be as reasonable with you, as you are trying to be.
- **Allow your manager the right to reply** – and listen to what you are being told rather than immediately reacting. It might be that you need to reach a compromise. You admit that you have been late from a break on the odd occasion and your manager admits to having over-reacted.
- **Try to find a way ahead.** Your manager might suggest another meeting in a month's time to see if matters have improved. You might even draw a set of rules or procedures that both of you agree to keep to during that period.

Grievance procedures

Sometimes talking about the problem clears the air and relationships improve. However, if this fails you might have to resort to more formal procedures. From 1 October 2004 all employers have had to have a written grievance procedure, reference to which should be included in your terms and conditions of employment. At this stage if you are a member of a union you might want to contact your representative for help and guidance and, if necessary, to accompany you to any subsequent meetings.

You are entitled to:
- a meeting in private between you and your line manager (you will normally have the right to be accompanied)
- a formal discussion at which written notes are taken
- either an immediate response from the manager or an undertaking that you will be informed in writing of any decision
- the right to appeal to a more senior line manager should the initial meeting not resolve the situation.

Find out

You can find out more about the disputes procedures on the Department of Trade and Industry website at www.dti.gov.uk/er/resolvingdisputes.htm and read the example memo that can be sent to employees informing them of their rights. Check to see whether such a memo has been sent in your workplace and, if so, what information it contains.

Find out

Find where details of your workplace grievance and disciplinary procedures are located, if they are not included in your terms and conditions of employment.

Find out

Check your staff handbook, contract of employment and disciplinary and grievance procedures to see what they say about how you could be dismissed and for what reasons.

Did you know?

If an employer does not follow the required procedures any dismissal becomes automatically unfair – no matter what the rights and wrongs of the case. A mandatory minimum award of four months' pay is awarded to the employee and any additional compensation is increased by a minimum of 10 per cent to a maximum of 50 per cent. Equally, if an employee fails to follow procedures any award he or she might receive is also reduced by a minimum of 10 per cent to a maximum of 50 per cent.

Disciplinary procedures

Unfortunately it sometimes happens that while you are thinking about bringing a grievance your line manager is thinking about taking disciplinary action against you. It may also be the case that you are subject to an independent Access disciplinary procedure. To comply with the new rules, the following steps should take place:

- Your employer should send you a letter informing you that there is a problem and arranging a meeting to discuss it. If the problem is regarded as sufficiently serious, and the disciplinary procedures provide for this, you may be suspended, normally on full pay, until the meeting is held. It might be, for instance, that there has been an incident in the office involving a number of employees and the employer needs to get statements from them before proceeding any further.
- Any action taken as a result of the meeting will depend on how serious the breach has been. You may be given a verbal warning for a first or minor offence (although it is likely that a written note of that warning will be put on your personnel file at least for a certain period of time).
- If this is not the first occasion on which you have been disciplined or if the breach is quite major, then you might be given a written warning. This could be followed by a final warning if your behaviour does not improve.
- The final step, of course, is dismissal.

You could be dismissed with notice, or summarily (instantly) dismissed without any notice. The latter normally happens only if an employee is guilty of very serious misconduct, such as assault, stealing or fighting in the workplace near dangerous machinery.

Constructive dismissal is where you are not actually dismissed but your employer makes life so miserable for you that you have no option but to leave.

Whatever disciplinary action is taken against you, you normally have the right of appeal against it to a more senior manager, or even to Acas if you are arguing that a dismissal is unfair.

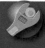

How to... Access information and seek guidance about your employment rights and responsibilities

- **Check your documents** to see that you have all the relevant information.

- **Ask within the organisation for advice.** You might want to talk to a senior colleague, someone in the human resources area or your trade union representative.

- **Look for external advice** – at the Citizens Advice Bureau either in person or online at www.adviceguide.org.uk or an online Community Legal Service Adviser on www.clsdirect.org.uk. If the matter is sufficiently important, you might want to consult a solicitor, most of whom now give clients a free first interview.

- **Go online.** Check, for instance, the TUC website at www.worksmart. org.uk or the Acas website at www.tiger.gov.uk.

Snapshot – When not to let your hair down!

Office Christmas parties can sound a good idea but can be quite hazardous for both employer and employee. Employers cannot afford to leave all the arrangements to one of the staff and just turn up on the night.

- They must check on health and safety issues (such as fire exits) and, ideally, the food to ensure there are choices for vegetarians and people with certain religious beliefs.

- They will also be held liable for staff behaviour even if the party is held off the works premises and outside working hours. In Canada, one employer was held partly responsible for a crash injury to a worker who drove home drunk from the Christmas party. The employer had offered to call her husband, and also to pay for a taxi, but this was not enough – he had a duty to take positive steps to stop her from driving.

- They must ensure that no one is sexually harassed. Younger members of staff may be particularly at risk and the employer should take steps to prevent this from happening. In one case an employer was held liable when an entertainer used blue and offensive material at the party because it was held that he should have put a stop to the act if it was causing too much embarrassment. The decision has been criticised but it is still important that the employer vets the material used by any entertainer.

- The employer may need to remember it might be incorrect to hold a Christmas party at all! The Employment Equality (Religion or Belief) Regulations 2003 outlaw certain discrimination, harassment

Snapshot Continued

and victimisation on the grounds of religion or belief. It has been suggested, therefore, that Christmas parties could discriminate against non-Christian staff if their religious festivals are not also celebrated.

On the other hand, all employees must avoid having so much to drink that they become offensive or, worse, start a fight. If employees have been warned in advance that they must not get tipsy, or if there are safety concerns, such as a requirement to operate machinery the next day, then disciplinary action could result. And if actions outside work affect the business, the same can apply. On one occasion some employees got into a fight outside the hotel where the party was being held. They were dismissed because the fight was reported in the papers and the firm said that its reputation had suffered as a result of it.

Employees are normally expected to turn up for work the following day and not phone in 'sick'. Some employers now have a policy of warning staff about a 'no show' before the party actually takes place.

Sometimes it's easier just to stay at home watching TV!

Witnessing or experiencing discrimination or bullying at work

One of your friends, Fatima, confides in you that although most people she works with are nice, her immediate line manager is not. Recently he has:

- made one or two disparaging remarks about her religion – she is a Muslim – and refused to even consider taking into account the extra stress she was under during Ramadan, a religious fasting period
- made generally critical remarks about women workers always becoming pregnant and going on maternity leave
- given her a below-average appraisal and made it clear that her male colleague, who is no better qualified or experienced, is next in line for promotion.

She has tried to talk to him about her concerns but since then he has become even more hostile and has isolated her from the rest of the group and given her all the low-level routine jobs.

If all this is true Fatima may have to consider taking a grievance out against him (see page 145). She may also be able to claim that her boss has been guilty of sex discrimination and discrimination on the grounds of her religion or belief.

Sex Discrimination Act 1975/Sex Discrimination Act 1975 (Amendment) Regulations 2003

The sex discrimination legislation prohibits discrimination against a woman on the grounds of her sex, or of a man on the grounds of his sex.

Examples of direct discrimination include refusing access to:
- jobs
- promotion opportunities
- training schemes
- opportunities to earn overtime, additional bonuses and benefits
- entitlement to paid time off for trade union duties
- eligibility for subsidised mortgages, occupational pensions, company cars and other perks
- equal choice of holiday dates.

Examples of indirect discrimination include:
- imposing a minimum height which could discriminate against women
- relocation around the country and/or work trips necessitating staying overnight away from home
- rotating shifts varying from day to day or week to week
- requiring a certain number of years of experience before being considered for promotion.

An employer does have certain defences to a claim of discrimination:
- **Genuine occupational qualification.** Examples include where the essential nature of the job calls for a man or woman for reasons of physical appearance (e.g. modelling), for reasons of authenticity (e.g. in dramatic performances), for reasons of privacy or decency (e.g. where members of the opposite sex are using toilet or washing facilities), in single-sex establishments, or work in a private home.
- **Positive action to change.** An example would be changing a traditionally all male workforce into one including women.
- **Justification on grounds other than sex.** That is, it corresponds to a real need for change on the part of the employer. For instance a man who was refused a job at a coffee shop because he had a beard was held to have been discriminated against but this discrimination was justifiable for health and safety reasons.

Did you know?

There are two types of sex discrimination:

Direct discrimination is where a person has received less favourable treatment on the grounds of his or her sex.

Indirect discrimination is where an employer applies a condition that would be far more difficult for one sex to comply with than the other and therefore is to the detriment of a considerably large proportion of women than of men (or vice versa).

Did you know?

Although a lot of discrimination is deliberate, on occasions some employers have argued that they were acting without malice. They may honestly believe, for instance, that a woman should not work in a warehouse because she is not physically capable, or that a man wouldn't want to work as a secretary and therefore wouldn't mind being deprived of the opportunity to do so. The end result is the same. It is still discrimination.

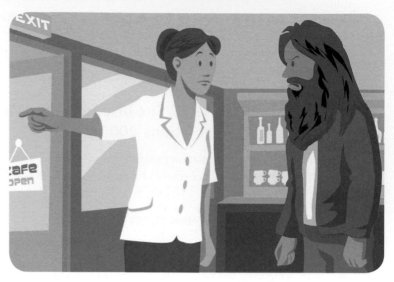

Sometimes discrimination is justified for health reasons!

Dress codes

Find out

Find out whether your organisation has a dress code and, if so, what it is. Find out also whether anyone has objected to it and, if so, why.

Appearance matters! Dress codes that have different rules for men and women may be directly discriminatory if more stringent requirements are imposed on one sex than the other. In one case a golf club had a policy that women were not allowed to wear trousers at work, which was obviously discriminatory. On the other hand a dress code that banned female shop assistants from wearing trousers but also banned male shop assistants from wearing T-shirts was held to be fair as both sexes had a similar requirement imposed on them. Similarly a supermarket's dress code that applied different rules to men and women about the permitted length of their hair was held to be non-discriminatory in that other dress and appearance provisions were imposed on the women. Note, however, that a dress code may be held discriminatory on the grounds of religion or belief, if, for example a requirement that women must wear skirts would discriminate against Muslim women.

Did you know?

The **Race Relations Act 1976** follows the same approach as the Sex Discrimination Act in deciding whether or not someone has been discriminated against because of his or her race. The website www.cre.gov.uk outlines the Act's main provisions and also the European Union's Article 13 proposals for combating racism. See also pages 161–7.

Employment Equality (Sexual Orientation) Regulations 2003

Recent legislation has concerned itself with gender bias. The **Employment Equality (Sexual Orientation) Regulations 2003** make it unlawful to harass, victimise or discriminate against workers because of their sexual orientation whether they are bisexual, lesbian, gay or heterosexual. The **Gender Recognition Act 2004** says that transsexual people must be treated as of their new sex for all legal purposes including in the workplace.

Employment Equality (Religion or Belief) Regulations 2003

As well as having a possible claim under the Sex Discrimination and Race Relations Acts, Fatima may be able to claim that she has been discriminated against on the grounds of her religion or belief. Again the regulations follow the same lines as the other discrimination legislation and cover areas such as religious observance in the workplace:

- Many religions or beliefs have special festivals or spiritual observance days and where it is reasonable an employee should be granted a request in order to celebrate them. Larger firms obviously tend to be in a better position than smaller firms to do this.
- Some religions or beliefs have specific dietary requirements and staff bringing food into the workplace may need to store and heat food separately. Where possible this should be allowed.
- Some religions require their followers to pray at specific times and staff may therefore request access to an appropriate quiet place. Employers are not required to do this but it is obviously good practice if they do.

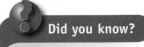

Did you know?

From October 2006, age discrimination in recruitment, promotion and training will be unlawful as well as forced retirement before age 65. All employees will also have the right to request working beyond 65.

Disability Discrimination Act 1995/2005

Robert has hearing difficulties and wears a hearing aid. He is also partially sighted. He has difficulty answering the telephone and takes a long time to read anything in written form, which hampers his work rate. He feels excluded in meetings as he frequently cannot follow what is going on in group discussions. His line manager isn't too sympathetic and tells him to do the best he can. His line manager might be guilty of breaking the law. The Disability Discrimination Act 1995 (as amended) tries to safeguard the interests of people who are physically or mentally disadvantaged and it is written in much the same terms as the Sex Discrimination and Race Relations Acts – although in this case discrimination is not divided into 'direct' and 'indirect' discrimination but is defined as 'less favourable treatment that cannot be justified'. Among other things it aims to prevent discrimination in employment and requires the employer to make reasonable adjustments to the workplace to enable a disabled person to do the job.

Bullying

Fatima and Robert have another problem to cope with. They are the newest and youngest members of staff in that particular department. The rest of the staff have worked there a long time and have known each other for years. A small group of them seem to have set out to make the new members of staff feel miserable or inadequate.

Did you know?

The House of Lords has now held that employers not only have a duty to protect employees from bullying if they know of that bullying but also if they could foresee that bullying might occur and that, if it did, it might cause physical or mental harm to an employee.

Did you know?

Harassment has been defined as attention from someone else that is unwelcome, causes alarm or distress. The **Protection from Harassment Act 1997** has made harassment and threats of violence a criminal offence with a maximum sentence of six months' imprisonment or a maximum £5000 fine.

- One of them has been spreading a rumour that Fatima isn't properly qualified for the job.
- She is also verbally insulting to both Fatima and Robert and refers to them openly as no-hopers.
- Sometimes she gives them jobs she knows they can't do because they have not sufficient experience.
- They are excluded from certain meetings and get-togethers. They are always given different tea breaks so that they cannot socialise with each other or anyone else.

All those instances constitute bullying and, particularly for a new employee, can cause a lot of unhappiness. Fortunately, however, employers now have a duty to protect employees from bullying and the last thing anyone should do is to suffer in silence. Even so it is not easy to tell tales, particularly if one of the people doing the bullying is your line manager.

How to... Assert your employment rights if you experience discrimination or bullying

- Don't keep things to yourself. Talk to a friend or a work colleague and ask for another opinion. If nothing else, the person should offer you moral support.

- If you can, talk on a one-to-one basis with the person doing the bullying to see whether you can persuade him or her to stop. Say how the treatment makes you feel and suggest that the other person may not realise how difficult he or she is making life for you.

- Keep a note of the incidents as they occur, including dates, times and details of anyone else who was present at the time.

- If you have a trade union representative, talk to him or her. Trade unions are used to dealing with this sort of situation.

- If the person bullying you is not your manager, talk to your manager and describe the type of treatment you have been receiving.

- If he or she is your manager you should try to see another manager – either a senior manager or perhaps the human resources manager.

- If no action is taken then you have to consider lodging a formal grievance.

- As a last resort you may have to look for another job, but in that case make sure you state in your letter of resignation why you are resigning and who you think is responsible (be careful, however, not to defame someone's character unless you are completely sure of your facts). Such a letter may help if you ultimately decide to take the employer to an employment tribunal.

How to... Support someone you witness being discriminated against or bullied

It is not easy. A lot of people keep silent if they see someone being bullied because they are frightened they might be bullied in turn. However, there is action you can take:

- Discuss the problem with the person concerned and check that they have their facts correct and are not being a bit too sensitive.

- Offer to accompany him or her to any meetings if procedures allow this.

- Ask other people to lend their support if relevant.

- Show them this page!

Find out

Find out more about bullying at work by checking Bully OnLine at www.successunlimited.co.uk.

Procedures you should follow when ill or needing time off

Sick leave

One of the terms in your contract of employment will almost certainly relate to the procedures you should follow if you are off sick and the amount of time off you are allowed. Most contracts state these things as a minimum:

- **Who you must tell.** Normally you have to let your employer know as soon as possible and certainly on the first day of your absence. If you are really too ill to do this, someone else should do it for you.
- **How soon you must complete a self-certification note** (if this is required). Some employers will expect you to do this for the first week and then to get a medical certificate from your doctor. If you

are going to be off sick for a number of weeks you might have to get repeat certificates.

If your illness is long-term you might also find that you will be visited by a doctor retained by your employer to check on the state of your health and determine how long your absence will be. You might also be invited to speak to a member of the HR department to discuss how you feel, when you think you might be able to return and any particular concerns you might have about returning. This in itself can be stressful but it would be unwise to refuse – unless you think you are being unfairly treated and put under pressure to return when you simply do not feel well enough. Remember, however, that under extreme circumstances an employer will be able to dismiss you on the grounds of ill-health, if he or she can prove that the dismissal is fair because you are no longer capable of doing the work.

Time off work

There are other times when you have a legitimate reason to want to be off work. In some cases you have a statutory right to take that time off. The table opposite states what they are.

Asking for time off

It's one thing being given a legal entitlement to time off, whether statutory or contractual. It's quite another to do so without causing irritation and annoyance to anyone. In principle most employees welcome the right to time off, whether it applies to them or anyone else. In practice, if one person is off at a very busy time of the year or

Find out

Many organisations allow employees time off in additional circumstances to those outlined in the table opposite. Check your own organisation's policies on paid or unpaid time off work and make a list of any differences you find.

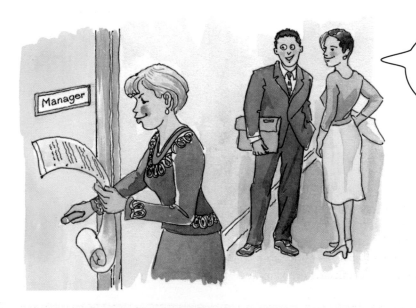

Well, she should do OK. At the last count, she had listed 34 reasons why she should have next Friday off.

Rights to time off work	
Reason for time off	**Statutory rights and eligibility**
Antenatal care	Yes, with pay. No need to have worked for employer for any particular length of time.
Maternity leave	Yes, paid. Length of maternity leave depends on length of service.
Parental leave (time off for parents to care for young children)	Yes, unpaid. Up to 13 weeks. Employee must have worked for employer for least one year.
Holidays	Yes, with pay, for most workers.
Jury service	No right to time off work and no right to pay unless in contract. Can only be excused from jury duty under certain circumstances.
Public duties (e.g. if a JP, a councillor, a school governor)	Yes, but no right to be paid. No need to have worked for employer for any particular length of time.
Study or training (16 to 18-year-olds)	Yes, reasonable time off with pay for relevant level 2 courses. No need to have worked for employer for any particular length of time.
Family emergencies	Yes, reasonable time off unpaid. No need to have worked for employer for any particular length of time.
Employees' representatives elected to be consulted in redundancy/transfer situations	Yes, reasonable time off with pay.
To look for work if in a redundancy situation	Yes, reasonable time off with pay but must have worked for employer for two years.
Trade union activities as a TU official or as a safety representative	Yes, reasonable time off with pay.
Trade union activities – taking part in TU activities	Yes, reasonable time off but without pay.
To attend a court as a witness	No, but if summoned or subpoenaed can be in contempt of court if do not attend. Need to negotiate with employer.

when a rush job must be done, it's harder to be tolerant. This does not mean you shouldn't have the time off due to you; it does mean that you should be aware of how to approach the topic. Dashing into your boss's office on Friday afternoon saying you want the following week off is not likely to win you any friends. It is much better to:

- Pick your time carefully.
- Raise the matter pleasantly. Even though you have a legal right to the time off it is still better to request than demand.
- Be prepared to discuss what should happen in your absence and whether or not you can ease the situation by working for a time alongside the colleague who might have to stand in for you. Obviously you cannot do this in an emergency situation.

- Where possible, prepare a file of relevant information for your stand in – useful telephone numbers, sources of reference, summary of work in progress, dates of meetings etc.
- Keep in touch, even on an informal basis, with your manager and colleagues throughout your period of absence if it is likely to be prolonged. This will probably help you as much as them and won't make the return to work as much of an ordeal.

Information recorded in personnel records, why these are needed and how to report changes

Most organisations today keep staff records electronically in a staff database – but not all of them. In either case, a new record is created each time a new member of staff is appointed and updated when required. The following information is normally entered:

- employee's name, address, telephone number and email address
- sex/ethnic background
- date of birth
- next of kin
- any disabilities
- National Insurance number and tax code
- schools/colleges/universities attended
- qualifications/training
- previous work history with dates
- date of joining the present organisation
- details of the current job, including where the employee will work, for what department or area, and for which line manager
- contract of employment details, including hours of work, details of wage/salary plus payroll reference number, holiday and sick pay entitlement, details of dispute procedures.

Information is then added relating to the following aspects of employment:

- additional training events or courses attended or relevant staff development activities
- disciplinary action taken or grievance procedures instituted
- sickness records and any occasions when leave from work has been taken
- performance appraisals
- promotions
- health and safety issues – such as accidents at work.

Why the information is needed

Personnel records are required for several reasons and by several people in the organisation:

- Line managers check the records of their staff if they are asked to provide a reference, if there is a disciplinary problem or other issue relating to a member of their own staff.
- The HR manager will monitor specific types of statistics, such as staffing levels, absence figures, sickness, lateness and staff turnover, and recommend appropriate action if there is a problem in any area.
- The health and safety officer or anyone responsible for risk assessments may wish to check that all staff have undertaken initial health and safety training and that those involved in higher risk activities have undergone further training.
- An organisation keen to promote diversity (see page 161) will want to analyse the workforce to assess the number of women, people from ethnic minorities and people with disabilities employed in the organisation.
- All organisations have a legal responsibility to keep full records relating to their workers, including the date they started and their salary for tax purposes. Health and safety law also requires them to keep records of accidents, injuries, diseases and dangerous occurrences.
- Individual staff may wish to refer to their own record from time to time, particularly if they are applying for internal or external promotion or if there is a dispute or problem.

How to report changes

In your own organisation, the method for reporting changes will depend on the system in use and whether staff records are kept in a central HR department, by your own line manager or by another member of staff in your department.

It is in your own interests to make sure that your record is up to date and accurate, particularly if you have been involved in training or staff development activities that would help your future promotion prospects.

In a large organisation your staff handbook will state who you should tell if your personal details change – for example if you move house, change your name or achieve a qualification. In a small business, you will need to tell your supervisor or boss. Changes to your job role and work record should be recorded automatically. If you want to check that these are accurate, don't forget that – for a small charge – you can ask to see your own record at any time.

Did you know?

If you work with personnel records then discussing these – or hinting what you know – to anyone not authorised to receive this information means that you would be in breach of confidentiality. Even if this is not an *express* term it is certainly an *implied* term of your contract of employment. It could result in disciplinary procedures being taken against you and possibly to your dismissal.

Remember

If you are taking the Technical Certificate you will need to know the main laws that relate to individual rights and responsibilities and the laws on discrimination, too.

Over to you

1 Your boss is giving a talk on equal opportunities at the next staff training day and wants to make it interesting. She has prepared some case studies to present and wants to try them out on you first. Look at the following examples and, in each case, make notes of what you think.

a A 35-year-old woman complained that she had been discriminated against because she applied for a job with the Civil Service but was not granted an interview because she did not meet the age requirements specified of between 18 and 29. The employer argued that there was no discrimination because the requirement applied equally to men and women. The woman won her case. Why do think she did?

b Because of health and safety concerns an organisation establishes the practice of allowing women to finish five minutes earlier than men so that there is less congestion at the factory exits. Is this discriminatory?

c An employer bans all part-time working because she doesn't feel it is cost effective. Can she do this?

d Susan is an administrator in the Sales Department. The all-male sales team is highly successful. They have worked together over the years, know each other very well and socialise together. Susan had some sales experience in her previous job and enjoyed it. She asks the sales manager if he will consider her for the next job that comes up. He says that, although he will consider her for promotion at some time, the sales team is not for her. The all-male atmosphere might make her uncomfortable and she would find it easier in an area where men and women were used to working together. Should she accept this decision?

2 Your friend Robert intends to talk to his boss direct about his difficulties in not hearing or seeing too well but wants as much information as possible before he makes an appointment to see him. On a recent training course you learned that much useful information is in Part II of the Disability Discrimination Act 1995 – employment provisions – and the Code of Practice for the elimination of discrimination in the field of employment against disabled persons or persons who have a disability.

Bearing in mind that Robert has sight difficulties, access the website www.disability.gov.uk and make a list of any provisions relating specifically to people with hearing or sight difficulties (including any adjustments an employer may have to make to equipment).

3   In your office there seems to be a bit of confusion about the right to time off and over the past few weeks you have had the following requests. In each case, say whether or not they are entitled to time off. If they are, state also whether or not they will be paid.

   a   David has been called for jury service.

   b   Halma's father has died.

   c   Geoff wants to go on a part-time course at the local college.

   d   Mary wants time off to look for other work as she has been told she is to be made redundant.

   e   Khalid's wife has just had a baby. He wants time off to help her.

   f   Robert has witnessed a fight outside a club. He doesn't want to testify against the people involved because he is frightened he may be at risk. The court has said he must attend.

4   One of your jobs is to make sure that you let the Personnel Department know of any changes that should be made to staff records. You try to fill in the appropriate form every month but you are having problems in getting some of the information you need. Decide what action you would take in each of the following cases.

   a   Halma is completely disorganised. She never keeps a record of anything and it is just a waste of time asking her what training courses she has been on.

   b   You know David has applied for another job because he has asked you for a reference. However, he doesn't want anyone else to know at present.

   c   Geoff dropped a heavy file on his foot and bruised it badly. He doesn't want anyone to know about it because he thinks he might get into trouble for not following the recognised safety procedures.

Evidence planning

1 Check that you know where your organisation's disciplinary and grievance procedures and any policies or procedures relating to discrimination, harassment, victimisation or bullying are kept and that you have included this information in your folder.

 If you need to find information yourself or seek guidance, make a note of what you did or keep copies of any emails you sent or printouts you made. Add these to your paper or electronic folder.

2 Add to your folder any information relating to the procedures you must follow to give notification if you are sick and/or if you want time off – unless this is already included in your contract of employment. Make a note of any procedures you must follow to book your holidays or if you need time off in an emergency. Then add any information you have been given relating to making changes to your staff record.

 If you follow any of these procedures at any time, keep a record. Alternatively you could ask the colleague you dealt with for witness testimony to say that you followed the procedure correctly.

3 You will need to prove to your assessor that you can assert your employment rights when necessary. If this type of situation occurs, record your own account of what happened and ask your line manager to countersign and date it to confirm it is correct. Put your account into your folder.

4 Keep your folder safely. You can use the information to help you answer questions from your assessor to prove that you can access information about many of your employment rights and responsibilities, carry out your responsibilities and assert your rights when necessary.

What if...?

What should you do if you don't need to ask for guidance on your rights and responsibilities while you are taking your award?

Your assessor can give you a dedicated task to cover the knowledge and understanding required. This will then be followed by a professional discussion where you can explain how you would perform in such a situation and what evidence you might bring forward.

Support diversity

When Julius Caesar crossed the English Channel and arrived in Britain around 54 BC he set something of a trend. Since then, people from all over the world have made similar journeys for a variety of reasons, sometimes fleeing from persecution or tyranny, at other times looking for work or to improve their standards of living.

The result today is a country with a hugely varied mix of peoples, with London now the world's most culturally diverse city. There are more than 50 ethnic communities of 10 000 or more people, who collectively speak more than 300 languages. Four out of every 10 people in the country, who were born outside the UK, live in the capital.

Diversity, of course, does not just relate to culture or ethnicity, it relates to any type of difference between people. In your own neighbourhood and in your social life you may mix, largely, with people of your own culture or age group. At work, the situation is different. You will mix with a far wider range of people. How you react and respond to them, and the business case for diversity, are the main topics of this section.

Find out

In September 2005, the BBC published its *Born Abroad* project, which shows that diversity in the UK is changing as people from a wider range of countries now migrate to Britain. Using 2001 census data, the project maps where the 7.5 per cent of people who were born outside the UK have come from, where they live and how well they do. Find out more at http://news.bbc.co.uk/1/shared/spl/hi/uk/05/born_abroad/html/overview.stm.

What diversity is and why it should be valued

While diversity is often taken to relate to race, ethnicity or culture, it actually means any type of difference – opinions, backgrounds,

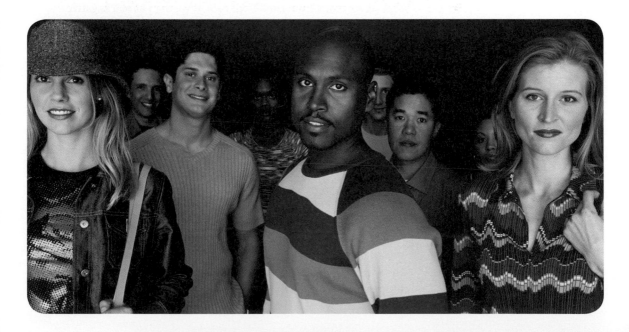

ages, genders, sexual orientation, health, fitness, religions, beliefs and wealth – to name but a few. In fact, if you take diversity at its broadest, it could be argued that there are hardly any two people the same!

From that point of view, it is arguable that social diversity helps to enrich our lives and makes the world far more interesting. People who travel the world usually do so because they enjoy seeing new sights and meeting people from other cultures. But not everyone responds so positively to diversity, especially when it is on their doorstep. Right-wing political parties actively protest against diversity and racial integration. 'Old boy' and 'male networks' still operate in some sectors of business to close ranks against women. People who are disabled or gay still have to fight open prejudice, often through ignorance. And there is still a tendency for many to regard anyone aged over 40 as 'past it' and ready for pensioning off.

The value of diversity

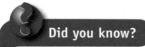

Did you know?

American research linked fear of differences among people to racism. Getting to know people and having positive experiences eliminated this fear.

Diversity brings other views and other perspectives to a situation, often through personal experience. You could not, for example, argue about famine in Africa, poverty in Bangladesh or political repression in Burma against someone who had witnessed these events at first hand. In that situation, if you were wise, you would listen and learn.

Mixing with a wide variety of other people also helps to overcome fear and prejudice. Research by New York and Harvard universities found that we are all inclined to be frightened of someone who is different, such as someone from a different race. If we then have a negative experience with this type of person – such as being mugged – this then reinforces our fear and contributes towards racism and racial prejudice towards the whole group. Conversely, a positive experience has the opposite effect. So, if you work closely with someone from another ethnic group, this helps to break down barriers and reduce or remove prejudice.

Advantages that diversity can bring to an organisation

You already know that it is illegal to discriminate against anyone in the workplace on grounds of sex, race, disability, sexual orientation, religion or belief and – from October 2006 – on grounds of age, too. Yet it is one thing to accept that diversity and equality is a legal requirement in Britain, and quite another to actively promote it. Yet there are very good business reasons for doing so.

Broadly, the main advantage of diversity is that organisations need to reflect their customers to be able to understand and satisfy their needs. This is as true of a small business in a multicultural neighbourhood as it is of global giants who trade internationally and public sector organisations – such as the police or ambulance service – who deal with people from all communities. A diverse workforce also helps to improve employee retention and gives customers more confidence in an organisation's ability to help them.

However, there are other more specific benefits that are identified in relation to specific types of diversity:

- **The Employers Forum on Age** argues that the UK workforce is growing steadily older as there are fewer young people entering the job market. This causes recruitment problems. By abandoning prejudices about older workers, employers can attract a wider pool of skilled talent and also benefit from lower staff costs, lower staff turnover and absenteeism and increased motivation and commitment from the staff.
- **Business in the Community's (BITC's) programme Opportunity Now** focuses on gender equality to reduce and remove prejudices against women and working mothers. The chairman argues that organisations that get it right reap the benefits and improve their business success – which is both good for them and good for women.
- **BITC's Race for Opportunity** campaign works with a network of private and public sector UK organisations who see reflecting their community and customer base in their workforce as a key to business success. These businesses monitor their performance across four key areas: employment, marketing to ethnic minority customers, using ethnic minority businesses as suppliers or business partners, and community involvement.
- **The Employers Forum on Disability** argues that they are the 'Cinderella' in relation to diversity practices. When they compared organisational performance they found that fewer organisations have an allocated budget or stated policies to promote disability equality rather than race or gender equality, and only 15 per cent check the impact of actions taken on reducing disability inequality. You can find out more at www.employers-forum.co.uk.

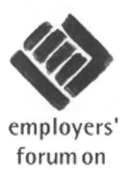

employers'
forum on
disability

Find out

How old is 'old'? According to the Employers Forum on Age, ideas vary wildly from 'a woman over 35' to 'a man over 42'. In many call centres, 'old' is seen as being more than 25! What are your views? Find out more at www.efa.org.uk.

Did you know?

According to the **Women and Equality Unit**, the gender pay gap between the hourly pay of part-time women workers and full-time men is 40 per cent, and 32 of the UK's top companies still have no woman on their board of directors. This is despite the fact that women make up 50 per cent of the population and make most of the consumer decisions!

Did you know?

A DTI report on diversity argues the business benefits of identifying more closely with customers. It estimates that the disabled population spends around £50 billion and minority ethnic communities spend around £15 billion a year.

Being sensitive to people's abilities, background, values, customs and beliefs

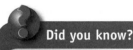

Find out

Compare media reports of professional men and women – such as in business, sports and politics. Reports about women often include a comment on her appearance and her age, those on men do not.

Did you know?

The Young Vic Theatre Company, along with several other theatres, is campaigning for more black and minority ethnic youngsters to work in the arts. Their survey showed many people thought that if they were not white and middle-class their CV would automatically be rejected.

If diversity has so many benefits – and is fundamentally a key aspect of equality and fairness to others – why do things go wrong? As you read earlier, fear of the unknown has a role to play – we find it safer to stick with people similar to ourselves rather than mix with other people. We may also find out information that reinforces these views. In some cases this may be because we listen to people who are prejudiced or ignorant, but more often we will be reacting to some of the stereotypical images promoted by the media.

When you watch a movie or television programme, read a magazine or newspaper or listen to the radio you are being bombarded with messages above and beyond the ones you think you are receiving! These usually include stereotypical images of different groups in society, for example:

- Successful women may be portrayed as ruthless and ambitious while men are shown as smart and fulfilling their potential.
- Television programmes and plays rarely reflect the ethnic mix we see around us.
- The strong, silent male and the action hero are often seen as masculine role models, whereas comedy programmes feature bumbling fathers.
- Reports about gays or lesbians are frequently negative.
- The word 'elderly' is often used to describe anyone over the age of 50.

More seriously, the media can create 'moral panics' by running scare stories on topics such as asylum-seekers or immigration which reinforce people's fears and prejudices.

Many people believe that the only way that different people can coexist peaceably in the future is through communication and understanding, and by integrating rather than living apart. Diversity in the workplace is an excellent starting point because by relating to other people as individuals we realise how ridiculous many of our fears, worries and prejudices are.

How to... Interact sensitively and respect other people's different backgrounds, abilities, values, customs and beliefs

- Always treat other people as you would like to be treated yourself.

- Never treat other people differently or assume they are happy to be excluded from the group because they are 'different'.

- Be aware of how prejudices, ignorance and stereotypes affect your own behaviour.

- Take a positive approach if you meet someone who is different – focus on the person, not the difference. Greet the person with a smile and assume he or she is friendly until you get positive proof you are wrong.

- Learn more about the cultures and beliefs of people you are likely to meet at work, whether they be Muslim, Jewish, Hindu, Buddhist or New Age. This is especially important if you offer light refreshments at work.

- If you work with someone who is from a different culture, religion or belief or who has overcome a disability, use this as an opportunity to find out more – without being intrusive.

- Learn how to deal sensibly and sensitively with someone who has a disability so that you are not nervous about approaching him or her. Then find out more at the Disability Rights Commission's website: www.drc-gb.org.

- Think about the words you use. Avoid racist language, slang or derogative phrases that ridicule groups of people – e.g. 'stop being an old woman', 'play the white man', or 'he's a right poof'.

- Don't be a snob! The office cleaner and security guard should think you are just as polite and friendly as your boss does!

- Be patient if you work with anyone who has learning difficulties or finds it harder than you to grasp certain tasks. Challenge yourself to give an explanation and/or demonstration that is appropriate and the person understands.

- If you feel that you would benefit from specific training to understand or communicate with different colleagues or customers better, talk to your supervisor.

- Remember, you stop noticing differences when you get to know people well and relate to them as individuals. This also gives you the confidence to relate to other people more easily.

Find out

The WW2 archive being created by the BBC – *The People's War* – has encouraged schools and colleges to 'adopt' a veteran and listen to stories from people of different nationalities who were personally involved and then type up their stories. These enable young people to learn more and break down generational barriers at the same time. Find out more at www.bbc.co.uk/dna/ww2.

Did you know?

If you work alongside Muslims you should know that the word 'halal' is not just used to describe meat. Its meaning is 'lawful' or 'permitted'. So halal meat is allowed, and so are halal mortgages. These comply with Sharia (Islamic) law which forbids the paying or earning of interest. They have been introduced by a number of UK finance firms such as HSBC. For more information go to www.hsbc.co.uk/1/2/amanah.

Ways in which you could learn from others

Diversity in the workplace shouldn't just mean being non-discriminatory. It should also mean learning from other people so that you improve your own knowledge and broaden your vision about the world in general. You may get some surprises! When Second World War veterans were encouraged to record their experiences for schools, many children were astounded at the tales of bravery they heard from elderly people, or even from their own great-grandparents.

At work you may have little time to sit listening to war stories, but there is a wealth of information you can find out in your workplace from people who are different from yourself. Here are some examples:

- What is it like living with a disability, such as being blind, deaf or needing to use a wheelchair? Which buildings are easy to enter and get around in your area, and which are not? How helpful (or otherwise) are other people, and what can you do that would give useful assistance?
- What are the main beliefs of someone of a different religion? How should you greet people from that religion? What do they eat, and what must they not eat? Why do they wear different types of clothes?
- What are the major cultural differences between yourself and someone else? Are there gestures that mean different things or are considered insulting (like showing the soles of the feet in Thailand)? What other cultural traditions are different?
- What is the history of your organisation? How has it changed since it was started? How was the work carried out then? What do people think was done better then – and what is done better now – and why?

As your knowledge increases you will find that you can use this to improve the way you work and how you interact with other people in the following ways:

- You will have greater understanding about how to deal with your colleagues, customers and other business contacts.
- You will know where to obtain advice if you have a serious problem or difficulty.
- You will be less inclined to make mistakes because you will not assume that you know everything without asking for the views of other people.

- You will have more confidence when you are dealing with other people.
- You will be nicer to know!

If you are open-minded and welcome the opportunity to constantly develop your knowledge and skills, then before too long you will find that you have stopped being just the learner and started to become the teacher, too!

Your organisation's procedures and legal requirements in relation to discrimination legislation

Your employer is almost certain to be aware of his or her legal obligations in relation to discrimination, which you read about on pages 148–53. If not, then there could be problems given the increase in the number of claims being taken to the employment tribunals.

Because of the growing importance of this legislation many employers now have detailed discrimination policies and procedures. A lot of them follow the Equal Opportunities Commission guidelines for employers:

- Gather information about the workforce to see how many women, people from ethnic minorities and disabled people are actually employed and in which areas and positions.
- Produce an equal opportunities policy, defining discrimination and stating the organisation's commitment to equal opportunities.
- Make someone responsible for equal opportunities in the organisation – normally a senior manager.
- Check that all employees know about the policy. No matter how good the policy is on paper it is useless if no one knows about it.
- Take steps to implement the policy. Again, if no one actually does anything about it, it might as well be torn up.
- Consider setting up an equal opportunities committee or working party to check that the policy is being put into practice and to monitor any possible breaches of it.
- Give equal opportunities training to all employees.
- Examine existing practices, policies and procedures to see that they all comply with the new policy. Some practices – such as always recruiting male apprentices – are so long-standing that managers sometimes do not realise they are discriminatory.

Did you know?

Between 2003 and 2005, sexual discrimination claims have increased by 41 per cent and more than a quarter of all claims settled in 2004 resulted in final payouts in excess of £10 000. The maximum recorded payout was £504 433!

Find out

Check to see what your organisation's equal opportunities policy is, who is responsible for seeing that it is carried out, and whether there is a budget or policy for promoting diversity in your workplace.

Over to you

1 Find out more about how the media stereotypes different groups at www.media-awareness.ca/english/issues/stereotyping/index.cfm. Although this is a Canadian website, much of the information is relevant as it includes many of the American movies, TV programmes and magazines that are shown in Britain. Then see what examples you can find yourself on TV and in magazines over the next two weeks. If possible, compare your findings with those of other members of your group.

2 Investigate the Women and Equality Unit at www.womenandequalityunit.gov.uk/about/index.htm. Download the brochure *Diversity Best Practice in the Corporate World: A Guide for Business* which includes a series of case studies on businesses that are actively championing diversity. Identify the one that inspires you the most and give your reasons. Note that these case studies are not restricted to gender equality but also include initiatives linked to other aspects of diversity.

3 *Either:* On your own, find out more about the work of at least two of the following groups of organisations. *Or:* If you are studying for your NVQ award in a group, allocate this task between you, with small groups investigating and giving a summary on the work of each of the organisations listed below.

- **On gender equality:** The Women's National Commission at www.thewnc.org.uk and Opportunity Now at www.opportunitynow.org.uk. At Opportunity Now find out which firms have won the latest workplace awards and why.

- **On age equality:** The Employers Forum on Age at www.efa.org.uk and Age Positive at www.agepositive.gov.uk.

- **On race equality:** Race for Opportunity at www.bitc.org.uk/programmes/programme_directory/race_for_opportunity/rfo_about.html and the Commission for Racial Equality at www.cre.gov.uk.

- **On disability equality:** The Employers Forum on Disability at www.employers-forum.co.uk and the Disability Rights Commission at www.drc-gb.org.

- **On equality and diversity issues:** The Equal Opportunities Commission at www.eoc.org.uk and Diversity Leaders at www.diversityleaders.org.uk.

Evidence planning

When you are gathering evidence for your option units you have to prove to your assessor that you interact with other people sensitively, respecting their diversity, and that you understand the advantages diversity can bring to an organisation. You can plan how to do this in the following way.

1   Make a list of the people you deal with on a regular basis. This list can include your colleagues, customers, suppliers and other business contacts. Make a note of those people who are different from you in any of the ways discussed in this section.

2   Think about the reasons why you interact with them and what you have learned from them and about them since you first knew them.

3   Make notes on diversity in relation to yourself and your own organisation. This should include the location of any equal opportunities or diversity policies, the benefits to your organisation of promoting diversity, and the practical steps you take to interact with other people sensitively and learn from them. These notes can then form the basis of a professional discussion with your assessor.

4   Identify the option unit(s) that would be most appropriate for including your evidence. This could be a log you keep of occasions when you deal with your business contacts or witness testimony from your colleagues. You should be aware that your assessor will probably want to watch you at some stage when you are dealing with other people.

What if...?

What should you do if your organisation does not have any procedures linked to diversity or discrimination that you have to follow?

If there are no procedures in place during the period you are being assessed, your assessor can give you a dedicated task to cover the knowledge and understanding required. This will then be followed by a professional discussion during which you can explain how you would perform in such a situation and what evidence you might bring forward.

Maintaining security and confidentiality

Not very long ago office security was concerned mainly with closing and locking windows, desk and filing cabinet drawers, office doors and going home! Today security is a far broader topic and relates to a wide range of issues, from physical theft of property to hacking into computer files. In addition, the legal responsibilities of organisations are far greater. The requirements of the Data Protection Act mean that organisations are responsible for information security. Copyright laws, too, prevent the distribution of original works without the creator's consent, and all employers have a duty of care to their employees to provide a safe place in which to work. Experts also argue that as well as precautions against theft, businesses also need to guard against malicious attacks from disgruntled employees and attacks from militant groups.

For all these reasons, security and confidentiality are not issues you can take lightly, particularly as your responsibilities in this area increase automatically with your seniority. If junior administrators and new trainees are given a little leeway and allowed to be slightly chatty or even careless at times, the same latitude is not allowed with more senior staff. Quite simply, the more you progress, the less this will be expected or even allowed.

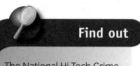

Find out

The National Hi-Tech Crime Unit estimates that British businesses lose £2.5 billion each year through computer-related fraud. Find out more at www.nhtcu.org.uk.

The importance of maintaining security and confidentiality

Maintaining security and confidentiality is just as important at the personal level as at the organisational level. If you divulge details of a colleague's home address, salary level, health or marital problems then you are likely to cause that person severe distress and anxiety if word gets out. If you are casual about security of information or security of the premises in general then you could cost your employer a great deal of money – either as a result of direct theft or through a successful prosecution for breach of confidentiality by a colleague, customer or client.

The security and confidentiality measures in place in an organisation vary depending on the nature of the work, but this does not mean that it is only in top-secret government establishments that strict security procedures are in place. Commercial organisations are just as sensitive about trade secrets being leaked, particularly when products are being developed – as anyone who works in the car, aerospace or pharmaceutical industry will tell you!

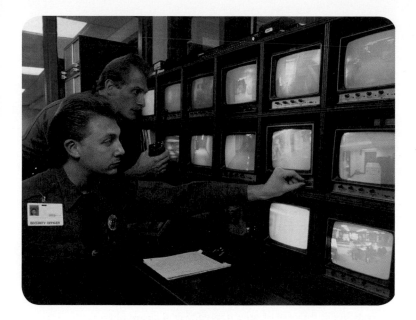

The usual way of assessing the security threat to an organisation is to carry out a **risk assessment**. This identifies the range of likely threats, based on factors such as the type of business, location, design and layout of the building, number of staff and visitors, type of goods, information handled and opening times. The aim is to:

- identify the main risks and threats to the organisation
- target security measures so that money is spent wisely
- decide basic standards that must be followed
- identify the measures required to consistently meet these standards
- draw up a security policy
- heighten awareness of security amongst the staff.

Security of physical property

One of the first steps in assessing security is to check the security of physical items. This relates to the following areas:

- **Buildings and the area around them**. Access points should be kept to a minimum and the visitor's entrance clearly signed. In a highly secure establishment a gatehouse prevents access to any area without permission. Even small firms benefit from an access control system to prevent uninvited visitors simply walking in. Access control can be through locks and keys, keypads or more sophisticated measures such as iris or thumbprint recognition. Signs that identify restricted areas help to increase staff vigilance and also give visitors fewer excuses to wander around. All areas, including car parks and storage areas, should be well lit at night.

Did you know?

Many organisations are very guarded about the information they give to prospective customers over the telephone. They are aware that some may be competitors, trying to find out their client list or their charges!

Find out

The 2004 Information Security Breaches Survey (ISBS) by PriceWaterhouseCoopers identified staff as a major security threat, yet only 43 per cent of organisations follow up references and carry out background checks on their staff. Twelve per cent never informed staff about their responsibilities in relation to information security, and only 36 per cent included security in staff inductions. Find out what vetting procedures for new staff are in place in your organisation and check how your colleagues are made aware of security issues.

Find out

If you wanted to break into your office, how would you do it? If you wanted to steal something, would it be easy or hard? If you can think of any weaknesses you could exploit, tell your employer now!

- **Equipment**. A list should be made of all valuable equipment on the premises, including the make, model and serial number. The equipment should be permanently marked or tagged. Computer equipment can be secured to the desk and alarms fitted. All portable equipment should be stored in a secure area overnight and access to the area should be restricted. The same applies to areas where any stock is kept, particularly if it is of high value.
- **Personal property**. This should be kept away from public areas and staff should be encouraged to guard their own property carefully and never take personal valuables to work unnecessarily.
- **Visitor checks**. All callers should be asked to prove their identity, including delivery people and contractors arriving to do maintenance work. A visitor pass/visitor book system can be used to authorise access to the building or to specific areas. In many organisations visitors are always accompanied – they are never allowed to roam around freely, or left alone in an office. Visitor details recorded in the book also help to ensure that a head count is possible in the case of an emergency evacuation.
- **Staff security**. Staff who handle cash or valuable goods should be kept separate (or screened off) from callers. Staff should not work alone without some safeguards such as a personal alarm or regular checks that there are no problems. Coded security locks on doors prevent visitors wandering into staff areas. Anyone who has to deal with potentially aggressive customers should receive special training and have specific protection relevant to the degree of threat. This can include personal alarm systems, CCTV, security guards and unbreakable glass screens.

Did you know?

If staff and visitors are required to wear ID badges at all times this makes intruders easier to spot.

Did you know?

IT security experts argue that protecting the information on a computer system is far more important than guarding the equipment, which is relatively cheap and easily replaced.

Did you know?

You can generally expect to find personnel records, customer details, product developments, organisational plans, financial information and security details to be treated as confidential.

Security of information

Information can be classified into that which is strictly confidential, that which is restricted to a department or kept within the organisation, and that which can be made publicly available. Assigning the correct category is important. If too high a level is assigned then over-elaborate precautions may be taken to protect information that is not in fact particularly important, and people who would find it useful may be prevented from receiving it. Conversely, failing to respect confidentiality requirements sufficiently can mean that both personal and commercially sensitive information is treated too casually by staff.

Information must be assessed in terms of the way it is held – in paper files and as computer files. In some establishments the telephone system would also be checked for security. The questions to ask are:

- Who should have access?
- What are the threats to information security?
- How the information can be protected against these threats?

The table below identifies the precautions that should be taken.

	Examples of threats	Access restrictions	Additional precautions
Paper-based information	Junior or temporary staff who may pass on information unwittingly; staff who have a grudge against their employer	Clear marking of confidential papers Restricted circulation Approved distribution lists Restrictions on photocopying Distribution in sealed envelopes Papers not taken off the premises Filing and file retrieval only done by nominated staff	Papers stored in security cabinet Copies made on desktop photocopiers in private office Copies/files destroyed in cross-cut shredder Personal fax machine used to send/receive confidential messages that holds them in memory until the correct password is entered.
Computer-based information	Malicious software (e.g. viruses, worms, spyware); hackers who gain unauthorised access; disgruntled employees	User IDs and passwords Additional access restrictions to confidential electronic files and records	Firewall Anti-virus software and 24-hour monitoring Critical data back-up nightly Website hosted offsite Encryption of data and financial transactions Special passwords to access wireless network Old CDs shredded Hard drives in obsolete computers destroyed Strict IT policy

Did you know?

Some firms insist that any employee who gives notice must clear his or her desk and leave immediately. The reason is to prevent sabotage and/ or confidential information being disclosed to competitors.

Did you know?

If your firm has a wireless network, watch out for delivery drivers or reps parking outside for long periods. They may be hitching a free ride on your network, if there are no security measures! If you work for a large firm the worry may be more about 'screen scraping'. This involves copying a computer screen to tempt customers to enter their security details on a bogus site.

Legal and organisational requirements for security and confidentiality

You already know that your employer has a legal responsibility to provide a safe place for you to work under the terms of the Health and Safety at Work etc. Act. This includes taking the necessary steps to protect you from violence in the workplace as well as monitoring or eliminating any security risks that could endanger you.

Complying with the law

Your organisation also needs to comply with the laws that relate to the security of information in the workplace.

Data Protection Act 1998

The main terms of this Act were described on pages 130–31. Employers who process personal information are classed as data controllers and included on a national register held by the Information Commissioner's Office. If an employer fails to comply with or contravenes the Act then an enforcement notice can be issued by the Information Commissioner stating what action must be taken, or what activities must be stopped. Alternatively an information notice may be issued which requests details of an activity. The Information Commissioner also has the power to search premises if there is evidence of contravention. An organisation that fails to comply with a notice or obstructs a search is guilty of a criminal offence.

Copyright, Designs and Patents Act 1988 (as amended)

This Act protects people who create original works by limiting the actions that other people can take with these. So you cannot legally photocopy this page five times for your friends! As a student you are allowed to take one copy of any written material, but this must be for your own private study or for research purposes. This does not apply to your employer – all businesses must obtain a licence from the appropriate agency, such as the Copyright Licensing Agency or the Newspaper Licensing Agency. If you read an article or book and quote from it, then you should make the reference clear. You will see how to do this in optional unit 310.

Find out

Copywatch, part of the Copyright Licensing Agency, offers rewards of up to £20 000 for people who report blatant systematic copying of literary material (e.g. books) without permission. Find out more at www.copywatch.org.

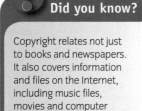

Did you know?

Copyright relates not just to books and newspapers. It also covers information and files on the Internet, including music files, movies and computer programs. Copyright is one type of **intellectual property**; other types include products, trademarks and brand names. You can find out more at www.intellectual-property.gov.uk.

Computer Misuse Act 1990

This Act is designed to protect businesses against computer hackers or anyone who tampers or alters data or software without permission. There are three criminal offences under this Act:

- gaining unauthorised access to computer material (i.e. hacking)
- gaining unauthorised access to computer material with the intent to commit or help to commit further offences
- making unauthorised modifications to computer material (this includes deliberately deleting or corrupting files and introducing a virus into the computer system).

Did you know?

Converting a Word document to pdf format before you circulate it means no one can alter it.

Organisational requirements

As you know, organisations can use policies and procedures to state the actions that are permitted by managers and staff.

- Security, IT and data processing policies explain the organisation's priorities in relation to the security of both premises and information.
- Security, IT and data processing procedures specify the actions that must be taken by staff to comply with the policies and with the law.

In addition, organisations may monitor the activities of their staff, such as by checking emails, monitoring websites visited and even by recording keystrokes.

Did you know?

The TUC (Trades Union Congress) is against staff monitoring and claims it is a breach of human rights. The Information Commissioner has therefore drawn up codes of practice relating to staff surveillance which state that organisational policies should make the stance on monitoring clear. Find out more at www.information-commissioner.org.uk.

Snapshot – A spooky kind of job!

Fans of the TV programme *Spooks* were delighted when MI6, the UK secret intelligence service (SIS), launched its own website in 2005. The aim, however, was not to give away state secrets but to provide basic information about the service. Its 'sister' organisation MI5 uses its website to give security advice. This includes top-ten guidelines as well as guides relating to physical security that all businesses can use to better protect their property and confidential information.

Both websites include information about admin careers and MI5's includes job vacancies. In October 2005, administrative assistants were required to work in London at salaries from £15 750, depending on experience. Duties involved creating files, maintaining the database, drafting documents and organising meetings. Excellent communications and team skills were vital as well as – unsurprisingly – integrity and a keen understanding of confidentiality. Needless to say, all applicants are carefully vetted!

Find out

The PriceWaterhouse Coopers ISB survey carried out in 2004 (see page 171) found that only 33 per cent of all companies and 66 per cent of large businesses had a security policy, and data protection procedures were in place in only 44 per cent of firms. Find out the policies and procedures that exist in your organisation.

Snapshot Continued

Find out more about security for businesses on the site at www.mi5.gov.uk, and more about admin jobs and profiles at www.mi6.gov.uk and job vacancies at www.mi5careers.info – where you can also read about the purpose and values of the service.

Did you know?

Many large organisations provide training for administrators and receptionists on the action to take if they receive a bomb threat. This is very important in organisations where members of the public would need to be evacuated quickly, such as tourist attractions and city centre department stores.

Procedures if you have concerns about security and confidentiality

Your first action, if you think there has been a breach of security, is to check whether there is a specific policy or procedure telling you what to do. If there is, you obviously follow instructions.

However, no policy or procedure can cover every possible eventuality so that are times when you have to use your common sense. You will have to do this all the time if there are no policies or procedures at all! The first point to assess is whether you can take action to eliminate the risk yourself, without putting yourself in any danger.

How to... Maintain security and confidentiality and report any concerns

Find out

The international standard for security is known as BS7799. This sets out the controls and procedures that are required to ensure that all types of information – no matter how it is stored or handled – is secure from internal, external, accidental or malicious threats. If your boss thinks more could be done in your organisation, investigate http://emea.bsi-global.com/InformationSecurity/Overview.

- **Check that you know and follow your organisation's policies** and procedures covering security, IT, confidentiality and data processing.

- **Follow the advice given on the MI5 website** to prevent yourself being a security risk to your employer.

- **Carry out routine security checks.** Keep money, confidential papers and valuables locked away. Check that windows and doors are locked at night. Keep keys safe. Make sure visitors are not left alone in an office, and query their presence in areas where they are not permitted.

- **Never disclose confidential work matters** to your colleagues, customers, friends or family.

- **Develop secure IT habits.** Commit your password to memory, and have a word/number combination that cannot be second-guessed. Switch screens (use Windows + D to return to desktop

How to... Continued

or Alt + Tab to switch documents) to avoid someone reading a document. Angle your screen away from visitors. Log out if you are leaving your desk. Lock away back-ups securely. Never open email attachments from unknown senders.

- **Watch for minor breaches by your colleagues** – a jacket on a chair (probably containing money or credit cards), confidential papers left on a desk – and take remedial action yourself.

- **Follow police advice** – be alert and observant and report any unusual or suspicious activity to the appropriate person or department. Trust your instincts – if you feel something is wrong, tell someone in charge!

Remember

Employment contracts often stop employees contacting or working for direct competitors for a certain length of time. Another clause may prevent them from getting grievances off their chest on the web. In the US, Ellen Simonetti was fired because of her blog. Joe Gordon, who worked for Waterstones, got into serious trouble for the same reason – so beware!

Over to you

1   The government is very keen that small business users are protected against IT threats. Find out more about the service it has launched, ITSafe, at its website www.itsafe.gov.uk. If you work for a small business, identify the benefits it could provide for your employer. If you work for a large business, check how your IT department has protected you against security threats.

2   On the same site you can access the IT glossary to find out about any term that baffles you – such as blog and bug under 'b'. Search the glossary to find the answers to the following:

   a   What is a denial of service attack?

   b   Why do firms encrypt data?

   c   What is a firewall?

   d   How does a keystroke logger work?

   e   What is a logic bomb?

   f   What is phishing?

   g   Can spyware ever be good?

   h   What is a Trojan?

   i   What is the difference between a virus and a worm?

   j   What is meant by the term 'payload'?

3   The government is keen to provide free advice to all businesses about actions to take to protect themselves from security risks,

Over to you Continued

largely in relation to information. Access the following information to find out more about the risks that are relevant to your industry and your sector.

a At the Department of Trade and Industry, check out advice and guidance on information security online at www.dti.gov.uk/industries/information_security.

b On the same site, access and save the latest version of the PriceWaterhouseCoopers Information Security Breaches survey and check out your own sector in more detail.

c At Business Link, under the IT and e-commerce heading, find out about IT security for businesses, both large and small.

d Download the Home Office booklet *Your Business: Keep Crime Out Of It* from www.crimereduction/business40htm. Then read how you can help your employer to keep the workplace safe at www.homeoffice.gov.uk/security/staying-safe/work/?version=1.

4 Your employer has decided to include security information in induction programmes for all new administrators in your organisation and has asked for your help. Based on your own organisation, decide on ten key items you would include. Prepare a prompt sheet for yourself which includes these item headings, with your reasons for their inclusion, to discuss with your employer to get his or her agreement.

Evidence planning

You will have to prove to your assessor that you preserve the security of property and the confidentiality of information in your own workplace. You will do this while you are gathering evidence for your optional units. However, start to plan this now, in the following way.

1 Make a list of any security guidance documents or security procedures that relate to your own workplace. These include computer or IT policies. If you work for a small firm where there are no policies, make a note of your key areas of responsibility. Your answers to question 4 in the section above should help you to do this.

2 Carry out a security check of your own office and workstation and any other office areas for which you are responsible. Then assess the actions of yourself and your colleagues and decide what specific security risks there may be related to your own job role and how you deal with these.

3   Keep safely any memos, emails or other instructions you receive that relate to either security or the confidentiality of information.

4   Decide which types of security and confidentiality issues, risks and actions apply to the option units you have chosen. As obvious examples, if you have chosen an IT unit, this will link to IT security risks/password procedures whereas the meetings unit links to confidentiality of information.

5   If you need to report any concerns about security or confidentiality, keep a record of the memo or email you sent and the result. If you make a verbal report, remember that you can ask for witness testimony to prove this.

What if...?

What should you do if you do not have any security concerns or worries about confidentiality during the time you are taking your award?

Your assessor can give you a dedicated task to cover the knowledge and understanding required. This will then be followed by a professional discussion during which you can explain how you would perform in such a situation and what evidence you might bring forward.

Assessing and managing risks

Taking risks is part of everyday life, although the type of risks – and the degree – differs from person to person. If you enjoy paragliding and bungee jumping then it is fair to say that you live life more dangerously than someone who spends their spare time listening to music or playing a Sony PS2. But how safe are those activities? Listening to loud music doesn't do your hearing any good, and one 15-year-old PS2 addict was diagnosed with hand–arm vibration syndrome after playing a driving game in vibration mode for up to seven hours a day. This is normally a

Find out

If you are a music fan then your hearing could be at risk. You can find out at www.dontlosethemusic.com/home, the microsite of the Royal National Institute for the Deaf (RNID) web campaign. If you like going to clubs or chilling out to loud CDs in your room then you might want to read it!

Remember

Further information on Health and Safety is contained in unit 110, on the CD-ROM that accompanies this book. It includes further guidance about risk assessments.

condition associated with miners and other users of heavy equipment. Other problems reported by computer gamers include joystick digit, mouse elbow and central palm blister.

So does this mean you should stop doing anything that might constitute a risk? Obviously not, or you would never travel anywhere, use a sharp knife or a pair of scissors, play any type of sport, eat food unless you had prepared and cooked it yourself – the list is endless! Quite simply you cannot eliminate risk from your life, or from anyone else's. Even a couch potato could be in danger of rolling over and falling off! What you can do is manage risk so that you reduce the chances of anyone being hurt or injured. Understanding how to do this is the aim of this section of the unit.

Sources of risk in the work that you do, including health and safety

The correct term for a source of risk is 'hazard', and a hazard is different to a risk:

- A **hazard** is anything that can cause harm – hot water, a sharp knife, a car, electricity, a flight of stairs.
- A **risk** is the chance, whether great or small, that someone will be harmed by the hazard.

The aim of identifying hazards, or sources of risk, is to decide the risk factor and whether this is high, medium or low. If it is high, then action must be taken to eliminate or minimise the risk to an acceptable level.

Specific risk assessments

Under Regulation 3 of the Management of Health and Safety at Work Regulations (see page 127), employers must carry out risk assessments on all types of work activity that may potentially cause harm or ill-health. There are five stages in a risk assessment. These are illustrated in the diagram.

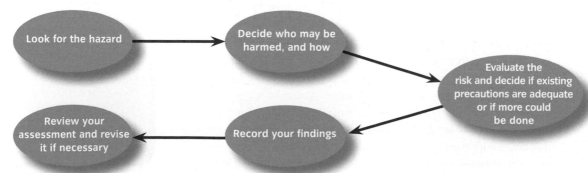

Look for the hazard → Decide who may be harmed, and how → Evaluate the risk and decide if existing precautions are adequate or if more could be done → Record your findings → Review your assessment and revise it if necessary

Additionally, specific risk assessments must also be carried out in the following areas:

- Under the **Fire Precautions (Workplace) Regulations**, all employers must carry out additional fire-risk assessments by identifying potential sources of ignition that could start a fire, identify who would be harmed and then evaluate existing fire precautions and check whether these could be improved.
- Under the **Health and Safety (First Aid) Regulations**, the employer must assess the risk level of the working environment when deciding on the level of facilities, equipment and staff to provide first aid.
- Under the **Health and Safety (Young Persons) Regulations**, special risk assessments must be carried out in respect of young or inexperienced workers. A separate set of regulations – the Health and Safety (Training for Employment) Regulations – also covers students or school pupils undertaking work experience in a company. Both of these groups are at increased risk and must receive proper training to minimise the risk.
- The risks to staff of using VDUs and workstations must be assessed under the **Display Screen Equipment Regulations** (see page 187).

Looking for hazards

The first step in carrying out a risk assessment is to look for hazards, but if you work on the basis that anything can be a hazard, you will end up with a very long list! So you need to be sensible. You should be noting only significant hazards. A useful way to start is shown in the 'How to...' box below.

Did you know?

Offices are usually classed as 'low risk', so a minimum of one first aider is required if there are between 50 and 100 employees. Above this number, an additional first aider is needed for every 100 workers. The situation would be different if the office was in a more dangerous environment, such as a chemical factory.

Find out

Find out the procedures that are in place in your organisation to make sure risk assessments are done regularly to comply with the law.

How to... Identify and agree possible sources of risk

- Identify whether you are carrying out a general risk assessment or one related to a specific area, such as display screen equipment or a young worker.

- Walk around your workplace and study the relevant areas to identify sources of risk.

- Check equipment manuals – particularly the safety notes and the 'troubleshooting' pages for information.

- Check the state of equipment that is used and how often it is maintained.

How to... Continued

Find out

Most accidents in an office are caused by slipping, tripping or falling. Find out whether any floors in your workplace are particularly slippery when they are wet. Check, too, when the cleaning takes place – ideally it should be done regularly but out of hours, warning signs put up if floors are wet and cleaners trained to use cleaning equipment and products safely.

- Check your accident book to find out the reasons for recent accidents.

- Talk to your colleagues and ask for their views and opinions. Find out, too, if anyone has had a 'near miss' accident recently and what caused it.

- Review your list and identify the hazards, or sources of risk, that may be significant.

- Agree your list with your tutor, trainer or supervisor.

Did you know?

Keeping keyboards clean can be very difficult. Eating biscuits, crisps or sandwiches at your desk contributes to bits of food between the keys. Now, instead of turning it upside down and giving it a shake, you can just give it a wash, if you persuade your boss you need the new Unotron SpillSeal keyboard. Find out more at www.unotron.com.

Did you know?

Age and gender are both relevant to risk. According to HSE statistics, even when job role and workplace differences are taken into account, men are 20 per cent more likely to be injured than women, and young men aged 16–24 face a 40 per cent higher risk of workplace injury than other men.

How to assess and monitor risk

For every hazard you have identified you need to assess whether the risk is high, medium, low or non-existent. This will depend on the following factors.

Who might be harmed?

The HSE lists the following groups as the most vulnerable:

- young workers, trainees, new and expectant mothers and others who may be at particular risk
- cleaners, visitors, contractors, maintenance workers and others who may not be in the workplace all the time
- members of the public or the people you work with, if they could be hurt by your activities.

How might they be harmed?

The next consideration is the type of injury that could occur. Paper can give a nasty cut but cannot result in a critical injury, such as could occur if someone fell down some steep slippery steps.

Other relevant factors

These can relate both to the people concerned and, in the case of your colleagues, to their job roles. Someone who often works alone in an office, especially at night, or regularly deals with strangers who walk in off the street, will be more at risk than someone who works in a communal area during the day and deals with callers only over the telephone. Similarly, everyone will be more at risk in a crowded, frenetic office with everyone trying to meet tight deadlines. In this situation many people may be tempted to take shortcuts, such as carrying too many files or forgetting to close a desk drawer.

The main factors you should consider in relation to yourself and your colleagues are identified below.

Factors which contribute to risk

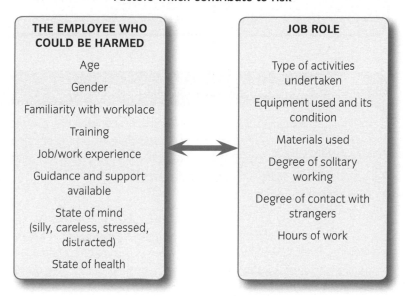

THE EMPLOYEE WHO COULD BE HARMED	JOB ROLE
Age	Type of activities undertaken
Gender	Equipment used and its condition
Familiarity with workplace	Materials used
Training	Degree of solitary working
Job/work experience	Degree of contact with strangers
Guidance and support available	Hours of work
State of mind (silly, careless, stressed, distracted)	
State of health	

Monitoring risk

Risk levels can change. A path or tiled floor may be perfectly safe on a sunny day but far different on an icy morning or when it is raining. A shelf is a zero-risk item until it suddenly becomes loose. There may be no risks from lifting because you have a useful little trolley for moving portable equipment, but things are different when it breaks.

You will also need to reassess the risks for a colleague who announces she is pregnant or if someone returns to work still recovering from an illness or injury. Monitoring risk means constantly staying alert to potential sources of risk and who could be harmed.

Remember

Stress and violence at work were all covered on pages 128–9. If you are regularly working in a hurry, or if you work for a business that regularly deals with irate members of the public then your risks are higher than if any or all of these factors are absent.

How to... Assess and confirm the level of risk

- For each significant hazard on your list, identify those people who might be harmed.

- Work through your list again, deciding how serious an injury could be.

How to... Continued

- Note down other relevant factors that could increase the level of risk at any time or to any particular groups of people.

- Consider how likely it is that someone will be harmed.

- Use your notes to decide whether the risk level is currently high, medium or low.

Snapshot – Room for improvement?

Just because an office looks beautiful does not mean that it is good to work in. According to international architects Gensler, poorly designed offices could be costing British businesses over £135 billion every year, because employees would be more productive in a better working environment.

The Gensler report, *These Four Walls: The Real British Office*, was based on answers from managers in the legal, financial services and media sectors. Fifty-eight per cent believed that their office had not been designed to support their company's business objectives or their own job function, and 19 per cent admitted to being embarrassed to take customers back to their office. Gensler argued that saving money by ignoring office design is a false economy because staff are demotivated and therefore far less effective at work.

If you struggle to work effectively because you are too hot, too cold, too cramped or are expected to spend hours every day in a tiny cubicle staring at a computer screen, download the full report from www.gensler.com/pdfs/WhitePaperSummary.pdf and leave a copy on your boss's desk!

Methods of minimising risk

Your aim now is to make all risks as low as possible. You can do this in two ways. You can get rid of the hazard completely, or minimise the risk as much as possible.

Getting rid of the hazard

This may be as simple as tidying up or rearranging the furniture. Or you may need the help of maintenance or specialist staff if, for example, the

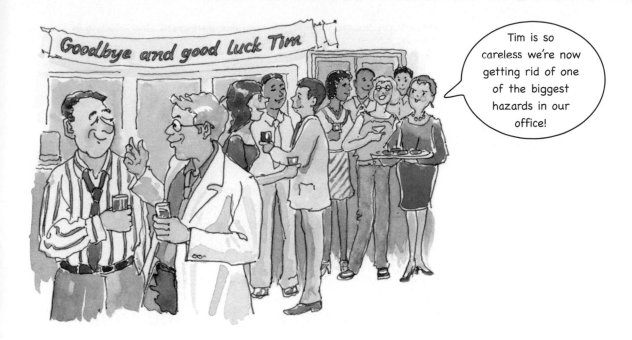

Tim is so careless we're now getting rid of one of the biggest hazards in our office!

water temperature is suddenly uncontrollable, a window has jammed or the wire connecting your VDU has started to crackle when it is moved.

Minimising the risk

This means assessing the current precautions to see if enough is being done.

- Start by checking whether the law is being broken. In this case action must be taken immediately.
- Next decide whether the hazard can be removed completely.
- If not, what other action can you take?
  - Is there a less risky option available?
  - Can access to the hazard be prevented, such as by a guard or other safety device?
  - Can work be reorganised to reduce the risk?
  - Can personal protective equipment reduce the risk?
  - Can better welfare facilities be provided?
  - Can special procedures be written and training given to staff who may be affected?

Managing risks

Assuming you have now minimised the identified risks as much as possible, can you truly claim that you are 'managing' risks? Not really – unless you keep a careful record of what you have done and review your assessment to take account of new risks.

Find out

Safety signs are used to warn people about risks that cannot be eliminated. Check the range available online at www.seton. co.uk.

If you are carrying out a formal risk assessment, then you will be given specific forms to complete. Otherwise you should still keep your own records to note down the following information:

- the date on which you made the assessment
- the items you checked and hazards you identified
- how you rated the risk at the time
- the action you took to eliminate or minimise the risk
- your conclusions that there is nothing else you can reasonably do and the remaining risk is low.

Review your records when significant changes take place – such as if you are asked to take on a new job (or someone else is) or if you work in a different location or when new equipment is purchased.

Routinely review your records from time to time to make sure that they are still up to date and effective.

The importance of learning from mistakes

If someone is injured from a risk you had identified as low or non-existent, you might then worry about your ability to do the job. You could then over-react and introduce so many precautions that you drive everyone insane!

You will be less likely to do this if you consult other people when you are assessing risks and if you remember that it is impossible to prevent every minor accident or injury that occurs. However, you also need to re-evaluate your approach to see whether your assessment could have been better or whether additional precautions are necessary if one does occur.

Remember

It is sensible to review your records if someone has an accident or is injured (or there is a 'near miss'), to check that this does not change your evaluation of any particular risk.

Did you know?

The Office Hours supplement in *The Guardian* carried the story of a global company that was so fixated with safety that it issued procedures on how staff should cope if they were attacked by a bear. It issued this worldwide – not just to offices in grizzly bear countries!

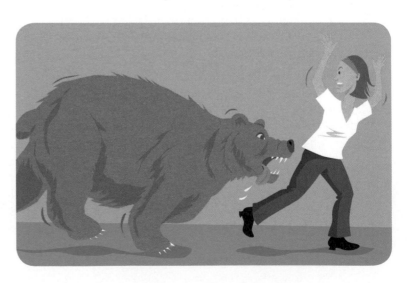

You also need to listen to feedback from your colleagues if they think that any precautions are too extreme. If your workplace is unionised, advice from your trade union safety rep will be invaluable if you are uncertain about a possible risk. Otherwise, there may be a staff or works committee responsible for safety that you can consult – or join. The point is to use any mistakes as a learning experience. The only time you should hang your head in shame is if you make exactly the same mistake again.

Find out

Some people argue that we must have lost our sense of proportion about risks if children are prevented from playing because they might be injured. The HSE started a debate on the topic in 2005 on its website at www.hse.gov.uk/riskdebate. The TUC, however, argued that taking a more casual approach was not appropriate in the workplace. Join the debate and see what you think.

Over to you

1 Your boss has read that 450 000 British workers now suffer from repetitive strain injury and 1.1 million suffered from a musculoskeletal disorder caused or worsened by work in 2004. As a result she wants you to reassess the risks to administrators in your office from using a computer.

   a Read the summary of the Health and Safety (Display Screen Equipment) Regulations below and find out more from the HSE by downloading and reading the booklet *Working with VDUs* from the HSE website at www.hse.gov.uk. You may also wish to consult unit 110 on the CD-ROM for further ideas. Then list the main points you would look for in your assessment.

Main aspects of the Health and Safety (Display Screen Equipment) Regulations 1992 (as amended)

These regulations relate to the use of VDUs and the design of workstations.

A workstation relates to all the equipment, furniture and work environment of the person using the computer; i.e. their desk, screen, keyboard, printer, chair, work surface, lighting, temperature, noise levels and space.

Employers must:

- Ensure all the workstations meet the minimum requirement as set out in the regulations (see below).
- Analyse workstations to reduce risks by examining the workstation and equipment and also the job being done and the special needs of individual staff. Employees and safety representatives should be encouraged to report any health problems. The employer must then take steps to reduce identified risks.
- Plan work so that there are frequent breaks or changes in activity. It is better if the user can choose when to take a break, but this is not a specific requirement.
- Arrange and pay for eye tests, on request, and provide special spectacles if the test shows these are needed.

Over to you Continued

- Provide users with relevant health and safety training and information.

Workstations must conform to specific standards:

- **Display screens** must have clear characters of adequate size, a stable image, adjustable brightness and contrast, be tiltable and swivel easily. There must be no reflective glare.

- **Keyboards** must be tiltable and separate from the screen with sufficient space in front to provide a 'rest' space. There should be a matt surface, the keyboard should be easy to use and the symbols must be clear on the keys.

- **Work surfaces** must be large enough to accommodate the work being done and must have a low reflective finish. It should be possible for users to rearrange the equipment to suit their individual needs.

- **Work chairs** must be stable and allow easy movement and a comfortable position. The seat height and back must be adjustable and there must be good back support. A footrest must be provided if requested.

- **Working environments** should have satisfactory lighting with minimal glare. Windows should have blinds or workstations be positioned to avoid reflections. Noise and heat levels should be comfortable. Radiation levels must be negligible and humidity controlled to a satisfactory level.

- **Software and systems** must be appropriate for the task, user-friendly and appropriate to the level of knowledge of the user.

b Obtain a copy of the HSE book *The Law on VDUs – An Easy Guide. Making sure your office complies with the Health and Safety (Display Screen Equipment) Regulations 1992 (as amended in 2002)* either from your college or local library. Alternatively your tutor, trainer or workplace safety officer may have a copy. Use the VDU workstation checklist it contains to assess your own workstation and the position of your VDU, chair and papers to see whether the arrangement can be improved. Make a note of your findings.

c Two of your younger colleagues ignore your constant reminders to sit properly, exercise their wrists and take regular breaks. They accuse you of nagging. Suggest how you could overcome this type of resistance.

2 A young student from a nearby school is coming into your office on two weeks' work placement.

a You want her to carry out some filing, photocopying and computer work as well as helping to reorganise the stationery cupboard. Identify the sources of risk to her that would exist in your own workplace and decide whether each one is high, medium or low. For each 'high' or 'medium' risk you identify, suggest how this could be eliminated or minimised.

b When she arrives on the first day she is wearing a short tight skirt, very high heels and long dangling earrings. As she totters towards reception you realise you made the mistake of not considering the girl herself and her personal preferences. Suggest how you would note, and minimise, this risk to prevent a recurrence.

3 The TUC issues a weekly online bulletin for safety reps and others called *Risks*. You can register to receive this by following the links on the TUC site at www.tuc.org.uk.

Evidence planning

Although you will be obtaining your evidence for this section through your option units, it is sensible to plan for this now in the following ways:

- Identify the sources of risk in the work that you do and areas of your work where it is appropriate or required to assess and manage risk.

- Decide which of your chosen option units relate to these areas. Remember that if you are involved with other areas of health and safety or if you have already completed unit 110, then you should discuss with your tutor or trainer any evidence you already have that may be cross-referenced to this unit.

- Keep records of all risk assessments you undertake, either for yourself or involving the work of others. Make sure these include information on how you assessed and confirmed the level of risk and the action you took to minimise this.

- Prepare brief notes that explain how you monitor risks, are alert to new risks and manage these when they occur. In particular, include any occasions when you reviewed your assessments for any reason. You can then use these notes as the basis of a professional discussion with your assessor.

Key skills reminder

If you are taking Key Skills awards, remember to discuss with your tutor or trainer how your evidence for this unit could also count towards those awards.

Supervise an office facility

Unit summary and overview

This option unit covers the activities required to provide, maintain and organise office equipment, resources and facilities to meet the needs of users. This is suitable for you if you are responsible for organising these aspects of an office – whether this is the sole office in a small firm or a departmental office in a large organisation. In both cases the smooth functioning of the office is essential to the efficient operation of the business.

The unit focuses on the provision and maintenance of office equipment, arranging for sufficient office resources and monitoring the use of office facilities.

The difficulty for administrators can be in efficiently and effectively carrying out day-to-day, routine operations while calmly coping with the variety of different demands from users. Good organisational and people skills are vital, as well as understanding the value of appropriate office systems and procedures, and having the ability to solve problems and agree priorities with users. Information on all these aspects of supervising an office facility is included in this unit.

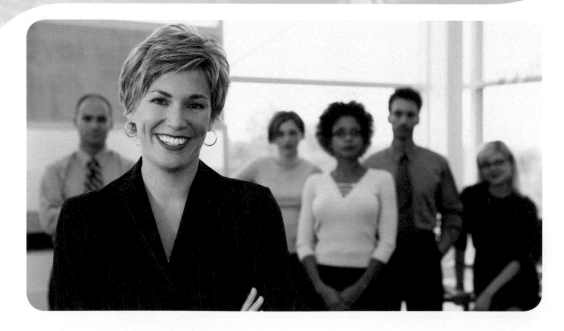

The importance of providing and maintaining an effective and efficient office facility

The role of an office facility is to provide support to its users. The users will usually include the managers of the organisation, any technical and/or sales staff and professional specialists as well as other people who come into contact with the organisation – such as customers and contractors.

For an office to be truly supportive it must be run efficiently and operated effectively. This has the following benefits:

- Managers are free to concentrate on managing the enterprise and staff without having to concern themselves about routine office maintenance issues and supplies. They also know that policies, systems and procedures that have been laid down are followed and regularly monitored.
- Other users can focus on their own job roles without worrying about whether equipment will be working or resources will be available. They can rely on administrative tasks being carried out promptly and efficiently to a high standard. They also know that they will be kept informed of proposed changes that will directly affect them.
- A professional image is given to everyone who comes into contact with the organisation – callers, visitors, customers or clients, contractors, delivery people and other business contacts. All are treated courteously and professionally and their needs are dealt with promptly and appropriately.
- Because the office runs smoothly and standards are high there are fewer mistakes, problems or misunderstandings to resolve.
- The costs of running the office are lower, because facilities, equipment and resources are well maintained and used effectively.

Range of office facilities, equipment and resources

Certain standard items are essential in all offices – such as desks, chairs, computers and photocopiers. Other facilities may be provided depending on the type of building, its design and layout and the size of the business. A large organisation may have a gatehouse or concierge, car park and staff dining room. A small firm may have a kitchen area and perhaps a staff 'rest room'. There may also be additional

Links to core units

As you gather your evidence for this unit you should also obtain evidence for your core units. Watch for the CU link logo which suggests how the evidence you may collect could count towards both this unit and your core units.

Remember that you might be able to identify other links yourself, because of your own job role and the evidence you have obtained.

Talk to your assessor if you need further guidance on how your evidence should be cross-referenced.

Special note

If you are unsure what, exactly, is meant by an office 'facility' and whether your role covers the types of task needed to obtain evidence for this unit, you may find it helpful to read the case study on page 216 and the changing places feature on pages 218–20 first. These give examples of the types of administrative job that relate to this unit and may help you to better understand what is required. If you still have concerns after reading these, discuss the matter with your tutor, trainer or assessor.

Did you know?

Efficiency relates to being productive and working quickly and cost-effectively. **Effectiveness** means doing high-quality work and prioritising correctly. Ideally you can do both!

facilities linked to the type of business, such as access to an electronic legal database in a law firm or large display boards to hold property advertisements in an estate agency. The table below includes many of the facilities, equipment and resources commonly found in offices today.

Did you know?

The term **facility** usually refers to a building or area – or services within a building – that are provided for a specific purpose, such as a lift or meeting room. However, other people may use the term more generally to refer to office services, such as carrying out photocopying, processing mail or taking messages for office users (e.g. 'Do you have the facility to do colour copying here?').

Standard office items	Additional items and facilities
Office furniture: desks/chairs/ filing cabinets etc. Reception area or reception desk Telephone system Answering machine/voicemail Computer network Computer software and email Computer workstations/VDUs Laptops Photocopier(s)/scanner(s)/ printer(s) Fax machine(s) Shredder(s) Laminators Binding machines Mailing equipment Stationery store with range of small equipment (calculators, staplers etc.) and stationery Audio equipment Mobile telephones	Kitchen area with microwave, fridge, jug kettle etc. Vending machine Water cooler Air conditioning Central heating Outside areas and car park Burglar alarm Meeting rooms Video conferencing Changing rooms and shower facilities Lockers
	Specialist items
	Facilities, equipment or resources specific to industry or sector; e.g. electronic whiteboards, OHPs, data projectors, flipcharts and textbooks in an educational establishment

You cannot supervise an office facility properly unless you know the range of facilities, equipment and resources for which you are responsible. The last thing you want is suddenly to find that it is your job to replace the portable television in the staff rest room when you had no idea that it had anything to do with you!

● **Monitoring facilities** can mean anything from spotting that a sink is blocked and arranging for a plumber to call, to checking that the reception area is tidy before some visitors arrive. In terms of office services, it means ensuring that quality and deadline targets are met.

● **Providing and maintaining office equipment** means checking that equipment is regularly serviced, arranging for it to be repaired when required and obtaining quotes for replacement or new items when necessary.

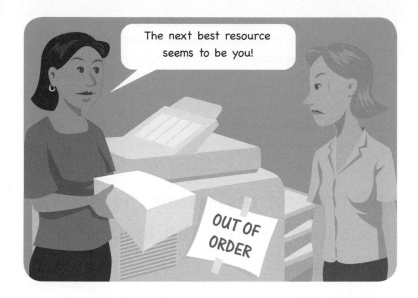

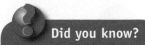

Did you know?

The term **resource** can be applied to anything or anyone that helps you or your colleagues to do or achieve something, from an item of equipment or member of staff to a flip chart or highlighter pen!

- **Arranging for resources** can include scheduling or allocating shared resources so that everyone is treated fairly or according to need, ordering small items of equipment and stationery, and arranging cash advances to staff travelling on business.

The use of facilities, equipment and resources

In addition to knowing the range of items for which you are responsible, you also need to know – or find out – why each item is used. Some will be common sense – it is quite obvious why the photocopier and the telephone system are needed. Others may be more difficult to establish, such as the small room at the top of the stairs that has three old filing cabinets in it, or the mysterious black box at the back of the IT storeroom!

If you cannot find out why something is used, then check whether it *is* used. Ways in which you can do this are given in the next section. You then need to check frequency of use. There is a huge difference between an item of equipment or a resource that is required once or twice a year and one that is used every day.

- **Facilities.** Some facilities may be very popular with everyone, others may be virtually ignored by some staff because of individual preferences. In most organisations, car parking facilities are usually in the greatest demand, which is why a reserved place is usually seen as a perk.
- **Equipment.** The potential use should be taken into account when equipment is being purchased, so that the model that is bought can cope with the demands that will be made on it. Otherwise

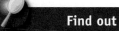

Find out

List the facilities, equipment and resources for which you think you are responsible and then agree this list with your line manager or supervisor. For each relevant item you should also know the name of the supplier and the cost.

you can expect more breakdowns and higher servicing and maintenance costs. Usage should also influence the type of service or maintenance contract that is agreed for expensive items.

- **Resources.** The minimum amount of stock assigned to consumable items should be based on frequency of use and the amount of time needed to obtain replacement stock. This means that there is always a 'buffer' stock available. If average usage increases then the minimum stock levels will need to be reviewed.

Identifying and reviewing the needs of office users – and the methods you can use

The needs of users determine the types of facility, equipment and resource that are required. An office with many visitors needs a reception area, one that deals only with callers on the telephone does not; but if sales or technical staff come into the office when they are not visiting clients there needs to be somewhere for them to work. Similarly, although some resources are commonly found in all offices – from staplers to calculators – others often relate to the type of work being undertaken by the organisation.

The needs of users will also influence the features that are required when new equipment is purchased, the type of resources that are stocked and the way in which supplies are issued. In a small firm where you are supplying a small team of staff there may be few formal systems in place and items may be available virtually on demand. This is both impractical and unwise in a large department and if you are supplying other users – such as casual workers or external contacts. Apart from anything else, you will need proper records of amounts you have spent and the items you have issued to satisfy your finance department and your auditors.

Changing needs of users

There are several reasons why the needs of users may change:
- **Technological developments** may mean that equipment is outdated and no longer serves its purpose, and new applications can result in different ways of working – such as sending documents by fax or email.
- **Work demands may increase** so that additional facilities or resources are required. If work levels fall then this may mean some existing facilities, equipment or resources are no longer needed.

- **New tasks and activities** may be undertaken for which there are currently no appropriate resources, equipment or facilities available.
- **Legal requirements, risk assessments or changes to office systems** and procedures may mean a review of current facilities or resources is required.

All users will normally welcome a change that is an obvious improvement. If an old copier is being replaced with a state-of-the-art digital model that produces better copies much faster than the old one then everyone will be pleased. However, it is not always possible to meet the changing needs of all users. There may not be sufficient money available to upgrade or replace equipment or purchase some types of resources. In this situation, the more information you have obtained the better. This is because you can support the final decision with facts and cannot be accused of deliberately ignoring the needs of some users.

First, of course, you need to obtain your information and there are several ways of doing this.

Asking people

This can be done formally or informally, individually or collectively.

Doing it formally means communicating in writing so that you have a record. You could issue a questionnaire or send an email to find out users' views. Informally means chatting to people in the office. Both methods have their advantages and disadvantages. If you communicate in writing then you have proof of what people said, which is useful if you are going to need to defend a decision. However, no one wants to be drowned in questionnaires or emails, so use this method sparingly. Talking to people should be part of an ongoing information gathering strategy anyway, so that you stay in touch with what your users think and want on a routine basis.

Rather than talk to people individually you can save time by talking to them as a group, such as during a team meeting, if there is an issue that you want to raise with several people at once. This is useful because it enables you to establish the majority view more easily.

Observation

Being observant will tell you a lot. If there is a queue at the photocopier and the water cooler every morning then, unless everyone is just standing around gossiping, you can be fairly certain that these items are well-used. Conversely, if the notices on the staff noticeboard are all over three months old because everyone now prefers to use email you can be fairly certain that this resource is no longer needed.

Remember

If you know the main users of an item then you will know who will be most affected if there is a problem and who to consult if you want to make a change.

Remember

Talking to users helps you to understand how they think and feel. You will also learn to differentiate between those who don't want to trouble you, even when something is important, and those who will always want more no matter what you do.

Remember

If usage of a resource increases, remember to differentiate between occasional or seasonal reasons and long-term trends.

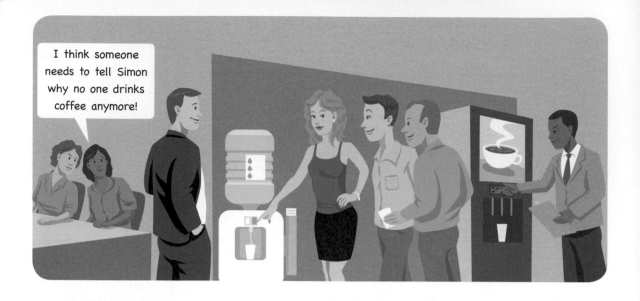

Find out

Many photocopiers have personal identity numbers (PINs) for different users or departments. This helps to monitor usage and check whether this is within target levels. Find out if this is the case in your workplace.

Record and monitor complaints by users

This enables you to check whether a problem is a 'one-off', is widespread or is the pet hate of one person who keeps telling you about it!

Check the records

These should tell you whether an item of equipment is breaking down more often or needing more frequent servicing; and whether a particular resource is required more. They should enable you to check whether concerns and complaints by users are justified.

How to... Identify, agree and maintain office facilities

- List the facilities, equipment and resources in your office.

- For each item on your list, check that you are clear about why it is used and who the users are.

- For all relevant items, check that you know the name of the supplier and the cost of the item.

- Check that you are aware of which items are routinely serviced or maintained, by whom and how frequently.

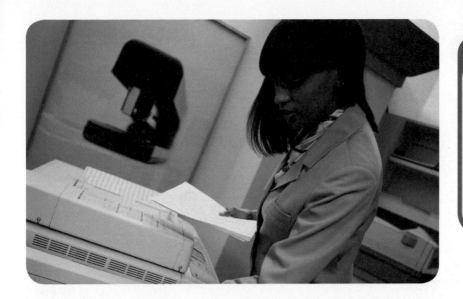

Did you know?

Parkinson's law states that work expands to fit the time available. Some people claim it can also apply to photocopiers! No matter how much a firm upgrades to bigger, flashier models, within a matter of weeks people are using the new one to maximum capacity!

How to... Continued

● Agree with your supervisor or line manager the items on the list that are your responsibility.

● For each item of equipment on your list, note who you should contact if it brakes down.

Why office systems and procedures are important

You first read about office systems and procedures in unit 302. If you have forgotten about these, turn back to page 113 and refresh your memory.

● **Systems** will help you to supervise an office facility because they will help you to obtain a specific and consistent result.

● **Procedures** will provide a list of (usually) step-by-step guidelines for all users to obtain that result.

Both are invaluable for coordinating the use of office resources between a number of users, for three main reasons. First, they ensure that everyone knows what to do to obtain a particular resource. Second, the system is then fair – and seen to be fair – because all users are treated in the same way. If there are any differences this will be on specific stated grounds. Therefore, your boss may be able to take a laptop abroad because it is necessary in her job, but you could not do the same thing because you wanted to take one on holiday! However, what no one can do is to pick and choose what individual users can or cannot have just on a whim. Third, if there are any problems then 'what happens next' will be covered by the procedures (see below). This can save a lot of arguments.

Office systems and procedures that are appropriate to your responsibilities

If you work in a departmental office in a large organisation, particularly in the public sector, then there are likely to be specific systems and procedures in place that cover many aspects of your work to ensure that all departments (and users) do the same thing. In a small firm, particularly in the private sector, there may be very few official systems or procedures to follow. However, you may find it useful to devise some of your own from the list below!

Typical office systems and procedures

- **Purchasing equipment and consumables** – such as the type of items that can be routinely replaced and those that cannot; the completion of official purchase orders and who can sign these; the limits on expenditure; whether specific suppliers must be used.

- **Damage, loss and equipment breakdowns** – such as how these must be reported; the action that must be taken; the forms to be completed; the replacement policies.

- **Taking valuable items off the premises** – such as who is allowed to do this; whether permission is required (and from whom); the forms that must be completed for insurance purposes; the length of time/ distance the item can be taken.

- **Allocating and coordinating the use of resources** – such as booking rooms or specific types of equipment; how this is done; the amount of notice that is required; what happens if there is a clash or a problem.

- **Monitoring and checking usage of equipment or resources** – such as inspecting facilities or equipment to check the condition; checking actual usage records against predicted use; monitoring requests for particular items.

- **Stock control** – such as the method staff must use to order stationery items from internal stores; how these are booked out; the minimum and maximum amounts kept in stock; how deliveries are checked and booked in; how often stock checks are carried out.

- **Mail processing** – such as the maintenance and use of mailroom equipment; times by which outgoing mail must be received; policy on use of first-class postage and so on.

- **Security issues** – such as the storage of valuable equipment and resources; access to confidential information; number of keys and named keyholders; the storage of key backup computer data off the premises; visitor procedures etc.

- **Carrying out risk assessments** (see page 179).

Identifying systems and procedures appropriate to your responsibilities

Your first step is to identify the relevant systems and procedures that exist in your own organisation. One way is to think about the type of questions asked by a new member of staff, and decide how easily you could answer these. Here are some examples:

- How can I get a car parking permit?
- How can I book a data projector?
- How does the photocopying system work?
- What do I do if my computer develops a fault?
- How do I book a meeting room and order refreshments?
- What must I do to get some printer paper, and can I have as much as I want?
- What do I do if I want to buy some special presentation folders?
- I've lost my office key. What do I do now?

You could probably add at least another ten questions to this list! Although your users will rarely use the terms 'systems' and 'procedures', in all these cases you could easily substitute these words: 'What's the system for...?' or 'What are the procedures for doing...?'

Remember

Procedures should be kept as simple as possible to achieve their objective. If you make them over-complicated or elaborate users will invent their own shortcuts to save time.

Remember

You can always tell when there is no proper system or that users don't understand it because you will be asked the same questions over and over again! In this case you might want to talk to your line manager about devising one.

Find out

Find out the systems and procedures that apply to your own responsibilities and check that you know where any reference documents are located.

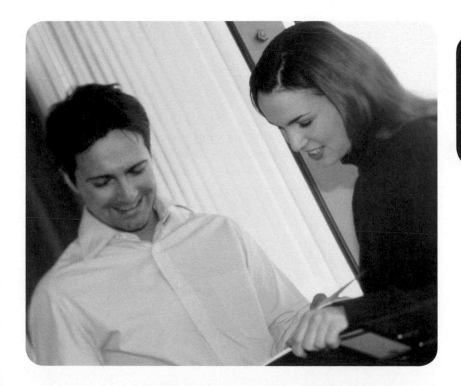

Communicating office systems and procedures and providing users with information, guidance and support

You cannot expect users to follow systems and procedures if they don't know they exist. Therefore, for every system or procedure that your users need to know, the first step is to make sure you communicate it. How you do this, and the type of information, guidance or support you provide, will depend on the system or procedure, its complexity and the particular types of users who need it.

Ideally, your existing systems and procedures already answer all the questions you are routinely asked and new members of staff are told about these at induction. However, you also need to remember the needs of other users, such as:

- existing staff who are not certain (or cannot remember) how some systems operate because they use them infrequently
- staff from other departments, if you have your own departmental systems and procedures in a large organisation
- people who frequently work off the premises, such as representatives or technical staff
- external contacts, such as your suppliers, who may enquire about your ordering or payment procedures and customers, who may be affected if there is a problem or delay
- all your users, if there is an unexpected problem or disruption that affects them.

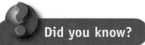

Did you know?

There are several ways of providing information, guidance and support. Your task is to select the most appropriate method for the procedures and your particular users.

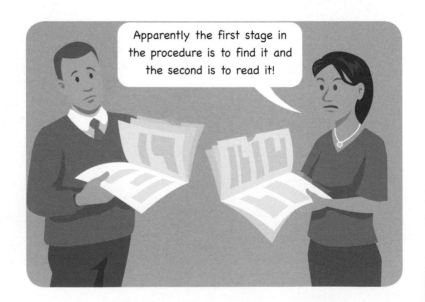

Providing users with information, guidance and support

User support needs to be appropriate for both the person and the procedures. No one wants to attend a training day to find out how to refill a paper tray, but neither is it realistic to expect people to read ten pages of information before they can fill in a form! The following are the most usual methods that may be used together with their advantages and disadvantages.

Remember

Users will always be more keen to follow a procedure if you spell out the benefits for them, not just for you!

Methods of communicating systems and procedures		
Method	**Advantages**	**Disadvantages**
Email	Useful to give basic information about new/updated procedures	May be ignored or not understood
Answering questions/ discussions	Provides quick clarification of queries	Answers may be forgotten. Continual interruptions are disturbing
Printed sheet	Useful to give basic information on simple or updated procedure	Easily lost or forgotten by casual users
Printed notice	Useful near office equipment and unsupervised areas; e.g. stationery or equipment store to say basic procedure and whom to contact if the user has an urgent request	Can be overdone. Too many notices are impersonal, untidy and give the impression of being dictatorial
User handbook	Can be kept with relevant equipment	Can soon become tatty or go missing – and be difficult to replace
Procedure documents and manuals	Ensures that related, complex procedures are stored safely	Too bulky/expensive for casual users to have own copy
Company Intranet	Ideal for holding information support pages on a variety of subjects	May not be available remotely to staff working off the premises
Demonstration	Ideal for showing how to do a particular task. Users remember what to do if given chance to practise	Only appropriate if the demonstrator is an expert at the task, otherwise bad habits are passed on
Training session	Enables complex procedures to be communicated properly and questions to be asked answered	Must be well organised and be the right length to retain interest

How to... Implement, communicate and review office systems and procedures

- Identify the system or procedure that you want to implement.

- Check that you are clear about the outcome you want to achieve.

- List the benefits to be gained by users – i.e. how their needs will be met.

- Check that the procedures you want users to follow are appropriate, easy to understand and achieve the desired outcome. If you have any doubts, test them on two or three users first, then take account of their feedback and revise them if necessary.

- Decide the best method to communicate the system or procedure to users, bearing in mind the type of users and their needs and the complexity of the system or procedure.

- Monitor its success by checking whether the system or procedure is being followed. If you are still answering lots of questions or users are complaining about problems or asking you continually for more information or for support, then you need to review either the type of information you provided, the way you provided it or the system or procedure itself.

- Stay alert to signs that a system or procedure should be reviewed, such as changing user needs, changing technology, changing activities or increased questions or complaints.

Snapshot – Virtually an office!

A relatively new venture in many towns and cities are business centres that provide a wide range of office services and facilities for their clients. They are ideal for anyone who is working away from home and needs office support services, or for business people who work from home but want an office address and meeting room facilities when they are having discussions with a client. These 'virtual offices', as they are called, also provide a wide range of administrative services as well as personalised telephone answering, voicemail and Internet access.

Sharing office space and facilities between multiple users is not restricted to business centres. Many businesses have reduced their need for additional, costly space as the organisation expanded by reviewing how their office space is used. Many so-called office staff often spend considerable periods of time away from the organisation – at meetings, visiting customers, at conferences or because they frequently work from home. This led to the concept of hot desking when a desk or workstation is used by more than one member of staff. In some firms, users have to follow certain procedures to pre-book the area and facilities required; in others they simply turn up with their laptop and mobile phone.

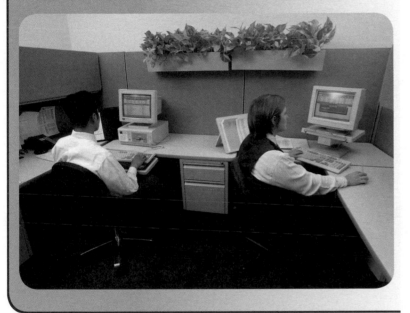

 Over to you

1 You are being interviewed for a job in a business centre in your area. As part of the preparation, find out more about the facilities, equipment and services available in virtual offices. You could try these links: www.bluesquareoffices.com, www.ukincorp.co.uk/s-1I-virtual-office-service.html and www.watfordoffice.co.uk/watford-office-facilities.htm. Use this information to suggest:

a four types of facilities you are likely to find in such a centre

b four types of equipment they will contain

c two examples of procedures that casual users will have to follow

Over to you Continued

> **d** two ways in which information and guidance may be given to new users.
>
> Check your ideas with your tutor or trainer or with the answers on the CD-ROM.
>
> **2** Your boss is considering including a slot in the induction programme for new staff to include a brief presentation of the main systems and procedures they will have to use in relation to office facilities, equipment and resources. He is also wondering whether a short staff handbook would also be useful.
>
> **a** For your own organisation, identify the systems and procedures you would want to include in your presentation.
>
> **b** For the systems and procedures you have identified, state how this information is normally communicated to users.
>
> **c** For any one system or procedure, identify other ways in which users are given support.
>
> Check your ideas with your tutor or trainer.

Core unit links

If you communicate information to your users and receive their comments and feedback, then this may link to unit 301, performance indicators 1–7. If you use this feedback to improve your own performance, then this may link to unit 301, PIs 16 and 17.

Setting high standards for your work, adapting readily to change (in this case the changing needs of your users) and behaving generally in a way that supports effective working may link to unit 301 PIs 22–28.

Working to achieve your organisation's purpose and following the systems and procedures relevant to your job may link to unit 302, PIs 1 and 2.

Evidence collection

1 Prepare a list of the office facilities, equipment and resources for which you are responsible. Against each item state why the item is used and the main needs of the users.

2 Write an account stating how you coordinate the use of office resources in your organisation. Include any systems and procedures that help you to do this. You do not need to include copies of these documents provided that you identify where they are located. Ask your line manager to countersign and date your account to confirm it is correct.

3 a Carry out a survey of your own users to check that they are satisfied with the information, guidance and support they currently receive. Check, too, that their needs are still being met. Do this by drawing up a brief questionnaire and issuing it to your users; then analyse their responses.

   b Produce an action plan to resolve any shortcomings that emerge.

Use both documents as the basis of a professional discussion with your assessor.

Building relationships with suppliers

Your 'suppliers' may include all the following groups of people:

- suppliers of office equipment and related maintenance services
- suppliers of consumable items
- contractors who are responsible for building repairs and maintenance – from a central heating contractor to the local glazier
- firms that provide other types of support and maintenance, such as for the burglar alarm or IT system.

Depending on where you are employed and your own job role, you may have some flexibility about choosing your suppliers. In other organisations you may be expected to use specific suppliers on an approved list, or you might have to submit all requests to a purchasing department for approval.

No matter which system you use, you should be aware that suppliers are only human – especially when you are dealing with a local service engineer or plumber rather than an online stationery store. A traditional rule about building up and maintaining relationships with a supplier is to find one who is trustworthy and then use that one time and again. The supplier will then be far more eager to help you if you have a problem than if you are a 'one off' customer.

However, this does depend on what you are buying. The more specialist your requirements, the more important it is that you have a good relationship with a supplier. So this can be crucial if you are ringing for

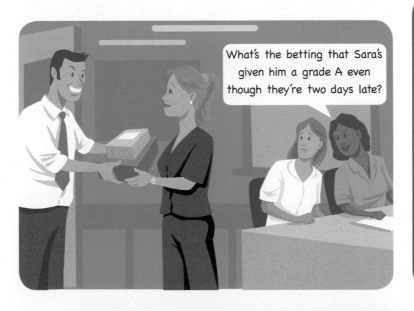

What's the betting that Sara's given him a grade A even though they're two days late?

Did you know?

One way of choosing suppliers is to grade them as follows:

A = trusted – quality and delivery excellent; competitive prices.

B = usually good service; may be rather pricey or sometimes deliver slightly late.

C = unreliable delivery; quality variable.

You would contact B and C suppliers only when A-grade suppliers cannot provide the goods.

IT support because your system has crashed but is far less important if you want a packet of paper or envelopes!

No matter who is your supplier, if you gain a reputation for panicking unnecessarily, expecting everyone to do your bidding immediately, being rude and abrupt to people or paying bills late then you can expect to be at the bottom of your supplier's list for attention in the future.

Key points to remember in your dealings with suppliers are given in the table below.

Dealing with suppliers		
Purchases of facilities and equipment	**Repairs to facilities and equipment**	**Resources**
Research the item required to identify the most appropriate features and facilities required for the users	Take care of equipment by following all recommended procedures and having it serviced regularly	Store items appropriately and securely
Agree the budget available and amount that can be spent	Make basic checks, if there is a problem or damage, before requesting assistance	Have a system for booking out resources to prevent problems and crises
Obtain quotes or discuss requirements with two or three known suppliers	Don't try to carry out 'home repairs' to equipment	Allow sufficient time for items to be replenished
Compare offers and accept 'best value' for price, features and delivery	Have a contingency plan in place in case the problem is serious	Submit official orders with all information accurately and clearly included
Submit official order with appropriate information accurately and clearly included	Report the problem accurately and concisely	Check items on delivery
Pay bill promptly	Accept there may be a short delay before a repair can be undertaken	Report accidental over-supply as well as under-supply!
	Be courteous to all supplier staff visiting the premises	Pay bill promptly
	Pay bill promptly	

How to... Make sure office equipment is serviceable

- Check that all equipment is sited and/or stored according to recommendations in the handbook.

- Check the recommended maintenance/servicing requirements. If these are part of a service contract, put the dates in your diary to remind you to check they are carried out.

- Read the instruction booklet – particularly the troubleshooting section – so that you know what to do if a problem occurs.

- Have procedures in place to ensure the equipment is used only for its intended purpose.

- Routinely check the condition of equipment for which you are responsible and note any problems.

- Carry out routine cleaning and maintenance operations yourself, as detailed in the user handbook. Alternatively, train users how to do this correctly.

- Make sure there is a proper procedure for all users to report promptly any problems they experience. They must never try to carry out repairs themselves unless they are qualified to do so.

- Devise a contingency plan that will enable you, so far as possible, to remain operational even if an important item of equipment is out of action for a short time.

Health, safety and security in the office environment

If you have already studied core unit 302, you will have learned about the importance of security in the workplace, and how this is achieved. You will also have found out how to assess and manage risk. If you have forgotten about these topics, refresh your memory by turning back to pages 170 and 179.

Security is vital to protect the people who work in the organisation as well as the information and the property that is kept there. Organisations have a duty of care to their employees to protect them from harm and must also comply with the requirements of the Health and Safety at Work etc. Act (see page 126) and other regulations that apply to the workplace.

Main health, safety and security requirements in an office environment

The health and safety requirements that apply to an office facility are covered by several regulations. The list below gives a summary of the main ones that you should know, given your responsibilities.

Health and Safety Regulations relevant to most workplaces

- **Control of Substances Hazardous to Health Regulations (COSHH).** All hazardous substances (such as toxic cleaning fluids) must be clearly labelled and stored in a special environment and users provided with protective clothing.
- **Electricity at Work Regulations.** These govern the design, construction, use and maintenance of electrical systems.
- **Employers' Liability (Compulsory Insurance) Regulations.** All limited companies must take out insurance so employees who are injured at work can claim compensation.
- **Fire Precautions Act and Regulations.** All business premises must possess a fire certificate and have suitable fire precautions – such as fire-resistant doors, fire extinguishers, break-glass alarms, a fire alarm system and a protected means of escape.
- **Health and Safety (First Aid) Regulations.** All organisations must provide adequate and appropriate first-aid equipment and facilities and trained first-aiders. The number of first-aiders must be appropriate to the risks in the workplace.
- **Health and Safety (Safety Sign and Signals) Regulations.** Safety signs must be displayed to identify risks and hazards that cannot be eliminated and written instructions must be provided on how to use fire-fighting equipment.
- **Manual Handling Operations Regulations.** These govern the way items should be lifted and handled. Preferably an automated process must be used, but if items are moved manually employees must be trained properly to minimise injury. This means not trying to lift too heavy weights and bending their knees to take the strain and keeping their back straight.
- **Noise at Work Regulations.** These require employers to check noise hazards and reduce these where possible and provide ear protectors if necessary.
- **Personal Protective Equipment at Work Regulations.** Protective clothing and equipment must be provided when risks cannot be eliminated. They must be free of charge, fit properly and be kept in good condition.
- **Provision and Use of Work Equipment Regulations (PUWER).** These relate to the maintenance and safety of all work equipment. Employers must make regular checks and inspections and provide appropriate training and instructions for users.
- **Reporting of Injuries, Diseases and Dangerous Occurrences Regulations (RIDDOR).** All organisations must notify the Health and Safety Executive (HSE) of any serious or fatal injuries and keep records of certain specific injuries, dangerous occurrences and diseases.

The security requirements that are important to an office environment were covered in core unit 302, on pages 170–79.

How to... Review the office environment in line with the health, safety and security policy

- Obtain a copy of your organisation's health, safety and security policy and check how this links to your own responsibilities.
- Carry out regular risk assessments which include checking:
  - that all equipment is sited safely and in accordance with manufacturers' instructions
  - that there are no trailing leads
  - that there are no signs of wear or damage to the premises, to other facilities or to equipment that could create a hazard
  - that stock and/or consumables are safely sited and stored
  - that all stock and other items are lifted, moved and transported safely
  - that hazardous items are stored in accordance with the requirements of COSHH
  - that those who operate equipment or undertake routine maintenance have undertaken appropriate training
  - that there is sufficient PPE (personal protective equipment) for those who need it.
- Carry out a separate risk assessment for every new item of equipment that is purchased or when other changes are made to the office facility.
- Routinely review security in terms of:
  - entrances and exits to the building
  - the storage and protection of valuable equipment, stock and resources
  - visitor access to the building and staff areas
  - information handling and the storage of confidential information
  - IT security procedures
  - staff leavers – to check they have returned office keys and no longer have access to the IT system.

Remember

Two other important regulations are the Management of Health and Safety at Work Regulations 1999 and the Health and Safety (Display Screen Equipment) Regulations 1992. You can find information on these in unit 302 on pages 127 and 187–8.

Dealing with problems that arise when supervising an office facility

Types of problem

These can be divided into three groups:

- supplier problems
- user problems
- damage, breakdowns and crises!

Supplier problems

If you have developed a good relationship with a supplier then these will usually be minimised. At the very least, if a problem is unavoidable, your supplier will tell you in advance and suggest alternatives. Problems can include:

- late delivery of goods you have ordered
- faulty goods being delivered
- the wrong goods being delivered
- poor or shoddy work by a supplier
- no one turning up to do the work as agreed
- the account for the work (or supplies) bearing very little relation to the quote you received.

User problems

If your communications with your users are good and if there are systems and procedures to control what they can and cannot do, then you are likely to prevent many of these problems. They can include:

- incorrect use of equipment – which breaks or damages it
- trying to correct problems – and making matters worse
- forgetting to book or order items in advance
- not following the correct procedure
- causing an injury to themselves or others
- having requirements that conflict with those of other users.

Damage, breakdowns and crises

Good maintenance procedures will minimise these types of problem, but that does not mean you can allow for every eventuality. And you can be sure that the most crucial item of equipment will always chose your busiest day on which to break down completely! So your problems may include:

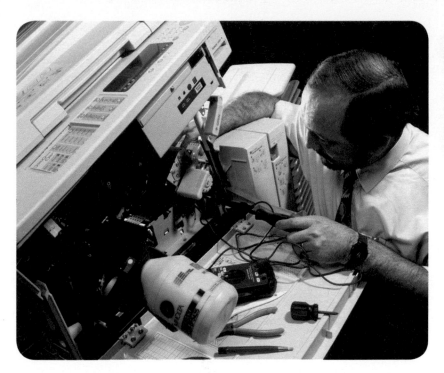

Routine maintenance minimises breakdowns

Find out

Good systems and procedures help to prevent conflict between users because they make it clear that everyone is treated the same. Do yours?

- vandalism, break-ins or theft
- equipment malfunction/breakdown
- IT security breaches
- indiscretion by a colleague
- major disruptions of a key service, such as your phone line or Internet connection.

Resolving problems

Not all problems will require your immediate and undivided attention. The key aspect is whether it is crucial because there is a safety risk, because the problem has the potential to disrupt or stop work, such as computer or phone line failure, or whether the problem can seriously affect the reputation of the business – such as a security breach that could result in confidential client information becoming public knowledge.

The next point to consider is how you found out about the problem. If it was because someone complained to you then you need to assess how accurate the account is likely to be, and check it for yourself.

Find out

Many organisations have **disaster recovery plans** so that the effect of emergency events – from IT failure to flood or fire – will not be totally catastrophic. Find out if your employer has one, otherwise do your boss a favour. Go to the Business Link website at www.businesslink.gov. uk/bdotg/action/layer?r. s=sl&topicId=1074458463 and find out more about the actions all businesses should take to prepare for emergencies and how to devise a business continuity plan.

Remember

Your users will assess problems differently from you – often in terms of their own personal inconvenience. So you will probably hear about a problem with the coffee machine or the photocopier in record time!

When you become aware of a problem, there are various decisions to make:

- What *exactly* is the real problem? Many reports you receive will be vague and unhelpful, such as 'I don't think the fan's working' or 'My computer's doing funny things'.
- How quickly must action be taken?
- How seriously could the problem affect the work situation or the business?
- What would be the consequences of delaying taking action?
- What alternatives are possible?

The table below should help you to assess how quickly to take action. Under normal circumstances, category A problems need dealing with urgently, category B problems fairly quickly and category C problems within a few days.

Finally, you need to consider why the problem occurred in the first place and identify whether there is any action you can take – such as reviewing the systems and procedures in place – to prevent a recurrence.

Guide to assessing the seriousness of a problem with facilities, equipment or resources	
Category	**Seriousness**
1 Health and safety	A – Could possibly cause serious injury or even death B – Could possibly cause a minor injury C – Very slight chance of minor injury
2 Disruption to work	A – One or more people will not work for some time B – One person will lose a couple of hours' work C – Hardly affects the work routine at all
3 Effect on business image/reputation	A – Serious consequences for future business prospects with some external contacts B – Some problems likely with certain external contacts C – No effect on external contacts
4 Consequences of delaying	A – Substantial further problems highly likely B – Some additional problems may emerge in a day or two C – No additional problems likely
5 Alternative actions/substitutes	A – No alternative action possible B – Temporary alternative solution possible C – Alternatives available

How to... Resolve problems effectively

- Check the information you have been given to make sure the facts are correct and ask appropriate questions to fill in any gaps or clarify any doubtful areas.

- Assess the seriousness of a problem by considering its impact on others and the business and the consequences of delaying or not taking action.

- Check if there are any procedures you should follow before you try to solve the problem – such as reporting it to your line manager or obtaining authorisation.

- Identify whether you and your colleagues can solve the problem yourselves or whether you need external help. Remember that if you are in any doubt about this, obtain expert advice.

- Consider the range of solutions that are possible. If you must act quickly, remember that you may have to settle for a compromise between what would be ideal and what you can live with.

- If you are struggling to get agreement amongst different users, try to identify any common ground or indisputable facts that can be used as a basis for negotiation. Then talk to the people concerned assertively but not aggressively. Focus on solving the problem rather than scoring points or winning the argument. Someone might have a better idea than you that works.

- If you can afford the time, remember that sleeping on a difficult problem often helps you to think of a solution.

- After the problem has been solved, think about why it occurred. What can you do now to prevent a recurrence?

Controlling office facilities – and the types of activities to monitor

All office facilities need to be controlled for the following reasons:
- to prevent theft or inappropriate use of equipment or resources
- to prevent damage
- to enable users' needs to be met as much as possible, even though these needs may conflict
- to enable scarce resources to be shared fairly amongst users

- to enable the office facilities to be maintained in good condition for as long as possible
- to conserve the budget – so money is not spent on unnecessary repairs and replacements.

Agreeing priorities with users

One problem with controlling office facilities is that the users will have different needs, so that what suits one person does not suit another.

- Some users may regularly need access to certain types of equipment and resources at the last minute, because of the nature of their jobs.
- Some are often disorganised, so forget to book essential items in advance.
- Others may frequently be asked to attend outside events at the last minute, for which they need special equipment and resources.
- Others may be senior staff who expect you to give their needs top priority at all times.
- Some may be very adept at using certain items of equipment, others may be walking disasters.
- Some may read a procedure carefully before starting work, others will scan or ignore it.

The only way to get the maximum benefit for everyone is to identify key priorities. These should relate to the aims and objectives of the business. They should also take into account the needs of users, or key user groups in a large organisation. Therefore, if there is a genuine need for an 'emergency' supplies system, it should state the reasons under which items can be obtained.

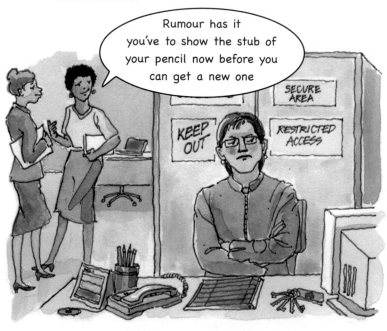

Remember

Everyone thinks their needs are paramount. If you appear to enjoy saying 'no', rather than trying to help, you can expect to have a few problems! In this case, 'it ain't what you say, it's the way that you say it!'

How to... Control the use of office facilities

- Identify the facilities that need to be controlled because of issues of safety, value, scarcity etc. This should enable you to identify the main aim(s) of introducing any particular 'control' system.

- Identify the users who will be affected by any system you introduce.

- Identify the needs of these users and prioritise them.

- Draft a system that will enable you to best meet your main aim(s).

- Check how the needs of your users may be affected if the system is introduced.

- Identify whether you need to introduce any flexibility into the system (e.g. emergency supplies, priority bookings).

- Check your ideas with your supervisor and/or line manager.

- If appropriate, consult with users or key user groups over the proposal and/or introduce the system for a limited time and ask for feedback.

- Take into account feedback and revise the system as required.

- Provide final information and guidance to users based on the final, agreed system.

Remember

Normally top priority will be given to items that can be used to generate more business, better customer relations or higher profits, rather than to items that are just an internal convenience or 'perks' for staff.

Find out

Check the information and guidance on office facilities that is currently given to users in your workplace. Find out whether your users are satisfied with this or if it could be improved.

Case study Another side of the school desk!

Read the case study below and then answer the questions that follow.

Kate Watkins is the office administrator in a primary school. She counts as 'users' of her office facility: the 420 pupils of the school; around 75 school staff including teachers, support workers, catering staff, cleaners and caretakers; and the numerous visitors to the school – such as family support workers, education welfare officers, the behavioural improvement team and parents – to name but a few.

Running the office efficiently and effectively enables the head and her staff to concentrate on doing their own jobs, safe in the knowledge that Kate will deal with all the administrative tasks

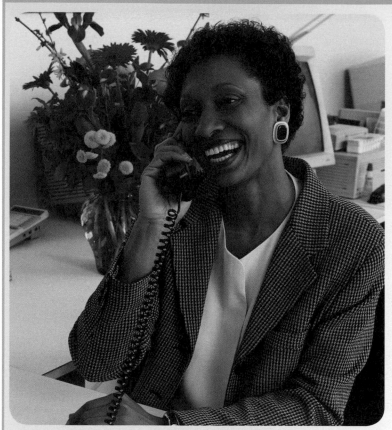

and challenges faced by a busy school each day. One of her tasks includes the scheduling of all the shared resources in the school, from TVs, laminators, laptops and data projectors to musical keyboards and other instruments. Maintenance at the school does not just mean checking whether the photocopier needs servicing, it also means buying replacement reeds for clarinets! Rooms are another resource Kate controls. It is part of her job to find rooms for visitors to use, from nurses arriving to carry out vision tests to SEN (special educational needs) advisers who want to assess a pupil.

The school office uses a wide range of equipment. The fax machine is a critical item. Its main use is to send out purchasing orders for stationery and to chase up absent pupils. Government initiatives to reduce truancy have resulted in a sophisticated electronic system which aims to trace any pupil who goes missing by tracking them through their UPN – unique pupil number. At 9.30 each morning class registers are checked. The names and UPNs of absent pupils are faxed to the agency responsible for finding out the reason for the absence. The agency faxes back the form later that day with comments against each pupil's name.

If truancy is suspected, the education welfare officer becomes involved. If the situation is potentially more serious – because a child has gone missing or is at risk – schools and education offices all over the country are automatically alerted over the Internet. This means that any child who is suddenly moved to another part of the country and then taken to a new school will be detected.

Kate is reliant on her computer both for producing documents and for keeping the school's accounts. She also counts the office telephone and photocopier as essential needs. She uses a risograph for longer print runs because the operating costs are cheaper than for a photocopier.

The electronic whiteboards in the classroom are another item on her equipment list. Kate arranges routine maintenance for all equipment covered by a service agreement. If any equipment develops a fault, she arranges for it to be repaired. When this is not possible she checks the budget to see whether the school can afford to buy a replacement.

Kate is also responsible for general building maintenance. Recently the school has had a new skylight installed and the hall floor has been re-laid. She chooses from an approved list of tried and tested suppliers on her database. The maintenance of the building and grounds is undertaken by the county council and the playground is the responsibility of a private firm. Kate also keeps a list of equipment and stationery suppliers and makes decisions on which firm to use based on price and delivery. For large orders she asks two or three to quote and then compares them.

Systems and security are two key aspects of Kate's job. There are specific procedures staff must follow to take children out of school and a special form to complete which must be signed by a member of the senior management team. If children have a minor accident, such as a bump on the head, they must take a letter home. Kate ensures that the correct procedures are followed by all staff in both cases. She must also make certain that all equipment is locked away when not in use and must abide by the rule that there must never be more than £200 in cash on the premises and that this must be kept locked in the safe.

Kate can have a problem allocating scarce but popular resources. Since teachers were awarded time for PPA (planning, preparation and assessment) they often request a quiet room in which to work. This can be difficult, if not impossible, on a busy day. In a crisis she prioritises the needs of external visitors and will use any vacant room, including the head's study when she is away. Kate's other main worries relate to finance. She must check that she is staying within the budget when she buys goods – but is also aware that any money that remains unspent at

Did you know?

A risograph is a modern digital printing system where the original is scanned to make a 'master' from which multiple copies are printed.

Case study Continued

the end of the year will be clawed back by the government. One of her responsibilities is to make sure that this type of problem doesn't occur – simply by monitoring the needs of the school and current spending levels and checking that there is no money left at the end of the financial year that could be spent on additional facilities, equipment or resources for the staff or pupils.

Questions

1   *Identify the sector in which Kate works and give a reason for your answer.*

2   *Kate divides her 'users' into three groups. Suggest two important needs of each particular group.*

3   *Give two benefits to the school of having both a photocopier and a risograph.*

4   *If you were Kate, suggest how you would control the use of shared facilities, such as the TV, laptops or data projectors.*

5   *Kate says that if the fax machine breaks down she would instantly replace it and wouldn't even think about having it repaired. Suggest three reasons to support this decision.*

6   **a**   *What is meant by the term 'tried and tested' suppliers?*

     b   *How might this phrase prove that Kate tries to build up good relationships with her suppliers?*

7   *Identify three actions taken by Kate that prove that safety and security are important at the school.*

8   *If Kate were undertaking a risk assessment, suggest four areas she should inspect.*

9   *Identify two problems Kate encounters and explain how she copes with these.*

10 *Identify one problem faced by Kate that would never be met by an administrator working in the private sector – and then suggest one that would!*

 Changing places

Your assessor will ask you how you would apply your skills if you changed your job in the future, where the office facility and the equipment and resources may be very different, as you can see opposite.

Jacqui Slater works as senior administrator for a group of IT consultants. They rent a suite of offices on the third floor of a large building in the city centre. The firm pays a service charge to have the building maintained and Jacqui is responsible for checking the equipment, buying resources and liaising with the building manager if there is a general problem, such as the central heating failing or the windows not being cleaned. Equipment maintenance isn't a problem – there is a new multifunction copier/fax/laser printer which is regularly serviced and the consultants themselves can resolve any computer issues. The main problems have occurred with building maintenance so the tenants have recently formed a group to put their concerns to the building manager en masse. Jacqui's boss has asked her to represent the firm on the tenants' group. Jacqui says the building manager is defensive and difficult to handle, but since the group formed it has been far easier to deal with him

Rubina Iqbal works as an administrator at the local leisure centre and assists the manager, Janet Kelly. The office is used by many of the staff who work at the centre and organise a range of sessions from swimming and judo to children's parties. There is also a beauty therapy salon as well as a café and a crèche. Rubina is responsible for ensuring that the office equipment is kept serviceable and for reporting any problems related to the office or reception areas to the centre manager. Building faults are reported to the building maintenance department of the local council. Recently this included reporting that new emergency doors didn't release automatically, as they should do, during a fire drill. Rubina's resource list can be as varied as membership forms for reprinting to leisure centre pens and towels or even inscribed trophies to be given as awards.

Rebecca Dawson runs the office of a local estate agent. There are four members of staff who are regularly out doing valuations or accompanying clients on viewings. Rebecca uses her computer to create the property information leaflets by merging the text with the downloaded digital photographs that are taken when a property is put on the agent's books. She then posts the leaflet on the website as well as sending it out to enquirers. Rebecca is responsible for ensuring that the fax machine, photocopier and her computer and printer are all well maintained as well as arranging for any basic repairs or maintenance required to the office. She also supervises the cleaning of the office and windows and buys all the resources that are required by the business.

Zaheda Shah is a departmental administrator in a college. She works in the Adult Centre, which is in a separate building from the sixth form

Changing places Continued

college. She liaises with the college safety officer when risk assessments are done for the building. She also carries out a weekly inspection of all the classroom areas to check that equipment such as OHPs are working. Where she can, she will remedy faults herself or report them to the facilities manager or the IT support department. Zaheda is responsible for ordering resources required by staff and ensuring that large equipment items are regularly maintained. The department has three photocopiers. One is a digital copier that is connected to the computer network so that documents can be sent direct from PCs for printing.

1   For any **one** person listed above, identify the differences he or she would find if moving to your organisation and doing your job.

2   For any **one** person listed above, say how you would need to adapt your skills if you did their job rather than your own.

Over to you

1   Identify the immediate action you would take if each of the following problems occurred. Also say what action you would take to prevent a recurrence. Check your ideas with the answers on the CD-ROM.

   a   Despite the fact that there is a clear stock control procedure for users, when you carry out a stock audit it is obvious that there is a considerable discrepancy between the amount on the records and the amount on the shelves.

   b   You have just received 5000 new letter headings and spot that the telephone code has a digit missing. When you check the sample copy you were sent, you realise that you did not spot it at the time, but agreed it as correct with the printer.

   c   A key supplier tells you that as the last three invoices to your organisation remain unpaid, no more goods can be delivered.

   d   Your only data projector, which sales staff regularly use for PowerPoint presentations at exhibitions, has stopped working.

   e   The painter who was contracted to redecorate the reception area last weekend did not turn up and is not answering his mobile phone.

2   Suggest ways in which you could allocate or control the following facilities. Compare your ideas with those of other members of your group or with the answers on the CD-ROM.

a The firm next door offers your staff five car parking spaces on their parking area, but you must name the staff who will use them and give the registration numbers for security purposes. There are 18 members of staff with cars in your organisation, all of whom would love a free parking space!

b There are two meeting rooms. One holds ten people, needs decorating, is furnished only with a large table and some chairs. The other holds 20 people, overlooks the garden and has state-of-the-art equipment. Everyone always wants to book the second one!

c The new marketing manager often wants to send out mailshots to prospective customers on letter-headed paper. This is causing you serious problems because your supplier needs two weeks' notice to reprint and replenish your stock.

Evidence collection

1 Keep a record of communications you have with suppliers that demonstrates how you strive to achieve and retain good relationships. These can include faxes, emails, letters or your accounts of telephone conversations, countersigned by your line manager. You do not need to keep separate copies of documents if you know where they are located and can show them to your assessor when he or she visits you.

2 Keep a log of all the occasions when you review the office environment to carry out a risk assessment or to check on other aspects of health, safety or security. Note any problems you identified and the action you took to solve them. Ask your supervisor or line manager to countersign and date your log and any written account to confirm they are correct.

3 Note the location of documentary evidence you can discuss with your assessor, such as the information and guidance that is given to users on office facilities, maintenance schedules of equipment and purchase orders for new equipment or resources. In addition, be prepared to demonstrate how you control the use of office facilities and take into account the needs and priorities of users. You can do this by asking one or two users for witness testimony to support your claims.

Core unit links

Putting your organisation's values into practice when you deal with suppliers and working with outside contacts to protect and improve the image of your organisation links to unit 302, performance indicators 3–5.

Working positively with your users and recognising different needs may link to unit 302, PIs 11 and 12, as well as to unit 301, PIs 27 and 28.

Providing information and guidance on office facilities and listening to feedback about new or proposed controls links to unit 301, PIs 1–7 and 16.

Maintaining health and safety and security may link to unit 302, PIs 14–22; and following procedures, policies and guidelines may be cross-referenced to unit 301, PI 15, and to unit 302, PIs 2, 5 and 6.

Solving problems, if necessary with the support of others, links to unit 301, PI 11.

What if...?

What should you do if no problems arise during your assessment period?

Your assessor will ask you to confirm your competence by explaining the action you would take if certain problems occurred. It is likely this will be as part of a professional discussion relating to other parts of this unit but, of course, your assessor may ask verbal questions.

 Key skills reminder

If you are taking Key Skills awards, remember to discuss with your tutor or trainer how your evidence for this unit could also count towards those awards.

Manage and evaluate customer relations

Unit summary and overview

This option unit is divided into three sections:

- identify customer needs and expectations
- deliver services
- monitor and evaluate services.

The importance of good working relationships with customers cannot be over-stated. Building these involves identifying and confirming customer needs, and delivering appropriate services promptly and to agreed quality standards. Monitoring and evaluating your services involves obtaining and analysing customer feedback and taking appropriate action where required to improve customer relations.

This unit covers all these areas. If you regularly interact with internal and external customers and are responsible for meeting their needs, then this unit will be suitable for you. It will provide you with useful information and development opportunities to improve your knowledge and skills.

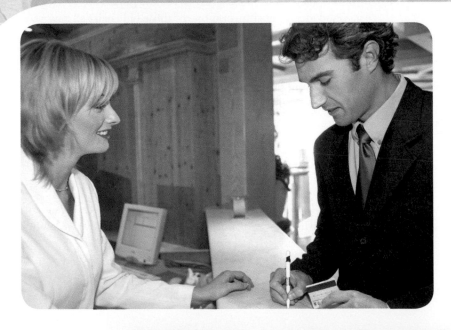

Identify customer needs and expectations

Link to core units

As you gather your evidence for this unit you should also obtain evidence for your core units. Watch for the CU link logo which suggests how the evidence you may collect could count towards both this unit and your core units.

Remember that you might be able to identify other links yourself, because of your own job role and the evidence you have obtained.

Talk to your assessor if you need further guidance on how your evidence should be cross-referenced.

Who are your 'customers'

If you walk into a shop and buy some food, it is pretty obvious that you are a customer. It is equally obvious that you are a customer if you book a holiday online or order some clothes from a catalogue. What is a bit less obvious perhaps is that if you are on a college course you are regarded as a customer of the college. If you need to contact your local council because your wheelie bin has not been emptied, you are regarded as a council customer – and so on.

At work it is normally quite easy to find out who your **external customers** are. They are those people who buy your goods or services. Even so, it is a good idea to remember that the person placing the order or asking for the service may not be the only one deciding to buy from you. Behind that person there might be a number of other people who have had some say in making that decision.

For instance you might see the order placers, who are the people who actually pick up the telephone. They, however, might be doing so as a result of discussions with:

Did you know?

Social service departments now call their reception staff 'customer care officers'. The reason for this is that they are dealing all day long with people the department thinks of as their customers or clients.

- **the initiator** – the person who makes the original suggestion (e.g. 'Let's get some new office furniture')
- **the user** – the person who is going to use the product or service (e.g. 'Good idea, after sitting on one of those old chairs all day, my back kills me')
- **the influencer** – the person who can give some specialist advice (e.g. 'We need to buy those ergonomically designed chairs that are meant to prevent people getting bad backs')
- **the gatekeeper** – the person who can give the go ahead or block the whole idea (e.g. 'We have enough left in the departmental budget to cover this').

In order to please the order placer, you have got to please everyone else!

Remember

You too are an internal customer. If you don't like the services other people are providing for you, you have a right to say something. In the interests of good office relations it might be as well to say it tactfully!

It is sometimes less easy to spot your **internal customers**. They can include people who want your word processing services, reprographic services, reception services, meetings skills etc. The same principle applies – you are providing a service and they are either satisfied or dissatisfied with it.

Why effective and efficient customer service is important

The major reason you should try to satisfy your customers is that you will not have any business if you don't. A number of surveys suggest that companies with good customer services are able to charge up to 9 per cent more for the goods and services they offer and grow twice as fast as the average. That is not only good for the customer, it is good for you as well.

Your organisation's customer service systems

One of the first tasks in making sure you deal with customers effectively and efficiently is to discover your own organisation's procedures for dealing with customers. You might find, for instance, that one of the following statements is true:

- There is a separate customer care unit.
- Customer care is a sub-section of the marketing department.
- One of the senior managers has a specific responsibility for customer care.
- Customer care staff report directly to a member of the senior management team.
- One person from each department or section is part of a cross-organisational team responsible for overseeing the way in which customers are dealt with.
- Everyone in the organisation takes individual responsibility for customer care.

You also need to know the various customer service **procedures** that are in operation. Examples are:

- how to deal with customers
  - personally
  - over the telephone
  - with appointments
  - without appointments
  - when there is a delay
- the methods of communication, including the period within which a response must be made to any customer
- how to prepare all the relevant paperwork – letters, customer records, complaint forms etc.
- how to access the computerised database and whether or not you can input any information

Find out

In your own organisation, check how your customer service operates and what procedures are in operation that you should follow.

- how to find out about and update the information you have about the products or services offered by the organisation
- how to deal with complaints
- how to obtain, analyse and act on customer feedback
- how and when to obtain help and support.

How to build positive working relationships with customers

Rae and Linzi work next to each other on the reception desk. Rae greets customers with a smile, remembers their names, knows who they want to see and why. She also knows enough about the firm's products to be able to give some basic information over the telephone to anyone who makes an initial enquiry. Linzi cannot be bothered. She wants to get rid of everyone as soon as possible, thinks it is someone else's job to tell customers about the product, and lets the phone ring in the hope that the person on the other end of the line will get fed up and put the phone down. Rae helps the firm to get business, Linzi doesn't.

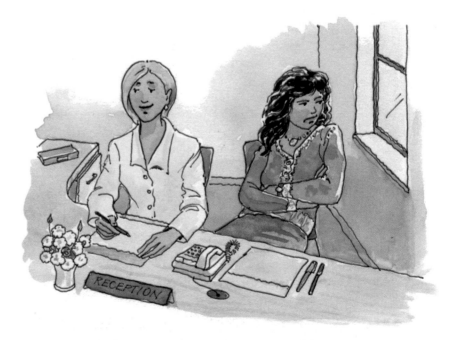

Assessing customer feelings

One of the most important ways to build up a positive working relationship with customers is by listening to them. Use your eyes and your ears to try to pick up all the messages your customer is sending

How to... Build positive working relationships with customers

Remember

You never get a second chance to make a first impression.

- **Be positive and proactive.** Customers want to deal with someone who is helpful and friendly rather than offhand and uninterested.

- **Know what you are talking about.** If you haven't a clue what to say about the product or know less than nothing about the service, your customers are going to lose faith in you.

- **Have customer-friendly systems.** Customers like paperwork that is easy to complete, simple payment systems, a clear brief about whether or not a product or service is available etc. They also like to be able to contact you virtually 24 hours a day!

- **Have a product that does what it is meant to do.** No matter how helpful you are, the customer is not going to come back to you if the washing machine keeps breaking down or the cleaning fluid doesn't actually clean.

- **Have a service that works.** Again, no matter how persuasive you are, if nothing is delivered on time or if the workpeople never turn up, then the customer will go somewhere else next time.

you – not just the direct one. If, for instance, a customer tells you that your prices are quite high, he or she might:

- be waiting for you to justify this
- be trying to find out whether you are in a position to negotiate a lower price
- be trying to let you know that the same product is sold at a lower price elsewhere.

Even if you cannot give a totally satisfactory response – such as offering to reduce the price – at least you will be aware that there may be more than one agenda.

Another useful way to assess what a customer is actually feeling is to observe his or her body language.

Remember

Look back to unit 301, pages 19–20, for information on negative and positive body language.

If the customer is smiling, nodding encouragement at what you say and making eye contact, you can assume that things are going well enough. If, on the other hand, you see negative body language – such as tapping of the feet, drumming of fingers on the desk or counter, avoidance of eye contact or its opposite, eye-balling, flicking through papers on the desk as you are talking, or shrugging at everything you say – stop and think how to handle the situation. Do not just plough on and hope for

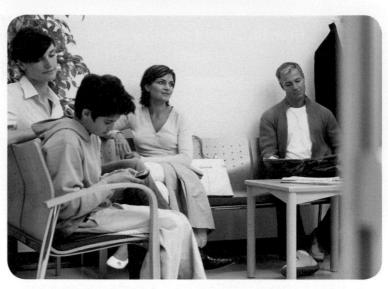

A pleasant waiting room makes the wait seem less long

the best. Sometimes a direct approach helps. You might say 'You seem to be a bit annoyed. What would you like me to do to help?' or, if you can, 'Shall we go back to the beginning. Would you like to have a cup of tea and talk about it in more detail.' You should get some response from the customer and then you can build on that.

The most regular customers are the ones you are most likely to be able to build up a good working relationship with – and to know immediately what sort of mood they are in.

The importance of identifying and confirming customer needs

If you work in the fashion industry one of your most important tasks is to keep up with the latest trends. If you stay with last year's fashions, never mind the fashions of a few years ago, you will lose business. Even if you are offering a product or service that does not change quite so often, you still need to make certain that you identify exactly what the customers want.

Customers *want* to deal with an organisation that:
- has a good reputation
- provides them with the product or service they want
- has a good customer service policy
- has helpful and well-informed staff
- makes it easy for them to contact it
- replies quickly to enquiries

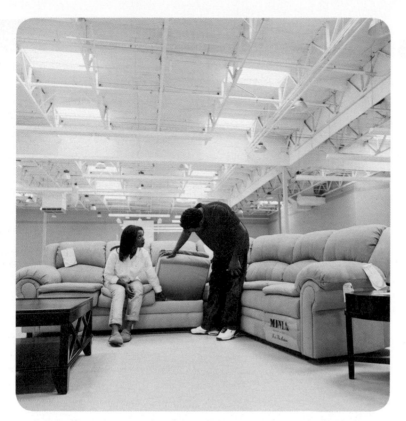

Customers expect high quality goods with value-added features

- has some value-added features – free service, additional discount etc.
- checks up on how satisfied they are with the product or service.

The organisation *needs* to provide that for them.

In addition to their general requirements, customers also have specific requirements. It all depends on what they want. If, for instance, a customer comes into your furniture showroom and asks to have a look at some sofas, she certainly wants good quality and reliable service. What she may also want, however, is a sofa that is 'child friendly' (one that doesn't stain or damage easily), that fits in with the rest of the furniture in the room, that is no longer than 1.5 metres and that can be delivered in the next two weeks. If you are the salesperson you can supply her with all that information. However, she may not say exactly what she wants all in one go. She might need you to talk to her for a while, to ask some questions, to offer a few alternatives etc.

Similarly, a customer might ring you up and say that he wants to order some stationery. Even if he has details of everything you offer you may still have to ask some relevant questions to make sure he is getting the best possible deal and will then come back to give you some repeat business.

Did you know?

It took only one silly remark by the managing director of a firm of jewellery manufacturers – that some of his stock was 'tat' – to bring about the collapse of the firm's reputation. It eventually closed down.

Did you know?

Companies such as General Electric, BMW and Staples are now actively involving their customers at the design stage of any of their products. What they say influences what the finished product is going to be.

How to... Identify and confirm customer needs

- Collect information about your existing customers:
    - their order history
    - records of their contacts with your business – phone calls, meetings etc.
    - direct feedback – anything they've already told you
    - changes in their order patterns – whether they have stopped/started ordering more frequently.
- Collect information about your product or service:
    - changes in the overall success – e.g. rise or fall in sales, number of people using the service
    - feedback about the existing product/service – 'It's not as good as last year's', 'I like it a lot better now'
    - number of enquiries about new products or services
    - feedback from customers about things they buy or services they get from other people
    - changes in goods or services made by your competitors.
- Manage the customer information by using a database system or customer relationship management (CRM) software.

Quality standards that are appropriate to your responsibilities

If you work in a large organisation you will have a number of policies and procedures in place telling you what your customer service standards are. Even if you work in a smaller organisation you are likely to be following the same standards even if they are a bit less formal.

Whatever the case, you will probably be expected to meet the following quality standards:
- to give professional, courteous and prompt service
- to be competent and well trained
- to pay attention to detail
- to give the customer your full and undivided attention
- to charge fair prices for quality products and services
- to provide opportunities to the customer to give feedback
- to make sure the customers know you appreciate their custom.

How to... Prepare customer service quality standards

Find out

Check to see what quality standards your organisation has in place and compare them with the list opposite.

- Involve customers and staff in preparing them.

- Make sure that the standards link to the overall targets of the organisation.

- Make all standards achievable.

- State the standards clearly and put them in writing.

- Make sure everyone knows what the standards are.

- Try to develop a culture where everyone knows that not following the standards is unacceptable.

- Review the standards regularly and add new ones as necessary

Over to you

In order to give quality service and information to customers you need to be well informed yourself. Using the guidance form below, check on the types of information and paperwork you can access in your own organisation to help you. Where you would answer 'no', discuss with your tutor or trainer whether or not having that information would be of use to you.

Customer information questionnaire

System/procedure in place

I can easily find:
- the customer database
- pre-printed forms for customers':
  - orders
  - complaints
  - queries
  - feedback
- other pre-printed forms (say what they are)
- product/service information that is regularly updated
- organisation chart and/or details of the main people who can give me any relevant information
- a helpline or emergency contact to a member or members of staff who can help me with urgent enquires or complaints
- a copy of the complaints procedure
- information on how to ask for customer feedback over the phone or in person
- the staff handbook.

Core unit links

Assess your communications with customers to check the links to unit 301, performance indicators 1–7. Then analyse your customer database or records to check whether you have evidence to cross-reference to supporting diversity – see unit 302, PIs 11–13.

You should also check whether you can link evidence relating to targets, guidelines and timescales and how these affect your working methods and performance to unit 301, PIs 8–15.

Identifying customer needs and fulfilling these also links to achieving your organisation's purpose and values. You should therefore check how your evidence on following guidelines and procedures links to unit 302, PIs 1–6, and to unit 302, PI 15.

Evidence collection

Your assessor will need to know how you identify the needs of your customers, how you identify and confirm these, how you agree timescales and quality standards, and the procedures you follow if these are not achieved.

1   Use the guidance form you have prepared and the information you have obtained on quality standards as the basis of a professional discussion you can have with your assessor about the procedures you follow in your workplace to assess and fulfil customer needs.

2   For five or six customers you deal with, summarise recent arrangements and transactions that illustrate how you have dealt with enquiries, requests or concerns and fulfilled their needs. Make a reference to any customer records or files that you can show to your assessor to prove your account, and ask your supervisor or line manager to countersign and date your claims to prove their authenticity.

3   Make a note of the location of any additional internal documentation that specifically refers to meeting customer needs – such as minutes of a meeting to discuss customer needs, or emails you received or sent to facilitate this.

Deliver services

Setting and meeting timescales and quality standards with customers

Did you know?

The law says that a customer must be given goods or services of satisfactory quality and that services must be carried out within a reasonable time and at a reasonable price. Otherwise the customer can claim compensation.

Have you ever waited in for someone to come and repair something and been very annoyed when no one turned up? Have you ever gone to a hair stylist and asked for a particular hair colour and been disappointed because it lasted only a few days? If so, you'll appreciate how customers feel if they don't think they have been given what they asked for.

Some of the problems are a bit beyond your control. If you have promised a customer that someone will repair a television on a particular day and the repairer either does not arrive at the time agreed or actually mend the television, that's up to your boss to sort out.

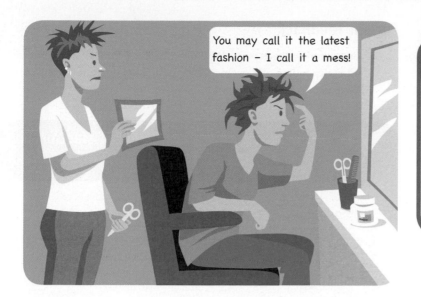

Did you know?

One London-based hair stylist now asks customers to sign a form stating not only what they have agreed to have done but also who is going to do it. This prevents dissatisfied customers from saying they were given a trainee when they expected someone fully qualified.

However, you can help. If you are responsible for taking the order and making arrangements for the product to be delivered or the work to be carried out, then you need to be sure that you know exactly what has been agreed and that your customer knows the same thing.

In the case of some repairs, you could make sure that the customer knows that, because the repairer cannot estimate exactly how long he or she will be with each customer, a precise time cannot be given. All you can promise is that he or she will be there on a particular day and between certain times.

If a customer asks for something that is a bit vague – 'I want some highlights in my hair' – you can discuss in more detail what is wanted and, if relevant, point out that that particular colour is not likely to last more than a week or two.

The importance of monitoring customer satisfaction – and how to do so

If you don't find out whether or not your customers like your products or service you are never going to be able to improve. That may be OK if you are the only maker of a product or deliverer of a service, but nowadays you are not likely to be in that position.

Did you know?

There is a difference between a customer being 'satisfied' and being 'not dissatisfied'. Research by Xerox has shown that customers who score an organisation 5 or 6 out of 7 on satisfaction are five times more likely to go to a competitor than a customer scoring a 'completely satisfied' 7.

Formal feedback

Customer feedback procedures differ between various organisations, often depending on how big they are and how much money there is available.

How to... Monitor customer satisfaction and obtain feedback

- Install a freecall telephone line, displayed very publicly on correspondence, the product itself, the delivery vans etc.

- Put comment cards and forms in places that are easy to get at, or send them to customers with a prepaid return slip.

- Have suggestion boxes for both external and internal customers.

- Have customer care desks with staff trained to talk to customers.

- Produce customer surveys or questionnaires, sent to both existing and possible new customers and/or sent by email or included on the firm's website.

- Conduct interviews in person or on the telephone, again by specially trained staff.

- Introduce 'customer happy calls' to check satisfaction over the telephone.

- Set up focus groups to obtain customer views on products, services, staff responses, store layouts, advertisements etc.

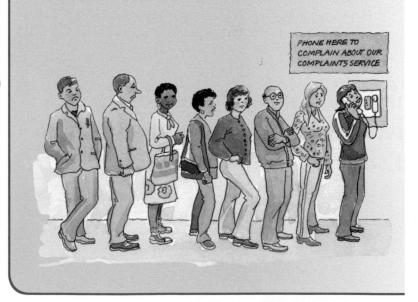

PHONE HERE TO COMPLAIN ABOUT OUR COMPLAINTS SERVICE

Did you know?

Many large organisations employ independent researchers to act as mystery shoppers or mystery callers to contact the firm and then score the service they receive. The researchers then send a report on the results to the firm at regular intervals. At Dixons, the chairman used to make these calls to staff himself!

Customer questionnaires and surveys

A very well used procedure to get customer feedback is to send existing customers a questionnaire. This has a lot of advantages.

- It is direct. You know that the customer knows who you are.
- You can get a lot of spin-off material from a questionnaire.
- It is another way of 'reselling' your product or service. A lot of questionnaires and surveys are done over the Internet, and organisations go to some trouble to make them not only useful to them but fun for the customers to complete – just as if they were doing a quiz in a magazine.

The information organisations want to get from the surveys differs depending on the product or service. Organisations offering a product, for instance, want to know how well the customer rates it in areas such as:

- price
- rapid delivery
- range
- the product itself
- packaging
- catalogue information
- returns procedure
- ease of access to the website.

Organisations offering a service tend to want to know what customers think about:

- speed of service
- the way in which the service was delivered
- the attitude of the staff
- the quality of the finished result.

Informal feedback

Even though most organisations have formal systems of finding out whether or not customers are satisfied, it is sometimes an equally good method to try to find out informally what customers think. If you sit in a reception area for a morning you will soon see whether or not the visitors think they have been well treated. If you are speaking to someone over the telephone and hear them sigh with exasperation as you explain that you cannot deliver the product ordered until the following week, you know the customer is not pleased. Similarly, if you get a bunch of flowers and a thank you card from a grateful customer, you know you have done your job.

Did you know?

Russell Hobbs, a firm of electrical suppliers, sends a customer survey to its existing customers asking questions not only about the purchase of the product but also about holiday destinations, leisure interests, newspapers read, number of cars, occupation, housing and salary range! This helps to give a picture of the 'typical' customer. Many people, though, object strongly to questionnaires that ask them about their earnings, so a lot of surveys now omit that question.

Did you know?

The IWOOT (I want one of those) Customer survey divides its questions into 'boring stuff' and 'less boring stuff'. It also puts its questions in fun format – e.g. 'The killer question … how old are you?' and 'Where do you live, roughly speaking'?

Did you know?

Even the method of scoring the results has changed over the past few years. Most surveys ask customers to score them on a points scale or on a range from 'excellent' to 'poor'. Some, however, ask customers to rate them on a score from 'excellent' to 'OK' to 'rubbish'!

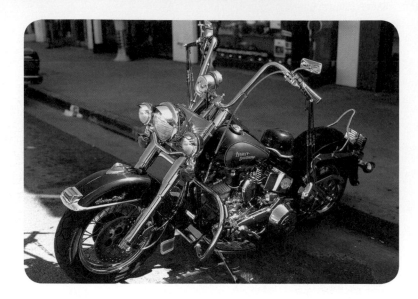

Indirect feedback

A lot of organisations check customer satisfaction through indirect as well as direct feedback. If, for instance, customer sales are falling, you know that something is wrong. If no one has ordered anything from your sales catalogue, again this needs investigating.

In addition you can get a lot of indirect feedback if you are looking at internal customer satisfaction. If you wander into your dining area and find that there are only two people sitting there at what should be the busiest time of the day, you might suspect there is something wrong with the food or service. If you keep advertising for staff and no one replies, you might think that word has spread that internal customers (i.e. the staff) are not treated too well.

Problems that customers may experience – and how to solve them

You work for a catalogue company that offers its products over the Internet but also has a number of direct sales outlets where customers can call in, check the catalogue and fill in an order form. They can either get the goods there and then or they are delivered to them within the next few days. One morning you are in the back office of one of these outlets where you can both see and hear Jaffaar, one of the new sales staff, dealing with customers. You are a bit alarmed.

- One customer says that there are no more order forms left. Jaffaar stares at her blankly. She repeats what she has said and, after a silence, he shrugs his shoulders. She goes away.

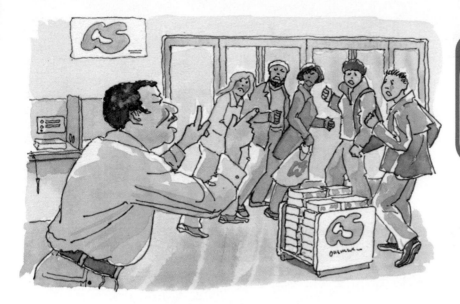

Did you know?

Research of one particular sales outlet over a period showed that only 20 per cent of customers ever returned if they had been asked to call back later.

- Another customer arrives at the counter to complain that a clock she bought yesterday is not working. She wants to return it. Jaffaar apparently knows that there is a returns policy. However, it is rather a long process and involves a bit of form filling. He moves at the pace of a rather slow snail.

- One customer is a bit of a ditherer and keeps asking questions. Jaffaar tells him that he's holding everyone up and can he speed up or come back later.

- A queue starts to build up. Jaffaar is bothered that he is not going to get a break and he therefore starts to speed up. However, in doing so, he makes a mistake and hands out the wrong articles to two customers. Fortunately they realise what has happened and swap round. They aren't too pleased but Jaffaar is dealing with another customer and does not acknowledge his mistake.

- Someone near the back of the queue starts complaining loudly and asking Jaffaar to speed up. Jaffaar shouts at him and tells him that he has only two hands and is doing the best he can – it's not his fault that the place is so under-staffed. He also tells him to go elsewhere if he doesn't like it here.

At this point you think you have to do something. You come out to the counter and start dealing with the customers. You also smooth down a number of rather ruffled customers.

Jaffaar is not a company asset at the moment. He has done just about everything he shouldn't have. He has not realised that when you are dealing with customers all day long there are almost bound to be problems:

- A customer doesn't like the quality of the product or service.

- The product or service is not what he or she expected it would be.
- The product or service has not arrived on time.
- The customer thinks the price is too high.
- The customer has not got enough information.
- The back-up service is not satisfactory.

At this point, as front-line staff, Jaffaar should have used a number of different skills in dealing with problems. First of all he should have listened to what was being said. He was so busy trying to get rid of the customers that he didn't take the time to find out what they wanted and to deal with them as individuals.

How to... Listen to customers

- Identify the tone of voice. Is it annoyed, frustrated, doubtful or furious?

- Decide exactly what the customer wants – straightforward information, to make a complaint, to be reassured, to confirm something etc.

- Identify any hidden purpose. Is the customer angry because he or she is worried etc.?

- Give a prompt if you think the customer is looking for one – e.g. 'Do you want to have a look at the catalogue to see if there's something else you prefer?'

- Ask short, relevant questions to make sure you've understood what the customer has said.

- Let silence fall before you reply. You are letting the customer know that you are thinking about what has been said.

- Don't interrupt no matter how much you want to.

- Don't keep asking the customer to repeat everything.

- Don't show impatience just because the customer is taking a long time explaining.

- Don't try to shut a customer up.

- Don't give an immediate negative response – 'I can't do anything about that.'

Jaaffar was equally hopeless at dealing with angry customers. He either tried to ignore them or started arguing. He also let the organisation

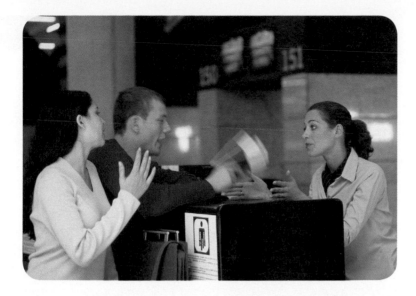

down by trying to put some of the blame on them. Angry people only get angrier if you start being aggressive with them.

How to... Deal with angry customers

- Don't get angry back.

- Use sympathetic body language.

- Use certain phrases to show that you are taking the matter seriously – e.g. 'Obviously something has gone very wrong.'

- Apologise for the fact that there is a problem, but at this stage don't admit any fault. You are not likely to have all the facts.

- Don't interrupt, however difficult that can be.

- Try to listen carefully to what is being said for both the direct and indirect message – what is actually being said and what the customer actually means. 'I'm absolutely furious that the computer is still not working' may mean 'I'm not absolutely sure how to work it but I don't want to look a fool in front of you.'

- Get all the facts. Customers tend to like it when you write down what they have been saying. They think it shows that you are taking them seriously.

- Try to be positive. Tell the customer what you are going to do about the problem.

Did you know?

One management writer, Armen Kabodian, found that it costs six times more to attract a new customer than it does to keep an old one and that service organisations in particular depend on existing customers for 85–95 per cent of their business.

Snapshot – No customers, no job!

A director of the painting and decorating division of a London-based construction company wanted to find a way of measuring how effectively the business was performing. He therefore devised a customer feedback programme as one of a number of key performance indicators the firm uses to measure its efficiency.

- In step 1, he sent out a customer questionnaire that was tightly focused on the areas he wanted to measure. In answer to one question, 'Did the painters tidy up to your satisfaction?', the customer could reply 'yes' or 'no' or give a satisfaction rating ranging from 1 to 10 and using faces going from smiles to scowls.

- In step 2, he looked at any negative feedback very carefully. For example, 30 per cent of customers said that the contractors were not tidying up very well. He therefore had a brainstorming session with the contract managers and supervisors and discovered that they could improve their image as being tidy by using throwaway protective materials with their logo on – to highlight to customers how tidy they actually were.

- In step 3, he reported his findings to the other directors to encourage them to introduce similar customer feedback schemes.

He learned as he went on. At first he expected 100 per cent response from the customers but got about 30 per cent. He realised eventually that that was not a bad response.

His top tips!

1 Start simply. You won't be able to get everything right at once.

2 Deal with any negative feedback right away. In the long run it could actually win more business.

3 Make it as easy as possible for customers to give feedback.

Did you know?

There is now a wide range of computer software on the market for handling complaints. It logs full details of the complaint, together with the action taken and the people involved. It also logs all acknowledgements and replies as well as keeping track of the correspondence. Various types of report can be produced, including specially customised ones.

Following complaints procedures

No one likes dealing with complaints. However, if you deal with a complaint properly then you are likely to keep the customer. As the director in the snapshot above says, you might actually get more business because of your prompt action.

Nearly every organisation has its own complaints procedure that it wants staff to follow. Normally this would expect you to do the following:

- Reassure the customer as much as possible and ask for details of the complaint.
- Listen carefully but ask questions when necessary.
- Check the details of the complaint to make sure you understand what it is.
- *Either* explain to the customer that you will look into the matter further and give him or her a date when you will reply; *or* agree what action should be taken there and then.
- If you can take action right away, go ahead and do so.

Find out

If you work in a large organisation you may have a customer complaints charter that tells customers how to complain and to whom. It may also tell the customers what to do next if they are not satisfied with how the complaint has been dealt with by the organisation – such as how to contact an Ombudsman. Check to see whether you have such a charter.

Over to you

1   Your boss has been getting a lot of complaints about the long queues at the reception desk. At a weekly staff meeting he asks for ideas on how to solve this problem. He does not mind how elaborate they are at this stage. Discuss your suggestions with your tutor or trainer, and check your ideas against those on the CD-ROM.

2   The following problems have occurred in your office recently:

   a   An important customer complains that the order he received was late and he now wants you to take the goods back.

   b   A customer complains about the rudeness of one of the reception staff. He says this isn't the first time it has happened.

   c   A customer rings up to say that the goods she ordered two weeks ago have not yet arrived.

   d   One of your 'internal customers', the marketing manager's chief administrator, complains about the quality of the photocopying done by someone in your department.

   In each case decide what you would do to improve things. Decide also what you could do yourself and what you need to discuss with your supervisor. Discuss your ideas with your tutor or trainer and check them against those on the CD-ROM.

Evidence collection

You need to prove to your assessor that you provide services to agreed timescales and quality standards, check customer needs and expectations are met and resolve or refer complaints in a professional manner and to a given timescale.

Core unit links

Evidence relating to checking customer satisfaction links to units 301, performance indicators 1 and 2, as well as to units 302, PIs 1–3.

Check the evidence from your internal customers to identify how you can cross-reference this to prove that you behave in a way that supports effective working – see unit 302, PIs 22–28.

If any of the information you are given is confidential, note that this will cross-reference to unit 302, PI 15.

Evidence collection Continued

1   Keep a log of follow-up calls or other methods you use to contact customers to check that their needs have been met. Include a note of the questions that you ask and other methods you use to seek confirmation. In particular, if any call resulted in a customer reporting dissatisfaction with a service, record the action you took as a result to resolve the problem and keep a copy of any relevant documents you created or completed.

2   Identify the way in which you log or record complaints as part of your organisational procedures. For a selected number of complaints, include the documents as evidence or note where these can be found to show them to your assessor. You should also keep copies of written notes you have made in response to any complaints or copies of any complaints forms you have completed. Attach details of what you did after you received the complaint or found out about the problem – for example, how you solved it or who you passed it to, the timescale you set and how you checked the complaint had been resolved.

3   Ask two or three of your internal customers for witness testimony in which they describe your working relationship with them. It is helpful if they can confirm that you always identify and confirm their needs, agree timescales, quality standards or the procedures you must follow, deliver services as promised and solve any problems as and when they occur. Your witnesses should include specific examples of services you have provided or problems you have solved to support their claims.

Note that you should not ask external customers for witness testimony without the specific agreement of your supervisor. However, should you receive a thank you letter or card, discuss this with your assessor who may agree that you can use it as evidence.

What if...?

What should you do if no problems occur within the time you are being assessed?

Your assessor can give you a dedicated task to cover the knowledge and understanding required. This will then be followed by a professional discussion during which you can explain how you would perform in such a situation (or the actions you have taken in the past) and what evidence you might bring forward.

Monitor and evaluate services

Techniques for collecting and analysing customer feedback

On pages 234–6 you read about a number of ways in which customer feedback can be obtained. Quite obviously, there is no point in obtaining this and then ignoring it! The next stage is to analyse the information you have received to see what it tells you about your services. This also includes noting what complaints have been received and why.

How to keep track of customer complaints

One complaint by one customer should always be taken seriously. However, the complaint could be:

- genuinely a 'one off' – the van driver delivering the goods having an accident on the way
- unreasonable – the customer expecting a high-quality product for a fraction of the normal price
- easily dealt with – the customer wanting a pen that works at the building society counter.

In these cases there is not much that can be learned from them – other than to remember that the customer is always right no matter what!

Did you know?

Business Link says that people willing to complain are rare. Those who do may be alerting you to a problem other customers have had but who have silently taken their custom elsewhere.

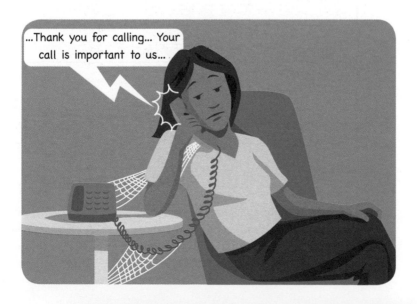

In most other cases, however, complaints are taken so seriously that a record has to be made of each one. Nowadays they are normally put on a computer database for ease of access, input and retrieval. An example of one customer complaints form is shown below.

JON WILKINSON RECRUITMENT CONSULTANTS
Customer complaint form
Customer's name: Organisation (if relevant): Address: Telephone no: Fax no: Email address: Customer reference number:
What the complaint is about:
When it happened:
Where it happened:
Staff involved:
Action taken so far:
Any follow-up action: (give dates)
No further action required: (document ready for filing)
Signature: Date:

Example of a customer complaints form

Obviously it is not much good collecting together all the complaint forms and simply putting them into a filing cabinet or letting them get lost on a computerised database. Somebody has to do something about them. That somebody is normally a senior manager. In most cases the number of complaints received is dealt with not only as an individual issue where a very prompt response is needed but also as part of the whole customer feedback issue when all aspects of customer service are considered.

How to... Analyse and evaluate customer feedback

- Decide on a timescale. Is the analysis going to be weekly, monthly etc?

- Decide on who is going to be involved in the analysis – an individual, a group, an outside agency?

- Decide on the categories into which you are going to put the complaints – about the product, about the staff, about the venue etc.

- Decide on what the finished format is to be – a written report, a set of figures, or a combination of both.

- Decide on what format the figures should take – tabular, graphic, pictorial etc.

- Decide on what is going to be done with the results – circulation to managers, staff etc.

- Decide on how any improvements are going to be recorded as a result of any action taken.

- Decide on what response is going to be made to the customers.

Feedback of results

It is pointless to analyse what customers like and don't like about your services if you then do nothing about it. What many organisations do is:
- produce information to be discussed by all levels of staff
- have procedures in place for feedback from the staff to either senior management or some named person who is responsible for taking follow-up action.

Then they use a number of ways to give feedback on what they have done. For instance, many organisations:
- display notices or posters in a public area where passers by are likely to read them (many big stores do this)
- send a personalised response to each customer – if the organisation is very small
- send all customers a summarised version of what action has been taken as a result of customer feedback, or publish the results online.

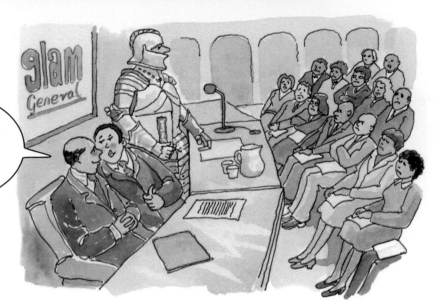

After last year's protest Bill said this was the only way he was prepared to attend.

In addition, in both public and private sectors, there is a growing tendency to make customer feedback reports a major item of discussion not only at board or chief executive level, but also at shareholder meetings or meetings to which the general public are invited. These are occasions that customer services managers dread. No matter how well they have prepared the feedback there is always likely to be someone who asks the awkward question (e.g. 'You say in your feedback that car parking facilities have improved. Not that anyone would notice. It took me 40 minutes to find a parking space before this meeting – and I missed the pre-meeting cup of tea. I'm going to send you a bill for my petrol costs.'). Quick wits are needed here – and a lot of experience in dealing with customers!

The importance of continuous improvement

You work with a senior colleague who is not very good at dealing with change. If anyone suggests any improvements she makes comments like "I've worked here for ages, I should know what I'm doing by now' or 'There's nothing you can tell me about how to deal with customers'. What a pity! She's like a dinosaur who keeps plodding along doing the same thing the same way, not noticing that the world about her is changing and not realising that if she's not careful she'll soon become extinct.

Wherever you work, you will probably have to deal with some type of competition. If you work for an organisation that manufactures electrical goods, you will know just how many other organisations make the same product. If you work in the retail industry, you are not likely to be the only shop in town. If you work in the town hall you might find that your department survives only by having put in the best tender for the work, in competition with outside bidders.

In order to stay ahead of the competition, you have to keep in touch with what the customers actually want. Not long ago most people were quite happy with videos. Now nearly everyone has changed over to DVDs, and the big video rental firms have changed too. Otherwise they would have soon been out of business.

If the product or service changes, so too should you. You need to be aware of the changes and be able to advise the customers accordingly. You also need to be able to reassure them if they are a bit unwilling to accept the changes. Persuading older people who have bought the same product for years that it is now not available but that they will like the new one just as well, if not better, is sometimes quite tricky!

It is not only the organisation that benefits if you keep yourself up to date. You do too. You may not always want to be in the job you now have. You might want promotion within your organisation. If you show that you are flexible and willing to take on board new ideas, you are more likely to be noticed and earmarked for a higher level job, than if you show no interest in making even the slightest change in the way you operate. Quoting a price out of last year's catalogue, misdirecting a customer to the wrong room, or saying that you have a product that is no longer on the shelves will not endear you to your customer or your supervisor.

Here are some other ways of making sure that you continuously improve your customer care skills:

- **Observe other people who are good at their jobs.** If some of your colleagues are absolutely brilliant at dealing with awkward customers on the phone, sit near to them to listen to what they say – or ask to pick their brains.
- **Observe those who are not as good** – for example a member of staff who is always snappy with customers or who cannot be bothered to give the right information – and make sure you don't fall into the same trap.
- **Learn by your mistakes.** Anyone can take the wrong approach with a customer once and most people will be sympathetic. Keep doing it and you'll get less sympathy – or job satisfaction.
- **Welcome training.** Make sure you know about what your organisation offers or whether your supervisor might let you undertake external training.
- **Welcome the challenge.** Every time you deal successfully with a difficult customer or get a word of thanks from a grateful one, give yourself a pat on the back and aim to make this happen more often!

Did you know?

Many small shops make extra income by stocking goods that are no longer offered by the major stores. For instance, the major children's clothes suppliers no longer sell frilly knickers for baby girls as nowadays most babies are put in baby-grows. However, the smaller shops still supply these knickers for doting but slightly old-fashioned grandparents to give to their newest granddaughter!

Did you know?

One firm has as its motto 'Customer satisfaction isn't our highest priority, it is our only priority.'

Case study Unfortunately, the customer is always right!

Read the case study below and then answer the questions that follow. Then check your answers with those on the CD-ROM

Carolyn Lee was good at maths at school. When she left school, therefore, she was pleased to get a job in a bank. She thought she would be adding up figures, counting money and doing other number-crunching activities. The reality was quite different.

First of all she was asked to wear the bank's uniform. She didn't mind this as the uniform was smart and it prevented her from having to think of what to wear each day. On the first day of her induction, however, she was told that the real reason for staff all being dressed alike was to promote the bank's image with the customer. Each branch of the bank had the same type of furniture and fittings for exactly the same reason.

A lot of the initial training Carolyn underwent was intended to make her aware of the bank's products and services. At a later date she went on a number of specialised courses on customer care, marketing and sales. She had not expected this. She also had not expected to go on IT courses to learn about packages specifically designed to record details of customer satisfaction with the bank's services.

As she became more experienced, Carolyn went on another specialised course on which she was taught how to do telephone surveys of customer satisfaction. She learned, for instance, never to ring at teatime because clients disturbed in the middle of making a meal tended to be annoyed.

Carolyn is now very aware of the importance the bank places on customer satisfaction. There are various ways in which she is expected to help in this. First of all she has to talk face to face with customers and to deal with any complaints they have. For instance, at one period when the bank was seriously under-staffed, nearly every customer complained to her about having to wait so long in a queue. She pacified each one as best she could but then raised the matter with the manager. He reorganised the lunch rota so that as many people as possible could be on the counter at busy times.

Carolyn also has to send out customer feedback surveys on a regular basis to check on customer level of satisfaction on various issues – not only waiting times but the knowledge displayed by the counter staff, their attitude, their willingness to go and get help and so on. The results of these surveys are sent to regional and then head office, analysed by them and the manager and his staff are then made aware of what they have achieved – and what they need to put right!

One morning Carolyn had a particularly demanding customer who wanted some detailed information on a fairly complicated type of investment. Carolyn had to try hard to satisfy her and also to remain pleasant. It's a good job she did because the customer turned out to be a 'mystery shopper' employed by the bank to check on the way counter staff deal with the awkward customers. Again the results were sent to head office.

Carolyn now has a very different view of her role. She is dealing with figures all day long but she is also dealing with people. Asked which is the harder of the two jobs, Carolyn replies without hesitation: 'I really like most of my customers, particularly my regulars, but I can't afford to relax for a minute when I'm dealing with them. Dealing with figures is simple in comparison!'

Questions

1   *Carolyn works side by side with a number of other staff on the counter. She is nearly always busy with her own customers but she can't help noticing that the newest member of staff is struggling a bit, particularly with awkward customers. What action do you think she could take to help her colleague?*

2   *Carolyn is doing some customer feedback work. One of the customers she telephones says that he is thinking about changing his bank because the hours are not customer-friendly. He works full-time and cannot often get out of work to come to the bank in person. Suggest what Carolyn could say to the customer and do afterwards.*

3   *Carolyn's manager gives her an urgent task to do by the end of the day. She is working on this when she notices the counter staff are a bit under pressure. What do you think she should do?*

4   *One of the staff is terrified about being faced with a 'mystery shopper' and tries to avoid going on the counter. How do you think that problem could be solved?*

5   *One day two customers start arguing with each other about a personal matter (nothing to do with the bank). However, they are disturbing the other customers. What can the bank staff do – if anything?*

Case study Continued

6   *A regular customer cashes a cheque. Half an hour later he returns and says that he hasn't been given the right amount. The member of staff who dealt with him is out at lunch and Carolyn is the one now dealing with him. What should she do?*

Changing places

Your assessor will ask you how you will adapt your knowledge of managing and evaluating customer relations if you change your job in the future. You will need to think about the way in which aspects of these tasks if you worked for a different organisation.

Carla works at the reception desk in the town hall. Her role is to back up the other reception staff by dealing with any complaints made by the general public. She has detailed information about the departmental structure and the names and job titles and telephone extension numbers of everyone in each department. Whenever she deals with a complaint she has to record it on a computer database and note whether she dealt with it herself or whether she passed it on to another person. She also operates a follow-up system to check whether any action has been taken and, if so, what. This information is then passed to the chief executive.

Dominic works for a large computer firm. His job is to give customer back-up if anyone has difficulty in setting up a computer or following the operating instructions. He has to have a certain amount of technical knowledge but he also has to know when to consult a technical expert.

Ephraim is an administrator in a small organisation. Customer care is only one of his responsibilities and he has to deal with complaints alongside all his other jobs. The approach to customer care is informal. Once Ephraim has dealt with a complaint all he has to do is to make sure that his boss has a note of what has happened. His boss then raises it at the weekly management meeting if he thinks it is a complaint that is likely to happen again.

Chlöe works in the customer service section of a large insurance company. Her boss is responsible for all aspects of customer care and she is frequently involved in sending out customer feedback forms, checking to see how many have been returned and doing a first-stage analysis of the results. She is then part of the team that makes a more detailed analysis of the results and produces the information in a report to the managing director and other senior managers.

1 For any **one** person listed above, identify the differences he or she would find if moving to your organisation and doing your job.

2 For any **one** person listed above, say how you would need to adapt your skills if you did their job rather than your own.

Over to you

1 You work in the customer services section of a large store. You have a number of different methods of checking on customer feedback (look back to pages 234–6 to remind yourself of them) and each week your boss and the whole customer services team sit down to analyse what feedback has been given. This week your boss is pleased that the store has received a number of compliments and you are asked to send emails thanking those staff who have been individually named. However, you then get on to the complaints that have been made as shown below.

Example of an analysis of weekly complaints received by the customer services section of a large store

Week ending: 23 July 200–

Complaints	Number
Rude staff	1
Not enough staff	2
Signs difficult to follow	1
Goods advertised not available	3
Poor car parking	8
Too hot	3
Restaurant dirty	4

a In some cases only one complaint has been made. Do you think therefore that it is safe to ignore? If not, say why.

b Some complaints are very difficult to satisfy straight away. Which do you think they are, and why?

c Are there any complaints that could be dealt with almost immediately? If so, what are they?

d Who else do you think should be aware of these complaints, and why?

Over to you Continued

2   The store manager is discussing whether or not to introduce a customer loyalty scheme and on what basis. Ideas include rewarding loyalty for repeat custom, amount spent, orders for large quantities, and prompt payment. There is also some discussion about what customers will get for being loyal:

- a points card with a monetary value that increases every time the customer buys something and which can be traded in for vouchers or used to buy goods more cheaply

- a percentage discount on certain items when the customer has a certain number of points

- invitations to wine tasting sessions, fashion shows etc.

- previews of the new season's goods

- early access to sales events.

Your boss knows that you are the youngest member of the team – and the one most keen on shopping! He asks you to put yourself in the place of a customer and to say what would attract you most, and why. He also asks you for any new ideas you might have. Discuss with your tutor or trainer how you would reply.

Core unit links

Evidence that you encourage and accept feedback from other people to improve your own performance links to unit 301, performance indicators 16–18.

Evidence collection

You will need to prove to your assessor that you obtain and record customer feedback, analyse and evaluate this and take action to improve customer relations.

1   List all the ways in which you obtain customer feedback in your workplace. Then check that you can easily access all documentary records relating to the feedback you have obtained and recorded. If this is not summarised in any way, it may be useful to create a short log of the key points that have been identified through feedback sessions. Alternatively, if you collect feedback through focus groups or by email responses, check that you have copies of minutes or summaries that you have prepared or received – and similarly if outside agencies prepare feedback for you. Remember to include details of the actions that were taken as a result.

2   Write your own account identifying three or four occasions when you have made or suggested improvements as a result of feedback you received, from your internal or external customers. Ideally you

should support your claims with documentary evidence, but an alternative would be to ask your line manager to countersign and date your account to confirm its authenticity.

 Key skills reminder

If you are taking Key Skills awards, remember to discuss with your tutor or trainer how your evidence for this unit could also count towards those awards.

Research, analyse and report information

Unit summary and overview

This option unit is in two sections:

- research information
- analyse and report information.

It covers the activities required to obtain, record, analyse and report on information required by colleagues at work. It is suitable for you if you are regularly expected to find out information, either electronically or using paper-based sources, and present it appropriately.

The difficulty for many administrators today is in selecting the most appropriate sources and types of information for a particular task, especially given the vast amount available online. The secret is in agreeing specific aims and objectives before undertaking a search, as well as understanding how to research efficiently and accurately. The skills of organising information appropriately so that it can be analysed effectively, and presenting the final information in an appropriate format, are all covered in this unit.

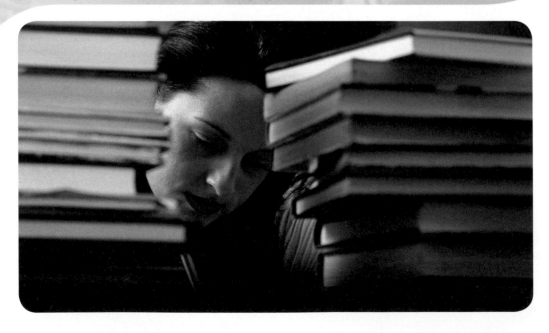

Research information

The importance of researching information efficiently and accurately

Your boss has been asked to chair a meeting to decide whether or not to introduce a new Intranet system. He asks you to do some initial research. You want to make a good impression, so you don't ask him too many questions. You also want to produce a quick result.

- You try to cut corners by accessing the Internet and running off a copy of any document that makes even a vague reference to an Intranet.
- You don't check how old the information is or whether it is just an attempt to sell a product.
- You don't check whether it is UK-based or for worldwide use.
- You put all the information into a folder without any explanation.

Your boss is not as pleased with your efforts as you thought he would be.

When researching you need to make sure that any information you produce is complete, to the point, current and understandable.

- **Completeness.** It is rare for all the information you want to be obtainable from one source only.
- **To the point.** Nearly anyone can download a document. What they don't want to do is to wade through pages of irrelevant information.
- **Current.** Out-of-date information can be downright dangerous in some instances – if, for example, you are checking legal rights and responsibilities.
- **Understandable.** Most people are very busy nowadays, so they want information that is easy to read.

The information must also be **accurate**. You don't get too many chances with this. If people suspect that the information you are giving them is not at least 99 per cent reliable then they are going to look elsewhere for help. At first sight this might seem quite simple. That is true in the case of downloading or photocopying material. Summarising it, however, is less simple. If, for instance, you are asked to summarise a set of figures, and you type 1000 instead of 10 000, you should not be surprised if your boss gets a bit snappy!

Links to core units

As you gather your evidence for this unit you should also obtain evidence for your core units. Watch for the CU link logo which suggests how the evidence you may collect could count towards both this unit and your core units.

Remember that you might be able to identify other links yourself, because of your own job role and the evidence you have obtained.

Talk to your assessor if you need further guidance on how your evidence should be cross-referenced.

Did you know?

In a recent survey of UK managers, over 80 per cent of them said that they valued accuracy above initiative.

Types of information you are required to obtain and analyse

What you are asked to do depends on your place of work. If you work for a university professor you will probably check through subject-related websites, academic journals and textbooks. If you work for a sales manager you may have to contact suppliers or manufacturers for product details, access relevant websites, check newspapers and journals for details of competitors' products and trawl through trade catalogues.

Agreeing aims, objectives and deadlines

You arrange to meet a friend. Your friend is not there when you arrive. Later on you found he had been there an hour earlier. When you finally meet you are dressed for a game of football, he's wearing a swimsuit. Neither of you is pleased. If you had planned the day from the outset it would have been a lot more enjoyable. The same applies to business – you need to establish right from the start exactly what is required. This is not always easy.

For instance, you may have a boss who is not quite sure what he wants. One day you find a note on your desk asking whether there is a first aider in the department. You find out that there is. You get a second note asking whether he is fully trained. He is. You get another few notes each asking for further information. You're beginning to get fed up.

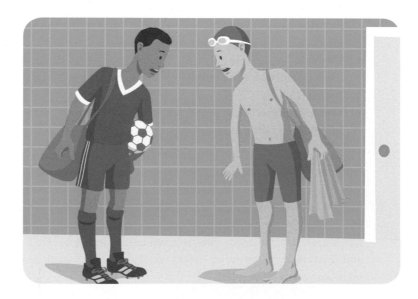

If your boss had sat down with you, you would have been able to get much further much more quickly.

How to... Agree aims and objectives

- **Find out *exactly* what is wanted.** If the information wanted is quite complex, you might want to summarise in writing what has been agreed so that there is less chance of any misunderstanding. See the table below.

- **If required, arrange a number of update meetings** to check that you are on the right lines and that your boss is still in agreement with what you are doing.

- **Sort out how you will go about finding the information required** – what sources you will use and in what order.

- **Allocate a specific period of time** to the research. If you don't get the full picture from the start you might have to carry out your research and present it bit by bit.

- **Put the information you find into a clear, concise document** rather than in a series of scrappy notes in response to your boss's equally scrappy notes.

Information requested	Date required	By whom	Date completed
• Number of trained first-aiders in the department	31 May 2007	(Initialled by person making request)	
• Review of the legal requirements			
• Check on whether any essential training is required			

Information sheet

Over to you

1   You may be surprised at how often you are called upon to do some research. Keep a diary of all sources of reference you use in a week. Copy the example below and complete it with the relevant information. Discuss with your tutor or trainer – or a colleague – whether this is a typical week.

Job title:			
Day/date:			
Information required and why (report, meeting etc.)	Outline of source used (website, personal contact etc.)	Time spent on research	How easy/ difficult it was to find
Details about Freedom of Information Act – required for seminar	Website – foi.gov.uk: email request for leaflet	15 minutes	Accessing website, easy. Seven days for leaflet to be sent from the Department of Constitutional Affairs

Diary information

2   You like your boss, but she can be a bit difficult. She travels a lot and many of your communications are via her mobile phone. When she asks for information she wants it virtually straight away. She doesn't like detail, saying that that's your job, and gets irritable if you ask too many questions. You're new to the job and sometimes when she wants some information you don't even know the right questions to ask to make sure you are doing the right thing.

Make some notes on how to cope with this and discuss them with your trainer or tutor and/or check your ideas with those on the CD-ROM.

Relevant information sources and search methods

The Internet

The Internet is now the main source of reference for many businesses. Suppose, for instance, you work in a firm that has recently had a computer system installed but it is not working properly. Your boss decides that legal action is required, but before going to a solicitor, which might be expensive, he asks you to find out whether there is anything else he can do. You access the Internet and type in the keywords 'legal disputes'. This leads you to 'mediation' and in turn to 'alternative dispute resolution' and an organisation, ADRnow.org.uk, that gives detailed information about the various approaches you can take when trying to solve a legal problem. It may not be the route you eventually take but it's given you a start.

Search engines

The Internet has tens of millions of sites but, unlike a library, has no index. That's where search engines come in.

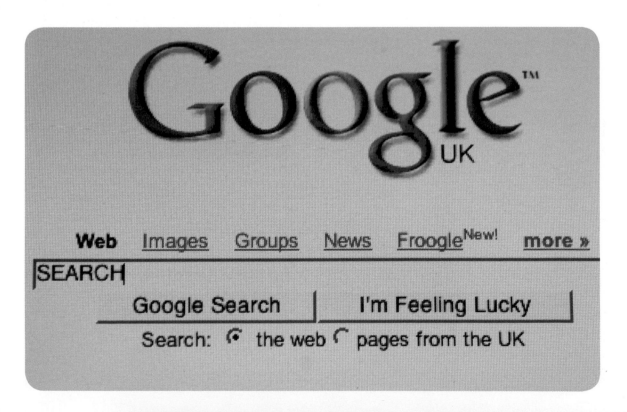

A search engine is a program that interrogates the Internet for fields or web pages containing or relating to words or phrases you enter into the search box. It involves a program called a 'spider' or 'robot' scouring all the websites it can get access to, recording all the information it finds and putting it in enormous databases.

Search engines vary in size, and work in different ways. However, they all allow for both simple and advanced level searches and usually include a help section listing the possible options for limiting your search – such as whether you want to trawl worldwide or limit your search to the UK. The table below has information on some of the more popular search engines.

Some of the most widely used search engines	
Altavista	One of the largest search engines on the web in terms of pages indexed. It has comprehensive coverage and a wide range of searching opportunities.
Ask Jeeves	A service that directs the user to the exact page to answer the question. If it can't find a match in its own database, it will give matching web pages from various search engines.
Excite	Another popular search service. It offers a medium-sized index and integrates non-web material such as company information into its results when appropriate. It has good news search services.
Google	Probably the most popular search engine. It is especially good at finding sites in response to general searches such as 'travel' or 'holidays'.
HotBot	Very like Altavista. It has a large index and good searching features.
Infoseek	A well-used search service. It has a small to medium-sized index so may not be totally suitable for a comprehensive search. However, it is very good for general searches.
Lycos	Features a very good directory of websites called Lycos Community Guides.
Northern Lights	A large index along with the ability to cluster documents by topics. It also has a set of 'special collection' documents from thousands of sources, including magazines.
WebCrawler	Because of its smaller index it is useful for people who might be overwhelmed by too many results of their initial search.
Yahoo!	A popular search service with a reputation for helping people to find information easily.

Did you know?

- **Search engines** such as Google and Yahoo! look for sites based on the information you enter in the search box.

- **Directories** put sites into categories instead of just listing them – e.g. the Yahoo Directory at http://uk.dir.yahoo.com or www.dmoz.org.

- **Portals** are sites that are used as a gateway either to the Internet or to a specialist topic – e.g. www.lycos.co.uk.

- **Forums** are sites where people give their views on an issue.

- **Business Directories** are lists of companies, products and services – e.g. www.kellysearch.com and www.applegate.co.uk.

Search terms (or key words)

Identifying your search terms can be quite easy. If you work in personnel (HR) and your boss asks you for information on the national minimum wage, those are the key words you would use. In other cases it is not quite as straightforward.

Suppose one of your friends phones and says she's pregnant. She picks your brains about a number of things but then floors you by saying that her partner is keen on taking paternity leave. She's heard that different companies offer different packages, but wants your advice. You need to think a bit more carefully about your search terms.

 How to... Find what you want on the Internet

- **Choose words that are key to your research**. In the case just mentioned, 'law' and 'paternity leave' would obviously be key. You might also identify 'other companies' as being relevant. The rest of the wording you can ignore for the time being.

- **'Explode' the relevant terms**. You can use 'paternity leave' right away. However, you might decide to explode 'law' into 'employment law' or even 'equal opportunities law'. If you use the word 'companies' you will get access to thousands of them. Therefore you might want to add some words such as 'light engineering companies' or 'companies in Lancashire' etc.

- **Combine your terms if required** by:

  - using the word AND – e.g. paternity leave AND light engineering businesses AND 'Lancashire'

  - using OR – e.g. Lancashire OR West Lancashire

  - putting the words in brackets – e.g. (Lancashire or West Lancashire)

  - putting the words in quotation marks – e.g. 'Lancashire' or 'West Lancashire'

  - decreasing the number of words by using the word NOT – e.g. Lancashire NOT West Lancashire.

 Did you know?

Have you ever typed in your own name as a search word to see what comes up? If you have, you're known as a 'vanity googler'!

Too much information?

Your boss asks you to get some information on the European Monetary Union. When you use the key words you find that the amount of information you have accessed is incredibly large. You therefore decide to place limits on your search.

- You start by restricting it to title only. If your key words appear in the title of an article or book then it is likely that the work will be relevant.
- You could restrict the search to material type. You might decide to limit it to journal articles only.
- You could restrict the search by year or date range (e.g. the most recent five years).

Too little information?

Your boss asks you to do some research on a very obscure sporting issue and your basic key word search does not produce anything relevant. You have either to admit defeat or do one last trawl.

- You can change the keywords or try alternatives, such as replacing 'sportspeople' with 'sportsmen' and/or 'sportswomen'.
- You can recheck the subject terms or descriptors that the database uses to describe any relevant material you happened to have found and using them as key words in your own search.
- You could check whether or not your database has a link to 'more references like this'.

Finding the information again

It is a good idea to **bookmark** your favourite websites so that you can access them directly, rather than going again through the search engine.

- With Netscape Navigator, for instance, you click on the 'Bookmarks' drop-down menu and click the 'Add Bookmark' option.
- With Microsoft's Internet Explorer, you click on the 'Favorites' drop-down menu and then click on 'Add to Favorites'. You can also click on the right mouse button while pointing at the page and you'll be offered the same option.

It is a good idea to make a regular check of these sites in exactly the same way that you do when you make a periodic update of your paper-based files. You can then weed out those that are no longer relevant and add in those that you are using more frequently.

Useful websites

Obviously, of the millions of sites available not all of them will interest you and you probably treat the Internet as a giant filing cabinet waiting for you to access it. Much depends, of course, on the nature of your work as to the websites you access most frequently – whether they be legal, commercial, educational etc. Many administrators, however, will at some time need to access government or official websites, and the table below gives some of the most useful addresses.

Official and Government websites	
The government information service	www.direct.gov.uk
Department of Trade and Industry	www.dti.gov.uk Among other things this site signposts you to: • Low Pay Commission • Equality Direct • Department for Education and Skills • Acas (Advisory, Conciliation and Arbitration Service) • Employment Tribunals Service • Business Link – Small Business Service • European Union • ILO (International Labour Organisation) • JobCentrePlus • Health and Safety Executive
Office of Fair Trading	www.oft.gov.uk
Department of Work and Pensions	www.dwp.gov.uk
Inland Revenue	www.hmrc.gov.uk
National Statistics Online	www.statistics.gov.uk
Official Labour Market Statistics	www.nomisweb.co.uk
Office for National Statistics	www.bized.ac.uk

Finding the site you want is only your first task. You then have to decide whether you can rely on the information it gives you. To do this you have to use the same skills as you would when reading a particular newspaper. Is it left- or right-wing? Is it eager to sensationalise? Does it want to entertain rather than to inform? and so on.

If you are not convinced that the information is reliable, don't use it!

Did you know?

There has been an explosion of online diaries (or 'blogs'), according to the web monitoring firm, Technorati. Cadbury's is now using 'blogs' from its existing employees as part of its campaign to attract new staff!

How to... Check on the quality of a website

Don't use it in these circumstances:

- You are not clear who has written the information.

- You do not fully understand the aims of the writer. Does he or she want to give an opinion, make a political statement, sell something?

- You cannot check out the information, because it is a statement of opinion rather than fact or is too general to be checked.

- You are looking at information that is undated or several years old.

- You are reading biased information with one point of view only being given.

Do use it if you think it is:

- truthful

- factual

- free from personal bias

- up to date.

Your organisation's Intranet

If you work in a big organisation and have easy access to the Internet you are likely also to have access to an Intranet, which is an in-house information network.

- **An Intranet is easy to access**. It is there at the press of a button. Long gone are the days when a vital update reaches your boss's desk and sits there without you even being aware of its existence.

- **An Intranet is easy to update**. If anyone wants to let you know of a change to the current health and safety regulations, previously they would have had to send a memo or email to everyone in the organisation – or to those they could trust to pass on the information. The master document would then have had to be manually amended by each individual. The Intranet achieves this in minutes.

However, because each system tends to be tailor-made for the individual organisation, you may find that the amount and type of information each contains varies widely.

Some Intranets are very basic. They give information about the organisational structure, the names, job titles and telephone numbers of all the staff and very little else. Others expand on this by giving details

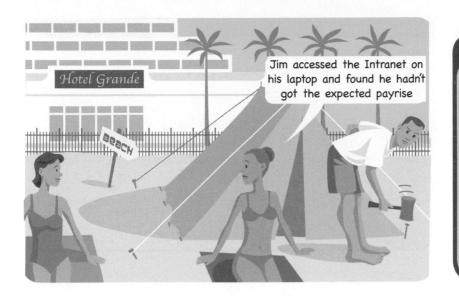

Jim accessed the Intranet on his laptop and found he hadn't got the expected payrise

of the organisation itself, its products and services and the work carried out by each department or section. Nowadays many concentrate on human resource issues such as staff terms and conditions, grievance and disciplinary procedures, training opportunities, health and safety requirements etc.

Snapshot – People before systems!

One organisation that specialises in setting up Intranet systems always starts by trying to get the staff on board. Without staff cooperation, it reasons, the Intranet is almost bound to fail. It asks questions like these:

- Is the organisation happy with the present setup? If so, go no further.

- Is it quite small and communications easy?

- Is it large and communications poor?

- Are all staff aware of what each area is doing?

- Do some work areas keep everything to themselves?

- Is there a good existing system of communication which an Intranet might improve upon?

- Does it have to start from scratch?

- Is any information 'shared' already.

- Are there any core documents that have to be included?

Snapshot Continued

● Is there going to be a named person responsible for it?

It then starts to 'sell' the idea to the staff.

● It does not rely on the Intranet to sell itself.

● It uses other media such as posters, memos, emails, meetings, training sessions etc. to make the advantages clear, as well as making it clear that staff will be expected to use this as a method of communication.

● It expects complaints and tries to handle the complainants gently!

Only then does it start on the actual installation!

Other sources of reference

Marvellous though the Internet is as a source of reference, it is not the only source. Talking to people both inside and outside the organisation, looking through your office files, using the library and checking journal articles can be equally useful.

People-based sources by personal contact

You are in the office one day and start listing the jobs you need to do.

● Your boss is going on a sales trip to Brussels and Antwerp next month and you need to start making the arrangements.

Did you know?

Research has shown that people pick up a lot more information first time round through talking to someone than they do when reading the same information – however simply it is written.

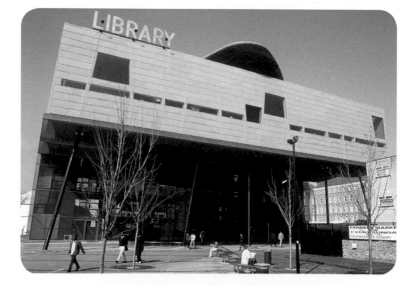

- You want to amend the terms and conditions of employment in a job description.
- Your boss wants some up-to-date information about the latest legislation on disciplinary and grievance procedures.

You can get the information you want from a number of sources. However, the easiest way in each of the above instances may be to ask someone. Someone in the office may have recently been to Brussels on holiday and be able to give you some travel tips. A member of staff in the HR department may be able to update you immediately about the terms and conditions of employment. Someone at Acas should be able to provide you with information about disciplinary and grievance procedures – and so on.

People know a lot. Think how often people consult *you* about something, and how often you ask other people for information both inside and outside the organisation. It's quick, easy and direct. If you don't understand something, you ask a question and it becomes clearer. If you don't get the information you want, the person you are asking may be able to direct you to someone who can tell you.

If you want further information you can go back to the original source – although it is not a good idea to keep approaching the same person with a variation on the same query. Make certain that you have a good idea of what you want to know before making the approach, otherwise you might wear out your welcome quickly.

It is good practice to warn people beforehand that you need some information. Bouncing in to see them just as they are in the middle of an important telephone conversation or writing a complicated report might not be the best idea, particularly if you want their full cooperation.

Obviously you have to know the person you are asking for information. If the person is notoriously slapdash or forgetful you will be less eager to accept what he or she says than if you know the person to be reliable and trustworthy. You have to use either your prior knowledge of that person – or remember good or bad experiences!

Telephone contact with people

Unless the person you want to speak to personally is in the next office, the best method of making contact is by telephone or email. Like every other source of reference, however, it can be frustrating if you do not have the telephone number immediately to hand. If you have access to an Intranet, that is useful. If not, you have to have your own telephone indexing system, either computer- or paper-based. Make sure it is up to date.

Did you know?

In a recent office survey, workers in an open-plan office were asked to list the five things that distracted them most from their work. Nearly everyone put the unexpected 'dropper in' at the top of their list.

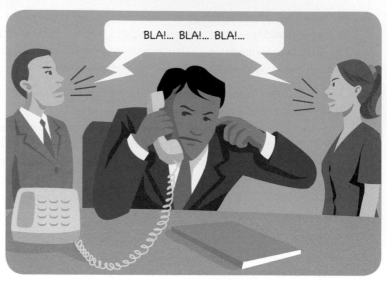

When making a phone call, make sure you will be able to hear the other end of the line!

The same rules apply when asking for information via the telephone as when talking to someone directly. However, it is a good idea to *practise your listening skills*. It is surprising what a difference personal contact makes. If, for instance, you are talking to someone face to face you are not just listening to what is being said, you are also observing body language, and possibly reading relevant documents or a computer screen together. You cannot do that over the telephone.

If you think you are going to have difficulty following what someone is saying on the phone, choose another form of communication or make certain that you write down as near as possible word for word what you are told. You can then sort it out later in your own time when you have more chance of understanding the information.

Make sure you can hear properly. The best listener in the world is helpless if he or she is making a phone call in a busy office with phones ringing, people talking, equipment being used etc.

Try to avoid being interrupted during the telephone call. If you keep breaking off to talk to someone else or to answer another phone, you are not improving your chances of being given total cooperation.

Paper-based sources

How many times a day do you open your filing cabinet? You probably do this more often than you think even if you do have a computer database. If, for instance, you work in a human resources section you might find during the course of one day that you need:

- documents to be used at job interviews, including lists of questions to be asked, how the candidates are going to be assessed and the letters of reference
- copies of the minutes of a previous meeting together with the handwritten notes made by the chair
- office equipment catalogues.

You may be able to access some of this information from a database, but it is equally probable that much of it will be stored in your paper-based filing system. A lot has been written about the 'paperless office', but even now, despite all the advances in computerised filing systems, many administrators still like to store at least some of their material in a filing cabinet. This includes:

- long documents
- catalogues, sales literature, promotional material etc.
- equipment instructions and handbooks

Useful contacts

- Internal staff – personnel, computer services, catering, security, accounts etc.
- External clients/customers
- Local/reference library
- Council departments (You may have contact with several departments. If so include the main telephone number together with the departmental extension number.)
- Local councillors/MP
- Police/fire brigade
- Individual advisers – solicitors, accountants, Inland Revenue, VAT, Health and Safety Executive, insurance companies etc.
- Security/burglar alarm personnel
- Maintenance personnel – plumbers, electricians, industrial cleaners etc.
- Office suppliers/computer services personnel
- Travel agencies/tour operators
- AA/RAC/National Breakdown
- Airline offices
- Local taxi/car hire firms
- Passport/immigration offices
- Professional bodies – Law Society, British Insurance Brokers' Association etc.
- Trade Associations, Horticultural, Glass and Glazing etc.
- Banks
- Trade unions
- JobCentrePlus (local branch)
- Department of Work and Pensions (local branch)
- Local college(s)
- Management/training consultants
- Local newspaper(s)

Find out

Check your computer database or paper files to see that you have a list of all relevant telephone numbers, names and addresses and email addresses of people and organisations that you contact on a regular basis. Compare it with the sample list of people/ services given in the table opposite.

- clients' files of correspondence – or any information sent to you from an external source
- all original documents.

If you do have such a system by now you have probably selected the filing classification that suits you best and have refined it to meet your exact requirements. However, every so often it is a good idea to check that the system still meets your requirements, and that no other system would be an improvement.

Libraries

You work for a firm specialising in renting out country cottages in Scotland. Your boss wants to produce a brochure outlining not only what type of properties are on offer but also details of their surroundings. You are asked to do some research on Scotland and to find out anything of romantic or historic interest about the places where the cottages are situated. You have a number of options:

- You can go to the Internet.
- You can contact the Scottish Tourist Information Board.
- You can have a look at some travel brochures.

However, you can also check in the local library. You might find there not only travel guides but also biographies of famous Scottish people, cookbooks with Scottish recipes for Aberdeen Angus beef or Loch Fyne salmon, and gardening books giving advice on how to grow a Scottish thistle! It should not take you long to gather enough snippets of information to make the brochure much more interesting and attractive.

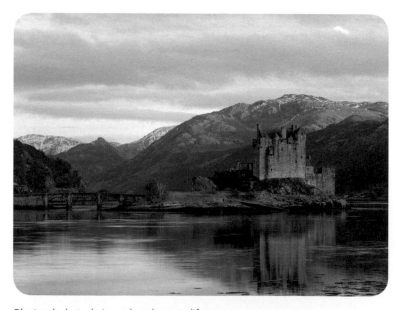

Photos help to bring a brochure to life

Nowadays most libraries:

- store information in a variety of different formats on site, which allows immediate access to a large body of information both via the Internet and its own online catalogues
- provide extensive local information on what is going on in the area
- offer back-up support to schools, colleges and businesses
- offer a service to the housebound
- give training in the use of email and/or the Internet.

Librarians are trained to help you. If you are in any doubt about how to find something, talk to one of them. In smaller libraries, however, you will probably be able to find the material you want directly by getting to know the layout, and in particular the areas housing the subjects you are most likely to need.

It is a good idea to familiarise yourself with the online library catalogue. As with the Internet, you may find yourself with just too much information at first and need to refine your search, but most libraries have now paid quite a bit of attention to website design and to making their online systems 'user-friendly'.

Magazines and journals

At work you may find that you need certain magazines or journals that relate particularly to the work of your organisation. Nowadays you can choose between ordering paper-based copies or using a subscription database on the Internet.

A quick scan through any of the Internet search engines will produce a number of sites offering you access to a wide range of journals that are available through subscription and relevant to your job. However, your library again comes in useful if you or your boss need to look at journals only occasionally.

- You can check its stock periodically without any hassle from a sales person.
- You can actually look through the journals on display to see whether they are what your boss really wants.
- Even with the financial restraints placed on libraries these days, you can still ask for a particular journal to be added to those in stock or at least to make arrangements for it to be loaned from another library. Obviously, the more mainstream the subject, the more successful you are likely to be. Asking for a journal on hand-weaving or trout farming to be added to the library stock might receive less attention than asking for one on business, accountancy or statistics!

Did you know?

Libri, a charity for libraries, says that although four out of five people visit a library for books, only 9 per cent of a library's budget is now spent on books. It maintains that this spending on other activities will eventually result in all books being destined for the skip!

Did you know?

Most libraries still use what is known as the Dewey Decimal System of classification. This is so precise that it allows you to find the exact location of a single book in a library containing thousands of them.

Did you know?

Sellers of subscription databases claim that online journals are better than paper-based ones because they allow:

- immediate access to the most current edition
- access by more than one person at a time
- access to back numbers.

They also avoid clutter in the office and the possibility that someone might lose a journal, take it home or put it in the bin by mistake!

The table below lists some of the major business-related periodicals.

Frequently used business-related periodicals

Accountancy	Industrial Relations Journal
British Accounting Review	Information Systems Journal
British Journal of Industrial Relations	Investor's Chronicle
Bulletin of the ECC	Journal of Business Finance &
Business	Accounting
Chartered Secretary	Journal of Management Studies
Company Lawyer	Journal of Marketing
Computers in Industry	Journal of Small Business &
Economic Journal	Enterprise Development
Economic Review	Labour Market Trends
Economist	Labour Research
European Business Review	Law Quarterly Review
European Industrial Relations Review	Management Accounting
European Journal of Industrial	Public Administration
Relations	Public Law
European Journal of Marketing	Quality Management Journal
European Law Review	Statistical News
Harvard Business Review	Strategic Management Journal
Health & Safety at Work	Tax Advisor
Human Relations	Total Quality Management
Human Resource Management	Training & Development
Journal	Training Journal
Industrial Law Journal	

Newspapers

Most newspapers have an online edition nowadays. They are useful for all sorts of up-to-the minute information. Among other things they can give you details of:

- any changes in the law that might affect your organisation
- activities of competitors
- financial trends
- employment issues
- the job market.

The importance of maintaining a record of sources – and how to do so

You work for the Leisure Services Department of your local council. There is to be a promotions week when a number of different sporting events will take place. Each of these events will be opened by a sports personality. Everyone taking part will be presented with a certificate of achievement, a short biography of each of the sporting personalities,

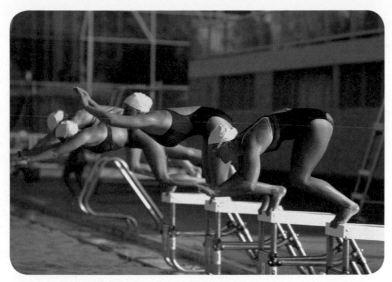

Sports personalities help to pull in the crowds

and a glossy colour brochure about the department. The week will end with a buffet to which a number of well-known local people will be invited. You are asked to research the following information:

- the background history of the sports personalities
- the history of all the sports and activities involved in the event
- the type and prices of brochures that could be produced both in-house and from external printers
- what the in-house catering facilities are like and what options they offer
- those people to whom you think invitations should be sent.

You spend a lot of time on this research and think you have done a good job, and so initially does your boss. Things then start to fall apart a bit when she asks you the following questions:

- 'Are you sure Glen is 65? I thought he was still playing first-team football.' – You think you must have made a typing error but you cannot find the note on which you scribbled the information.
- 'I liked what you said about the first Olympic Games but could you give me a bit more?' – You would if you could think which website you accessed on the Internet.
- 'Are you sure you've contacted all the schools in the area? Surely there are more than four.' – You don't know off the top of your head.
- 'Are all the caterers willing to provide vegetarian food?' – You threw away the initial correspondence after you had summarised it.

All is not lost. You can start again and find answers to your boss's questions. However, you've created a lot of extra work for yourself.

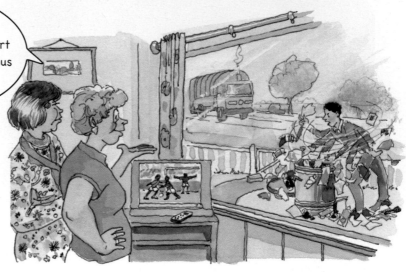

It's an interesting conflict – the receipt to support his expenses claim versus the World Cup live.

Did you know?

One local authority reports that its refuse collection department receives a number of desperate telephone calls each year from people who have thrown away important papers and who are trying to get them back. Normally by that time it's too late to do anything about it.

Ideally, every time you are asked to carry out any research, you should try to remember to keep hold of any original documents – letters, quotes, photocopies of articles etc. – and also make a note of where you found the information.

How to... Keep a record of your sources

- If you ask someone for information, make sure that you note the name, job title if relevant, telephone number and email address.

- If you've consulted someone in a large organisation, make sure that you have not only the organisation's telephone number but also the individual's extension number.

- If you email for information and receive an emailed reply, keep copies of both of them.

- If you write to someone, make sure that you have a copy of what you send and the reply.

- If you access the Internet, write down details of the relevant sites.

- If you find the information you require from a journal or book, make a note of the title, author and page number – and where the original is stored – office, library etc.

Over to you

1   The table lists the features of a good filing system. Check it against your own filing system and discuss with your tutor or trainer *either* why you think your system meets your own particular needs *or* if and why you are thinking of changing it to another one.

Features of a good filing system

How does your filing system shape up? Decide whether you can tick Yes or No against each item given below.

- Simple
- Useful for miscellaneous papers
- Able to introduce new headings without disturbing the entire system
- Extremely accurate
- Able to allow you to use the file number as a reference on correspondence
- Able to allow you to classify a document by location
- Able to keep all documents on one topic together
- Direct (with no index needed)
- Capable of unlimited expansion
- Useful in specialist research areas
- Linked with an index that is used for other purposes
- Easy to use without cross-reference
- Easy to forecast in terms of space requirements
- Less time-consuming to set up
- Free from difficulties in deciding on a subject title and from the possibility that more than one file might be opened for the same subject

2   Visit your local or college library and check that you understand how the books are ordered so that you can find both books you can borrow and reference books you can access on the premises. Then check the electronic sources of information that are available as well as the newspapers and business journals kept in the library. List six items that will be of help to you in your job, based on the type of information searches you are asked to make.

Evidence collection

Prepare a form that will enable you to record and summarise the information for each search you make and the outcome. This will make it easier to talk about the scope of your job with your assessor during a professional discussion, and will make it easier to provide appropriate product evidence as requested.

Core unit links

Focusing on information you are asked to provide and selecting and reading written material and identifying and extracting the main points links to unit 301, performance indicators 1, 6 and 7. Planning and agreeing appropriate targets and being accountable for your work may link to unit 301 PIs 8–15.

If any of the information you handle is confidential, then this may link to unit 302, PI 15.

Evidence collection Continued

Start by allowing space for your name and the person who has asked for the information. Below this you will include the aims, objectives and deadlines for the search and then the relevant sources of information you have identified. You will then summarise the appropriate information you have obtained, record the source in each case and, if you have copied or downloaded information, include its current location for reference. Finally, you need space to state the format in which you will present the information and any feedback you receive.

Retain any written instructions or information you are given by your colleagues in relation to searches you are asked to make, as well as any notes you make yourself, and attach these to the appropriate search forms.

Analyse and report information

Getting organised

When you first start researching something it is very tempting to print reams of information from the Internet, take lots of photocopies, note down the results of telephone calls etc., putting each one into a filing tray as you go along. That's fine. The danger arises when you sit down to try to make sense of it and find that it's a bit overwhelming. At that stage you might find yourself picking up each document in turn, looking at it vaguely and then returning it to the basket having done nothing about it. You *can* make life easier for yourself!

How to... Organise your information

- **Examine** the material you have gathered together and make a list of all the various categories of information. If you have prepared a special filing system for yourself, that should be quite simple. In the case of the leisure department promotion, for instance, you might decide to:

- have categories – catering, printing etc.

- list all documents belonging to each category in date order

- make out an index of all names, telephone numbers and email addresses of those people you think you may need to contact more than once during your research.

- **Interpret** the material by taking each category at a time, checking the information you have gathered under that heading, and, if it's rather long or complicated, make a brief summary of it.

- **Extract** the relevant material by:

  - looking through it again and crossing or taking out any information that is irrelevant or that you already have

  - drafting out a first paragraph of the document you have been asked to prepare and checking it against your originals to see that you have included everything

  - repeating the exercise with all the categories

  - checking the final result.

At this stage you might find that you have too much information, or that some of it is very repetitive. If so, be ruthless and cut it down. In contrast, there may be some definite gaps. If so, go back to the Internet, library, helpful colleague etc.

Preparing the final document

Remember the basic rules for the preparation of any document.

- Look at your draft information. At this stage do not be too bothered about detail but concentrate on the general framework. Make a note at the appropriate place of any charts etc. that will be required. Then take another look at it and decide whether you are pleased with the initial effect.

- Start preparing the final version, bearing in mind the basic summarising principles.

- Use short rather than long sentences, and simple rather than complicated sentence and paragraph structures.

- Keep reminding yourself of your audience. Is it for senior management, is it for new trainees, or is it for your boss's eyes only?

- Check that your vocabulary is clear and easy to understand. Do not use jargon or initials that might not be familiar to all your readers.

- Check that it is properly punctuated and grammatically correct.

Remember

Check unit 301, pages 27–9, if you want to remind yourself how to summarise!

- Check that it is not too long – or so short that some vital information is squeezed out.
- Check the numbering system.
- Check the general layout for these points:
  - correct typeface (Arial, Times New Roman etc.)
  - good use of formatting (italic, bold etc.)
  - consistent use of line spacing
  - appropriate use of graphic symbols (bullets, asterisks, leader dots etc.)
  - appropriate use of capitals/underscore/boxes etc.

Acknowledging where you found your material

Sometimes you might be asked to say where you found the information in case anyone wants to have a look at that source for further details. You can do this in a number of ways, using footnotes, appendices or a bibliography.

There are two basic ways of including footnotes. One is to put a small superscript number (e.g. [1]) at the end of the sentence or word in which a quotation or reference is included. The full reference is then displayed either at the bottom of the page or in a list at the end of the section or chapter.

Another method is to use what is known as the Harvard system. Instead of entering a footnote number in the text, put a basic reference in brackets (e.g. Carysforth, Rawlinson & Chadwick, 2006, pp. 22–25) and then display the full details at the end of the document.

You can create an appendix if you want to refer to more detailed information that is too extensive for a footnote. In one document, for instance, you might have summarised some information from the staff handbook. Your boss might ask you to put the full version in an appendix, to be consulted by anyone who is interested in having more detail.

In some documents you might be asked to include details of any journal articles, books etc. you have used. In that case a bibliography, normally in alphabetical order, can be placed at the end of the document. This book might be referenced thus: e.g. Carysforth, Rawlinson & Chadwick, *Business and Administration NVQ Level 3*, Heinemann, Oxford, 2006.

Responding to feedback

If you have spent a lot of time preparing a document it is difficult to step back from it and see it objectively. Try to let someone else give you feedback at this stage. The other person can give you answers to these questions:

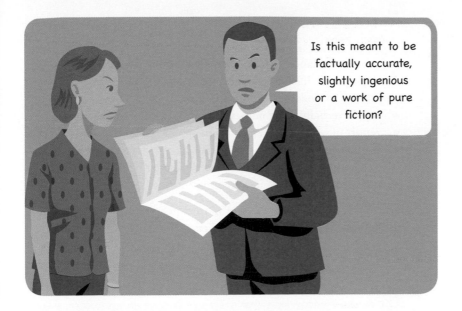

- Have you kept to your terms of reference, or have you strayed off into other areas by mistake – or because you happen to be particularly interested in them?
- Have you covered everything necessary?
- Have you been factually accurate? You can look at something time after time and not notice a mistake whereas someone else might spot it straight away.
- Have you put equal emphasis on each area and not been carried away with something that is particularly interesting, leaving out the boring stuff?
- Have you not been too subjective? If you feel very strongly about something you might have unconsciously let your feelings show too clearly.

Sometimes, you can 'play about' with the research too much, trying to get it perfect or constantly finding something else to include. If you are not careful you can start missing deadlines just because you want to put in that little bit extra. If you make arrangements with a colleague or a line manager to check through the first draft, you are forcing yourself to get it ready on time.

Formats of reporting that may be required

You have had a busy time researching over the past few weeks, but now you must concentrate on the finished result. The format you will use will probably depend on the type of information you have been asked to research, as well as its purpose.

Suppose, for instance, your boss has asked you to research the latest developments in the unauthorised use of email in the office. You could report back in a number of different ways:

- **report verbally** using notes you've prepared for yourself
- **report in writing** – in an email, memo or more formally as a report
- **summarise the information** to include only the very basic points to be put on the staff noticeboard, newsletter or bulletin or to be included as an agenda item at a meeting.

You might, of course, have to reproduce it in a number of different formats, each one for a different audience.

Remember

For fuller details of how to prepare information in various formats, see unit 301, pages 7–13.

Case study Seek and you shall find!

Read the case study below and then answer the questions that follow. Then check your answers with those on the CD-ROM.

Parveen Dhala works in the Citizens Advice Bureau as an adviser. She sees a large number of clients each week and advises them on a wide range of issues.

On one day, for instance, she might deal with a client who wants a divorce, a client whose new washing machine keeps breaking down, a client who wants details about emigrating to Australia and a client who has just been made redundant. On the day after she might be faced with an equally wide variety of issues. No wonder her head is spinning at the end of each day.

Obviously she cannot rely on her memory or general knowledge to solve all these problems. On each occasion she has to check the Internet, the in-house information system or one of a number of handbooks – on employment law, welfare benefits, fuel rights, consumer remedies etc. She frequently has to contact a number of specialist services – the local council, social services, electricity, gas and water suppliers, the Inland Revenue, Acas and so on. She also taps into her colleagues' experience wherever she can.

Parveen is now training to become a specialist adviser. She enjoys dealing with employment queries and is going on a number of courses aimed at training her to help clients with employment problems. She is even being trained to help clients prepare for and take a case to an employment tribunal. When her training has finished she will see clients by appointment only and will be able to spend much more time with them.

She really enjoys her job because she likes meeting people and the sense of satisfaction she gets when she feels she has helped someone. The downside, of course, is that she cannot always help and she then feels a sense of failure. She also gets a bit frustrated when she cannot get a client the information he or she needs. One day she sat at the end of the phone for at least 45 minutes before someone at a debt management firm actually picked up the receiver.

Parveen also likes the research part of her job. She loves trawling through the Net and hunting through books and leaflets and has a real sense of achievement when she finds what she wants.

Parveen's advice to anyone who wants to be a researcher is: 'Take your time, be thorough and always double check!'

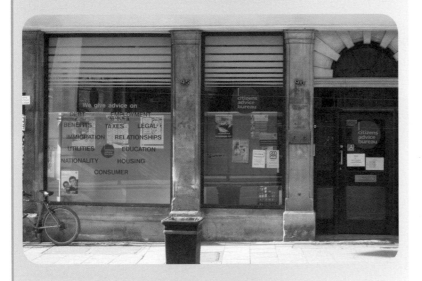

Questions

1 *Parveen not only has to find the information for her clients, she also has to explain it to them. How do you think she can check that they understand what she has said to them?*

2 *Parveen often has to try to get some information via the telephone. Nowadays, however, particularly when she is dealing with a large organisation, she is frequently put into a queuing system and it is some time before anyone answers. How do you think she can get around that problem?*

Case study Continued

3   *Occasionally Parveen finds a leaflet or a booklet on the shelves that is out of date and therefore unreliable. How can she make sure that her written sources of information are up to date?*

4   *The case sheets Parveen writes up after seeing each client are put on to a computer database and checked by a supervisor. If the supervisor thinks some further action should be taken she sends a note. Parveen is always busy with clients and tends to put answering the notes at the bottom of her 'to do' list. However, the notes start piling up and the supervisor becomes more insistent. How would you advise Parveen to make time to answer the notes?*

5   *A lot of information Parveen deals with is very confidential and she knows not to discuss it even with family and friends. She shouldn't even say who has called in to the bureau, never mind what they want. However, one day a friend calls in to ask whether her mother is there. She's noticed her car outside and the parking time has nearly expired. What should Parveen do?*

Discuss your ideas with your tutor or trainer and check your ideas with the suggestions on the CD-ROM.

Changing places

Your assessor will ask you how you will adapt your knowledge of researching, analysing and reporting information if you change your job in the future. You will need to think about the way in which aspects of these tasks would change if you worked for a different organisation.

Faizal works in the reference section of a public library. He has to access a wide variety of information via the library's online system, the Internet and the book and journal collection. He has a particular responsibility for helping school children with local history projects and often has to contact local museums and heritage centres for information for them. He also helps them produce their finished documents.

Randall works in a local authority housing department and has to deal with clients claiming various welfare benefits. He therefore has to make sure that he is fully aware of all the up-to-date legislation and current benefit rates. He does this by checking the latest editions of the welfare rights handbooks and keeping in telephone contact with the Department of Social Security, Department of Work and Pensions and the Disability Benefits Unit.

Mel works for a sales director who spends most of her time travelling in the UK and abroad. She has bookmarked all the relevant travel sites on the Internet and uses them virtually daily. She has a personal folder of travel tips including information about good hotels, the most efficient rail services, local travel agencies, details about various airports etc. She updates this at the end of each trip.

Jillian's boss is a research physicist. She has to make sure that he has online access to the latest scientific journals including subscription access to those sites not available to the general public. She has to make regular checks of the stock in various specialist libraries. She has to check that all his articles have the correct references and has to be particularly careful to remind him about copyright when he is preparing various articles for publication.

1   For any *one* person listed above, identify the differences he or she would find if moving to your organisation and doing your job.

2   For any *one* person listed above, say how you would need to adapt your skills if you did their job rather than your own.

 Over to you

You work for a public relations (PR) officer who is a very busy person.

● She travels a lot in the UK. She sometimes uses her car. Where rail travel is convenient she uses the train. She also has to spend some time travelling abroad.

● She has to keep an eye on what is going on in the media, particularly the newspapers.

● She has to prepare all the press releases and other publicity documents and must make sure they are grammatically correct and properly spelled.

● She is responsible to her boss for keeping her up to date on employment law issues.

She asks you to 'bookmark' a number of useful websites in each area. Discuss with your tutor or trainer which websites you would choose, and check your ideas with those on the CD-ROM.

Core unit links

Remember that information is normally needed for a purpose and this is likely to relate to your organisation's main purpose and values. This may link to unit 302, performance indicators 1–5.

Communicating information to others clearly and accurately is likely to link to unit 301, PIs 2–7, and taking account of feedback links to unit 301 PIs 16–18.

Working cooperatively with colleagues to meet their needs may link to unit 301, PIs 22–28, and to unit 302, PIs 11 and 12.

Note that if you are asked to carry out a specific information search related to employment responsibilities and rights or risk management, this may link to unit 302, PIs 7 and 21.

Evidence collection

1   Record the results of any searches you have undertaken on the appropriate search forms that you prepared on page 275. Attach any analysis summaries you prepared. Remember that you do not need to attach all the information you copied or downloaded, nor do you need to attach your final summary document provided that you note down the location where these can be found so that you can show them to your assessor on request.

2   Attach to the search form any written feedback you received from your colleagues as a result of the search you made and the information you obtained.

3   Prepare a personal statement that says how you have carried out specific searches. Ask the colleague who gave you the work to countersign and date both this and the related search form to confirm that your statement is correct.

What if...?

What should you do if no feedback is necessary during the assessment period?

Your assessor can give you a dedicated task to cover the knowledge and understanding required. This will then be followed by a professional discussion where you can explain how you would perform in such a situation and what evidence you might bring forward.

Key skills reminder

If you are taking Key Skills awards, remember to discuss with your tutor or trainer how your evidence for this unit could also count towards those awards.

Plan, organise and support meetings

Unit summary and overview

This option unit is divided into three sections:

- prepare for a meeting
- at the meeting
- after the meeting.

This option unit relates to the responsibilities of an administrator for arranging and ensuring the smooth running of meetings at work. This is suitable for you if, as part of your job, you plan and prepare meetings, support meetings and undertake follow-up activities. The meetings you arrange may be formal or informal, but to satisfy the requirements of the unit you will need to be involved in preparing an agenda and meeting papers as well as preparing a record of the meeting afterwards. If the meetings at your workplace are very informal then it would be wise to check the full specification of the unit with your assessor to confirm that this unit will be appropriate for you.

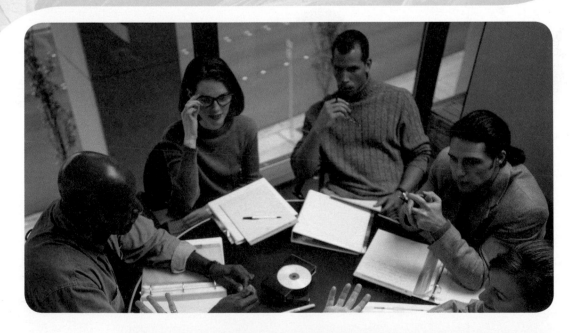

Link to core units

As you gather your evidence for this unit you should also obtain evidence for your core units. Watch for the CU link logo which suggests how the evidence you may collect could count towards both this unit and your core units.

Remember that you might be able to identify other links yourself, because of your own job role and the evidence you have obtained.

Talk to your assessor if you need further guidance on how your evidence should be cross-referenced.

The unit focuses on your role in relation to the way you prepare for meetings, support meetings, produce minutes of meetings and follow up action points. While this role can be unnerving for many people until they become familiar with the tasks involved, the skills required are invaluable for all administrators as meetings are so commonly held in every type of organisation. This unit includes hints and tips to help you to support all types of meetings with confidence.

Prepare for a meeting

The role of the person organising and supporting the meeting

It is hard to avoid meetings even if you work in the smallest of offices. At one end of the scale you might find yourself sitting with a few colleagues organising next week's diary. At the other end you might be sitting next to your manager in a management meeting assisting him or her by taking notes.

Meetings can be wonderful or dreadful. If you have just come out of a meeting where everyone has contributed and you've made a lot of progress you'll feel great. If you come out of one that has lasted for ever, where everyone has fallen out, nothing has been decided – and you

Did you know?

Apologies to male readers! Research has found that women are better than men at doing more than one thing at once and that at work they can keep track of a whole range of small 'to do' jobs. That's what makes them particularly good at organising meetings.

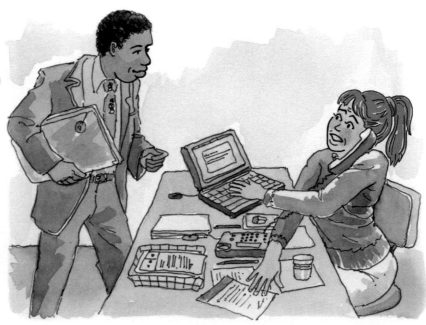

didn't even get a cup of tea and biscuit – you'll try every which way not to attend the next one.

Meetings need to be organised, and if you're a good organiser you can make all the difference to their success.

 How to... Organise and support meetings

- **Before the meeting**:
  - Circulate all the relevant paperwork.
  - Check that the chairperson is fully informed.
  - Check on who is coming and who has sent apologies.
  - Book the meeting place.
  - Check that the reception staff know about the meeting and any visitors who may arrive.
  - Remind smokers of any no-smoking policy.
  - Check on any equipment required – power points etc.
  - See that refreshments are available.
  - Check on car parking if necessary.
  - Get there before anyone else!
- **During the meeting**:
  - Have a supply of spare agendas, notes of previous meetings, etc. – someone is sure to have forgotten them.
  - Check the room itself, for tidiness, warmth, space etc.
  - Keep a look out for any new members so that you can welcome them – and remind the chairperson to do the same.
  - Take notes.
  - Be ready to provide back-up information.
- **After the meeting**:
  - Check that the date of the next meeting is entered in everyone's diary – particularly the chairperson's.
  - Draft out the notes and let the chairperson have them.
  - Send a copy to all the members.
  - Deal with any other paperwork – letters, memos, emails etc. – that have been asked for at the meeting and carry out any other follow-up action.
  - Bring the meetings file up to date.
  - Assess what went well and what needs improving, even down to the quality of the refreshments served by the canteen staff!

Planning and supporting meetings effectively and efficiently

Kerry dreads organising staff meetings. She knows that something will go wrong:

- She always forgets to plan ahead. The staff are never told until the very last minute where and when the meeting will take place. She even forgets to order tea.
- She leaves preparing the agenda until the very last minute.
- She never asks anyone if they want an item putting on the agenda.
- She never checks the notes of the previous meeting to see what various people have agreed to do – and, if necessary, give them a reminder.
- She doesn't consult her boss who is chairing the meeting until the day of the meeting itself, and doesn't tell her of any possible problems that might arise – such as a key member not being able to attend.
- She is often the last to arrive.
- She tries to do too much at the meeting – take the notes, serve the tea, answer telephone calls on her mobile etc.
- She is so relieved when it is over that she stuffs all the notes into her filing tray and tries to forget about them. By the time she gets round to looking at them she really has forgotten what has gone on and has to start phoning people to find out what they can remember.

Tamsin loves organising meetings – because she does the exact opposite of Kerry!

Did you know?

It's an old management saying that if you are the last to arrive at a meeting you'll be the first to leave. It's all to do with mindset. If you're the notetaker of course, you can't leave, however much you may want to!

Types of meeting and their main features

A lot of American soaps feature rich and successful people who are constantly warring with each other over the boardroom table. That is one type of meeting. You can see another type in the Rovers Return in *Coronation Street* where there is nearly always a group of characters meeting to discuss what to do about something going on in the street.

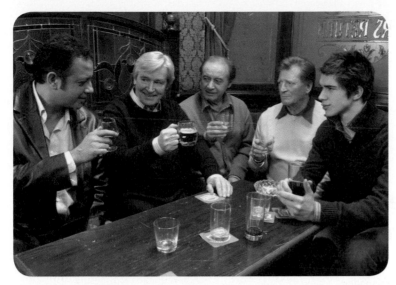

An informal meeting in Coronation Street's *The Rover's Return*

Did you know?

Why 'soaps'? It goes back to the 1930s when a lot of advertisers and sponsors of popular radio programmes were soap manufacturers.

You can have a meeting that is entirely formal and one that is so informal that you hardly recognise it as a meeting. The table below shows some of the differences.

> **Differences between formal and informal meetings**
>
> **Informal meetings include:**
>
> - **Regular meetings** – held by small groups of staff normally chaired by the team leader or manager
> - **Briefing meetings** – where, for instance, the manager or an organisation representative such as the health and safety officer talks to staff about a particular issue
> - **Progress meetings** – where a group of staff working on the same project get together to check where they are
> - **Working parties** – set up for a particular purpose, such as the introduction of a new computer system, and ended when the job is complete
>
> **Formal meetings include:**
>
> - **Meetings of the board** of directors or senior executives
> - **Committee and sub-committee** meetings reporting to the board or senior executives
> - **Annual general meetings**
> - **Meetings of shareholders**

Find out

In your own organisation, check what types of meeting are held. Check in particular what types of meeting you attend or organise.

The main features

Whether meetings are formal or informal, they have certain features in common.

- They have a number of people attending them. It is hard to have a meeting by yourself!
- Someone is in charge of them. In formal meetings he or she is normally called the chairperson.
- Someone is responsible for organising them and/or taking notes.
- There is an agenda, either written or unwritten.
- There is an end result – a decision taken, a job completed etc.
- There is a record of what went on – either a formal set of minutes or a more informal summary.

The importance of planning and agreeing a meeting brief

Did you know?

Many managers these days will not read anything other than bullet points that fit on to one side of an A4 sheet of paper. This makes it very difficult for administrators to brief their managers on important issues.

You open your email one morning and find this message from your manager:

Remind me (a) to talk to the staff about the staff appraisal procedures, and (b) to find out whether they want to join the new pension scheme.

He is out of the office at the moment so you decide to use your initiative and book a full staff meeting for the end of the week. When your boss arrives back he is surprised. He wanted to talk to the new staff individually about the organisation's appraisal and pension schemes. It is partly his fault in giving you a garbled message – but you should have checked with him before inconveniencing both yourself and the rest of the staff.

How to... Plan and agree a brief for a meeting

Make sure you are:

- perfectly clear about what you have to do
- able to go back to your boss to check that you are doing the right thing
- able to ask the right questions.

Here are examples of the types of question you might need to ask:

- What is the purpose of the meeting? Is it just a briefing meeting to give staff some information? Is it going to be a brainstorming session? Is it a formal meeting requiring formal paperwork etc.?
- Are you expected simply to organise the meeting, or will you be expected to be there? If so, what will your role be – as a member of the meeting, as a note-taker, or as both?

- Who should attend?

- How long is it likely to be? Is there going to be fixed start and end times?

- Where should it be held?

- What papers need to be prepared?

- Who needs to be informed even if they don't need to attend? For example, the managing director might want to know about all meetings taking place in the organisation even if he or she doesn't attend all of them.

- Do the car parking, security and/or reception staff need to be informed?

- Is anyone coming from outside the organisation? If so, are there any special arrangements to be made for them?

- Are refreshments required? If so, have the catering staff to be involved?

Find out

Think of the meetings you organise and the way in which you plan and agree a brief with your boss. Try to find out whether people in other parts of your organisation plan in the same way. If they do anything different, make a note of any examples of good practice.

Main points that should be covered by an agenda and meeting papers

Did you know?

One London-based firm of solicitors is so keen to keep its experienced meetings staff that it gives them extra perks, such as a free car parking space in the heart of the city!

Some meetings are so informal that all you need to do is pick up the telephone and ask people to turn up at a particular place and time to talk about a particular issue. Others are so formal that a full-time meetings secretary is appointed to oversee all the very complicated documentation involved.

Most meetings in an office come somewhere in between these extremes. If you have a regular staff meeting every month, for instance, you will probably have a meetings file in which you keep all the relevant paperwork – both of what has gone on in previous meetings and what is planned for the next.

Notice of the meeting

The first document you might have to prepare is a notice telling people when and where the meeting is to be held. Make sure you ask them to reply to you telling you whether or not they are going to attend, otherwise you will not know whether to expect two or twenty!

Below is an example of a document sent to call a meeting. Today, however, many meetings may be called by email instead.

WILKINSON RECRUITMENT CONSULTANTS

Memorandum

To: All recruitment personnel
From: Jon Wilkinson
Date: 10 June 2007

Monthly progress meeting

The next meeting will be held in my office at 10 a.m. on Monday 4 July. Please let me know if you cannot attend.

JW

Example of a notice of an informal meeting

Agenda

You then need to produce an agenda. No matter how informal the meeting is, you have to give people at least an idea of what it is about. Below an example of one is given. The normal contents are as follows:

WILKINSON RECRUITMENT CONSULTANTS

10 June 2007 at 10 a.m.

AGENDA

1   Apologies for absence

2   Minutes of the previous meeting

3   Matters arising

4   Update on

- new applicants
- employer requests for staff
- job placements

5   Appointment of new receptionist

6   Health and safety issues

7   Any other business

8   Date and time of next meeting

Example of an agenda for a meeting

- **Heading** – normally the name of the organisation.
- **Apologies for absence** – the names of those who cannot attend.
- **Minutes of the previous meeting** – to give anyone the chance to correct any mistakes made in the previous minutes. Otherwise everyone agrees that they are correct.
- **Matters arising.** Sometimes someone wants to report on any action they have taken as a result of a discussion at the last meeting or to give an update on some issue.
- **Main business** – the real reason for the meeting.
- **Any other business.** If someone has been too late in asking for something to go on the agenda, the chair might agree to it being discussed under any other business rather than it having to wait until the next meeting.
- **Date and time of next meeting.**

Did you know?

One businessman automatically puts a line through the last three agenda items of any meeting he chairs, because he thinks that all the really important stuff will have been put at the beginning!

How to... Agree an agenda

- **Ask the chairperson** for any items he or she wants on the agenda.
- **Ask the other members** whether they want anything on the agenda.
- **Look back at the notes of the last meeting** to check whether you were asked to include anything specific on the next agenda.
- **Don't make the agenda too long.** If it seems a bit overloaded try to persuade someone to keep his or her item for the next meeting.
- **Don't produce the agenda right at the last minute** so that the chairperson does not have a chance to agree it.

Did you know?

Some chairpersons want their own 'special' **chairperson's agenda** to remind them of what they are going to say about each agenda item. If that's the case, make sure that only you and the chair see that copy – some of the comments about other members of the meeting can get a bit personal! (See also page 302.)

Other papers

Up to this point you know where you are with the documents you have to prepare. From now on, however, anything else you produce depends on what is going to be discussed. You may have to check with the chairperson or with anyone else who has put an item on the agenda. It is not a bad idea to check also the notes of the last meeting to find out whether anything else is required.

It is difficult to hit the right balance. If you produce a mound of paper for every item on the agenda, not only will you be there until midnight, people won't have enough time to read it. If you produce nothing, then your chair might start complaining that there is not enough information available.

One solution is to send the information to the members before the meeting – particularly if it is a long report, complicated set of figures etc. People then have the chance to read it and pick out any points they want to raise. The only problem there, of course, is that some members will not even glance at it and some will forget to bring it to the meeting.

Types of information that attendees will need

There are some situations that you must avoid at all costs. For instance, you don't want half the members sitting waiting in one room while the other half are sitting waiting in another for the meeting to start! You don't want the chairperson stamping into the room in a fury because nothing had been said about the temporary car parking arrangements – and so on. Essential information for all attendees is:

● the practical arrangements – the date, time and place of the meeting, where they can park etc.
● what type of meeting it is, and roughly how long it will last
● who has been sent all the relevant papers
● whether or not they can send a deputy if they cannot attend in person.

You also need to let certain individuals know:

● the facilities for disabled people – access, lifts, loos etc.
● that there will be vegetarian refreshments available
● that there is a loop hearing system/ paperwork available in large print etc.

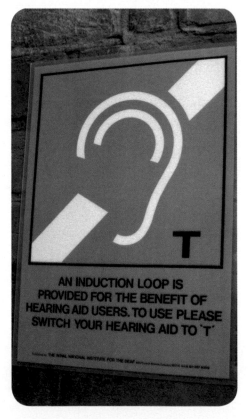

AN INDUCTION LOOP IS PROVIDED FOR THE BENEFIT OF HEARING AID USERS. TO USE PLEASE SWITCH YOUR HEARING AID TO 'T'

Identifying suitable venues for different types of meetings

You might not have any say in what venue you use. If you always meet in the boss's office that's OK – provided there is enough room. If you are always expected to use the meetings room, again that's fine provided you book it in time.

It is a bit more complicated when you are expected to research different types of venue and assess whether they are suitable for a particular meeting.

 How to... Identify suitable meetings venues

- **For internal venues**, check:
  - whether there is a meetings or conference room you can book
  - how you should book it and whether there a centralised booking system.
- **For external venues**, check:
  - whether it is company policy always to book one particular venue
  - whether arrangements for booking outside venues are always carried out centrally
  - the budget (if you are expected to do your own bookings).
- **For facilities**, check:
  - how many rooms are needed – one, a main room plus seminar rooms etc.
  - that the room is well lit, the right size and has a temperature that can be controlled
  - that there are enough chairs and tables
  - that the furniture can be arranged in a way that suits the needs of the meeting
  - that other equipment is available – projector, flip chart, computers
  - access to a telephones, fax machines, Internet, email etc.
  - the CCTV facilities
  - the car parking facilities
  - the catering facilities

How to... Continued

- reception arrangements, including arrangements for leaving coats, briefcases etc.
- any secretarial backup
- whether any overnight accommodation is wanted for visitors travelling long distances.

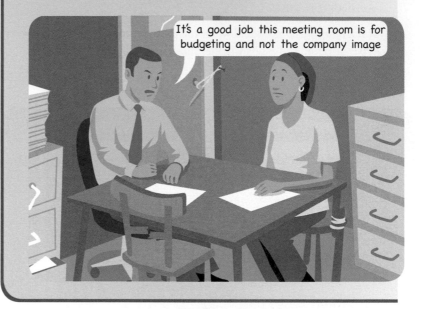

> It's a good job this meeting room is for budgeting and not the company image

Snapshot – Major league meetings!

Meetings are big business. One hotel chain, Le Meridien, goes to great lengths to make sure they are successful. Not only are prospective clients given detailed information about all the meeting facilities, they are also encouraged to ask much wider questions, including questions about the location, the facility and the food and drink.

- The location:
  - How easy is it to get to? Is it costly to travel to?
  - Is there a good taxi service?
  - Is there sufficient parking space?
  - How near is it to the airport/railway station?
- The facility:
  - Are the front-of-house staff efficient and friendly?
  - Is the lobby attractive and clean? Is there a doorman/woman?

- Is the registration desk easy to find? Are there sufficient staff to handle busy check in/out times?
- Are there any other services – shops, bars etc.?
- How many rooms are available for early arrivals and late departures?
- What are check-in and check-out times?
- What is the cut-off date for a room block?
- What is the refund policy for cancellations?
- Are there any planned renovations that may be in progress at the time of the meeting?

● Food and drink:
- What's the quality and service like?
- How much does it cost?
- What is the cash bar policy?
- Are any special services such as tailored menus, theme meals, table arrangements etc. required?
- Is there room service?

And you thought you only had to book a room and a few sandwiches!

If you want to see the full range of services offered, look on the website at www.lemeridien.com.com/meetings.

Types of resource that will be needed for different types of meeting

Your boss has a busy few months ahead of her. She has to attend all the usual management meetings. She is the chair of the health and safety meeting. She is also going to a number of meetings held outside the organisation. Your job is to make sure that she has everything she needs for each different type of meeting.

For regular/cross-organisational meetings she needs:
- notice and agenda
- notes or minutes from the last meeting
- any other information sent with the meetings papers
- her diary/planner
- notes of anything she wants to say
- her mobile phone – for use outside the meeting room!

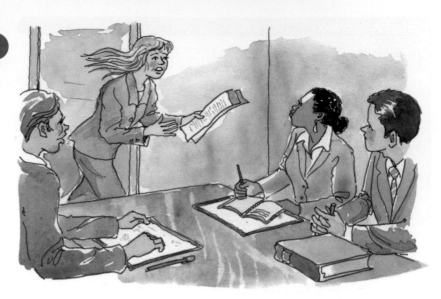

Finding last minute information can be stressful

For external meetings she needs all of the above, plus:

- directions (by car, rail etc.)
- information about the hotel/venue – where to park, what entrance to use etc.
- identity card/conference badge etc.

For any meetings she chairs she needs everything as for regular meetings, plus her chair's agenda and/or details of what she wants to say and what other people might say.

Other resources

Other resources required will depend on the meeting. However, whatever the meeting, you will need to provide:

- a suitable room and furniture layout
- appropriate equipment
- all the relevant paperwork
- pens, pencils and notepaper
- water/boiled sweets etc.
- back-up staff – even if that just means you!

From then on the resources required tend to increase the bigger and more formal the meeting becomes. Look back to pages 295–6 for information on some of them.

Providing for special requirements that attendees may have

You are making arrangements for a regular monthly meeting of a management committee, all of whose members come from outside:

- You know that one of the members is a vegetarian, so you make sure that some of the sandwiches do not contain any meat.
- You know that one of the members is a Muslim. Again, you make sure that there is a vegetarian alternative.
- You know that one of the members cannot hear very well. If the room is not equipped with a loop system you need to have a quiet word with the chairperson and, if possible, tactfully steer the member to a seat where he or she has the best chance of hearing everything that is said. If the meeting is a large formal meeting, such as an annual general meeting, you may have to consider using a sign language specialist.
- You know that one of the members cannot see very well. You make sure that his or her copy of the paperwork is printed in large type.
- You know that one of the members is frightened of lifts, so you need to let him or her know how to reach the meeting room by the stairs.
- You know that one of the members needs wheelchair access. You make certain that you either arrange for the meeting to take place on the ground floor or that there is access via a lift capable of taking a wheelchair. Check also the availability of suitable car parking spaces and suitable toilets.
- You know that one of the members needs a taxi home, so you should make the appropriate arrangements with the reception staff.
- You know that one of the members always arrives late because of family commitments. Normally this is a matter for the chairperson to deal with by discussing the problem direct with the member. In the meantime you can help by sorting out the agenda so that the most important items are not dealt with in the first 15 minutes.
- You know that one of the members dislikes another member. You need to sort out the seating arrangements so that the two of them are not sitting next to each other!

A successful meeting is one where everyone feels comfortable. If they don't, they become so fixated by what they don't have that at best they don't listen to what is going on and at worst they become a bit awkward. If at all possible, it is best to try to meet their individual requirements.

Did you know?

One survey found that changing a meeting place from the ground floor to the top floor of a building cut down the numbers attending by 10 per cent. Some members said that they didn't want to use the lift and couldn't face the stairs. Others said they just couldn't be bothered to make the trip!

Health, safety and security requirements when organising meetings

It is very tempting to forget health and safety requirements when you are involved in an important meeting. It is also quite easy to forget about them when you are actually planning the meeting. When arranging an in-house meeting you should be able to assume that the room will be covered by the same health and safety regulations as the rest of the building.

If the health and safety officer has not already done this, you should check:

- the lighting, ventilation/heating, and noise level
- the arrangement of the equipment and furniture to make sure that there are no trailing cables, unsafe mats, or steps that are hard to see
- the fire precautions, such as signs indicating specifically marked fire exits and escape routes and arrangements for disabled people
- no smoking signs.

Immediately before the meeting it is also a good idea to check its cleanliness – emptied wastepaper baskets, clean floors etc.

If the meeting is held at an external venue it is even more essential that you check first of all with the hotel or conference health and safety officer and then personally that all safety precautions have been taken. You might also want to remind the chairperson right at the beginning of the meeting to let members know where the fire exits are and what to

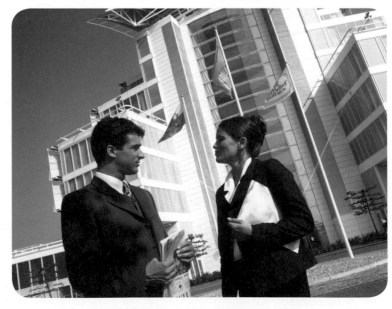

External venues need to be checked for health and safety standards too

do if the fire alarm sounds. They should know what to do in their own organisation, but they need to be given more information if they are in an unfamiliar place.

The importance of briefing the chairperson in advance of the meeting

A chairperson can make a meeting effective or sheer chaos – and equally make your life easy or very difficult.

How to... Be a good chairperson

- Be well prepared.
- Know the rules.
- Know who everyone is.
- Start and end the meeting on time.
- Allow discussion but keep it to the point.
- Encourage everyone to speak.
- Summarise the discussion.
- Get a decision.

However, do not:

- dash in at the last moment scattering papers all over the place
- ignore new members
- let one member speak all the time
- let the meeting go on for ever
- let the meeting end without anyone knowing what's going to happen next.

Remember

Some chairpersons can use their body language negatively. One local council survey found that some committee members felt their chairperson never needed to speak. When he was pleased he smiled and made eye contact. When he wanted someone to shut up he stared out of the window or looked pointedly at his watch. The meetings didn't last very long. Look back to unit 301, page 20, to see what he should be doing!

However good or bad your chairperson is, it is part of your role to give support. The first thing you can do is to make sure that he or she is properly briefed before the meeting actually begins.

One method you can use is to prepare some additional notes for each agenda item so that the chair is ready for any awkward questions or remembers what to say about a particular topic. For instance, in the case of the Wilkinson Recruitment Consultants meeting you might decide to prepare a longer version of the main agenda – sometimes referred to as the 'Chair's agenda' – reminding Jon of things he wants to say or what questions he may have to answer. See the example below.

WILKINSON RECRUITMENT CONSULTANTS

10 June 2007 at 10 a.m.

1 Apologies for absence

   Khalid has sent his apologies. He's in London for the day.

2 Minutes of the previous meeting

   Shouldn't be any problem here unless someone raises something at the meeting.

3 Matters arising

   Perveen might want to bring up the sales brochure. I'll make sure you have a copy of it with your other meeting papers.

4 Update on:

   ● new applicants

      No problem: numbers are up

   ● employer requests for staff

      Again, no problem

   ● job placements

      Numbers have dipped but Linda is going to come up with some ideas.

5 Appointment of new receptionist

   Franz and Sue have all the information about this – they'll be able to brief the others.

6 Health and safety issues

   You want to raise the question of switching computers etc. off last thing at night – remember the cleaner's complaint.

7 Any other business

   You want to remind them of the financial audit.

8 Date and time of next meeting

   Suggest 6 August at 10 a.m.– or the week following that: 13 August.

An example of a chairperson's agenda

1 You have just received this notice and agenda and can see a number of things wrong with it. List what they are and discuss them with your tutor or trainer, or check your ideas with the answers on the CD-ROM.

> To: All staff
>
> From: Jon
>
> Date: 23 June 2006
>
> The next staff meeting will be held on 25 June to discuss
>
> – The new selection tests
> – Changes to maternity leave
>
> Let me know if you can't come.

2 A recent survey has found that, out of 150 meetings in 50 companies, almost half did not have a prepared agenda. Discuss with your tutor or trainer why you think those meetings might not have gone as well as the meetings that did have an agenda. Check your ideas with the answer on the CD-ROM.

3 Karen Parker, the sales director, wants to hold a half-day meeting for the 15 regional sales staff to discuss the new product range for the autumn. Ten of the sales staff will require overnight accommodation because of the distances they are travelling. Karen has decided that she wants to hold the meeting at an external venue, starting at 2 p.m., after a brief buffet lunch. At 6 p.m. they will be joined by the MD and his deputy for the final part of the meeting, followed by an evening meal.

Investigate and suggest two possible venues in your own area, with reasons for your choices. Your reasons should link to the types of resource and facility that you think will be needed. Check your ideas either with other members of your group or with your tutor or trainer.

Evidence collection

Keep a log of the meetings you plan and prepare during the assessment period as this can form the basis of a professional discussion with your assessor. Your log should include the type of meeting, the meeting brief that was agreed, the arrangements you had to make, the number of attendees and any particular needs, the papers that you prepared, the

Core unit links

Providing accurate, clear and structured written information links to unit 301, performance indicators 2 and 7. Taking responsibility for the arrangements you make, keeping people informed of progress, meeting deadlines and following procedures may relate to unit 301, PIs 8–10 and 12–15. Helping and supporting other people and treating them with respect and consideration links to unit 301, PIs 27 and 28.

If your meetings involve you interacting with other people and showing sensitivity to individual needs and backgrounds, this may link to unit 302, PIs 11 and 12. Equally, if making arrangements involves you working with outside organisations and individuals, this may contribute evidence towards unit 302, PI 4. If you undertake risk assessments related to meeting venues, then this may link to unit 302, PIs 17–22.

Evidence collection Continued

equipment and resources that were required, and any other relevant tasks you carried out.

Make sure that your agendas and other meeting papers are retained so that you can show these to your assessor. There is no need to take additional copies if you keep standard meeting files and have these available.

On occasions when you check attendees' needs, keep the notes you make and ask at least two attendees to countersign and date these to confirm that you checked that their needs were met.

At the meeting

Types of information, advice and support you might have to provide during a meeting

'Ask me what I don't do!' is the answer you might like to give if someone asks you what you have to do during the course of a meeting. Consider the following scenario. You are sitting in the meeting room and the meeting begins:

- Just as the chairperson starts to speak, Jess raises her hand apologetically and says she's forgotten her agenda and the notes from the last meeting. You have spare copies and you give her these.
- The fire bell goes. The chairperson asks you whether this is a drill or a real alarm. You've taken the precaution of checking with the health and safety officer beforehand and you have special permission to remain where you are.
- Tashki starts to argue about a particular issue and says that he is sure that something different had been agreed a few months ago. You have your meetings file with you and can refer back right away to what was said.
- Aaron begins to give a report and finds he has not got some back-up figures. He's left them on his desk. You make a quick phone call to his PA to bring them to the meeting room as quickly as possible.
- The room gets too hot. You are the only one who knows how to turn on the air conditioning.

- During the break you have to tell everyone where the nearest loo is, remind them to check the time if they have parked on a pay car park, and show them where the tea, coffee and soft drinks are being served. You might even have time for a drink yourself!

Problems that may occur during meetings – and how to solve them

'Expect the unexpected' is the best motto you can follow if you are sitting in a meeting, no matter how well prepared you think you are. All sorts of things can happen, and it is normally your job to do something about them. Consider these scenarios:

- Five minutes before the meeting is due to start, four out of eight members have not yet arrived. You start making urgent phone calls. You decide that in future you'll remember to contact those who are likely to be late to remind them of the meeting on the day of the meeting itself.
- Half an hour after the meeting starts, other people start wandering in and look surprised that you are there. The room has been double-booked. You think about asking the other administrator to toss for it but instead phone a colleague and get her to check for other empty rooms. In future you make a note to check right up to the last minute that you have the sole right to the room.
- The meeting is dragging on because one of the members will not stop speaking. The others are getting very restless. Eventually

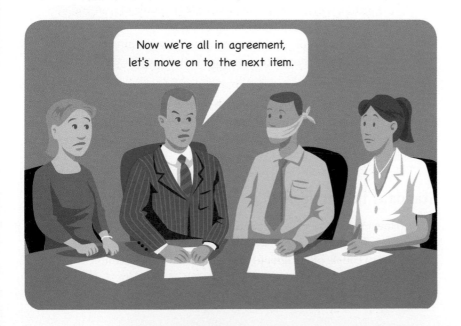

Now we're all in agreement, let's move on to the next item.

the chairperson manages to stop him. You hope that she will have a quiet word with him afterwards to avoid this happening again.

- You cannot hear what one of the members is saying. She is very quietly spoken and you are sitting where you can hardly see her. It makes note-taking difficult. Next time you decide to make sure that the you sit directly opposite her or as near to her as possible.

- The chairperson starts to speak and finds that she has left her reading glasses in her car. After everything else that has happened this hardly seems a problem. You get her car keys and persuade one of the reception staff to fetch the glasses.

After the meeting

What to include in the record of a meeting

You would normally keep a record of what was said at a meeting no matter how informal it might be:

- to make sure that all the important information discussed at the meeting is there for members and other people to read and, it is hoped, agree to at the following meeting
- to remind people who have agreed to do something exactly what it was, and to stop them from saying that they have not agreed to anything!

If you are using an agenda, your job is made easier. All you have to do is to make a note of what has been said under each agenda heading. If you do not have an agenda you will need to make up your own headings.

Standard information

How you have to write up your notes depends on the type of meeting. You might have to summarise them as a list of numbered points or write a couple of paragraphs to put in an email. An example is shown opposite.

> **WILKINSON RECRUITMENT CONSULTANTS**
>
> Notes of the monthly staff meeting held on 4 July 2007 in the training room of the Herriot Building.
>
> - Everyone was present except Khalid Javed who was away in London.
> - Perveen Lorca gave a progress update on the sales brochure.
> - Rab Howson and Linda Salazar gave an update on the statistics. The number of job applicants and employer enquiries had increased. There had been a slight fall in the number of job placements. Linda would circulate the exact figures.
> - Franz Kessler and Sue Treadwell were drawing up a shortlist for the new receptionist's job. The interviews would be held on 2 August 2007.
> - Everyone was reminded to check that all equipment was switched off at the end of each day.
> - There was going to be a financial audit at the end of the year. Everyone should start checking that they were following correct procedures.
> - The next meeting would be at 10 a.m. on 6 August.

Example of a summary of a meeting

You might have to produce a set of more formal minutes in which you follow the order of the agenda items. An example of this is shown below.

> **WILKINSON RECRUITMENT CONSULTANTS**
>
> Minutes of the monthly staff meeting held on 4 July 2007 in the training room of the Herriot Building.
>
> **Present:**
>
> Jon Wilkinson (Chair)
> Rab Howson
> Franz Kessler
> Perveen Lorca
> Linda Salazar
> Sue Treadwell (note taker)
>
> | Agenda Item | Action |
> | --- | --- |
>
> **1 Apologies for absence**
>
> Khalid Javed sent his apologies.
>
> **2 Minutes of the previous meeting**
>
> These were agreed as correct.

Agenda Item	Action

3 Matters arising

Perveen Lorca said that the new sales brochure was almost ready and should be back from the printers next week.

4 Updates

Rab Howson said there had been a 10% increase in the number of job applicants and employer enquiries.

Linda Salazar said there had been a slight fall in the number of job placements. She would get the exact figures by the end of the day and circulate them to everyone.   **LS**

5 Appointment of new receptionist

Franz Kessler and Sue Treadwell were looking through all the applications and drawing up a shortlist. The interviews were going to be held on 2 August 2007.

6 Health and safety issues

Jon Wilkinson reminded everyone to check that all equipment was switched off at the end of each day. The cleaner had recently found several computers and photo copiers that had been left on overnight.

7 Any other business

Jon Wilkinson reminded everyone that a financial audit was due at the end of the year and that they should start checking that all the correct procedures were in place.

8 Date and time of next meeting

The next meeting would be held at 10 a.m. on 6 August 2007.

Signed   Date

Example of the minutes of a meeting

Whatever format you use, there is certain information that you will almost certainly have to include:

- name of the organisation
- date of the meeting
- names of those present
- names of those who could not attend
- notes of what has been discussed or decided
- date and time of the next meeting.

Taking notes

Note-taking scares some people. This is unnecessary, particularly if the person chairing the meeting is on your side. All you need to remember are certain basic tips:

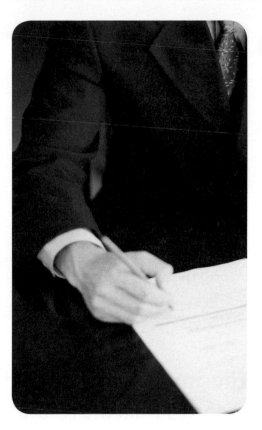

- Unless the meeting is very informal, write in sentences.
- Use the past tense in formal meetings – e.g. 'Jon said that...' rather than 'Jon says that...'.
- Change questions around. Translate 'What are we going to do about the Christmas party?' to 'Rachel asked what was happening about the Christmas party.'
- Spell everyone's name correctly!

Remember

You may have to write a summary. Look back to unit 301, pages 27–9, if you need to jog your memory about how to appoach this.

 How to... Take accurate notes of a meeting

- **Be prepared.** The more you can do before the meeting the better. Prepare an A4 lined pad by pencilling in the initial headings and leaving a suitable space for your notes (or a wide right-hand margin).

- **Collect together all relevant documents.** An example is an attendance sheet for members to sign so that you are not scribbling names down as each member arrives.

- **Listen.** That sounds easy, but it isn't when you're trying to follow what everyone is saying and the chair is allowing more than one person to talk at once.

- **Summarise.** Even if you can use shorthand, do not rely on it too much in a meeting. You don't need to write down every word, just the main points.

Did you know?

A top PA said that when she started taking notes she found it difficult to remember to change the time. She kept writing things like 'the interviews are taking place today' instead of 'the interviews took place on the 21st' – forgetting that her notes were going to be being read at a later date.

Find out

Think about how you prepare your meeting notes – and what differences, if any, there are between the way you prepare them and the methods suggested here.

How to... Continued

- **Don't panic.** If you miss something it is not the end of the world. Leave a gap in your notes and, if you can, note down the name of the person speaking. Have a word with him or her afterwards or, if that is not possible, talk to the chairperson. He or she should have a good idea of what has been said.

- **Follow a routine.** Get into the habit of drawing a line or leaving a space between each item. Get used to abbreviations – provided you can read them afterwards. Don't write something like 'M to see P on T in B' unless you are absolutely sure you can translate it afterwards.

- **Write up as soon as possible.** You will have a much better chance of remembering what has been said if you write up your notes as soon as possible after the meeting, even if the notes are not too good at this point.

The importance of making sure the record is accurate and is approved

You are at a meeting when an argument starts about what has been written in the notes of the last meeting. That is for your chairperson to sort out, of course, but it can be a bit embarrassing if it turns out that

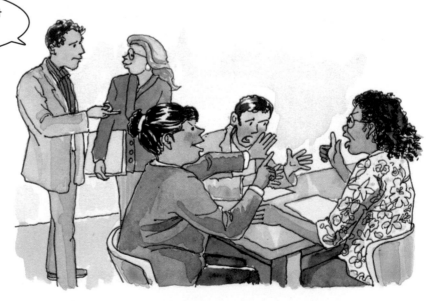

So the decision wasn't unanimous, then.

you misheard something or made a mistake. If you have, you need not feel too dreadful – everyone makes mistakes. However, you obviously want to prevent it from happening again.

The major thing to remember is to work closely with the chairperson. Prepare everything in draft form first of all and let him or her look at it before sending out the final version. It's a bit unfair, however, if you rely totally on your chairperson. If it has been a very long meeting or one where some important issues were discussed, he or she might easily forget what has happened on some occasions – that's when your good note taking can help.

It is sometimes a good idea to go through your draft first of all and mark any points where you have some queries or where there was a particularly long discussion so that you can talk them over together.

It is also helpful to the chairperson if you can point out any issues that may be a bit controversial. He or she might want you to alter the wording of that particular item to avoid offending some of the more sensitive or argumentative members!

How to record and follow up actions

People agree to do things at meetings for a variety of reasons:
- They genuinely want to help.
- They want to please the boss!
- They cannot think of a way to say no!

It is your job to make sure that what they have agreed to do is put on record. The easiest way to do this is to organise your notes in such a way that there is an action column in which you can put the names or initials of the person agreeing to do something against the relevant item. In the minutes of the Jon Wilkinson meeting, for instance, Linda agreed to circulate some figures to the rest of the members, so her initials were put against that item. If she forgets to do it, she has some explaining to do at the next meeting.

In reality, of course, you are not going to let that happen. When you start preparing for the next meeting you will realise that she has forgotten to provide the figures and tactfully remind her to do so as quickly as possible.

Sometimes, however, you cannot afford to wait, particularly if the action needed is quite urgent. It is a good idea, therefore, when you are preparing the summary or minutes, to keep a separate list of everything anyone has promised to do. You can then judge how important it is that the action is taken quickly and make a note in your diary or planner system to check that it has been done – and to give gentle 'nudges' where needed.

How to evaluate external services

After a meeting it is very tempting to get back to your office, put your feet up, complain loudly about that idiot in reception who kept directing people to the wrong room, and then get on with the next job. You are then really busy for the next week or two and it is only when you are on your way into the meeting room that you realise the same receptionist is on duty and you have not taken any action to avoid the same thing happening this time.

If you are relying on other people to help you to run a successful meeting you need to keep a check on how good they are at doing this. It is essential, therefore, that at the end of each meeting you evaluate what they have done:

- **Use your eyes**. If the paperwork has come back from central reprographics and is badly collated and photocopied, you can soon tell.
- **Use your taste buds**. If the coffee is cold and the sandwiches dry, the catering staff may not have done their job properly.
- **Use your ears**. If all the members are coming into the meeting grumbling about the receptionist, you can make a mental note of this.

You can then take steps to improve things for next time.

What you might also want to do is ask other people for their views. It's better than second-guessing them. You might find it useful to prepare a small questionnaire to be given out at regular intervals to members of various meetings – with your chairperson's permission of course – asking for their views on:

- the room – heating, lighting, furniture arrangement
- the quality of the paperwork
- the length of the meetings
- the intervals at which they are held
- whether or not members are given their papers in good time
- the catering arrangements
- the reception arrangements etc.

Case study Let's have a meeting!

*Read the case study below and then answer the questions that follow.
Then check your answers with those on the CD-ROM.*

When Alison Henderson started work as an administrator for a firm
of pharmaceutical suppliers she had no idea of what lay ahead. She
thought she would be responsible for the smooth running of the
office and for the work of her small team. What she didn't know
was that very soon she would be transferred to the HR department
and would eventually be encouraged to become a fully qualified HR
manager.

Obviously she knew that the job would involve talking to people a lot
of the time. What she didn't at first realise, however, were the different
ways in which she would be communicating with them. Not only did
she have to talk to them individually and in small groups, she also had
to have meetings with them. For instance she now has on a regular
basis to:

- attend the weekly staff meetings of each shift (sometimes at 6
  a.m. and sometimes at 11 p.m., before the start of each shift)

- assist her boss at all the management meetings

- attend the weekly meetings of the HR staff chaired by her boss

- chair the HR staff equal-opportunities meetings.

She also has to take part in other meetings, sometimes called at short
notice. For example, with her boss, she has to:

- be present at the meetings of all the trade union representatives

- attend any disciplinary or grievance procedure meetings

- attend meetings with Acas, the government body set up to advise,
  conciliate and arbitrate between employer and employees

- attend any pre-meetings if an employee has taken a case to the
  Employment Tribunal.

She has to spend hours collecting together paperwork before any of
these meetings.

Last month, for instance, when a female employee said that her male
supervisor had made a sexist remark to her and wanted to take out
a grievance against him, Alison had to take statements from her,
from the supervisor, from staff working alongside her and from staff
wanting to support the supervisor. She then had to check what the

Case study Continued

law said about sexual harassment. She had to let her boss know that a serious problem had arisen.

Her next step was to go with her boss to meet the union representative and employee to see what they wanted. At all times she had to make sure they were following the correct procedures.

After a meeting, which Alison's boss chaired, the problem was resolved. The supervisor admitted making an 'uncalled for remark' and apologised. The employee accepted the apology. Alison then had to write up the notes of the meeting and make sure everyone had a copy of them. She also had to make sure that a note of this was made on the supervisor's personnel record.

Recently Alison was asked what 'personal' as distinct from 'personnel' skills she thought she should have. She thought about it and then came up with the following list:

● liking to be with people

● knowing how they tick

● unflappability

● persistence

● thoroughness

● patience

● fairness.

When asked whether or not she thought she had all these skills, she replied 'ask me again in 20 years' time!'.

Questions

1 Alison is often involved in a number of different types of meeting. How would you suggest that she keeps track of the paperwork involved in each one?

2 Suggest how she might make sure that she keeps everyone informed of the outcomes of all these meetings.

3 Why is it particularly important that she keeps her boss informed about the sexual harassment complaint?

4 If she isn't careful, Alison will spend virtually all her time in meetings – with no time to do anything else. Suggest what she should do to make sure she has time for her other work.

5 If Alison had an administrative assistant, what duties do you think she should delegate in respect to the arranging and running of all the meetings?

6 *State how you think Alison should respond to a situation in a meeting where:*

   a *the trade union representatives are being very angry and awkward*

   b *one of the staff never attends the equal-opportunities meetings because 'she always has something more important to do'*

   c *the evening staff say that they are not kept as well informed as the day staff*

   d *she is accused of being the boss's friend and not dealing independently with the issues being raised.*

7 *What particular problems do you think she might encounter when attending either very early morning or late at night meetings with the staff – both from her point of view and that of the staff?*

Changing places

Your assessor will ask you how you will adapt your knowledge of arranging meetings if you change your job in the future. You will need to think about the way in which aspects of these tasks would change if you worked for a different organisation.

Zara works in a small firm of accountants. There are two senior partners, a newly qualified accountant and a trainee. The newly qualified accountant and trainee spend a lot of time out of the office doing audits. Zara has to make sure that everyone has the chance to meet as a group to discuss various issues. She therefore plans very short briefing meetings at least twice a week lasting no more than 20 minutes. She makes brief notes and circulates them by email.

Tomas works for the local council as a committee secretary. He makes arrangements for all council committee and sub-committee meetings which include preparing very formal paperwork. He has to follow detailed procedures as to the types of documents he prepares, the language he uses, the numbering systems he adopts and the times at which he sends everything out to committee members. He has to take minutes at each meeting and again has to follow very specific procedures in the way he writes them up.

Shazia works for the owner of a small garage. He never has any meetings but expects her to make sure that all the rest of the office staff

Changing places Continued

and the mechanics are kept fully informed about what's happening. She does this by having a meeting with him each day, making some notes and then going round to talk to everyone personally.

Derren works in a very large organisation and the only meeting he attends is the weekly staff meeting. He knows what an agenda and set of minutes looks like but he has never had to prepare one. All he has to do is word process a summary of the notes his boss makes. He has no idea of all the work that goes on behind the scenes to make sure the meetings are successful.

1   For any *one* person listed above, identify the differences he or she would find if moving to your organisation and doing your job.

2   For any *one* person listed above, say how you would need to adapt your skills if you did their job rather than your own.

 Over to you

1   You are sitting in a meeting when the following discussion takes place.

Chair: We need to make a decision on where we should put an advertisement for the new receptionist post.

Tracy: Why do we need an advert? Why can't we just go to the Job Centre as normal?

Baz: Because last time they only sent us two candidates and they were both awful.

Tracy: Lena wasn't awful.

Baz: You're only saying that because she's a friend of yours.

Tracey: That's just not true.

Chair: Can we get back to the point please. We've already decided that we will advertise – we need to decide where.

Karina: Why not the local paper? Everyone reads it on jobs night.

Chair: When is jobs night?

Karina: Thursday I think.

Chair: Has anyone else got any comments.
     (Silence)

Chair: Shall we agree to putting in an advert on the next available Thursday slot? (*Everyone nods*.) Good, that's settled. Karina, go ahead and make all the arrangements please.

Make a note of what has been said to be included in the written notes of the meeting. Discuss with your tutor or trainer and/or check your ideas with the answer on the CD-ROM.

2 A US survey found that a quarter of the workers interviewed said they would rather go to the dentist than attend a meeting. Discuss with your tutor or trainer why they might think that and/or check your ideas with the answer on the CD-ROM.

Evidence collection

1 During the period of your assessment, keep any written notes you take a meetings. Check that these include an attendance record. Make sure the notes are dates so that you can clearly link them to the meeting notes or minutes you prepared.

2 On the meetings log you started on page 303, note down any papers that were 'tabled' (i.e. given out during the meeting) and any specific information, advice or support that you gave at the meeting.

3 Check that your files of meeting notes or minutes are complete and available to show to your assessor. There is no need to make an extra copy for your portfolio provided you can produce the filed evidence to prove your competence.

4 Write your own account to describe how you prepared for two or three meetings. This should include how you briefed the chair, the type of meeting record you produced and that you circulated it within agreed timescales, how you followed up the action points and the results of your evaluation of external services you used. Ask your chair to countersign and date your account to validate it.

5 Finally, if you need to make amendments to a meeting record, keep a copy of the amendments you made as well as the original copy to show your assessor.

Core unit links

Many of the communications you will undertake during and after a meeting (e.g. focusing on information other people are communicating, contributing to discussions, using written material selectively and extracting the main points) link to unit 301, performance indicators 1–7.

Achieving agreed timescales for circulating the meeting record and carrying out other tasks link to unit 301, PIs 8–10 and 13. Solving any problems that occur and keeping other people informed link to unit 301, PIs 11 and 12.

Maintaining security and confidentiality may link to unit 302, PIs 15 and 16.

If you set high standards for your work and behave generally to support effective working at all meetings, check the way in which your evidence may link to unit 301, PIs 22–28.

What if...?

What should you do if either

- no information or support is required during the assessment period

- no amendments to a meeting record are necessary during the assessment period?

In either case, your assessor can give you a dedicated task to cover the knowledge and understanding required. This will then be followed by a professional discussion where you can explain how you would perform in such a situation and what evidence you might bring forward.

Key skills reminder

If you are taking Key Skills awards, remember to discuss with your tutor or trainer how your evidence for this unit could also count towards those awards.

Develop productive working relationships with colleagues

Unit summary and overview

This option unit relates to the working relationships you have with colleagues, both within your own organisation and within other organisations. It covers the way in which you behave towards other people and how you establish working relationships with them, as well as how you take their needs into account and fulfil agreements you have made. It also focuses on how you identify and resolve conflicts and disagreements, and how you exchange information and feedback with others.

Good working relationships between colleagues are essential for an organisation to flourish. This is why good 'people' skills are considered such an asset and frequently sought by employers. If you regularly interact with other people at work, this unit provides you with an invaluable opportunity to develop your skills and abilities to work productively with all your colleagues and to deal diplomatically and tactfully with difficult situations.

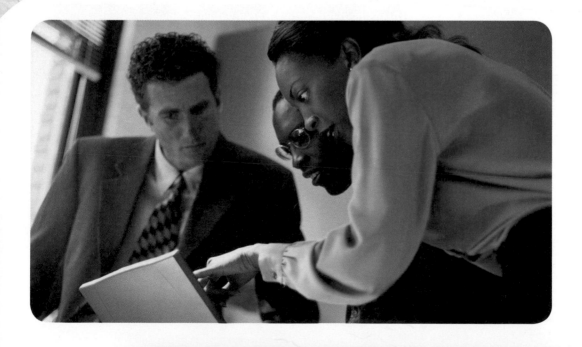

Links to core units

As you gather your evidence for this unit you should also obtain evidence for your core units. Watch for the CU link logo which suggests how the evidence you may collect could count towards both this unit and your core units.

Remember that you might be able to identify other links yourself, because of your own job role and the evidence you have obtained.

Talk to your assessor if you need further guidance on how your evidence should be cross-referenced.

Special note

This unit is imported from the Management Standards Centre's standards and has a slightly different structure. The management standards include ten specified behaviours that you must demonstrate as well as additional knowledge relating to your own industry/sector and to the context in which you work. Therefore, your evidence will need to include these additional aspects.

You will find a summary relating to the required behaviours on page 321 and margin note reminders at key points in the text. Specific sections on understanding your organisation, on pages 324, 341 and 351, cover all the additional knowledge items. Further guidance is also given in the evidence collection sections of the unit.

Benefits of developing productive working relationships with colleagues

Few people work completely on their own, with little or no contact with anyone else. Even the freelance IT consultant, who may spend most of the time interacting with computers, will need to liaise with clients at some stage. As an administrator, unless you are employed in a very small firm where the managers are out most of the time, you are likely to be interacting with a variety of colleagues every day.

Colleagues can often be classified into four types:
- those who are senior to you, such as your own line manager, other departmental managers and their managers
- those who work on the same level as yourself, although they may be employed in different sections or departments.
- those who are junior to you, even if you do not have any direct control over them or their work
- those whose job gives them a professional power over you, such as a security guard or refectory supervisor, because they have authority in their own areas.

Your relationships with all these people are extremely important because they impact on you, your colleagues and your employer. Quite simply, everyone benefits if working relationships are productive.

Benefits of productive working relationships	
To you and your colleagues	<ul><li>Work is far more enjoyable</li><li>You feel supported and appreciated</li><li>You can concentrate on the job in hand, rather than personal issues</li><li>You can share expertise and information</li><li>You learn from each other</li><li>You help each other</li></ul>
To your manager or employer	<ul><li>Time isn't wasted on disputes and conflict resolution</li><li>Productivity is high</li><li>Staff motivation is high</li><li>Collaboration and cooperation produces top-level results</li></ul>

Working relationships and organisations

Given all the benefits of productive working relationships you would think that everyone would work hard to achieve these in all organisations. In reality, this is not always the case. The culture of the organisation (see pages 328–9), the management style and the behaviour of individuals will all affect working relationships. In an organisation where the management is good and fair and where staff appreciate and respect one another, working relationships will usually be effective and productive. Other key factors are shown in the table below.

Features of the organisation	Behaviours exhibited by staff
Communications are clear and accurate; idle rumours or scaremongering is discouraged	They present information clearly, concisely, accurately and in ways that promote understanding 4
Decisions are fair and reasons for them are explained	They seek to understand other people's needs and motivations 2
The focus is on the job to be done; internal politics and gossip is discouraged	They make time to support 5 others
Staff are praised for effort and encouraged to develop their skills	They clearly agree what is expected of others and hold 8 them to account
Staff are respected and supported, even if they make mistakes	They work to develop an atmosphere of professionalism and mutual support 7
Differences of opinion are openly discussed in a positive manner	Their behaviour shows respect, helpfulness and cooperation 1.
Staff have the freedom to be open and assertive in relation to their rights	They keep promises and honour commitments 6
People respect each other, regardless of status or title	They consider the impact of their actions on other people 3
Productive working relationships are given high priority, and their importance is recognised by management and staff	They know how to say 'no' to unreasonable requests. They show respect for the views and actions of others 9

Remember

A key feature of the table is that it includes the **ten behaviours** that your assessor will expect you to demonstrate as part of your evidence for this unit.

Find out

A **hierarchical organisation** is one where there are several levels of authority. Often its shape is likened to a pyramid, because the higher you go the fewer people you will find at each level. Other organisations are much flatter, with perhaps only two or three levels – such as directors, managers and staff. Which applies to your firm?

It is fairly obvious, therefore, that productive working relationships don't just happen automatically. Each person contributes to the process through his or her behaviour. That is why the behaviours listed in the table are those that you are expected to demonstrate to your assessor.

However, it is one thing realising that productive working relationships have benefits and you have a role to play in this process in your workplace; it is quite another establishing and maintaining these – especially with colleagues with whom you have little in common. As a first step, it is sensible to think about the key features of a working relationship, and how these differ from the social relationships you have with your friends outside work. When you examine these you can see that it is no wonder that you have to work harder to establish good relationships with other people at work!

Features of working and social relationships	
Working relationships	Social relationships
Contact is often daily; no choice	Frequency of contact is a matter of choice
People may have disparate interests, ages, backgrounds and views	Usually formed with people with common interests
Usually temporary – often contact ceases with a change of job	May be long-term or lifelong
Often hierarchical – involves one person having power and authority over another	In a 'healthy' relationship, friends have equal say in decisions
May take time to establish rapport	May be formed quickly but superficially at a social event
Frequency of contact and pressure can result in conflict	Conflict more likely to be through different views rather than pressure
Focus is on task achievement	Focus is on enjoyment
Individuals are paid to act professionally at all times	Individuals can display emotions more freely
Major conflict must be resolved unless one person is willing to change job	Major conflict can mean end of relationship by mutual agreement

Establishing a productive relationship

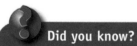

Some people seem to find it far easier than others to form social relationships. At a party they mix easily, laughing and chatting with a variety of people. If you struggle in that type of situation then you may find it comforting to realise that just because someone is socially confident it doesn't necessarily follow that they will be great to work with. In fact, the opposite could easily be true. If people are too confident they can become overbearing and arrogant – both irritating traits in the workplace.

When you meet someone for the first time, the most important factor affecting your behaviour is your attitude towards the person. This is influenced by your **perception** based on:

- your own history and personal experience
- your beliefs, values and attitudes
- the amount of confidence (or insecurity) that you have
- your personal history of that particular person.

Even if you have no personal history of someone you may have a positive or negative reaction towards the person for superficial reasons – such as his or her appearance, accent or age, or even because he or she reminds you of someone you didn't like very much! Or you may be influenced by the remarks other people make which influence your judgement.

In a social situation your perceptions do not matter too much because you can simply keep away from people who don't appeal to you. At work this is not an option. Whether you like it or not you will have to work productively alongside a variety of people, some of whom you would not choose to have as friends. The first stage in this process is to work at developing a rapport between you. The hints below should help.

Did you know?

You may form opinions of people before you get to know them – or even before you meet them. You might judge someone on a letter he or she has written, their manner on the telephone or because of rumours or gossip you hear from other people.

How to... Establish working relationships with colleagues

- Stay open-minded when you meet a new colleague or have to work with someone for the first time. Don't be overly influenced by appearance, looks or manner. Someone who seems remote may just be shy.

- Don't take it personally if someone seems uninterested in you. He or she may be distracted by work or personal worries.

- Talk about general, neutral topics at the start – preferably about your jobs and the task in hand. It takes time before work colleagues share personal information – and some never do.

- Don't talk too much – or retreat into a shell. Either extreme does not help other people to relate to you.

- Don't expect to have the same views and opinions as your colleagues or to be close personal friends with everyone you work with!

- Develop your listening skills, especially with those who are older or more senior than you are, so that they are aware that you value their comments.

How to... Continued

- Appreciate that other people have their own needs, pressures and problems, many of which may be unknown to you.

- Be supportive and uncritical of your colleagues and the chances are that they will be the same with you.

- Be positive and cheerful, even on a bad day. No one likes working with a moaner!

- Don't do anything to destroy other people's trust in you, such as divulging a secret they have told you, otherwise you may destroy the relationship for ever.

Understanding your organisation – 1

The more you know about your colleagues, both as people and in terms of their own job roles and responsibilities, the more likely it is that you will communicate with them sensitively and manage your working relationships successfully. This also means understanding how their priorities, expectations and authority differ. Similarly, understanding how your organisation is structured and how decisions are made helps you to work more effectively. This often depends on the line management responsibilities and relationships in an organisation, as you will see below. Understanding the main areas of work that are carried out and future work plans also enables you to recognise how your relationships with your colleagues may change and/or evolve depending on your job role.

Work roles and responsibilities

Understanding the work roles and responsibilities of your colleagues is important for the following reasons:

- You understand who has the authority and the power to make certain decisions, and who has not.
- You know who to contact – quickly – with the right query or information.
- You can understand what each of your colleagues expects from you.
- You can appreciate why your priorities and theirs may sometimes be quite different.
- You can empathise more with the problems and pressures your colleagues are experiencing.
- You are better able to offer assistance and support to colleagues, even without being asked.

- If you are responsible for staff, you can allocate work to them fairly.
- You don't unwittingly add to people's problems when they are having a bad day or are under extreme pressure to do critical work to a tight deadline.
- When you hear about future developments or work plans you will have a good idea who is most likely to be affected.

In most organisations, the work roles and responsibilities of staff are specified in a job description and their place in the hierarchy may be shown on an organisation chart. When you study an organisation chart you should remember that there are both benefits and drawbacks with it as a method of finding out more about your organisation.

Benefits of an organisation chart

- You can see immediately how the organisation is organised, the areas or departments into which it is divided and the formal relationships between people.
- The job titles in each area will show you the types of activity that take place and the work roles.
- You can see:
  - which staff are the most senior (they are at the top of the chart)
  - which staff are at the same level
  - which people manage other staff
  - who each person reports to.
- You can see how many staff each manager has to supervise:
  - The job titles of managers will identify their general area of responsibility and the way they are linked to each other.

Did you know?

Job roles have two elements. The **prescribed elements** are the tasks you must do and your responsibilities, as listed in your job description. The **discretionary** elements relate to the actions you take and the way you do the job. These are often linked to the values of the organisation and its culture. This means that if you change your job you may do the same types of task but be told to do them in a different way.

Role negotiation occurs when you discuss with someone what actions you can both do (or stop doing) to help each other to work more productively, such as sending copies of documents, stop forwarding unnecessary emails etc.

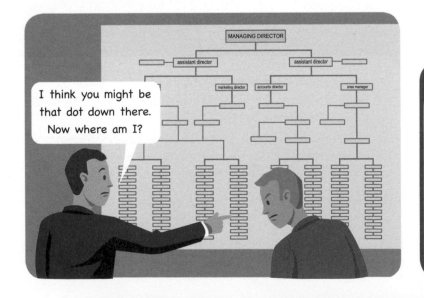

Did you know?

Organisation charts show only the formal relationships in an organisation. They show you who has official power, but do not show you the informal or social links or which members of staff have the most influence. Neither do they tell you anything about the office politics (see page 343).

Did you know?

Wise administrators know that it is not only good manners but also good sense to respect people at all levels in the organisation. You may want to impress the boss but you'll never do that if neither the caretaker nor the cleaner will cooperate with you in a crisis because they think you have no time for them.

Did you know?

Power is not the same as influence. **Power** relates to official authority, such as that held by a director, manager or a professional expert like a doctor or solicitor. **Influence** is the ability to act persuasively to change events. Power may not be something you associate with the managing director's PA, but in some cases he or she may have a huge amount of influence.

■ You can see how many levels there are in the organisation. As you saw on page 321, an organisation with many levels is said to be hierarchical, one with only two or three levels has a 'flat' structure. This may give you some clues as to how the organisation operates (see page 328).

Limitations of an organisation chart

● The organisation chart may not be up to date. Job roles frequently change, especially when people leave. This is why many do not include the names of the job holders.

● The chart cannot take account of future plans or developments. It will always be updated retrospectively.

● You cannot see *informal* links between people and departments – who is friends with whom, which people meet socially, who is popular with the boss and who the boss listens to or ignores.

● You cannot see the links between departments nor why they communicate.

● You cannot see from the chart whether the style of the organisation is formal or informal, whether management is fair or harsh, or what a particular manager is like to work for.

● The chart does not show the power held by certain people or groups of staff in certain situations. For example, the IT staff can close down the system if there is a virus threat, and the security staff can evacuate the building in an emergency. It is not only the people at the top of the chart who can make decisions and give instructions!

How to... Recognise, agree and respect the roles and responsibilities of colleagues

● Don't assume you automatically know the job roles and responsibilities of your colleagues simply because you work near them or have frequent contact with them.   4

● Check your organisation chart to identify people's roles and responsibilities – or sketch it out for yourself and check your assumptions with your line manager.   2

● Watch and listen to people at work to find out more about their responsibilities and areas of expertise.   1

● Find out how you can help colleagues to work more productively through role negotiation.

- Never think that the only people worth knowing are those high up in the organisation or who have an important-sounding job title. ⌐3

- Always be aware that people have roles and responsibilities outside work as well as within it.

- If you have to liaise with a new colleague because of changes at work, make it your job to find out about this person's roles and responsibilities so that you can relate more sensitively.

Decision-making processes in your organisation

Decision-making is a vital activity in all organisations. Some decisions will be very minor, others will be far more critical:

- Senior managers/directors will make strategic decisions that will affect the future of the organisation, such as the way in which it is structured, the range of goods or services to produce, the markets, the budgets available and staff resources.

- Line managers will take operational decisions related to their own sections or departments. This includes solving basic problems that arise.

- All staff should be encouraged to make appropriate decisions that relate to their job role and responsibilities.

However, other factors affect the decision-making processes in an organisation, as you can see below.

Did you know?

You can judge the importance of a decision by its complexity and potential impact. If the effect could be wide-ranging or have a potentially disastrous result, then this is normally an executive decision.

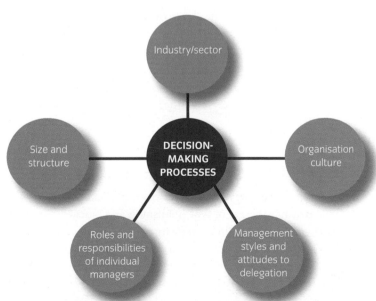

Factors that influence the decision-making process

Find out

Your assessor will expect you to know the regulations and codes of practice that apply to your industry or sector. Check that you understand what is meant by these terms by looking back at pages 51–2 and 112, and then find this information for your own workplace.

The industry or sector

Industries and sectors were first covered in unit 302, pages 96–9. If you have forgotten about them, turn back to those pages and refresh your memory. Public sector organisations, charities and public limited companies are all publicly accountable, and this affects the way in which they make important decisions. Usually these will be agreed by a committee or by the board of directors and may be based on similar past cases and organisational rules, regulations and codes of practice so that they can easily be justified if necessary.

In a smaller, privately owned organisation – particularly one operating in an industry where rapid decisions are essential and risk-taking encouraged – managers may be expected to be adventurous and have more scope for being innovative.

Size and structure

The larger the organisation, the more likely it is to be hierarchical and display certain characteristics, many of which affect the way in which decisions are made:

Did you know?

The number of staff for whom each manager is responsible is called the **span of control**. It is generally accepted that the optimum number is between six and twelve for a manager to operate effectively. This is why additional managers are needed when an organisation grows in size.

- There is likely to be more formality in areas such as internal and external communications, written policies relating to ways of working, deference to senior staff, official job titles, specific salary scales etc.
- There will be more written policies and procedures, to ensure that standards are the same throughout the organisation and that all employees are treated fairly.
- There could be less flexibility or scope for individual actions or decisions.
- Several people or groups may have to be consulted before certain decisions can be made.
- The greater distance between senior management and staff might mean that the latter have little idea why many formal decisions have been taken.

Organisation culture

This refers to the way in which the organisation operates. It is partly influenced by the size or type of business and industry. For example, you would expect to find a more formal culture in a solicitor's office or a bank than in a local radio station. However, working culture can vary even within an industry – you would probably find quite a difference if you moved from working for the *Sun* newspaper to the *Financial Times*!

Culture is influenced also by the attitude, beliefs and values of the founder(s) or boss. Charles Handy, a management specialist, identified four main organisational cultures, which are shown in the diagram below.

Find out

Your assessor will expect you to know about the **working culture** of your industry or sector as well as your organisation's culture. Find out more about organisational cultures by researching online, then study Handy's examples and see whether you can describe yours.

Power or club culture
(The web)

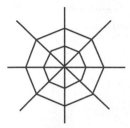

Usually a central figure in control and often started as a one-person/family business.

Few rules. Main ingredient is trust. Long-serving staff valued and often employed in key roles.

Role culture
(Greek temple)

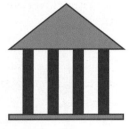

Pillars identify specialist areas (finance, production, sales, etc.). Many procedures and rules coordinated by senior managers at the top.

Usually specific job descriptions, predictable career path. Often a bureaucracy or public sector organisation.

Task culture
(A net)

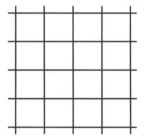

Concerned with getting the job done – no overall boss. The right people are put together for a specific job or task. The outcome is the main issue – may be achieved by groups or project teams.

Decision-making and control delegated downwards. Flexible and fast-moving enterprise.

Person or existential culture
(The cluster)

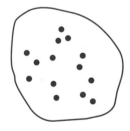

Individuals are most important ingredient – often highly trained professionals (e.g. barristers, medical consultants).

Each individual has power above and beyond the organisation. Each allowed to do his/her 'own thing' and further his/her own career.

Organisational cultures quoted from Understanding Organisations and Gods of Management *Charles Handy*

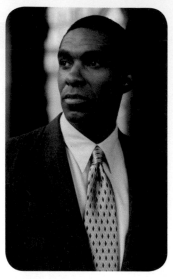
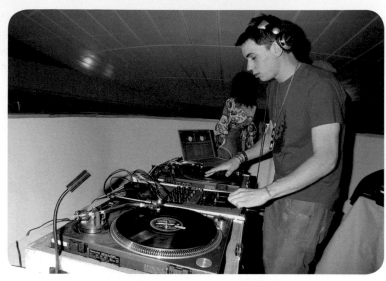

Which of these dress codes is most like the style in your place of work?

Remember

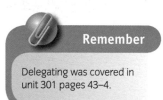

Delegating was covered in unit 301 pages 43–4.

Management styles and attitudes to delegation

Good managers delegate authority when they give people responsibility. This means that if you are responsible for doing a task you don't have to keep checking back each time you want to make a decision. Instead, you make all the relevant decisions related to that task yourself and ask for help when you need it.

Unfortunately, not everyone is good at delegating. Charles Handy's power culture is often described as the spider in a web – who pulls all the strings! In this case very few staff may be trusted to do everything and the owner of the organisation may even burn out under the pressure of trying to make every single decision. Or you may find a manager who is good at delegating, but a member of staff who finds it very difficult to make a decision without agreement or reassurance from above.

Find out

In your organisation, what decisions can you and your colleagues make for yourselves and which are you expected to refer to your line manager(s). Identify the **types** of decision that can be made by individuals and those that are usually made by groups of people in a meeting.

Line management responsibilities and relationships within the organisation

As an organisation grows, delegation of responsibility becomes more and more important, otherwise the burden on individual managers is too great. Important decisions may then be overlooked or not made quickly enough. Similarly, no matter how informal and friendly the culture, eventually a few basic policies and procedures become essential to prevent everyone 'doing their own thing'. Managers are allocated specific responsibilities, usually in relation to running key areas of the enterprise such as finance and sales.

The main areas of the enterprise and the way it is structured will affect relationships in the organisation, both between managers and their staff and laterally between departments. Look back at unit 302, pages 109–10, to refresh your memory about some types of structure you may find in organisations.

Priorities, expectations and authority of your colleagues

When you make decisions yourself or take action, you need to be aware that the people affected may respond differently, depending on their own priorities, expectations and authority:

- People's priorities normally relate to their own job roles and responsibilities. They will be more concerned, quite naturally, with meeting their own targets than meeting yours! They will also have priorities relating to their personal situations. You therefore cannot assume that if someone cannot stay late or assist you that this is merely because they are unhelpful or idle.
- Each of your colleagues will also have different expectations, both of you and everyone else. Some of these will be appropriate, others may be unrealistic. You should be able to correct unrealistic expectations by providing clear, accurate information about what you can and cannot do as part of your job. You should also be prepared to refuse unreasonable requests politely but assertively.
- If you understand how decisions are made in your organisation then you will also know who you must consult because they have authority either over you or over a particular area of work. This is important. You are likely to find yourself rebuked if you make a decision that is outside your area of authority without prior agreement.

If you sketch out your role set then you put the people with whom you have the most contact nearest to you – as you will see in the 'Over to you' section on page 334. These are the people who have the most potential to affect your personal effectiveness and happiness at work. It is important that you understand (and take into account) the different priorities, expectations and authority of all these people when you are making decisions or taking any actions.

Your role set may change depending on the work you are carrying out. Your assessor will expect you to know what this is and to be able to identify those colleagues who are relevant to this work, as well as their work roles and their responsibilities.

Did you know?

The culture of the organisation and the style of management will determine whether departments work cooperatively or competitively.

Remember

One of the behaviours you will need to demonstrate to your assessor is your skill at saying 'no' to unreasonable requests.

Did you know?

Your **role set** at work comprises all the colleagues who have a vested interest in what you do at work and have expectations of you in relation to your own work and behaviour. They are likely to include your line manager, any staff for whom you are responsible, your immediate colleagues, and other contacts in the organisation whose help or assistance is important for you to be able to do your job effectively.

Remember

One of the behaviours you must demonstrate to your assessor is your ability to consider the impact of your own actions on others.

How to... Understand and take account of the priorities, expectations and authority of colleagues

- For the people in your role set, identify the priorities that you think they have related to their job roles and responsibilities. Then check whether you are right by talking to them or discussing your ideas with your line manager.

- Note down the expectations that you think your line manager and your immediate colleagues have of you and your work. You can check these out by assessing feedback you receive (see unit 301, pages 56–7).

- Identify which decisions you can make yourself and which you have to refer to your line manager or to a colleague with particular expertise or authority for a certain area.

- Identify how decisions are made in your organisation and the processes you have to follow if a decision is outside your area of authority.

- For decisions you make or actions you plan to take, consider how colleagues in your role set will be affected. In particular, consider how their own priorities, expectations and areas of authority will affect their response.

Effective communication with colleagues

Unit 301 covered the importance of effective communication, how to communicate verbally and in writing, and the importance of good listening skills.

Good communications are obviously essential to productive working relationships. You are hardly likely to sustain a good working relationship with anyone if you cannot understand or are forever irritating each other. In fact, the quick test whether your communications are effective is to check how often you achieve the desired effect at the first attempt and don't upset anyone in the process!

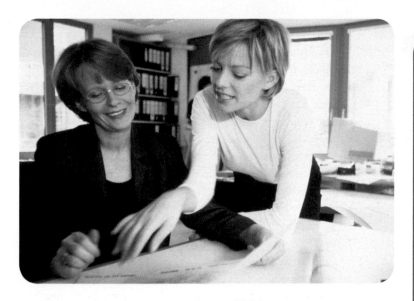

Did you know?

Communications are also affected by the industry, sector and culture of an organisation. In public sector organisations, large charities and large public limited companies there will be more written, formal communications and official meetings. In a small, privately owned firm, there are likely to be more face-to-face discussions and greater freedom for more frank exchanges between staff, especially if quick thinking and innovative ideas are important for success. Similarly, if an organisation encourages and rewards effective people, even if they make the odd mistake, communications will be more open. If a 'blame' culture operates, people will just want to tell the boss what he/she wants to hear!

This is more likely if you observe the principles identified in the table below when you communicate with your colleagues.

Main principles of effective communications	
DO	**DON'T**
Think about the needs of your audience, their possible reaction and the occasion.	Leave it until the last minute to contact people.
Pick an appropriate time, place and method of communicating.	Include your opinions unless these are relevant.
Give facts accurately, clearly, concisely and in a logical order.	Imply you know more than you are telling.
Use appropriate body language.	Make it a guessing game.
Listen carefully to the feedback you receive and check the body language of your recipients (if you can) to see if this supports what they are saying.	Disclose confidential information.
	Deny someone the right to an opinion just because it doesn't match yours.
Allow people time to respond. They may need extra time or 'space' if they are upset or annoyed by the information.	Over-communicate. If your messages are too long or too frequent people will ignore them.
	Gossip, spread rumours, speculate, tell lies or exaggerate!

Remember

One of the behaviours you will need to demonstrate to your assessor is that you present information clearly, concisely, accurately and in ways that promote understanding.

Did you know?

It is wiser, kinder and fairer to remind someone who is busy about an agreement he or she made while there is still time to take action, rather than leave it until it's too late, do the job yourself and then be aggrieved, angry or use it to get them into trouble.

Remember

You will need to provide evidence to your assessor that you fulfil the agreements you make with colleagues and let them know and advise them promptly of any difficulties or where it will be impossible to do so. You will also need to demonstrate two behaviours related to this:

- you clearly agree what is expected of others and hold them to account

- you keep promises and honour your commitments.

Making agreements with colleagues

Good communications are vital if you are making agreements with colleagues, for the following reasons:

- Any agreement is useless unless both parties understand exactly what has been agreed.

- The whole idea of making an agreement is that it will be honoured unless something happens unexpectedly to prevent this – in which case prompt and urgent notification is essential. The importance of advising colleagues promptly of any difficulties that mean it is impossible to fulfil agreements was covered in unit 301, page 47.

- You may have to negotiate with your colleagues to make an agreement that is mutually acceptable. This may relate to the way in which work will be done, the deadlines for completion or the main areas of responsibility. They will have their views and you will have yours. This is where considering and discussing different priorities and expectations is vital. Similarly, if someone has greater authority than you, then you will have to be more persuasive to reach an agreement you want. You certainly cannot insist on your own conditions! You will find out what to do if you cannot reach an agreement on page 338.

Over to you

1   Alex works in an office with five other people in addition to Jan, her line manager. She has drawn the following role set diagram:

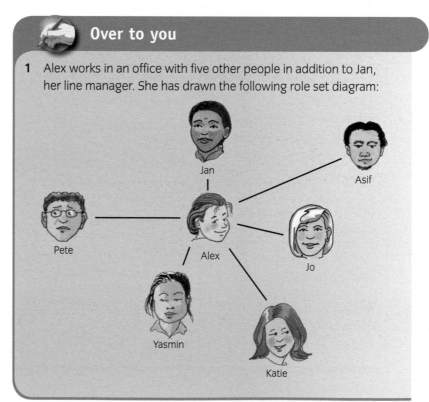

Study the diagram and then answer the following questions:

a Why has Alex placed Jan immediately above her on the diagram?

b With which colleagues does Alex have the most contact on a daily basis?

c With whom does she have the least contact?

d Which of the following two situations is likely to affect Alex the most – and why?

   i Jo and Yasmin arrange to go out to lunch together and don't invite her.

   ii Asif and Pete arrange to go out to lunch together and don't invite her.

e If Alex is having a bad day and takes it out on her colleagues, who will be most affected by her behaviour – and why?

f If a new member joins the group, suggest three ways in which Alex can find out that person's needs and motivations.

Check your ideas and suggestions against the answers on the CD-ROM.

2 a Obtain a copy of your firm's organisation chart or sketch out your own position in the firm. Make sure that you can easily identify those people who have authority over you, those who are at the same level as yourself and anyone for whom you have authority.

b Supplement your chart with a diagram that shows your own role set and then identify the main priorities and expectations of each of the colleagues you have included in your diagram.

3 Identify three people in your organisation who have power and three people who have influence. Discuss with your tutor or trainer the differences between these people and how their behaviour can influence the decision-making processes in your own workplace.

Evidence collection

1 Write a personal statement describing the actions you have taken to develop productive working relationships with at least two people in your role set. Your statement should include reference to the roles

Core unit links

Your communications with colleagues may link to unit 301, performance indicators 1–7. Similarly your overall behaviour that supports effective working may link to unit 301, PIs 22–28.

Your knowledge of your organisation's sector and main purpose and how your relationships with others relates to this may link to unit 302, PIs 1, 2 and 4. Your knowledge of the codes of practice that relate to your work links to unit 301, PI 15.

Evidence collection Continued

and responsibilities of your colleagues and your recognition of their needs and expectations and how you seek to meet these.

2　Keep records of communications you receive and send to colleagues which show that you communicate effectively and take account of their views and needs. These may include your own records of verbal communications as well as written documents such as memos, emails or minutes of meetings.

3　Prepare a document summarising the work roles and responsibilities of yourself and your colleagues as well as any future work plans that are proposed and how these may affect your working relationships or role set. In addition, include other relevant information that you can discuss with your assessor to demonstrate your knowledge of your own organisation, such as the decision-making processes that exist and the line management responsibilities and relationships within your organisation.

Identifying and dealing with disagreements with colleagues

Did you know?

Some disagreements and conflicts are constructive because they encourage people to think of new ways of solving problems. It is only when they become prolonged, bitter and people start to take sides that they become destructive instead.

Disagreements at work can be between teams, departments, individuals and their managers. An individual may have a dispute with a colleague, with his or her manager or with the organisation as a whole. In unit 302, pages 144–5, you saw how formal grievances and disputes are dealt with. This unit focuses more on the everyday disagreements that frequently occur at work.

The first thing to recognise is that disagreements at work are perfectly normal. Within any group of people there will always be occasions when individuals disagree. This may be a relatively minor incident and over in a few moments. On other occasions it may be quite serious and can escalate quickly. Then the productivity of all staff is threatened as more energy is expended on the conflict itself than on the work to be done.

Many experts consider that it is impossible for any organisation to operate without some conflict, mainly because of the different roles people have to undertake and the fact that they are often competing for both resources and rewards – whether it is the same promotion, an increase in the budget or who should have priority at the photocopier! Some of the main reasons are shown in the table opposite. For this reason you need to know how to identify disagreements and the action to take when they occur.

Reasons for disagreements and conflict at work	
Reasons	**Result**
Personality clashes	Disagreements about facts, goals, methods of working or values between two people.
Competition for limited pool of resources	Arguments about allocation between departments, teams or individuals.
Integrating/sharing work	Annoyance about doing more than others, doing better work than others, others not doing their fair share or fulfilling agreements.
Group values	Loyalty to a particular department or group can result in misunderstandings and disputes
Territorial possessiveness	Individuals will fight to retain ownership over what they consider 'theirs' including working space, resources they use, their current job role and responsibilities.
Fear of change	Arguments to keep things as they are when ideas for change are discussed Can result in serious conflict if change is imposed without agreement.
Perceived injustice	One person or group feels unfairly treated or discriminated against because of a decision. This may relate to working hours or conditions, time allocation, holiday entitlement etc.
Role conflict	A person holds two roles that are mutually conflicting. An example would be a supervisor on a staff committee who is asked to defend a colleague's grievance against their mutual boss.
Role ambiguity	In this case someone is unsure of his/her role and responsibilities and what he or she is expected to do. This can result in arguments and disagreements.

Identifying disagreements

When some people are annoyed or upset they go quiet, become uncooperative or even take a few days off. There may also be those who enjoy a good argument and treat it like a sport – which can be stressful

KQ3

to more peaceful individuals who will be tempted to agree to anything for a quiet life. You will identify disagreements more quickly if you follow four simple 'rules'.

- Know and understand your colleagues and appreciate their needs and motivations.
- Know and understand the situations that are likely to act as a trigger (these are listed in the table on page 337).
- Practice reading body language as well as developing your listening skills. Someone who is upset or dejected will have a completely different posture and demeanour from someone who is happy and confident.
- Watch people at work. If people are muttering in corners rather than doing their work, or looking for ways to get back at someone, then you need to find out what is happening.

Techniques for resolving disagreements

Several techniques are used by organisations, managers and individuals to resolve disagreements and reduce or manage conflict. Although all these tactics can be used appropriately in certain situations, collaboration is considered to be the most beneficial. This involves bringing the reason for the disagreement out into the open, discussing the reasons for it and aiming to find a solution that suits both parties.

Strategies for solving disagreements			
Tactic	**Aim**	**Disadvantages**	**Appropriate if...**
Do nothing	If the problem is ignored completely it will go away	It might not go away and it could get worse	Time is short, the disagreement is very minor and the outcome doesn't matter
Act the peacemaker	To appeal to people to ignore individual differences for the greater good	It ignores the root cause of the disagreement	The issue is far more important to one person than another
Order or threaten	To make people do as they are told	Threats often don't work, the problem could escalate or re-emerge in the future	The situation is critical, urgent and threatening the existence of the organisation or the needs and wishes of the majority of people

Strategies for solving disagreements			
Tactic	Aim	Disadvantages	Appropriate if...
Aim for a compromise	To find a solution acceptable to both parties; e.g. 'split the difference'	Neither person has won so neither feels very happy about the outcome	No other solution can be found, particularly if the disagreement is over resource allocation or rewards to staff
Facilitate collaboration	To negotiate a mutually beneficial outcome where both parties 'win' something	Takes time and skill to do it properly	You want to investigate possible alternatives with those concerned openly and positively

(handwritten beside table: 2 ... 1)

Identifying and resolving conflicts of interest with colleagues

A conflict of interest with a colleague occurs when you have aims, beliefs or targets that are incompatible. At an individual level it would occur if you cannot complete a task by a deadline without using up all the folders in the stationery cupboard and having uninterrupted access to the photocopier for the rest of the day. If one of your colleagues has exactly the same problem, with the resources you currently have at your disposal only one of you can succeed.

In many organisations a common conflict of interest is between departments. Sales want the customers to have all their needs met promptly, production want steady production runs, and finance want everyone to keep to their budgets. So at inter-departmental meetings everyone has a different agenda. If satisfying the needs of an important customer will mean a change to production schedules and an overrun on the sales budget, you can expect a fair amount of disagreement!

The way in which conflicts of interest are managed will depend on the type of organisation, its culture and its priorities. Most managers will aim to resolve these types of conflict by making their preferences or expectations clear. When there is a genuine quandary the issue is referred to a senior manager who will make a final decision based on the interests of the organisation, rather than the individuals. Another tactic is to work towards a 'win/win' outcome of any dispute.

This is based on the theory that there are potentially different outcomes of any conflict depending on the degree of cooperation and assertiveness shown by the parties. Both may 'lose' (I lose, you lose) so

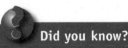

Did you know?

Someone's agenda can be known or hidden. A **hidden agenda** means that someone has an ulterior motive for saying or doing something. You can find out more about organisational and office politics on pages 343–4.

Remember

Win/win is a state of mind. It takes openness, creativity and a willingness to find a jointly acceptable solution. It is the ideal outcome because both people are pleased with the result and both have achieved something.

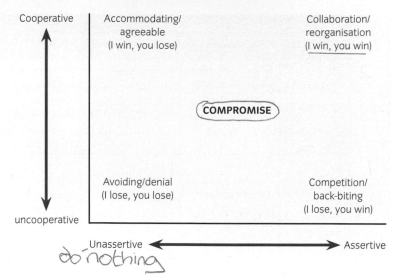

Cooperative

Accommodating/
agreeable
(I win, you lose)

Collaboration/
reorganisation
(I win, you win)

COMPROMISE

Avoiding/denial
(I lose, you lose)

Competition/
back-biting
(I lose, you win)

uncooperative

Unassertive ← → Assertive

both are unhappy, or one may give in or compromise (I win, you lose; or you win, I lose). However, the aim should be for both sides to win.

How can you achieve this? Suppose I need four days to do a task because I am very busy, but you want me to do it immediately. If you insist and I make a mess of it then we both lose. If you insist but I then have problems because my other work suffers then you win and I lose. If I stick to my guns then I win and you lose. We both win if:

- one of us finds someone else who can do the task more quickly for you
- we both find a way of rescheduling my other jobs so that I can do the task in the next day or so
- I suggest ways in which it can be done more quickly and you agree to this.

How to ... Resolve conflicts and disagreements to minimise damage to work being carried out

- Be alert to situations where conflicts of interest and disagreements can arise..

- Try to solve disagreements with colleagues quickly, through collaboration, whenever you can.

- Be aware of your own perceptions of other people and how these may influence your behaviour. If you have a personality clash with someone, try changing the way you respond to see what happens.

- If you are involved with trying to resolve a disagreement, follow these guidelines:

  - Start by establishing the reason for the conflict and get the issue out into the open.

  - Aim to help both parties to save face by going for a 'win/win' outcome.

  - Focus on finding a positive outcome – not necessarily the 'best possible' but 'what each can live with'.

  - Encourage people to express their feelings honestly and assertively.

  - Don't accept (or make) accusations or opinions unsupported by facts or evidence.

  - Try to identify areas where change or compromise is possible.

  - If necessary, suggest a change over a trial period and monitor progress.

- If you are involved in a disagreement that someone else is trying to resolve, work positively towards finding an acceptable solution.

Understanding your organisation – 2

The types of disagreement and conflict of interest that are experienced in organisations can depend on several factors. These are shown in the diagram below.

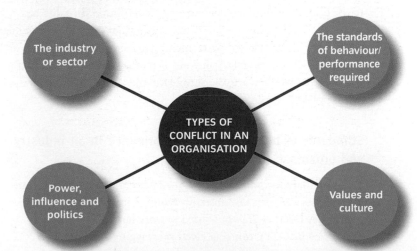

- The industry or sector
- The standards of behaviour/ performance required
- TYPES OF CONFLICT IN AN ORGANISATION
- Power, influence and politics
- Values and culture

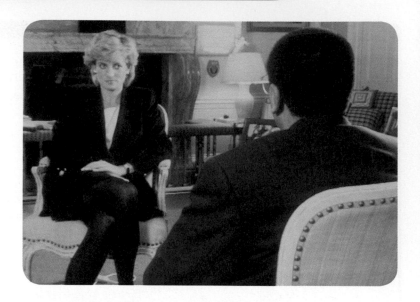

Find out

The conflicts of interest and disagreements your boss has to cope with, and how he or she handles these.

The industry or sector

Most people are aware that when the late Princess Diana wanted to make her problems public, she secretly agreed for the BBC interviewer Martin Bashir to record her feelings for a *Panorama* television programme. This caused a sensation when it was aired – and several problems for the then Chairman of the BBC, Marmaduke Hussey, who was a personal friend of the Queen. To say that he had a conflict of interest at the time between the wishes of his staff, the aims of the BBC and his personal loyalties is an understatement!

Such a problem is unlikely to exist for your local doctor or estate agent, but they will have similar issues related to their own jobs. Doctors may have a conflict of interest between budget allocations and the needs of some patients; an estate agent may have problems related to the diverse needs of a seller and a particular buyer. In a different sector, manufacturing, you have already seen that there may be regular conflicts of interests and disagreements between sales, production and finance departments. In fact, in your own organisation, it is doubtful whether the staff who are responsible for sales and marketing always see eye to eye with the finance section!

Standards of behaviour and performance in an industry and organisation

The potential for conflict and disagreement is greater when staff are stressed because they are constantly working towards tight deadlines – or if they feel they are not trusted to work hard without being monitored by CCTV cameras, electronic tagging and computer technology. Generally this type of activity is more likely to take place in the private sector than in the public or voluntary sectors. However, even in the professions, telephone monitoring can take place. Many service industries, such as legal and accountancy firms, have installed sophisticated systems that record the number of voicemails left for each person and the time taken to respond to these.

The values and culture of the organisation

Organisational culture was discussed on page 328 and the values of an organisation were first covered in unit 302 on pages 111–18. Turn back to those pages now if you have forgotten what is meant by terms like 'values' and 'ethics'.

These link to the types of behaviour by the people in the organisation that will be encouraged or discouraged. Where views differ on the values that should be adopted there is the potential for disagreement and conflict.

The power, influence and politics in the organisation

The difference between power and influence was described on page 326, and organisational politics were mentioned on page 339 in relation to hidden agendas. There is a link between the two, because individuals who are politically clever may use various methods to achieve their own goals, often by trying to influence other people to gain power or other benefits. Examples include lobbying other people for support for an idea (which may include picking a time when objectors cannot be present), negotiating behind closed doors for benefits or scarce resources (even if this means only telling a partial tale to acquire them), taking the credit for other people's ideas or successes, and damning colleagues by faint praise rather than (obvious) open criticism – e.g. 'It's such a shame, she tries so hard, we're all hoping she'll get better in time.'

In an organisation that is highly political, there may be almost as much going on under the surface as there is on it! Unless you are a political animal yourself, and enjoy the cut and thrust, you could find it hard to cope and become stressed and demotivated, particularly if you work in an organisation where only those who are clever at using office politics for their own ends are successful.

Eric Berne was a famous authority on the political games people play – sometimes without realising it. He argued they are all played for a 'pay-off' for the player and he recommended that the best way to deal with these is to recognise the game and to call it. To give you an idea of what he meant, some of the most prevalent are explained in the table below, together with the action to take to avoid open conflict.

Did you know?

In 2004, the AA announced that it was going to monitor its 3000 call centre staff by computer to ensure they kept to a new pay deal allowing them a maximum of 82 minutes free time – which included all breaks, including visits to the toilet. The GMB union was furious, equating it to treating workers like battery hens. The inventors of the sensors at Cambridge firm Ubisense were surprised, saying they were never designed to act as spies but to increase security.

Did you know?

Organisational politics refers to the various activities undertaken by individuals mainly for their own ends, rather than the good of the organisation or their colleagues. These activities may be subversive, devious or manipulative and may be encouraged, discouraged or tacitly accepted by management.

Find out

Find other ideas for coping with office politics online at www.officepolitics.com (an American site) and at www.ivillage.co.uk/workcareer/survive/archive/0,,156475,00.html.

The name of the game!			
The game	The tactic	The payoff	Call the game by saying...
Yes, but	All suggestions are countered with 'yes, but...' and a reason why it is impossible to do it	The game-player doesn't have to do it but never actually says 'no'!	If you don't want to do it, just say so
Harried	The game-player is permanently harassed, looks fraught and is forever complaining about his or her workload	No one dare ask the game-player to do anything extra	You are obviously really struggling to cope. Let's talk about it
Now I've caught you	The victim is given harder and harder jobs, tighter deadlines and poor guidance until a mistake is made	The game-player (the boss, in this case) can prove the victim is a poor worker	Here's a list of all the jobs I've got and how long each will take. Please prioritise them for me
Let him and you fight	This person tells you what he or she would do in your shoes – and encourages you to take action that he or she wouldn't dare!	The game-player has caused trouble without actually being involved in it	What a good idea. Can I say you suggested it?

Adapted from Eric Berne's book Games People Play

Snapshot – When it's time to call in the professionals

Most people can work productively alongside their colleagues fairly easily when times are relaxed and they are not under pressure. The situation is very different if there is rapid and continuous change or tight deadlines to achieve, particularly with scarce resources, or if business prospects are poor, so jobs are threatened. In these types of situation any minor niggles or problems can easily escalate into major rows or conflict.

Because of this a number of specialist companies offer Employment Assistance Programmes (EAPs) which include stress management, individual counselling (on the phone and/or online), and trauma support for employees. In addition, they will run training courses for staff as well as offering dispute or conflict resolution services as well as professional consultants who will investigate sensitive issues, such as diversity and equality, and recommend areas for improvement. Organisations that retain professionals to provide staff counselling prove that they recognise the value of staff harmony and demonstrate that they take the needs of their employees seriously. You can find out more at www. righcorecare.co.uk, www.workplacemediation.co.uk, www.validium.com and www.conflictmanagementplus.com.

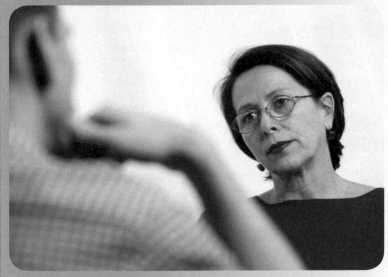

Professional counselling can help resolve disputes

Did you know?

In the UK, diversity policies are still more commonly found in the public and voluntary sectors than in the private sector, unlike in the USA where many directors of large companies, such as Wall-Mart, receive bonuses if they meet diversity targets. In October 2005, the British civil service published its ten-point plan to promote diversity with similar incentives for senior officials. There is a long way to go – in the senior civil service only 3.2 per cent of staff are from ethnic minorities, only 35 per cent are women (with fewer than a quarter in top posts) and fewer than 3 per cent of staff are disabled in some way.

Diversity issues when developing working relationships with colleagues

The issue of diversity was covered fully in unit 302, pages 161–9. This includes interacting and learning from people who are different from you, whether they be colleagues or customers. Turn back to those pages now and refresh your memory.

Exchanging information and resources with colleagues

Everyone in an organisation handles a tremendous amount of information every day. It arrives in the mail, electronically, through customer visits and over the telephone. More is received during meetings, team briefings and even during the lunch break. Much of this may be trivia, some routine, but other items may be very important or even essential – but perhaps to one of your colleagues rather than to you.

There are various ways to ensure that you remain alert to information that your colleagues may find useful. Here are three:

- Cultivate a good memory, so that you know the type of work different people are involved in.
- Make links between information you receive and the work to which this relates – whether this work is being done by you or your colleagues.
- Have a mental alarm clock that warns you when information is urgently needed so that you respond appropriately.

The value of exchanging information, rather than simply passing it on, is that by virtue of participating in a discussion or negotiation the value of the information increases. This occurs with a colleague when you exchange ideas or suggest making additions of amendments. The whole purpose is that an open and friendly exchange helps to consolidate a positive and productive working relationship.

The same applies when you agree how to allocate or exchange resources. In an ideal world there would be more than enough for everyone. In reality there are rarely sufficient resources for everyone in an organisation, especially during busy times. Rather than 'share and share alike', it is more sensible to apportion resources according to the priorities and the main objectives of the organisation and the current work pressures and deadlines of your colleagues.

KQ6

How to... Exchange information and resourc with colleagues to ensure all part can work effectively

- Be aware of how the roles and responsibilities of colleagues will influence the type of information and resources they need.

- Stay alert to changing needs – through new types of work, changing roles or urgent deadlines – that may affect colleagues' requirements.

- Cultivate a good memory for making connections between old and new items of information, topics and work issues, so that you know instinctively which information to share and with whom.

- Be aware of areas of overlap with your own work, so that you can share appropriate information.

- When in doubt, tell someone else. Don't keep important information to yourself.

- Focus on the needs of the group as a whole, rather than on your own priorities.

- Practise your assertiveness skills if you find someone else is ignoring your own needs and rights.

Obtaining and using feedback on your own performance

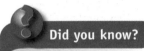

Did you know?

360-degree appraisals are so called because feedback is given by all colleagues – senior, junior and at the same level.

In unit 301 you learned about the importance of encouraging feedback from other people, including your colleagues, and how to use this to identify ways in which you can improve. Turn back to pages 56–7 now and refresh your memory – including how to cope if you receive negative feedback at any time.

Providing colleagues with useful feedback on their performance

It is bad management to give only 'official' feedback on infrequent, formal occasions, so that often the news may come as something of a shock to the recipient. Ideally informal feedback should occur frequently, for several reasons:

- Feedback always has more impact when it is immediate, so people are not scratching their heads to remember what happened.

- Feedback should be positive far more than it is negative, if you want to motivate and encourage your colleagues – and you should give praise freely and openly, when it is due.

- Prompt feedback means that any errors or mistakes can be rectified quickly, without becoming a serious issue. Sometimes these may be

Q7 use b

Remember

For feedback to be useful it has to be couched in terms that the recipient will accept. If you annoy someone at the start, he or she switches off and it is pointless carrying on. The person will merely be defensive or even aggressive in response.

caused by poor guidance or sloppy instructions, misunderstandings or a lack of knowledge so that the root cause of a problem is slightly different from what was first thought. Making an immediate query – in a positive way – will help to identify this far better than accusatory statements or hunting around to pin the blame on someone.

How to... Provide feedback on performance to colleagues

- Give positive feedback regularly and informally. Don't store it up for a special occasion!

- Prepare in advance when you are giving formal feedback and choose your time carefully – not when someone is busy or distracted and never in front of an audience if the feedback is critical.

- Always focus on the positive points of someone's performance and use these as a model for developing weaker areas.

- Get to the point quickly and focus on the issues and work aspects involved rather than the person.

- Give clear, specific examples to support your opinions. This is just as important if you are giving positive feedback as negative.

- Don't expect the listener to agree with everything you say, whether you are talking about a weakness or suggesting that a colleague could take on additional responsibilities. Remember you can only second-guess other people's thoughts and feelings – and you may be very wrong!

- Give your colleague time to respond to your feedback and listen to his or her views carefully.

- Don't penalise a good performer by giving extra work or tougher targets as a reward! It's only too easy to overburden a willing workhorse.

- Check that you both agree on the outcome of the discussion and what happens next by asking your colleague to sum up the session at the end.

- Check that you have given equal time to all your colleagues. It is tempting to give shorter feedback to those whose results are positive and not spend as much time discussing the person's individual needs. This is unfair on the person and may also lead to everyone guessing the outcome of each session simply by its length.

Case study Developing your own 'people' skills

Did you know?

Members of the IQPS can use a specific designation after their names. Linda is a Fellow, so can use FIQPS. Other designations include AffIQPS, MIQPS, LIQPS and FIQPS. You can find out more on the IQPS website at www.iqps.org.

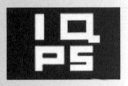

Read the case study below and then answer the questions that follow.

Linda Barton FIQPS is the national chairperson of the Institute of Qualified Professional Secretaries (IQPS) as well as being PA to the chief executive of Universities UK. She has considerable experience at developing productive working relationships with her colleagues. In fact, without this skill, it is very doubtful she would have such a glittering career. So what hints and tips can Linda offer you at this stage of your working life?

First, what does Linda do when she meets someone new – and how does she work to develop a productive working relationship? Linda suggests that when you meet a new colleague you should be polite and friendly but not over-familiar. This means being prepared to take your time to develop a relationship and concentrating on putting the other person at ease by being helpful and non-threatening. Do this by asking questions about his or her background – but remember this does not mean interrogation! As an example, meet a new recruit in reception and take him or her around the building. Give background information about the company to introduce the person to the new environment and to calm any butterflies. Introduce the person also to his or her new colleagues and explain who does what. This may be part of the company's official induction process but, if not, it is still helpful to someone just starting out in a job in your organisation.

Despite your best efforts, though, some people may still be difficult to deal with. Linda suggests that it helps if you get to know a person before you come to any conclusions, simply because there is often common ground you can establish. It is then just a short step to finding a basis for agreement. As an example, chat to an older colleague in the office kitchen about his or her family – you may find you have similar thoughts and views to the colleague's children. Finding out what makes someone 'tick' is just the first stage in understanding how he or she thinks and what makes the person react in particular ways.

If you start work for a new employer and think the whole organisation is against you or so different from what you are used to that you cannot stay for one moment longer, Linda suggests you give it time. It is unwise to make a judgement about a new workplace or a new group of colleagues in a matter of days. Allow yourself time to adapt and find out more about each person as an individual. This doesn't mean, of course, that everyone you work with will eventually turn out to be an angel! Remember that you don't have to like everyone you work with to do a good job. As long as you both have your employer's interests at heart then you should be able to work together cooperatively. If you still have problems reaching agreement, ask the person concerned to explain exactly what it is he or she wants, in detail, and to specify his or her ultimate goal. Then you will be clear about exactly what it is you have to achieve.

Everyone has a mental picture of their ideal colleague. Linda's would be patient, with a sense of humour, flexible and sensitive – someone who knows instinctively which subjects are 'discussable' and which are not! All this is, of course, in addition to putting in effort to achieve success.

Such colleagues deserve fair treatment in return. This means being fair and honest and always ensuring that any feedback you give is constructive, rather than destructive, and never critical. It is important to find a positive aspect in someone's performance and to build on this to encourage him or her to do even better.

This does not mean, of course, that you might be immune to criticism yourself. If you receive negative feedback, Linda's suggestion for coping is to think about the information you have received and then ask to discuss the matter further when you have got over the shock! By then the person concerned may have second thoughts and want to moderate the critical opinions.

Her final tip in relation to building productive working relationships is to develop your communication skills. This means providing honest and accurate information and being able to listen carefully to what other people have to say. If you work hard to do this and adopt a mature attitude that allows for and accepts the differences between yourself and other people at work, then you are on the first step to developing a wide range of productive working relationships, many of which may last for many years to come.

To find out more about IQPS, how you can become a member and the benefits it can offer, send your CV to IQPS, Suite 464, 24–28 St Leonard's Road, Windsor, Berks SL4 3BB, or by email to office@iqps.org.

Questions

1   *Suggest two reasons why Linda recommends that you should not become over-familiar with someone new at work.*

2   *Identify the key aspects of your organisation's induction programme, and/or suggest how you can help new recruits to your own section or department to settle down quickly.*

3 *Identify one person with whom you superficially have little in common and engage him or her in conversation over the next week. Identify one fact that could be a basis for knowing the person better, and develop this. Then describe the results.*

4 *Compare the culture of your employer's organisation with one other working environment, such as your school or college or that of a previous employer. Identify the main differences and explain how you have coped with the changes. Discuss your ideas with your tutor or trainer.*

5 *Suggest three strategies you would use to cope with a new boss who, at first sight, appeared to be overly demanding and unreasonable.*

6 *Write down five attributes in your own ideal colleague. Then try to assess objectively whether you possess these yourself! If you are in doubt, ask a trusted friend or colleague for feedback.*

7 *Your best friend is taking advantage of your friendship to arrive late in the morning, extend her lunch hour and do sloppy work. Explain how you would cope with the situation.*

Understanding your organisation – 3

Find out

Investigate the types of information and resources that apply to your own organisation, as well as how the work undertaken affects the type of agreements you make with colleagues.

On pages 324–41 you read that the type of organisation you work for, your job role and those of your colleagues and many other aspects of the workplace mean that there are differences between the aspects of work such as decision-making and the types of disagreement you might encounter. Two other areas that may be different are:

● the types of information and resources that colleagues might need
● the types of agreements you might make with your colleagues – which links with the information you read on page 334.

By now you should be able to investigate these areas yourself, as suggested below.

Changing places

Your assessor will ask you how you might adapt your approach to forming relationships at work if you change your job. You will need to think about how this would change if you worked for a different organisation.

Sean works for a small firm of software designers. The culture is very informal and there are few hard and fast rules. People speak frankly to one another and arguments can be fierce and heated but over in seconds. Many working relationships are continued outside work. There is a five-a-side soccer team that plays every Monday, and Friday nights normally end with 'happy hour' in the local bar until 7 p.m. Sean enjoys the relaxed, open and friendly relationships he has with his colleagues.

Michelle works for a large insurance company in a city centre. She rarely sees anyone outside her own immediate section and relates mainly to a small group of colleagues around her own age. One or two older staff can be rather prickly and difficult to deal with, so Michelle always takes extra care when she communicates with them. There are many formal procedures Michelle has to follow when she is processing claims, but the working atmosphere is positive and the resources are excellent. There has rarely, if ever, been any open conflict between staff.

Razia works as an administrator in a large company, producing clothing, run by a father and his son. The relationship between father and son is fairly stormy, especially when they disagree on major aspects of business. On these occasions, Razia keeps her head down and just gets on with her work – as do the rest of the staff. Razia is happy there because the staff work well as a group as they all have the interests of the business at heart.

Heather works as a senior administrator in a local health centre. Relationships between all the staff are good, although she relates on a personal level more to other administrators and nursing staff than she does to the GPs. She is keen to promote harmony and cooperation between all the staff for whom she is responsible and holds regular staff briefings to keep them informed of developments. This is particularly helpful for the part-time reception staff who may otherwise feel left out of the team. Heather is liked and respected by her staff for her open, friendly attitude and the fact that she is quick to praise good work.

1   For any *one* person listed above, identify the differences he or she would find if moving to your organisation and doing your job.

2   For any *one* person listed above, say how you would need to adapt your skills if you did their job rather than your own.

Over to you

1   Suggest how you would deal with each of the following situations. Ideally your answers should include an analysis of why each person may be behaving in this way and how this would or could influence your reactions. Check your ideas against the suggestions on the CD-ROM.

   a   Jasper, in finance, is frequently terse and abrupt when you contact him for information and often tells you that work will take longer than you think it should.

   b   Geraldine, a colleague in your office, is perpetually disorganised, rarely gives you information when you need it and – you think – often criticises you behind your back.

   c   Julie, a colleague at a more junior level, is desperately keen to do well but often makes appalling mistakes because she rushes jobs.

2   You are responsible for giving feedback to three members of staff: Kerry, who bursts into tears at the drop of a hat; Darren, who sulks if he receives information he doesn't want to hear; and Julian, who believes that attack is the best form of defence. Yesterday you returned unexpectedly from a training event to find that all three had gone home half an hour early leaving several jobs unfinished. Say what action you would take in this situation, and suggest how you would deal with each person's individual characteristics. Check your ideas with the suggestions on the CD-ROM.

Evidence collection

1   Analyse your own behaviour at work by starting a behaviour diary or log which records, in particular, key events when you have demonstrated a particular behaviour – either deliberately or as a reaction to an event. In each case, write a note that reflects on the event and identifies the appropriateness, or otherwise, of your behaviour and the outcome(s). You can use this log as a basis to prepare personal statements to analyse and summarise specific events that you can describe to your assessor as part of a professional discussion.

2   Keep records of communications that prove you have fulfilled agreements with your colleagues (or notified them promptly if this is impossible) and have exchanged information and resources to

All your communications with colleagues may link to unit 301, performance indicators 1–7. Accepting feedback from others and using this to improve your work links to unit 301, PIs 16–18.

Being assertive in relation to your own employment rights may link to unit 302, PI 9. Evidence to show that you support diversity by interacting with other people in a way that is sensitive to their individual needs links to unit 302, PIs 11 and 12.

If you deal with information about your colleagues that is confidential, then this links to unit 302, PIs 15 and 16.

Evidence collection Continued

facilitate effective working. Supplement your claims with witness testimony, or a personal account, countersigned and dated by your line manager, which supports this claim.

3 Make a note of the location of feedback records that you wish to discuss with your assessor. For any official appraisal records relating to your colleagues, make sure that you have their agreement before you show these to a third party. For unofficial verbal feedback situations record these yourself and ask your line manager or colleague to countersign your account.

4 Prepare an account describing the culture and ethos of your organisation and explaining how this affects staff behaviour. Include an account of any conflicts you have witnessed or in which you have been involved, and explain the action you took to resolve the issue – and why.

 What if...?

What should you do if, during the assessment period, no occasions occur when you encounter difficulties that will mean you cannot fulfil your agreements?

Your assessor can give you a dedicated task to cover the knowledge and understanding required. This will then be followed by a professional discussion during which you can explain how you would perform in such a situation and what evidence you might bring forward.

 Key skills reminder

If you are taking Key Skills awards, remember to discuss with your tutor or trainer how your evidence for this unit could also count towards those awards.

Unit 321

Provide leadership for your team

Unit summary and overview

This option unit relates to the way in which you provide direction for members of your team and motivate and support them to achieve both the objectives of the team and their personal work objectives. It covers the way in which team members are involved in planning and setting their objectives and how you help to steer and motivate your team members, particularly when they face difficulties, challenges or conflict.

Good team leaders are prized by organisations and staff alike. They know how to motivate members of their team, how and when to give support and encouragement and when non-interference would be preferred. They also know how to engender a positive team spirit to get the best out of individual members, bearing in mind their similarities and differences and complementary skills. If you are responsible for a team in your workplace then this unit will enable you to develop your leadership skills to the benefit of both yourself and your team members.

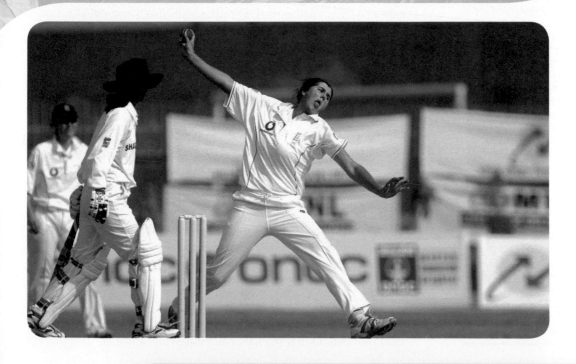

Ways of communicating effectively with team members

In unit 301 you learned about the skills required to communicate effectively with other people and the different ways in which information can be presented. You were also made aware that unless you are a good communicator and carefully consider the needs of your audience, you may sometimes give the wrong message or impression quite accidentally.

All of the lessons you learned in that unit apply equally to communications with your team – plus a few more. This is because each team member may easily put his or her own interpretation on what you say – and how you say it – based on a personal viewpoint and perceptions. In some cases, team members may then try to convince other members of the group that their interpretation is the correct one. So if you inadvertently miss out a piece of information, one person thinks you did it by accident, someone else considers that you just decided you don't want to overload them with details, and a third suspects there is a sinister meaning behind your motives. For these reasons, thinking in advance about what you say to your team, how you say it and how it may be received by each person becomes doubly important!

This does not mean that effective communications with a team are impossible. As you will see throughout this unit, if you and your team have a positive, trusting working relationship, then suspicion and misinterpretation of communications is less likely to occur. Despite this, there are some key points you should bear in mind.

There are two aspects to any communication with your team – the medium and the message. You need to consider both.

The **medium** relates to the method you choose. Whenever your team may have concerns or questions about the information they will receive you should always choose a method that facilitates interaction and feedback – such as a team briefing or meeting – rather than an email or notice. That way you can clarify issues, answer questions and address concerns immediately.

The **message** refers to the words you use and the attitude you adopt. Your words should be simple and straightforward and focus on the facts and not your opinion, unless this is relevant. It is your responsibility to reduce the potential for disharmony and misinterpretation, not add to it!

Your attitude must inspire confidence and trust within and between team members. Even if you have inner misgivings about an organisational policy or objective you are discussing with the team, it is your job to inspire them to meet their targets – not foster misgivings or disenchantment.

Be prepared to answer questions and discuss difficult issues if these concern team members. A major and valuable skill of team leaders is to be able to influence and inspire team members through a process of rational argument and mutual respect.

Be prepared to admit defeat on issues where you are out-voted by your team. Collective decisions are always more powerful than those imposed by a leader – as you will see on page 359.

Setting objectives

Team objectives provide a focus for the team that links their efforts to the goals and purpose of the organisation and/or department. They also enable resources to be allocated effectively relating to the types of task that need to be carried out and their importance. Setting objectives also means that the overall performance of the team is measurable, in addition to the performance of individuals. This is invaluable information for when you are giving feedback to team members, either informally or formally. Setting objectives and then measuring performance against them also highlights the need for any additional training or development that the team may need, either individually or as a group. All these benefits will be lost, however, unless the objectives are clear, appropriate and clearly understood by all members of the team.

Setting SMART objectives

There is a skill to setting objectives with a team because you will have to take into account individual differences between team members. Some people may love a challenge or may be over-ambitious about what they can achieve. Others may be far more nervous about their own abilities and need a lot of encouragement to take on anything new. Your aim is to help your team members to set objectives that are challenging enough to help them to develop and for the team to meet its targets while, at the same time, making sure that the objectives are realistic. For this reason you should aim to ensure that all the objectives are SMART.

You first learned about these in unit 301, page 34. SMART objectives means that they are:

- **S**pecific – each objective deals with one particular aspect of performance

Did you know?

Generally, it is wiser to communicate major events and developments to the whole team at once, rather than to individuals. This prevents anyone thinking that you have 'favourites' who you tell first, or anyone getting an unofficial version of the information from someone else.

Did you know?

A **group of people** comprises individuals each with their own aims. They may, or may not, have a common purpose or leader. A **team** is different. It uses the complementary skills of its members to achieve a common purpose for which all the members are collectively accountable.

Remember

Always be aware of the grapevine. It will pass on interesting titbits of information and speculative guesses far quicker than you can!

Remember

Team members communicate not only with you but also between themselves – often when you are not there.

- **M**easurable – achievement can be checked against a specific target
- **A**chievable – they are sensible and not over-optimistic or over-ambitious
- **R**ealistic – they are within the reach of the team, given its resources
- **T**ime-related – you have a deadline for completion.

Team objectives are different from individual objectives because they usually require the combined cooperation of everyone for them to be achieved. It is sometimes possible for a team to do well even though one or two members are not working effectively – as many sporting teams prove every week – but this does not mean that those people who are the good performers are happy about the situation, particularly if it lasts for any length of time.

How to... Set out and positively communicate the purpose and objectives of the team to all members

- Work with your own line manager to decide and agree the objectives for your team based on the aims of the business (or your department), its strategic and operational plans and the role of your team.

- Check that the objectives of the team match the priorities of the business (or your department) and the overall purpose of the team.

- Check that all the objectives listed are SMART and that you, yourself, understand why they have been set, are clear about each one and know how achievement will be measured.

- Involve team members in discussions relating to agreeing team objectives and check that these are demanding but realistic.

- Assist your team members to set individual objectives, linked to the team objectives. Remember that some may need support and encouragement to stretch themselves, others may be enthusiastic or even too optimistic about what they might achieve.

- Think about the likely questions you may be asked to clarify particular issues or provide further information.

- Make sure that the final list of agreed objectives is known by all the team. Provide a written list for future reference.

Achievement of team objectives involving team members

Achieving team objectives means making decisions related to coordinating and integrating the efforts of individual team members. Your role, as team leader, is to ensure that all the team members are pulling in the same direction and all the activities being carried out link together within an agreed timescale to enable a specific objective to be achieved. You cannot do this without the cooperation of your team, and this means involving them in planning how team objectives can and will be achieved.

These are major questions to discuss with the team for each objective:

- What, exactly, is the goal that must be achieved?
- By when is achievement required?
- How can this be done?
- What resources will be required?
- How will performance or achievement be measured?

Measurement of the performance is often done by deciding key result areas (KRAs) for each member of the team and then identifying performance indicators (PIs) which measure achievement.

It is also important to discuss the priority of different objectives, if all of them cannot be achieved simultaneously.

Showing how personal work objectives contribute to achieving team objectives

It is always easier to lead a team if the goals and objectives of the individual members are aligned with the team's objectives. Similarly, it is always easier for an organisation to be effective and successful if the goals and objectives of the teams, departments and managers are linked to the main purpose and goals of the organisation as a whole.

As a simple example, take an organisation that aims to grow large and expand. If all the managers are keen on the idea of working for a larger organisation then they will be more committed to achieving these goals. They will want their departments to be more profitable and to expand and they will see benefits for themselves in this process. They will work to achieve their own goals and, in doing so, will help the organisation to attain its goals also.

The same applies to you and your team. Your team may have an objective to generate more sales, provide better customer service or to do work more quickly. If this links to the personal objectives of the team members then they will be more motivated to be successful. If the two

Did you know?

Collective responsibility means that, once a decision is made or a plan is agreed by a team, everyone is committed to it. However, for this to work, everyone must have had their say in the process – otherwise they can, quite fairly, argue that the decision has been imposed on them.

Did you know?

Key result areas focus on the specific role and contributions of each member of a team. So a goalkeeper in a football team would be responsible for stopping goals whereas the key task of a striker is to shoot to score. Most people can cope with only three to five KRAs, otherwise they feel overloaded.

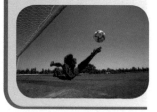

Did you know?

Some organisations offer team members a financial bonus based on the performance of the team. The aim is to give all members a personal incentive to attain the team goal.

are unrelated then you may end up with team members with two totally separate sets of objectives. If the two are in conflict then you have a problem. This would occur, for example, if you set a personal objective for someone to work more carefully and produce higher quality work when achieving the team objective requires him or her to work more quickly to meet certain deadlines.

Your job involves making sure that:

- each member of your team has personal work objectives linked to his or her job role
- these objectives complement the team objectives and don't cause conflict for individuals
- each member of your team understands the link between the two
- each member of the team is encouraged and supported to achieve both sets of objectives
- praise and recognition is given when objectives have been achieved.

Did you know?

There is an argument that people are motivated by achieving tough but realistic objectives. Therefore objectives should be demanding enough to provide a challenge but realistic enough to be achievable. One that is too easy will be disregarded and does nothing to improve performance; but if it is too difficult it may cause anxiety and stress for the person concerned.

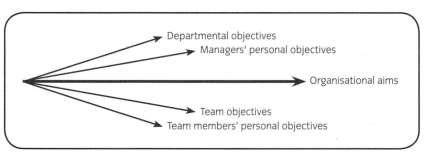

The productive organisation in which all goals are related to one another

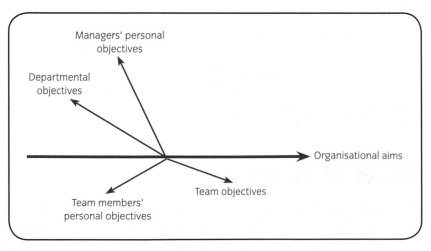

The non-productive organisation in which goals are not in alignment

Snapshot – A good place to work

In March each year the *Sunday Times* produces its Best Companies to Work For lists. These include the 100 best small companies to work for in the UK (with 50–249 employees); the 100 best companies to work for (with 250– 4999 employees) and the ten best large companies to work for (with over 5000 employees). In each case these organisations are nominated by their employees for inclusion and scored on specific criteria that include leadership and the feelings of employees about their immediate colleagues and how well they work together. In 2005, the top-ranked large organisation to work for was Nationwide, second was Asda, third was KPMG (a large firm of accountants), Carphone Warehouse was fourth and Mothercare fifth.

In 2005, top place in the small company list went to Pareto Law, a training and recruitment agency in Cheshire with 53 staff. Noticeable among all the winners, however, was the value that staff put on leadership and teamwork in their organisations. At Hart Worldwide, number two in the list, there is a 'one team' approach and 91 per cent of staff care about their team-mates, enjoy each other's company and work well together. At Lansons Communications, number 21 in the list, teams are close-knit and four out of five employees say working in their team gives them a buzz. Even more say they are confident in the abilities of their team-mates. At number eight in the rankings, Lexis Public Relations, 93 per cent of staff said they laugh a lot with their team, their team is fun to work with, and 86 per cent of staff said people in their team go out of their way to help them. At number seven, the chairman of advertising agency Miles Calcraft Briginshaw Duffy welcomes all staff personally; there is a welcome team lunch and 88 per cent of staff say that people in their teams go out of their way to help them.

You can read the latest reviews for yourself on the *Times Online* website at http://business.timesonline.co.uk/section/0,,12190,00.html. If you are impressed with the leadership and team spirit where you work, why not nominate your own organisation for inclusion next year at https://secure.bestcompanies.co.uk/BCOnline/overview1.aspx?

Styles of leadership

How important is the team leader to creating and maintaining an effective and motivated team? Most people would consider the attitude and style of the leader to be one of the most critical factors – often more important than the style or culture of the organisation (which has less

Did you know?

Many experts argue that, whereas the function of a manager is to get things done through leading people and achieving organisation goals, the function of a team leader is to act as a **facilitator**. This means motivating and encouraging team members to work productively through personal influence and enthusiasm.

impact on staff on a day-to-day basis), the attitude of senior managers (who are more distant) or the content of the actual job (which may be difficult to change). A good team leader should:

- concentrate on developing and harnessing the skills of the team
- know individual members and their strengths, weaknesses and needs
- work at fostering interrelationships between team members and achieving shared goals.

Leadership studies

Many studies have attempted to define the ability to lead other people. The main ones are summarised in the table below.

Leadership theories		
Theory	**Strengths**	**Weaknesses**
Charismatic leadership (good leaders are born, not made)	Easy to identify charismatic leaders: Hitler, Branson, Thatcher	Does not account for why many charismatic leaders are later changed or rejected
Situational leadership (choose leader who will be most effective in a given situation)	Explains war leaders and those chosen for specific situations: Churchill, Bob Geldof	Implies no specific leadership skills required and in different situation leader would be ineffective
Behavioural leadership (skills can be taught and adapted for different situations)	Focuses on what leaders do, rather than who they are or the situation	There is no known way to train people to become effective leaders

Did you know?

Studies have shown that, in critical environments, task-based, authoritarian leadership is often preferred. Examples include the armed or emergency services, air traffic control and some industrial production environments. In employee-centred and creative environments, people-based leaders are preferred as this encourages group interaction and supportive, open relationships. However, both types of skill are important and effective leadership involves balancing both.

Researchers Tannenbaum and Schmidt contributed to behavioural leadership studies by identifying different leadership styles and describing the choices that managers and leaders had when they were managing others:

- Leadership styles can be task-based, where the focus is on task-completion, and people-based, where the focus is on motivation and job satisfaction. In reality an effective leader needs to be able to operate both styles, although one is usually prominent in any one person.
- The leader can range from being autocratic or authoritarian at one extreme (where the leader makes all the decisions), to allowing the team to decide at the other extreme. Successful leaders will vary their style according to the situation, the team and the nature of the problem they are addressing.

Leadership styles						
Autocratic ◄—						—► Participatory
1	2	3	4	5	6	7
Leader makes decision and gives instruction	Leader 'sells' decision or idea to the team	Leader presents decision and answers questions to reassure the team	Leader suggests decision but may modify this after team give views	Leader states problem, asks team for ideas, then makes decision	Leader gives team the problem to solve but sets limits for type of ideas	Leader and team discuss problem and decide jointly

Leadership behaviours

Writing a list of qualities that a good leader should possess normally convinces most people they would never be able to do the job! A simpler way is often to identify someone whose leadership you admire and respect and use this person as your role model. In particular, analyse how he or she deals with difficult problems or people and under what situations the person varies the approach. You may also wish to compare his or her approach with people whose leadership does not impress you and think about why there was such a difference.

The table below identifies the behaviours that you must demonstrate to achieve this award. Quite obviously there is a purpose behind each of these behaviours and one suggested aim or outcome is shown alongside each behaviour in the list.

Team leader behaviours	
Behaviour	**Aim**
You create a sense of common purpose	… to give the team a common set of goals to which they aspire
You take personal responsibility for making things happen	… to set a clear, consistent model for others
You encourage and support others to take decisions autonomously	… to help team members to believe in what they do and do it successfully
You act within the limits of your authority	… to define clear areas of responsibility and boundaries for the team
You make time available to support others	… to provide an atmosphere whereby all members know they are valued

Team leader behaviours

Behaviour	Aim
You show integrity, fairness and consistency in decision-making	... to foster team spirit and appropriate values and ethics within the team
You seek to understand people's needs and motivations	... to be sensitive to the needs and expectations of team members
You model behaviour that shows respect, helpfulness and cooperation	... to encourage team members to perform well and gain fulfilment in their roles

How to... Win, through your performance, the trust and support of the team for your leadership

- Set high standards and clear objectives for yourself as well as your team.
- Provide a positive sense of direction so that your team can be confident in what they are doing and why they are doing it.
- Make sure each team member is clear about his/her role and responsibilities, so that team efforts are enhanced and not hindered.
- Identify the best way to motivate each team member and use this knowledge to help to achieve individual and team objectives.
- Take responsibility for team performance in meeting tomorrow's challenges, solving problems and coping with change.
- Consider problems and possible solutions carefully, choose the right time to make decisions and then act decisively.
- Communicate clearly with your team and involve them in all appropriate decisions and discussions.
- Be fair and consistent in your manner, attitude and judgements, regardless of how you feel that day or what is happening in your personal life.
- Treat all members of your team with respect and consideration.
- Be totally loyal to all your team members at all times and expect the same degree of solidarity between team members, too.
- Take personal responsibility if one of your team members makes a mistake.

Remember

You will need to demonstrate to your assessor that you can create a sense of common purpose in your team.

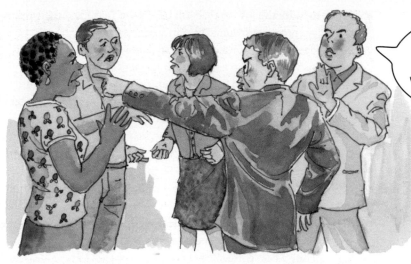

Now we've all decided we have a sense of common purpose, can we stop arguing about who suggested it first.

Motivating, supporting and encouraging team members and recognising their achievements

There is absolutely no point in helping your team members to set realistic – if demanding – objectives and then either letting them struggle to achieve them or ignoring the outcome. Your continual support is vital to keep your team motivated and regular, positive, feedback will encourage them to continue to get results.

Actually it is rare to find a high-performing team whose members are unhappy or demotivated. Therefore one key element for motivating your team is to try to ensure it is successful. This is more likely to be the case if the team is well organised and work is well coordinated so that each person knows exactly what he or she is supposed to be doing and also knows the responsibilities of other members of the team and how all the activities link together. You can help to ensure that all your team members are pulling in the same direction by planning ahead, being well organised and keeping all members of the team constantly informed about progress and any developments or changes that are required.

However, you cannot ignore the importance of team spirit or the needs of individual members who may encounter difficulties or sometimes feel they are being dominated by more forceful colleagues. In some cases this can lead to open conflict, and you will learn more about this on page 377. More fundamentally you need to work at developing strategies that keep you fully aware of what is going on in your team and how individual members are coping. Here are some methods you can use:

Did you know?

Nothing succeeds like success! Because people get a 'buzz' out of being successful, they normally want to repeat the experience. Good team leaders use this to their advantage by rewarding their team whenever they can – even if only in fun, informal ways.

Did you know?

An excellent example of team coordination is the Red Arrows, the flying display team. This involves careful planning, scheduling, practice, endless refinement and excellent communications. Meeting the challenge and achieving the goal both act as motivators for team members.

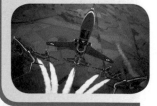

- **Learn to 'walk the job'** so that you observe at first hand the work your team is carrying out. This means you will have a greater knowledge of how your team operates and will be more aware of situations where support and encouragement are required.

- **Get to know your team as individuals** with their own strengths, weaknesses and preferences. Identify the team members who might need extra support and encouragement to take on new challenges, and discuss with them the best ways to help them.

- **Listen carefully to team conversations** and check that the views of all members are being considered. Be prepared to support anyone who has a useful opinion but finds it difficult to hold the attention of other members.

- **Be aware of key performance indicators** that denote levels of team spirit and job satisfaction. These include low rates of absenteeism, high-quality work, enthusiastic, positive responses to new ideas, and an enjoyable 'buzz' in team meetings. Take action if any of these factors seem to be lacking.

- **Cultivate an 'open door' approach** so that team members feel relaxed about talking to you informally about their own problems or difficulties and will alert you to those being experienced by their colleagues.

- **Acknowledge both small and great achievements**. Praise team members who meet a tight deadline or carry out a difficult task promptly. Give formal recognition to team members who achieve a higher level qualification or learn a new skill.

Remember

You need to demonstrate to your assessor that you make time available to support others.

Over to you

1 Summarise the difference between a group and a team in your own words. Check your answer with the suggestion on the CD-ROM.

2 Over the course of two weeks you have three types of information to communicate to your team or its members. For each one, state the method of communication you would use and why. Check your answer with the suggestions on the CD-ROM.

a The instructions for a complicated piece of work being done by three members of your team have changed.

b An important customer has complained to your boss about the way she was dealt with by a member of your team. You have been asked to investigate this.

c Your team will be involved in a new project next month. You have just received the details and been asked to suggest several ideas relating to its completion as well as a proposed deadline.

3 a Identify which of the leadership styles (numbered 1–7) shown in the chart on page 363 you would choose to use in each of the following situations, and give reasons for your choices. Check your ideas with the suggestions on the CD-ROM.

i Your boss has told you that there is £500 available for new resources and wants to know what your team needs most.

ii New security procedures have been introduced which all staff must follow.

iii You are trying to change the staff rota to meet various requests and are finding it impossible to suit everyone.

iv Your team want to arrange a night out to celebrate the engagement of one of the members.

v Your organisation is moving to new premises and you and your team have the choice of two different offices in which you can work.

b To what degree do you think your choices reflect your own leadership style?

Core unit links

Communicating with your team, both verbally and in writing, focusing on information they give to you, leading discussions and encouraging others to contribute link to unit 301, performance indicators 1–7.

Agreeing realistic targets and achieving these, keeping people informed of progress and taking responsibility for your work (and that of your team) may link to unit 301, PIs 8–15.

Helping your team to achieve its objectives, related to your organisation's purpose and values, may link to unit 302, PIs 1–6. Setting high standards and providing support and encouragement links to unit 301, PIs 22 and 28.

Evidence collection

You will need to prove to your assessor that you communicate the purpose and objectives of the team to all members, involve members in planning how to achieve these and encourage and support team members throughout this process.

1 Start by writing a personal statement that describes the objective-setting process for your team and your own involvement. This should include the way in which you involve team members in agreeing demanding yet realistic team and individual objectives. Either attach copies of the agreed objectives, work plans and/or meetings notes relating to these or include a note of their location.

2 Include a description of how your team's objectives are reviewed by your own boss and attach, or note the location of, any relevant documents. Explain the methods you adopt to provide support and encouragement and acknowledge individual and team achievements. Ask your line manager to countersign and date your statement to confirm that it is correct.

Evidence collection Continued

3   Obtain witness statements from two or three team members that confirm the process and state how you create a sense of common purpose in the team and encourage and support each member, both when they are deciding their objectives and when they are working to achieve them.

Understanding your organisation and team

You have already seen that the overall preferred leadership style of a team leader may vary depending on the situation, the type of team being managed and the natural style of the team leader. This is only one of the benefits of understanding your team, how it operates and its role in relation to your organisation. In this section you will cover the additional contextual knowledge elements of the unit that focus in more depth on this area and help you to learn more about teams and how they function.

Legal, regulatory and ethical requirements in your industry

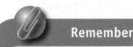

Remember

You will need to demonstrate to your assessor that you act within the limits of your authority.

These were covered in unit 302. Turn back to pages 139 and 118–22 to refresh your memory.

The specific requirements of your industry will affect the limits of your authority, the types of decision your team can make on its own, the style of team leadership you are most likely to adopt, and the scope your team has for deciding how to do particular tasks.

Members, purpose, objectives and plans of your team

If you have been a member of a team yourself, you will know that the way it operates depends on many factors. These include the style of the leader, the different members of the team, the length of time it has worked together and its main purpose and plans. If any of these factors change then the team itself is likely to be affected, for better or worse.

The members of the team

There have been many studies relating to the role of different team members. One of the best known was undertaken by Meredith Belbin who identified certain key roles that must be filled by members of a team. In small teams, some members would need to take over more than one role. An effective team, therefore, is not one containing the cleverest people or those with the same strengths or attributes, but one where members complement each other so that there is a balance of skills and abilities.

In a more recent study, Dr Cary Cooper argued that three ingredients are essential:

- There must be a **social emotional leader** who cares about the others, acts as peacemaker, arranges social activities and brings balance into a hard-working team. This does not have to be the official leader.
- There must be **task people** who are focused on achieving the objectives and goals that have been set. They are essential if the team is to fulfil its responsibilities.
- There must be at least one **communicator** who keeps everyone informed – both within and outside the team.

Other experts have proposed that, overall, five main personality types are required in an effective team:

- an **action person** who continually pushes ahead and is willing to take risks
- a **caring person** who is sensitive to the moods and feelings in the group, can mediate in an argument and promote harmony
- a **detail person** who is concerned with task completing, getting the details right and producing work of high quality
- a **coordinator** who can lead discussions, involve everyone and check that all team members are performing effectively
- a **creative thinker** who comes up with good or unusual ideas that give the team new ways of thinking about a problem.

Team relationships

Members of teams have two concerns. First they have to meet team goals. Second, they need to maintain good relationships with each other. These two areas are likely to be interlinked because if goals are not met this puts pressure on working relationships – particularly if it creates stress and some members of the group then blame the others for the problem.

This is less likely to occur if the team has been together for some time because teams are known to mature. A recent team, suddenly put under

Find out

Dr Meredith Belbin, an expert on teams, argued that 'although one person can't be perfect, a team can be'. He meant that, given the right mix of people, a team can collectively possess more strengths than can ever be found in one person. Find out more about Belbin's team roles by visiting your library, obtaining one of his books and using his questionnaire to find your own dominant style.

Find out

Check out your own team and decide which members are 'task-based' or action people and which are 'people-based' and more concerned with team relationships. Remember, you need a balance if your team is to be effective.

pressure, is unlikely to cope as well as an experienced team that has been in this situation before and whose members know each other well.

Team development was studied by B. W. Tuckmann who argued that teams go through five stages. These are shown in the table below, in addition to the type of role you should adopt, as leader, to facilitate team development.

Did you know?

There are literally dozens of team-building activities to help build cohesive teams – from paint balling and orienteering to problem-solving and adventure games. Find out more at www.businessballs.com/teambuilding.htm, www.wildevents.co.uk and www.buildingteams.com, or use a search engine such as Google to find alternatives.

Stages in team development and the role of the team leader		
Stage	**Behaviour**	**Role of team leader**
Forming	Team is new and members don't know each other. They look to the leader to tell them how they should behave, what rules must be followed and what the team goals are	Explain goals and how team will operate. Encourage social interactions between members through ice-breaking activities
Storming	Differences between team members start to emerge. Some may be disappointed or disillusioned and there may be arguments between team members as people voice different opinions	Make sure team members know their own responsibilities and their own role and place in the team. Allow dissent so long as team members respect each other's views
Norming	Team members have started to accept their roles and accept each other. Problems are discussed more openly and there is a more open exchange of opinions and greater camaraderie and closer group relationships	Encourage and foster open communications between team members so that all members contribute to discussions and feel their views are valued and important
Performing	Working relationships between team members are good and the team is mutually supportive. The team is now 'free' to focus on task performance. Each member feels secure and valued. The team is operating at maximum effectiveness	Encourage flexibility between team members to achieve joint needs or goals. Bear in mind individual differences between members
Mourning	The final stage for a team which is disbanding when members will go their separate ways. This is often traumatic for long-established teams and there may be a ritual ending ('last night out') and promises of future reunions	In some cases to keep in contact with team members for either social reasons or to recruit high performers into future teams

After B W Tuckmann

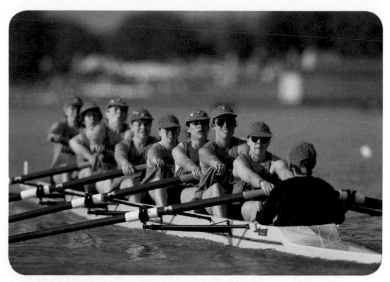

A winning team is one that pulls together

Objectives, purpose and plans

Teams should be formed for a reason. They should have a common purpose, shared objectives and a future plan to which all team members are committed. It is generally a mistake to try to form a team whose members will have different objectives or who are committed to different future plans, such as a group made up of departmental representatives all of whom have their own department's interests at heart! Similarly, the team should be treated as a unit. It is no use forming a team and then appraising and rewarding members on an individual basis that has no relationship to the team's objectives or purpose.

You should be fully aware of the objectives, purpose and plans that relate to your own team, the commitment of individual members to achieving these and the best way to encourage and support your team to achieve its goals.

Personal work objectives of members of your team

There are advantages and disadvantages to working in a team. A major benefit is that life is usually more fun and the team relationships and support networks found in a team meet many people's personal needs to socialise and make friends at work. However, being an effective team member can also mean sacrificing personal aims or objectives for the good of the team – and that does not suit everyone. So a 'loner', who has no particular desire to develop close relationships at work, or someone who is keenly ambitious and fixated only on meeting personal objectives, is unlikely to make a good team member.

Did you know?

Team leaders are more likely to be able to lead effectively if they are able to obtain benefits or negotiate better conditions for their team members. This is because they are then seen as strong leaders with power and influence rather than weak leaders who may be kind and have useful ideas but cannot get these accepted at a higher level. This means that you really need your own boss's support to be effective as a team leader.

Remember

Team work isn't for everyone. Individualists, loners and anyone who is ruthlessly ambitious are usually better working alone.

You can usually expect team members whose objectives and values accord with those of the team as a whole to be positive and helpful and an asset to the group. However, you will be very lucky if you never meet a team member whose behaviour causes problems, sometimes because his or her personal objectives or values do not match those of the team. Sometimes these objectives will be known, at other times the motives may be less obvious. No one is perfect, though, so it is important to be able to differentiate between the personal work objectives and motivations of a team member that may cause serious problems in your team and those that can be irritating but solvable. These include the type of behaviours shown in the table below.

Did you know?

Team members who put their individual career goals and objectives ahead of those of the team will normally have far less interest in team performance and achievements than those who are committed team members.

Dysfunctional behaviour by team members to meet own (hidden) objectives		
Objective	**Behaviour**	**Team leader response**
To prevent change/ new ideas	Constantly disparages other people's ideas and views	Ask for solutions, not problems. No one can criticise without suggesting a solution or a better one idea
To keep expert knowledge to self to stay ahead of rest of team	Despite having expert knowledge, refuses to share knowledge or insight with others	Avoid allowing one person too much control over a task. Insist on sharing in case of crises and emergencies
To be the leader's favourite	Flatters the leader to get attention and tries to do 'deals' with the leader when the others aren't present	Check that you don't respond to this and that people don't benefit by flattering you! Be aware of the risks of making private agreements with individuals
To do as little work as possible	Agrees to do tasks but fails to fulfil promises, normally with 'excellent' reason	Offer support and training to improve work skills and monitor non-achievement for regular appraisal and review sessions
To disrupt the team or become the next team leader	Often bossy or argumentative, and hostile and critical of you and others	Put this person in charge of quality monitoring and control to keep him/her busy, and give the person something official to check up on
To do 'own thing'	Rarely listens and often ignores team suggestions and objectives	Check that individual and team goals are aligned. Try to find jobs that need someone to be specifically responsible for. Tolerate if rest of team unaffected

Types of support and advice team members are likely to need – and how to provide them

The type of support and advice your team may need will depend on several factors:

- the type of organisation you work for
- the organisational culture and policies
- the type of rewards and benefits provided to staff in general and teams in particular
- team success in meeting team goals
- the overall mix of personalities in your team
- the degree of competitiveness and/or support between team members
- personal circumstances of team members.

In other words, if you and your team get on well together, work in an organisation where you feel highly valued and fairly rewarded, and if you regularly meet team goals successfully, then the only time you may need to provide support and advice is when team members suffer personal problems or difficulties. However, if you work in a competitive, cut-throat environment and have the misfortune to be trying to manage a quite dysfunctional team that is struggling to meet its targets, then you will need to take immediate steps to help your team to improve its performance and provide support and advice at the same time.

How you provide support and advice will depend on whether the matter concerns the whole team or one individual, and whether it is of general interest. You have a choice whether to provide advice and support formally and informally, to individuals or collectively to the team as a whole.

- **Support and advice to the team as a whole** can be provided during team briefings, team-building sessions and specific problem-solving meetings. These would be appropriate for advising on ways to carry out work, to clarify instructions, to discuss resource allocation or problems, to discuss demands being made on the team or to plan for the acquisition of new skills.
- **Support and advice to individual team members** can be provided formally in one-to-one appraisal or counselling sessions and informally in one-to-one discussions. They would be appropriate for discussing conflicting instructions or requests, for clarifying future work objectives, for discussing development opportunities, and for resolving personality clashes, personal issues or concerns.

Standard of performance for the work of your team

There may be specific ways in which you are expected to monitor the performance of your team. Here are some possibilities:

Remember

As team leader you may be called on to provide both moral support if someone has personal problems or difficulties, and practical support if someone is struggling to complete work by a deadline.

Remember

There is a big difference between offering support and interfering. Unless a problem involves work performance, you cannot – and should not – insist on providing support if your offer is rejected.

Remember

You will need to demonstrate to your assessor that you model behaviour that shows respect, helpfulness and cooperation.

- **By achievement of team goals or results.** In this case, all team members should know what is expected. You should know how often team goals are reviewed, whether you regularly achieve team goals, whether (and to what extent) team goals are surpassed, and what happens if team goals are not met.

- **By the way the team functions.** How effectively does your team work together? Do team members trust each other and discuss matters openly? Do they help and support each other? Has any change occurred that may have affected the way the team functions?

- **By the use of resources.** Do you have sufficient resources to meet your team goals? If the goals have been changed, have resources been provided to match? Could new equipment or the adoption of new technology help you to reach goals more easily?

- **Team knowledge and skills.** Does the team have the knowledge and skills required to carry out operations using current equipment and technology? What new skills are needed to meet future challenges? Are any new skills emerging that the team could usefully use? Can the team consistently achieve the quality of work required? Are there any particular skills or abilities the team lacks?

It is important, of course, that any discussion on the standard team performance includes the views of team members themselves. The focus should then be on dealing with any concerns or problems that are identified.

Remember

You will have to demonstrate to your assessor that you take personal responsibility for making things happen and seek to understand people's needs and motivations.

Over to you

1 Read the checklist for effective team performance below and identify the characteristics possessed by your own team. For each characteristic you feel that your team is lacking, suggest how you would remedy this deficiency.

Checklist for effective team performance

How many of the following characteristics apply to your team?

1 All members know and understand the team's goals.

2 Members are happy to identify with the team and describe their roles in it.

3 Members support and appreciate each other.

4 Members of your team willingly share their knowledge and opinions.

5 The team is far more interested in solving problems than blaming someone for any mistakes made.

6 Team members trust each other.

7 People tolerate and show respect for each other's views and opinions.

8 Working in the team is fun.

9 Team members have confidence in each other's skills and abilities.

10 There is team support for you, as leader.

11 Team members work together to achieve a task.

12 Team members put the team's aims before personal gain.

13 Conflict is open and focuses on the issue, not the people.

14 All members contribute to team discussions and making team decisions.

15 Communications are open and friendly.

16 Relationships with other teams are positive and cooperative.

2 You have been asked to lead a team of six administrative staff. Pete and Cathy are lively members of staff – fun, extroverted but also good at their jobs. Cathy is also very creative with lots of good ideas. Parveen, the third member of the group, is far quieter but she is also a very caring person who is the first to notice if someone is out of sorts or upset about something. Ben is a bit of a loner. He is the IT expert and often speaks in a language all of his own! However, he has a reputation for solving difficult problems, has a keen eye for detail and an excellent sense of humour once he relaxes. Liam and Nicola have worked for the organisation the longest. In fact, you know Nicola hoped to be team leader herself. They are both very hard workers and Liam is highly competitive, always wanting to push forward and do new things.

a You decide to check your team against the five recommended personality types listed on page 369. To what extent is your team 'complete', given its membership, and what strengths will you need as leader to balance the team profile?

b Suggest three dysfunctional behaviours that certain people in your team might display and state how you could handle these.

c Your team is relatively new. How might this affect its behaviour and what can you do as leader to help it to develop effectively?

d You decide that a useful way of improving team performance would be to arrange a team-building session. You have the choice of:

Over to you Continued

    i   a one-day training activity in-house, with a sandwich lunch

    ii an away day as a group.

    Research both alternatives online and list three types of activities you could undertake as a team, either in-house or on an away day, and identify how these may help your particular team to function effectively more quickly.

Check your ideas about team-building activities for your own team with your tutor or trainer, and compare your other answers with the suggestions on the CD-ROM.

Core unit links

Evidence that your team works to achieve your organisation's main purpose and puts its values into practice links to unit 302, performance indicators 1–5.

Interacting with other people in a way that is sensitive to their individual needs and learning from people with different backgrounds, abilities and beliefs links to unit 302, PIs 11 and 12.

Identifying ways to improve your work and testing their effectiveness may link to unit 301, PI 18.

Evidence collection

Prepare a personal statement that provides a description of your organisation and the role of your team to use as a basis for a professional discussion with your assessor to confirm your contextual knowledge. This should show that you are fully aware of the needs and motivations of individual team members as well as their personal work objectives and the best way to deal with them as individuals. You should also include information about the role of your team in the organisation, as well as the standards of performance for the work of your team and how these affect the type of support and advice that team members are likely to need.

Include in your statement the location of records that give a brief history of the team to explain its development as well as the objectives and plans that have been achieved in the past. If you and your team have been involved in team-building activities, then include details, including the type of activity and the benefits that were gained. You may also wish to attach documentary evidence and photographs (or even video clips). Remember to ask your own line manager to countersign and date your statement for authenticity.

You may also wish to ask individual team members for witness statements to state how you have advised them and given them support in the past to help them to overcome a particular problem and to give their own account of team-building activities they have attended.

Identifying and overcoming difficulties and challenges

Despite your best efforts to promote team harmony you may find that you still have to deal with disagreements and/or conflicts, either within the team or between your team and other groups. This can occur for various reasons but is usually either task-based or people-based. Understanding the difference is important because task-based problems are normally easier to define and solve than people problems, which can be more complex:

- **Task-based difficulties.** These relate to problems with doing the job, such as tight deadlines, the absence of some team members, lack of other resources, lack of skills, conflicting or complex instructions, equipment breakdown etc. You are most likely to meet this type of problem if you are operating to tight time limits, if the tasks undertaken are complex, if a high degree of skill is required, if tasks or instructions are frequently changing, if you and your team are short of resources, or if some of your team do not have all the skills they need.

- **People-based difficulties.** These relate to personality clashes, problems over allocation of roles, team members blaming each other when things go wrong, team members failing to help or support one another etc. You are likely to meet this type of problem if you are trying to lead a large team, if the team is newly formed, if members of the team feel taken for granted or under-valued, if decisions are imposed on the team rather than collectively agreed, if some members of the team are not committed to the team goals, if some team members display dysfunctional behaviour (see page 372), or if there is a 'blame-culture' in the team if anything goes wrong.

There are three stages to coping with this type of situation. The first is to recognise when a problem may occur. The second is to identify the reason for the problem. The third is to take appropriate action – as you will see below.

Did you know?

Teams can be too small or too large. If there are only a few members there may not be a wide enough range of personalities and knowledge. If the team is too large, people will not be able to get to know each other well enough and may tend to spit into sub-groups. There is no 'perfect' size, but most people think that between five and ten is about right.

Did you know?

Group dynamics relates to the interactions of a group or team and is Influenced by the personalities of the members and their beliefs. You cannot control the personal attitudes and feelings of group members, but you can insist on common courtesies, support for each other and good communications between team members.

How to... Steer the team successfully through difficulties and challenges, including conflict within the team

- Recognise that difficulties and challenges are part of the working life of a team and, where possible, should be openly discussed to find a solution that is acceptable to all members.

How to... Continued

- Identify issues that may create task-based difficulties at the outset, such as scarce resources or problematic deadlines, so that these can be resolved or minimised at the planning stage.

- Foster an ethos where 'moaning' is banned and the team collectively aim to find creative ways to overcome difficulties.

- Insist that the focus of a problem is 'how do we solve it?', not 'who caused it?'

- Be aware that some members of your team will opt for peace at any price, while others might love the cut and thrust of an argument. You may need to be assertive on behalf of the more passive members of your team at times.

- Know the difference between constructive and destructive conflict. Conflict is constructive when people openly but good-humouredly disagree with each other. This often produces excellent ideas (see page 381) and should be encouraged. Destructive conflict involves individuals insulting or criticising each other or refusing to communicate and must be stopped.

- Insist on negotiation and respect between team members when they hold different views and introduce them to the value of win/win – where both parties in a dispute benefit from the outcome. (For a full description of this tactic, see unit 320, pages 338–41.)

- Learn some useful team manager strategies for resolving conflict, such as:

  - adjusting resources so that both parties get something

  - agreeing that if a team member concedes something now they will get something of more value in the future

  - suggesting a completely different alternative to diffuse an argument

  - keeping a mental score sheet so that 'winning' is shared fairly between team members over time

  - renegotiating a solution so that the 'cost' to the loser is minimised.

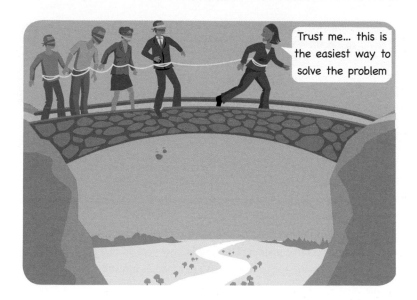

Trust me... this is the easiest way to solve the problem

Remember

You will need to demonstrate to your assessor that you show integrity, fairness and consistency in decision-making.

Encouraging others to lead – and how to achieve this

There are several advantages to allowing others to lead the team at times. As an obvious example, you may be too busy to become very involved in a minor issue that will affect your team far more than you. This is then a golden opportunity to empower your team to make its own decision. Or you may have an expert on a particular topic in the team. It would be downright silly to insist that you have the final word in this situation, if you don't know very much about the subject.

That said, when you do hand over the reins you then have to be prepared to go along with the outcome, otherwise you will completely undermine the efforts of the person to whom you gave the lead. For that reason, you need to give careful thought to the situations in which handing over leadership would be both beneficial and appropriate. These are outlined in the table below.

Did you know?

A **self-managed team** is one that collectively makes its own decisions. Even if your team cannot manage itself you can foster the empowerment of individual members by encouraging them to take the lead in appropriate situations.

Remember

Being team leader does not mean you know best (or most) about everything. Wise leaders earn respect by deferring to the team member(s) who know more about a particular topic or issue.

Encourage someone else to take the lead when...	Think twice about relinquishing the lead when...
... the outcome will affect him/her more than anyone else.	... the outcome will affect you more than anyone else.
... he/she is an expert on the topic or issue.	... you know more than your team about the topic.
... he/she has had had recent relevant experience.	... you have recent relevant experience.

Encourage someone else to take the lead when...	Think twice about relinquishing the lead when...
... the topic relates to his/her own work or area of interest.	... many people will be affected by the outcome.
... you want to foster and encourage that person's self-development.	... your boss will hold you personally accountable for the result.
... the issue is a useful one for the team to debate on their own.	... the issue is complex, tricky and beyond the scope of your team.

Did you know?

Even in informal groups a leader often emerges. In some ways human beings behave a little like pack animals – they prefer to have a leader to give them a steer rather than to make all decisions jointly.

Even if you happily hand over the lead when it is appropriate, there are two other aspects to consider. The first is how you do this. The second is your response to the suggestions that are made as a result.

Handing over the lead

How you hand over the lead to a team member should depend on the issue concerned. It is quite acceptable to say in a team meeting: 'Nina, you're our PowerPoint expert, what do you think is possible in the time we have available?' However, it is not appropriate to suddenly throw someone in the deep end by telling him or her to run an entire meeting for you at a moment's notice, without any guidance or preparation. The amount of notice and degree of guidance you give should match the importance and complexity of the issue. You will also need to give support and encouragement to those in your team who may be good at leading but may feel faint at the very idea, as well as advice to those who may be very keen but could upset others if they are too bombastic or determined to have their own way.

Did you know?

A useful way to develop **new leaders** is to sub-divide your team into smaller groups on a training or development day and nominate leaders for each group.

Following the lead

You can be certain that your responses to the suggestions made by your team with a temporary leader in charge will be watched very closely – not least by that leader! If you visibly shudder when you hear what has been proposed and then spend the next ten minutes giving reasons why these ideas won't work, you may see some 'knowing' looks passing between your team. If you habitually pour cold water on ideas you have not thought of yourself, it is also likely to be some time before anyone else offers to take over the lead from you.

If you are worried that some of the suggestions might be a bit outlandish, and you may be committed to actions you will later regret, it is sensible to set some boundaries beforehand. Quite simply, make sure your temporary team leader – or the team as a whole – are aware of the type of suggestions that will be acceptable and those that will not. As long as they stick to this brief then you have a duty to be loyal and support them in return. You never know – you may find that a quite different approach pays dividends when you try it!

Creativity and innovation in a team – and how to achieve this

One of the main benefits of a team, as you saw on pags 358 and 369, is that outcomes are possible that could not be achieved by one individual. This is particularly the case with creative teams who work together to suggest new ideas. The main benefit for the organisation – and for the team – is that once creative ideas start to be generated, and once team members realise that these are not only appreciated but actively encouraged, then team dynamics come into play. As team confidence grows and members believe in their own ability to take risks within the group, a wider range of ideas and suggestions is likely to emerge.

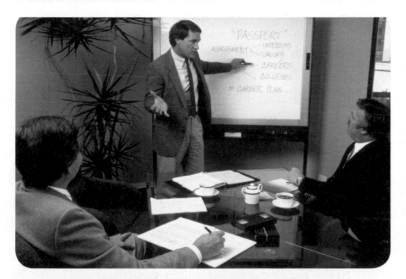

Remember

You will need to demonstrate to your assessor that you encourage and support others to take decisions autonomously.

Find out

Brainstorming is used by many creative teams, including those given the task of finding new product names. No ideas can be criticised and everything is written down. The team then identify those that are sensible, possible or far-fetched – and then try to link some of the far-fetched to the other categories to see what new ideas this generates. Try it yourself and see!

How to... Encourage and recognise creativity and innovation within a team

- Remember that your team will respond to requests for new ideas only as long as their suggestions are appreciated and never mocked or disparaged.

- Develop an ethos where taking risks is encouraged and where there is always approval and praise for making suggestions.

How to... Continued

- At the start of a creative session, encourage team members to keep bouncing ideas off each other without reaching any firm conclusion.

- If you value creativity, give team members time and space in which they can think without expecting immediate, time-constrained results.

- Stimulate creative thinking by dividing a large team into smaller groups. Then encourage members of each group to express their ideas and then compare results.

- Suggest different ways of looking at a problem or encourage team members to look at issues 'outside the box'. If no one can do this, arrange a team training day which will focus on developing creativity.

- Foster innovation and creativity by encouraging lateral thinking and highlighting interesting examples of different and ingenious ideas.

- If an original idea is approved, make sure your team member has the support and resources to put it into practice.

Did you know?

Paul Birch and Brian Clegg who co-wrote *Crash Course in Creativity* identified three different types of creativity that result in 'aaahh', 'ah ha' and 'ha ha'. 'Aaahh' is the response given to the Artist who creates beauty or challenge, whereas the Sage creates ideas or solutions ('ah ha') and the Jester creates humour ('ha ha'). According to them, companies need all three elements to be present to be successful.

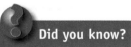

Did you know?

The Internet service provider AOL used small teams to decide new product developments. Each team was empowered to focus on specific targets and results and many achieved amazing results.

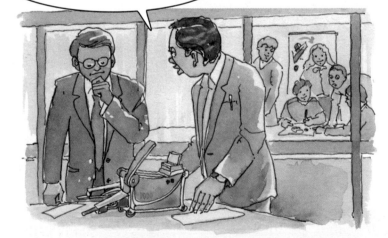

> I didn't like to ask them what it does, in case it undermined their confidence.

Case study If you can't stand the heat...

Gemma Walker was one of a team of four administrators in the departmental office of a large college. Their roles involved dealing with callers and carrying out all the administrative support activities for the staff and students.

Two years ago, when the department was growing rapidly and two new staff were being appointed, the head decided there would be several benefits in appointing a team leader to organise the work of the admin staff. This should benefit both the department and the staff themselves. The strengths and skills of team members could be maximised, there would be greater flexibility as team members could cover for each other and less duplication of work or effort if it was coordinated through a team leader. From the team's point of view, there would be help, advice and support available when they needed it and more opportunity to influence decisions that affected them. Gemma considered applying for the job but felt that with only two years' experience she might not be able to cope with the responsibility. The successful applicant, Jackie, impressed the interview panel because she had introduced strict quality procedures in her last workplace.

It was soon apparent that quality procedures didn't have much in common with leading a team. Jackie liked to be chummy with everyone in the office – as well as laughing and joking with everyone who passed by. This irritated the departmental head who felt that Jackie should set a more mature example. The administrators in the office – including Gemma – said nothing but did acknowledge that there was not much difference since Jackie arrived. They all still got on with their own jobs. They rarely received specific instructions or guidance – and although they liked Jackie and knew she meant well she rarely seemed interested enough in them or their jobs to give them advice or support. Her encouragement was focused more on how to stay up until 2 a.m. on a Saturday night rather than how to work effectively! Even on a team away day Jackie was more interested in beating everyone else rather than helping the team to achieve its goals.

Unsurprisingly Jackie didn't stay too long at the college. She was replaced by the oldest member of the office staff – Kath – somewhat against her will. This time the departmental head decided to take no chances. He felt that a far more sensible team leader was needed and persuaded Kath to apply on grounds of seniority.

What the head didn't know was that although Kath was efficient and conscientious she was also a tremendous worrier. The night before she started in her new job she lay awake for hours, fretting about how she would cope. She was aware that she would now have to behave differently. She could no longer treat the other members of the team as close friends with whom she could share moans and groans about the workload or joke about some of the contradictory or ambiguous instructions received from some members of staff. She now had her own office and was expected to stay apart from the others, in case there were occasions when she had to give them instructions (or worse) tell them off. The very thought made her blood run cold. These were her friends – how could she now order them around?

Kath's first day in the job didn't go too well. A key task of the senior administrator was to take the minutes of the departmental meetings. Kath's English skills weren't too good and she became so interested in one discussion that she forgot to write anything down. In the end, it was the deputy head who helped her out, so that her minutes were at least intelligible. In the meantime she brooded in her little office, missing the usual banter with the team in the main office. Every day seemed twice as long as it had done in the past.

Kath's friends told her it would take her time to adapt, so for several months she persevered. The crunch came when a member of the team left and, because of financial problems, she was told there would not be a replacement. It was her job to make sure the team met its targets even though they were one person short. Kath couldn't face the idea of trying to make her little group work any harder and asked if she could take over the team member's job and be demoted. Let someone else worry about achieving the targets!

By now Gemma had worked at the college for over four years, watching Jackie and Kath in their efforts to manage the team. In her view, good leadership didn't have to be so problematic. A leader is still a member of the team but just has different responsibilities – work could still be interesting and fun! The important thing was to lead by example, never to ask someone to do something you wouldn't be prepared to do yourself, and foster loyalty and good communications within the group. In her view, her colleagues were a super team – hard working and conscientious – although it would be better if they had regular informal team briefings on their own rather than the rather 'stiff' formal meetings they now had each month with the departmental head present – and they really did need some faster computer printers!

Today Gemma is leading that team. She has done so successfully for the last three years. Are you surprised?

Questions

1   *The departmental head appointed a team leader because he considered there would be several benefits if the admin staff worked as a team. Identify four of these.*

2   *Arguably, under Jackie's leadership, the administrators didn't benefit very much from having a team leader. Identify three ways in which Jackie's leadership was lacking.*

3 a *Why did Kath have reservations about becoming team leader?*

 b *To what degree do you think these were justified?*

4 a *In your view, what skills was Kath lacking when she took over the job?*

 b *How could the departmental head have helped Kath in this situation?*

5 *When Gemma took over the leadership of the team, one of the team members for whom she was responsible was Kath.*

 a *To what extent do you think this could present problems for Gemma?*

 b *What could Gemma do to help prevent problems occurring?*

6 *To what degree do you think the departmental head's support is important for Gemma to lead the team successfully?*

7 *Suggest four reasons why Gemma's leadership of the team is successful.*

Changing places

Your assessor will ask you how you will adapt your knowledge of leading a team if you change your job in the future. You will need to think about the way in which aspects of these tasks would change if you worked for a different organisation.

Jolanta works as administrator at a communications agency that produces a wide range of booklets, leaflets and technical documents for clients. She leads a small team of four admin staff who work together on various projects. They are collectively responsible for producing the documents required, ensuring that illustrations and photographs are provided, arranging for particular documents to be translated into different languages and scheduling the printing and distributing of the information. Meeting deadlines and quality targets is absolutely critical. Jolanta is personally responsible for liaising with the overall project leader and holds daily team briefings to ensure that she and her team are constantly kept up to date about progress and can support each other as and when needed.

Changing places Continued

Kate leads the team of administrators and receptionists for a large medical practice as well as assisting the practice manager. She says that she focuses on the long term, because there will constantly be new arrivals and departures in the team but it must always function as effectively as possible. She aims to integrate new members quickly and to ensure that communications are excellent, particularly as many staff work part-time and may be unable to make team meetings on a regular basis.

Zenobia works in a legal practice and heads the administrative team. Her staff may be assigned to work for any of the solicitors or legal executives employed by the firm. The senior partners consider this method to be more efficient than having secretaries and PAs permanently assigned to different members of staff. Zenobia is involved in agreeing the objectives of individual members of her team and all are assured of her support at all times, particularly if they feel they are struggling to cope with a project or need additional resources to meet specific targets.

Kelly's admin team support the sales staff of an international organisation who travel all around the world. Three members of the scheme are bilingual and one speaks three languages. They are totally committed to the overall objectives even if this means being woken up at 6 a.m. to note urgent instructions! Kelly is well aware that she needs to balance the workload of individual team members when they are particularly busy by assigning them assistance and support. She is also a great believer in the importance of team results and insists that team achievements are rewarded rather than individual efforts.

Julia works for a large charity. Her team provides support, advice and information to external clients and contacts. Two members of her team are voluntary workers, the others are salaried staff members who have more responsibility and work longer hours. Julia is constantly in touch by email and telephone and considers that good communications between team members, as well as shared goals, are vital to their success.

1   For any *one* person listed above, identify the differences he or she would find if moving to your organisation and doing your job.

2   For any *one* person listed above, say how you would need to adapt your skills if you did their job rather than your own.

Over to you

1   An organisation decides to pay its successful teams a bonus. Answer the following questions and then compare these to the suggestions on the CD-ROM.

   a   What advantages and disadvantages do you think there would be for team members?

   b   What would you do if you were placed in a team that didn't perform well?

   c   How do you think the idea would affect you if you were leading a team?

   d   What do you think might happen if your team was particularly successful for the next two years?

2   Suggest how you would deal with each of the following problems or challenges. Compare your ideas with the suggestions on the CD-ROM.

   a   A new team member is proving unpopular with the rest because she is far more laid back about achieving targets or producing good quality work to a deadline. You have only just found out about this because the rest of the team have been covering for her until now.

   b   You are on holiday next week and your own boss wants a member of your team to take the lead temporarily. When you asked for a volunteer, all you heard was silence.

   c   Your team has been asked to help at a customer services event that will be held on Wednesday and Thursday evenings next week. You are allowed to give time off in lieu. Two members of your five-strong team are happy to do Wednesday, no one wants to do Thursday, and Dan is arguing that staff should be offered overtime instead.

   d   Your boss has asked your team to suggest cost-cutting measures because of budget problems. You divided them into two groups and asked for ideas. One group listed 'using cheaper paper', 'reducing photocopying', 're-using file folders.' The other group criticised these as being worse than useless because they will cause more problems than they solve.

Core unit links

Behaving in a way that supports effective working, including coping with pressure, overcoming difficulties and treating other people with consideration, links to unit 301, performance indicators 22–28.

If you are involved in resolving problems that require discretion because you must maintain confidentiality of information, this may link to unit 302, PIs 15 and 16.

Evidence collection

1   Keep records of problems and challenges faced by your team, how they were discussed and the solutions that were agreed, as well as your own role in this process.

2   Keep notes or minutes of team meetings or other events when you were encouraging your team to be creative or innovative. These should include the suggestions that were made and further details of any innovative ideas agreed and later adopted. Ask the team members who made these suggestions to support your statement by providing witness testimony which confirms your role.

3   Write a personal statement that includes a record of occasions when you encouraged other members of your team to take the lead in discussions and the outcomes. Ask the relevant team members to either provide witness testimony to confirm your claims or to countersign and date your statement.

What if...?

What should you do if either:

●   no difficulties or challenges occur during the assessment period

●   there is no need for support and advice during the assessment period?

In either case your assessor can give you a dedicated task to cover the knowledge and understanding required. This will then be followed by a professional discussion during which you can explain how you would perform in such a situation and what evidence you might bring forward.

Key skills reminder

If you are taking Key Skills awards, remember to discuss with your tutor or trainer how your evidence for this unit could also count towards those awards.

Index

Note: page numbers with the prefixes 314. and 315. refer to units on the CD-ROM.

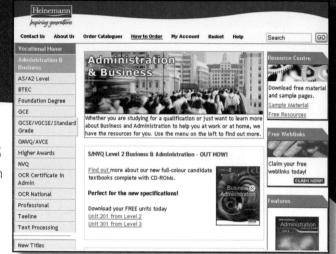
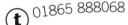 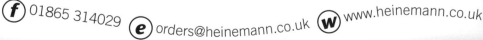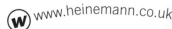
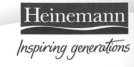